DATE DUE

~~JY 10 98~~			
~~MY 24 '99~~			
~~MR 22 '02~~			

DEMCO 38-296

Third Edition

Training for Sport and Activity
The Physiological Basis
of the Conditioning Process

Jack H. Wilmore
University of Texas at Austin

David L. Costill
Ball State University

Human Kinetics Publishers

ıgress Cataloging-in-Publication Data

ial basis of the
ostill. -- 3rd ed.

Includes bibliographical references and index.
ISBN 0-87322-557-0
1. Exercise--Physiological aspects.   2. Physical fitness-
-Physiological aspects.   3. Physical education and training.
I. Costill, David L.   II. Title.
QP301.W675   1993
612'.044--dc20   93-2145
                                        CIP

ISBN: 0-87322-557-0

Copyright © 1988 by Jack H. Wilmore and David L. Costill

Copyright © 1982, 1977 by Allyn and Bacon, Inc.

Training for Sport and Activity (3rd ed.) previously was published by Wm. C. Brown Publishers. Starting in 1993, this book is available exclusively from Human Kinetics Publishers.

Cover Design: Ben Neff
Printer: Versa Press

Printed in the United States of America

10   9   8   7   6   5   4

Human Kinetics
Web site: http://www.humankinetics.com/

United States: Human Kinetics, P.O. Box 5076, Champaign, IL 61825-5076
1-800-747-4457

Canada: Human Kinetics, Box 24040, Windsor, ON N8Y 4Y9
1-800-465-7301 (in Canada only)

Europe: Human Kinetics, P.O. Box IW14, Leeds LS16 6TR, United Kingdom
(44) 1132 781708

Australia: Human Kinetics, 57A Price Avenue, Lower Mitcham, South Australia 5062
(08) 277 1555

New Zealand: Human Kinetics, P.O. Box 105-231, Auckland 1
(09) 523 3462

To those who have made the greatest impact on my life: to Dottie, my lovely wife, and our three beautiful daughters, Wendy, Kristi, and Melissa, for their patience and love; to Mom and Dad, for their love, direction, and encouragement; to my students who are a continual source of joy and inspiration; and to my Lord, Jesus Christ, who is always there providing for every one of my needs.

Jack H. Wilmore

To the three most important women in my life, Judy, Jill, and Holly, for their patience and understanding; to Bill Fink, my friend and confidant; and to my students, who are the pride of my professional effort.

David L. Costill

Contents

SECTION B *Physiological Adaptations to Physical Training 110*

SECTION C *Optimizing Sports Performance 214*

SECTION D   *Special Considerations* 286

Preface

Like the previous two editions, the third edition of this book is dedicated to providing the sport practitioner—the coach, the athlete, the team trainer, and the team physician—with a basic understanding of the physiological principles underlying the physical conditioning process that is so important to athletic performance and physical fitness. This third edition has been greatly expanded to provide for the growing needs of the undergraduate major in physical education and related disciplines, with the intent to provide a clear understanding of the fundamental principles of exercise physiology as applied to sport and physical activity.

Over the years, research in the exercise and sport sciences has provided the practitioner with relatively little information of practical value. In addition, the information that has been provided has been poorly utilized, if not ignored. Unfortunately, there is a large chasm between the researcher in the laboratory and the practitioner in the gym, beside the pool, or on the field. They live in two different worlds, neither completely understanding the language, complexities, or problems of the other. On the positive side, however, during the past few years research has taken a turn toward problems of a more practical nature, and a wealth of information is now available to the practitioner. To achieve maximum utilization of this information, you must have or acquire a basic understanding of the scientific foundations of exercise and sport.

The third edition of *Training for Sport and Activity* has assumed a totally new dimension! First, and most importantly, this third edition has a coauthor. Dr. David L. Costill, Director of the Human Performance Laboratory at Ball State University, a distinguished scientist, well-known author and lecturer, and an accomplished Masters athlete, has added his knowledge-base along with writing and illustrative talent to this book. Second, and largely due to the fact that two can work twice as hard as one, the book has been greatly expanded into areas not covered in previous editions. Also, much of the original material has been expanded and reorganized to accommodate the many changes in this field over the past five years. The result is a totally new book—well, almost totally new! We hope you like it!

JHW

SECTION A

Physiological Responses to Acute Exercise

The human body is an amazing creation! At rest, countless events are occurring simultaneously, in perfect coordination, allowing complex functions such as hearing, seeing, smelling, tasting, breathing, and thinking to continue without conscious effort. The transition from rest to exercise is accompanied by substantial changes in a number of bodily functions, allowing the body to successfully adapt to additional stress. As the body experiences repeated bouts of exercise, such as in a physical conditioning program, long-term adaptations occur in the body allowing higher performance levels without undue fatigue, as well as providing the body with a feeling and/or sense of well-being.

People have been able to achieve rather remarkable physical feats in the realm of sport. Some have been able to sprint 100 meters in less than 10 seconds, run a sub-four-minute mile, and complete a 26.2-mile marathon in less than two hours, eight minutes. Others have jumped over 29 feet horizontally, nearly 8 feet vertically, and pole vaulted almost 20 feet. Still others can skate, ski, swim, and cycle for both speed and distance, and perform many other feats requiring high levels of skill and coordination.

Such feats can be accomplished only through a series of complex interactions within the body involving nearly all of the body's systems. The bones provide the basic skeletal framework through which the muscles can perform. The heart and blood vessels deliver nutrients via the blood to the various cells of the body, and provide oxygen to and remove carbon dioxide

from these same cells with the help of the lungs. Practically no cell, tissue, or organ escapes involvement in even the simplest movement. At the cellular level, various enzymes are activated and energy is generated to enable muscles to contract. The skin plays a vital role in maintaining body temperature, mediating both heat loss and heat gain. The kidneys assist in maintaining fluid balance and provide long-term regulation of blood pressure. Finally, the nervous and endocrine systems integrate all of this activity into a meaningful performance.

The major purpose of this section is to provide you with a basic understanding of how the body responds to an acute or single bout of exercise. The next section will then review those changes the body undergoes in response to either chronic exercise or a long-term program of physical training. The first chapter describes the musculoskeletal system, providing a basis for understanding how the body moves. The second chapter focuses on metabolism and energy systems, explaining how the body is able to convert food into energy which provides the fuel for muscular activity. The third chapter details how respiration is controlled during exercise, and how the body is able to maintain an acid-base balance within the muscle. The fourth chapter describes the regulation of the heart and blood flow with increasing levels of exercise. Finally, the fifth and sixth chapters review how the body systems communicate through neural and hormonal control.

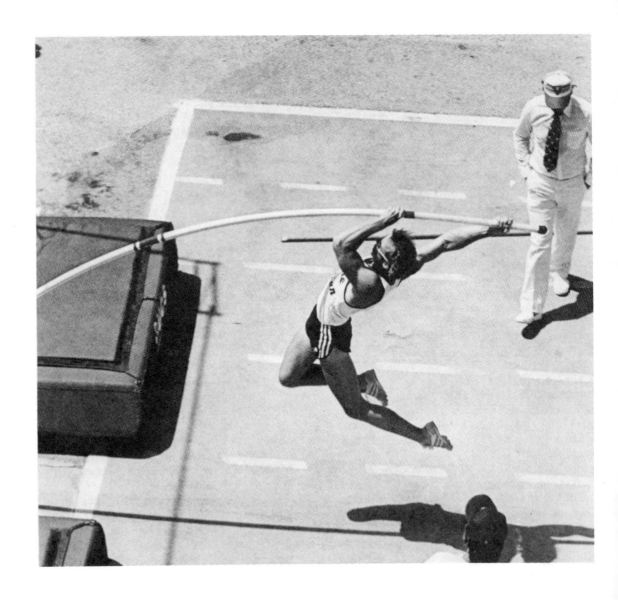

1

Essentials of Movement: The Musculoskeletal System

INTRODUCTION

All human movement, from the blinking of your eye to the running of a marathon, depends on the contractile or shortening qualities of muscles. But the muscles do not work alone. Muscular forces and the movements they create depend on activation by the nervous system and the structural support of the skeletal system. Added assistance is provided by a series of complex interactions involving nearly all of the body's systems. The circulatory system delivers oxygen and nutrients to the various cells of the body, while removing carbon dioxide and waste materials. Hormones, such as adrenalin, enhance the muscle's force production and assist in the process of energy production within the body.

In this and the following chapters, attention will be given to the anatomical and physiological systems that are essential to the optimal function of the muscles during acute exercise and the adaptation of the muscles to periods of intense training. Since the bones and muscles serve as the framework for body motion, our immediate attention will be directed toward these structures and their roles in producing movement.

BONE DEVELOPMENT

The bones, joints, cartilage, and ligaments form the structural support for the body. The bones provide points of attachment for the muscles and protection for delicate tissues, act as a reservoir for calcium within the body, and aid in the formation of red blood cells. Early in the development of the fetus, bones begin to develop from soft cartilage (elastic tissue). Flat bones, such as those of the face and skull, develop from fibrous membranes, while the remaining bones, which include most of the bones of the body, develop from **hyaline cartilage**. This cartilage covers the surface of bones within joints and forms the rib cartilages and many of the other types of cartilage found in the body. During fetal development, as well as during the initial 14 to 22 years of life, some membranes and cartilage are transformed from elastic tissue into hard bony tissue through the process of **ossification,** or hardening.

The ossification process is illustrated in Figure 1-1 on page 4. The general contour of the cartilage during embryonic development resembles the future shape of the mature bone. The central shaft of the long bone, the **diaphysis,** is where the initial

3

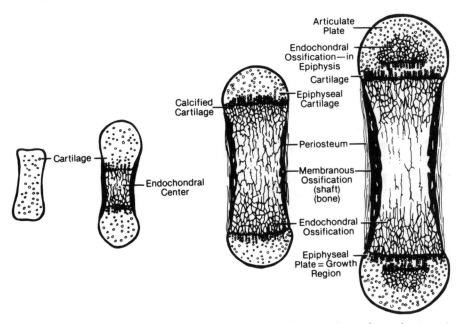

Figure 1-1 Bone formation and growth from a cartilagenous form in the embryonic stage to an almost mature bone.

hardening or transformation from cartilage to bone begins. The enlarged ends of the long bone are referred to as the **epiphyses.** The **periosteum,** the external or outer covering of bone, is the first part to develop, forming a ring or collar of bone around the diaphysis. At the same time, the cartilage cells in the diaphysis undergo a series of complex changes that eventually result in the formation of bone. As the cartilage cells continue to grow in length and thickness, the periosteum and bone formation from the center of the diaphysis continue towards the ends of the bone, the epiphysis. Eventually, the periosteum joins the epiphysis, establishing secondary centers of ossification at each end of the bone in each epiphysis. This allows bone formation from cartilage to continue at the ends of the long bones. Once this occurs, plates of cartilage develop between the diaphysis and the epiphyses that persist until full maturation, allowing for growth in the length of the bone. These plates of cartilage are known as **epiphyseal plate.** Cartilage continues to grow on the epiphyseal border of these plates, while on the diaphyseal

border cartilage is replaced, so that the plates or discs of cartilage will remain approximately the same thickness. Ossification is complete and bone growth discontinues when the cells of cartilage cease to grow and the entire discs are replaced by bone. This results in uniting the diaphysis with each epiphysis, making growth in bone length no longer possible.

The bone illustrated in Figure 1-1 is the shin bone, or tibia. Ossification is complete in the distal epiphysis (near the ankle) by the age of seventeen years and in the proximal epiphysis (near the knee) by the age of twenty years, although the exact ages will vary considerably from one individual to the next.

The structure of the mature long bone is surprisingly complex. Since bone is a living tissue that requires essential nutrients, it must have a good blood supply. The interior of the long bones is a cavity containing special tissue referred to as bone marrow. This center provides nutrients to the bone and is responsible for red and white blood cell production. Epiphysis bone tissue consists of cells that are distributed throughout a matrix or lattice-type of arrangement. Bone tissue is dense and hard due to deposits of lime salts, mainly calcium phosphate and calcium carbonate, and is referred to as spongy bone. Calcium is therefore an essential nutrient, particularly during growth periods, and the latter years of life, to prevent bones from becoming brittle with age.

Articulations: The Joints

Whenever two or more bones meet, joints or articulations are formed. The femur articulates with the tibia to form the knee joint; the humerus articulates with the radius and ulna to form the elbow joint; and the three phalanges of each finger articulate with one another to form several joints for each finger.

Essentially there are three primary classifications of joints: fibrous, cartilaginous, and synovial. **Fibrous joints** are those joints in which bones are joined together by fibrous-like elastic connective tissue, allowing little or no movement. The bones of the cranium or skull cap are joined together in this fashion. **Cartilaginous joints** are similar in characteristic, but there is limited motion. The vertebrae are joined in this manner. **Synovial joints** are formed by the articulating bones, a thin layer of cartilage on the ends of the bones, and a fibrous capsule that encloses the joint. All the joints of the extremities are synovial joints.

The fibrous joint capsule is lined on the inside with a membrane, referred to as the synovial membrane, that has a rich capillary network of blood vessels. The synovial membrane produces a viscous or relatively thick fluid, synovial fluid, that provides a natural lubrication for all joint movement. The smooth hyaline cartilage on the ends of those bones involved in the articulation, provides a surface that greatly reduces friction, and when combined with synovial fluid, allows for relatively free motion within the joint. Figure 1-2 illustrates a synovial joint.

A disc of fibrous cartilage is present in some joints, dividing the joint cavity and providing a smoother surface for joint action. The knee joint has several of these discs, or menisci, allowing for better articulation of the femur with the tibia. Frequently, when the knee is injured in athletics, the meniscus is damaged and must be surgically removed. Loss of one or both menisci in a single knee joint does not greatly limit joint movement, although the articulation is not as smooth. Joint swelling and pain often result in the possibility of arthritis in later years.

Ligaments are cords or bands of fibrous tissue that cross the joint, holding together one bone to another. Ligaments also provide strength to the joint capsule so that it can resist strain and irritation. Ligaments typically lie outside the joint capsule, but are also found within the joint capsule for certain joints, for example, cruciate ligaments

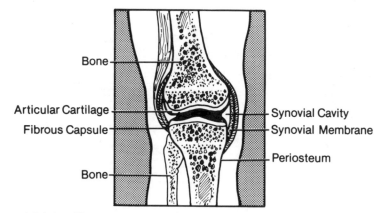

Figure 1-2 A synovial joint, illustrating the articular cartilage, synovial membrane, articular capsule, and ligamentous support.

inside the knee joint. **Tendons** are formed of connective tissue and provide the means by which muscles are attached to bones. Tendons cross joints and thus provide additional support for that specific joint. **Bursae** are small sacs filled with synovial fluid and are present in the area of joints where tendons are likely to rub against other supporting tissues. Their function is to reduce friction at these points of movement.

MUSCLES: STRUCTURE AND FUNCTION

There are basically three kinds of muscle tissue: smooth, cardiac, and skeletal. **Smooth muscle,** also referred to as involuntary muscle because it is not usually under the conscious control of the individual, has its contractions automatically controlled through the **autonomic nervous system.** Smooth muscle is found in the walls of the internal or visceral organs—blood vessels, stomach, and intestines. **Cardiac muscle,** found only in the heart, has

characteristics similar to skeletal muscle, but like smooth muscle, is not under direct voluntary control. **Skeletal muscle,** also referred to as voluntary muscle, is muscle the individual is consciously aware of and is able to control. The skeletal muscle attaches to and causes movement of the skeleton.

Skeletal muscle, in combination with the bones and joints, is responsible for all human movement. Obviously, any one single **muscle fiber,** or cell, does not function alone, contracting at will, independent of other muscles in the body. All skeletal muscles are coordinated simultaneously by a master network of nerve cells, both inside and outside the brain. The nervous system and its controls on muscular activity will be detailed in Chapter 5.

Figure 1–3 illustrates the basic structure of muscle. A single muscle is composed of a number of individual muscle fibers. Each muscle fiber is composed of many nuclei and is the structural unit of muscle. The number of muscle fibers per whole muscle varies considerably, depending on the size and function of the muscle. Within a given muscle,

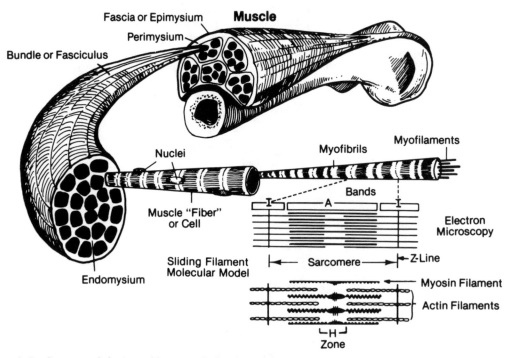

Figure 1–3 Structural design of human skeletal muscle.

the individual muscle fibers are grouped into bundles of fibers termed **fasciculi.** The **endomysium** is connective tissue that surrounds and binds together individual fibers to form the fasciculi. The **perimysium** is a white fibrous connective tissue that binds adjacent fasciculi together. The **epimysium** is the external connective tissue that surrounds the entire muscle, binding all of the fasciculi together into a unit. Each muscle fiber has a protective covering or membrane that surrounds it, the **sarcolemma.** Inside each muscle fiber, or cell, are numerous **myofibrils** that are comparable to numerous wires which comprise a large cable (fiber). **Sarcoplasm,** the protoplasm of the muscle fiber, is a gelatin-like substance that surrounds the myofibrils within each fiber. The **mitochondria** are the small rod-shaped bodies in the sarcoplasm that serve as the powerhouses of the cell, and are involved in providing energy for muscular contraction.

Individual myofibrils are aligned in columns with adjacent myofibrils. The myofibrils have distinct markings. A closer look at these markings indicate a definite repetitive pattern. These markings are referred to as striations, and skeletal muscle has been referred to as **striated muscle,** although this is a characteristic common to cardiac muscle as well. The repetitive pattern defines the contractile unit of muscle, the **sarcomere.** The sarcomere is bound on each end by a Z-line (see Figure 1–3). Between each pair of Z-lines are, in sequence, a light, or isotropic zone, referred to as the I-band; a dark, or anisotrophic zone, referred to as the A-band; an H-zone of slightly lighter contrast, that divides the middle of the A-band; and a second I-band. Each myofibril is composed of numerous sarcomeres which are joined end-to-end at the Z-line.

Scientists believe these variations in light and dark patterns are the result of the alignment of individual myofilaments that comprise the myofibrils. Looking through an electron microscope, it is possible to differentiate two small protein filaments, **actin** and **myosin.** The thinner of the two filaments is the protein actin, while the protein myosin forms the thicker filament. The I-band reflects that region of the sarcomere where there are only thin, or actin filaments; the A-band reflects that region where there are both thick, myosin, as well as thin, actin, protein filaments. The H-zone is the central portion of the A-band occupied only by the thick filaments when the sarcomere is in a resting state. The H-zone will disappear as the muscle contracts, since the thin filaments from the A-zone extend into it.

The precise mechanism used to shorten the sarcomere is not fully understood, but there is sufficient evidence to indicate that when stimulated the actin and myosin filaments slide past one another. This motion is accomplished by the pulling action of cross-bridges that reach out from the myosin filaments and attach themselves to the actin filament. After binding, the cross-bridges suddenly shorten, drawing the two protein threads past one another (see Figure 1–4 on page 8). This action is taking place simultaneously in thousands of muscle fibers, resulting in a forceful pull on the tendons.

The mechanism responsible for triggering this contractile process is quite complex. A nerve impulse from the specific nerve serving that muscle fiber travels along the sarcolemma, which is the cell membrane or outer cover of the muscle fiber, sending a weak electrical charge over the length of the fiber. A series of tubules enter this individual muscle fiber through pores in the sarcolemma. These tubules are referred to as **T-tubules,** and they conduct the impulse from the outer surface toward the center of the fiber, connecting with the **sarcoplasmic reticulum,** a system of channels that spread throughout the fiber (see Figure 1–5 on page 8). The nerve impulse travels along the sarcolemma and down the T-tubules to the sarcoplasmic reticulum. Calcium ions are stored within the sarcoplasmic reticulum and are released once the nerve impulse reaches the sarcoplasmic reticulum. It is the release of these calcium ions that allows the process of contraction to begin.

There are two regulatory proteins that are part of the actin filament that serve to keep the actin and myosin filaments from interacting with one another, resulting in contraction or shortening of the myofibril. These proteins, **troponin** and **tropomyosin,** work in an intricate fashion, along with the calcium ions, to maintain relaxation or initiate contraction (see Figure 1–6 on page 9). Once calcium ions are released from the sarcoplasmic reticulum, they bind troponin, blocking the function of

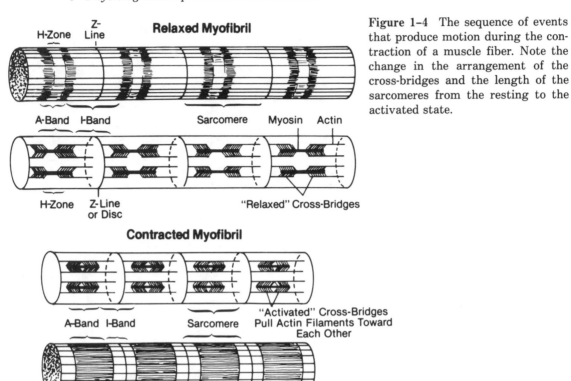

Relaxed Myofibril

H-Zone
Z-Line

A-Band I-Band Sarcomere Myosin Actin

H-Zone Z-Line or Disc "Relaxed" Cross-Bridges

Contracted Myofibril

A-Band I-Band Sarcomere "Activated" Cross-Bridges Pull Actin Filaments Toward Each Other

Figure 1–4 The sequence of events that produce motion during the contraction of a muscle fiber. Note the change in the arrangement of the cross-bridges and the length of the sarcomeres from the resting to the activated state.

Figure 1–5 Nerve impulse transmission from the sarcolemma to the sarcoplasmic reticulum.

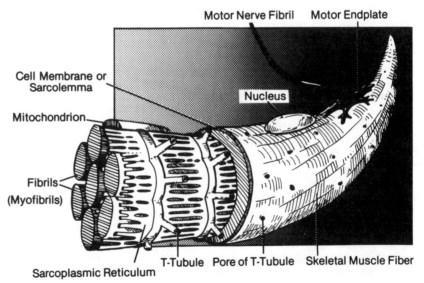

Motor Nerve Fibril Motor Endplate

Cell Membrane or Sarcolemma

Nucleus

Mitochondrion

Fibrils (Myofibrils)

Sarcoplasmic Reticulum T-Tubule Pore of T-Tubule Skeletal Muscle Fiber

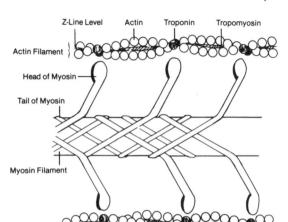

Figure 1-6 The molecular structure of the actin and myosin filaments and their interaction in contraction.

tropomyosin, which keeps the actin and myosin filaments from interacting. The enzyme **ATPase,** located on the head of the cross-bridge of the myosin filament, is then freed to act on **ATP (adenosine triphosphate),** causing it to breakdown to **ADP (adenosine diphosphate),** phosphate, and energy release. ATP is the chemical molecule in the body most available for energy release, and is the primary source of energy for muscular contraction. When ATP breaks down to ADP, releasing energy for contraction, there is an interaction between the myosin filament and the actin filament, resulting from the specific action of the cross-bridges. The extent of contraction of the individual sarcomeres appears to be limited by the myosin filaments and the Z-lines—the contraction will be complete when the myosin filaments reach the Z-lines. It has recently been hypothesized, however, that the myosin filaments can buckle during very intense contraction, allowing even greater shortening of the sarcomere.

Muscle Characteristics: Practical Implications

The athlete's endurance and speed during competition depends to a large part on the muscles' ability to produce energy and force. Individual differences in performance can, in some ways, be related to these characteristics in arm and leg muscles.

Thanks to technological advances over the past 15 years it is now possible to obtain samples of muscle tissue from subjects before, during, and after exercise. Through a muscle biopsy, a very small piece of muscle is extracted from the belly of a muscle for subsequent analysis. The area where the biopsy is to be taken is deadened with a local anesthetic. Once anesthetized, a scalpel is used to make a small, approximately quarter-inch, incision through the skin and outer connective tissue of the muscle. A biopsy needle is then inserted into this incision and is pushed into the belly of the muscle to the appropriate depth. A small plunger is pushed through the center of the needle, snipping off a very small sample of the muscle. The sample is removed from the needle, cleaned of blood and connective tissue, mounted, and quickly frozen. It is then thinly sliced, stained, and examined under a microscope. Figure 1-7 shows a close-up of a muscle biopsy needle. Figure 1-8 on page 10 illustrates in two parts: (A) the insertion of the needle to obtain a sample of tissue from the leg muscle of an elite female runner and (B) the resulting muscle specimen. This method has allowed us to study the make-up of the muscle cells (fibers) and gauge the effects of exercise and training. Microscopic and biochemical analyses are used to identify the muscle's machinery for energy production.

One characteristic of muscle that has gained considerable attention from the "world of sports"

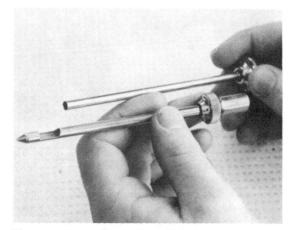

Figure 1-7 A muscle biopsy needle.

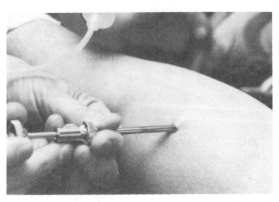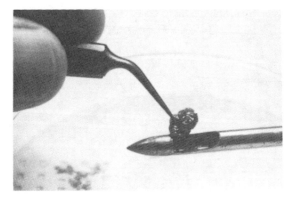

Figure 1–8 Obtaining a muscle specimen from the calf (gastrocnemius) of an elite female runner.

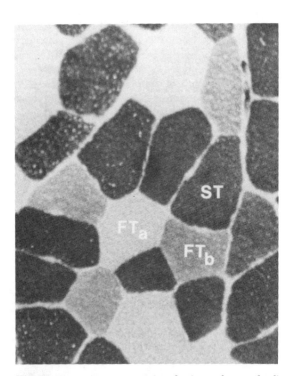

Figure 1–9 A cross-sectional view of muscle fibers from the thigh of an untrained man. The black-stained fibers are the slow-twitch (ST), while the fast-twitch type "a" (FT$_a$) fibers are unstained. The gray fibers are the fast-twitch "b" (FT$_b$) type. In general, slow-twitch fibers demonstrate higher aerobic and lower anaerobic capacity than do the fast-twitch fibers.

is the muscle composition of **fast- and slow-twitch fibers.** The following discussion will focus on the fiber "types" and their relationship to distance-running performance. The microscopic photograph of human muscle in Figure 1–9 illustrates the different types of fibers. Those fibers that stain black in this histochemical method are the slow-twitch type (ST). There are two types of fast-twitch fibers—fast-twitch type "a" (FT$_a$) and fast-twitch type "b" (FT$_b$). In this photograph, the FT$_a$ fibers are unstained and the FT$_b$ fibers appear gray. Although not shown in Figure 1–9, a third subtype of fast-twitch fibers has also been identified, type "c" (FT$_c$). On the average, roughly 50 percent of the fibers in a muscle are slow twitch, whereas the fast-twitch "a" fibers constitute about 25 percent of the muscle. The remaining 25 percent of the fibers are mostly fast-twitch "b", with the "c" fibers making up one to three percent of the muscle. The nerves controlling these fibers determine whether they will be ST or FT. The muscle fiber and its connecting nerve system are referred to as a **motor unit.** ST motor units may include one relatively small nerve cell connected to a cluster of 10 to 180 fibers (see Figure 1–10). FT motor units, on the other hand, comprise a larger nerve cell and have between 300 and 800 fibers per nerve cell.

In general, the ST motor units are characterized as having good aerobic endurance and are, therefore, recruited most often during low-intensity endurance events. The FT$_a$ motor units develop considerably more force than an ST motor unit,

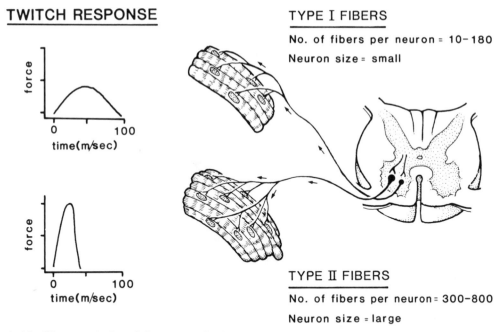

TWITCH RESPONSE

TYPE I FIBERS

No. of fibers per neuron = 10-180

Neuron size = small

TYPE II FIBERS

No. of fibers per neuron = 300-800

Neuron size = large

Figure 1-10 Characteristics of the type I (slow-twitch) and type II (fast-twitch) motor units. Each motor unit consists of a nerve cell and the muscle fibers it innervates. Note the difference between the duration and height of a muscle twitch for the type I and II motor units (from Costill, 1986).

although they fatigue rather easily. Thus, these FT_a fibers are used during shorter, faster races. Although the significance of the FT_b fibers is not fully understood, it appears these fibers are not easily turned on by the nervous system and are, therefore, used rather infrequently in normal, low-intensity activity.

It is not the speed of contraction, however, that determines the pattern of muscle fiber recruitment. Rather, it is the level of force that is demanded of the muscle that causes the motor nerves to selectively activate the slow- and fast-twitch fibers. Figure 1-11 on page 12 illustrates the relationship between force development by a muscle and the recruitment of ST, FT_a, and FT_b fibers. During slow, low-intensity exercise, most of the muscle force is generated by the ST fibers. As the muscle tension requirements increase at heavier loads, the FT_a fibers are added to the work force. Finally, in events where maximal strength is needed, the FT_b fibers are also turned on. Muscle

fiber recruitment will be discussed in greater detail in Chapter 5.

During events lasting several hours, athletes are forced to perform at a submaximal pace, where the nervous system recruits the muscle fibers best adapted to endurance activity; that is, ST and some FT_a fibers. During the event, as these fibers become depleted of energy, the nervous system recruits more FT_a fibers to maintain muscle tension. As more ST and FT_a fibers become exhausted, the FT_b fibers are called upon in a final effort to continue moving. This may explain why fatigue seems to come in stages during events like the marathon, and why it takes great conscious effort to maintain a given pace near the finish of the event. Much of that mental effort is probably used to activate muscle fibers that are not easily recruited.

Such information is of practical importance to our understanding of the specific requirements for training and competition. It suggests that all training done at a slow pace, or with light force,

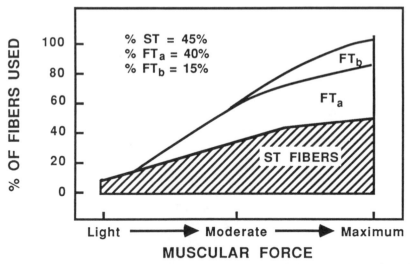

Figure 1-11 The ramp-like recruitment of muscle fibers in varied levels of muscular effort. Whereas light force requirements only use the slow-twitch fibers, heavy loads on the muscle will result in the recruitment of all three types of muscle fibers.

Table 1-1 Percentage of slow-twitch (%ST) and fast-twitch (%FT) fibers in selected muscles of male (M) and female (F) athlete. Also shown are the average cross-sectional areas of muscle fibers.

					Fiber size (μ^2)	
Athletes	*Sex*	*Muscle*	*%ST*	*%FT*	*ST*	*FT*
Sprint (runners)	M	Gastrocnemius	24	76	5,878	6,034
	F	Gastrocnemius	27	73	3,752	3,930
Distance (runners)	M	Gastrocnemius	79	21	8,342	6,485
	F	Gastrocnemius	69	31	4,441	4,128
Cyclists	M	Vastus lateralis	57	43	6,333	6,116
	F	Vastus lateralis	51	49	5,487	5,216
Swimmers	M	Posterior Deltoid	67	33	—	—
Weight lifters	M	Gastrocnemius	44	56	5,060	8,910
	M	Deltoid	53	47	5,010	8,450
Triathletes	M	Posterior Deltoid	60	40	—	—
	M	Vastus lateralis	63	37	—	—
	M	Gastrocnemius	59	41	—	—
Canoeists	M	Posterior Deltoid	71	29	4,920	7,040
Shot-putters	M	Gastrocnemius	38	62	6,367	6,441
Non-athletes	M	Vastus lateralis	47	53	4,722	4,709

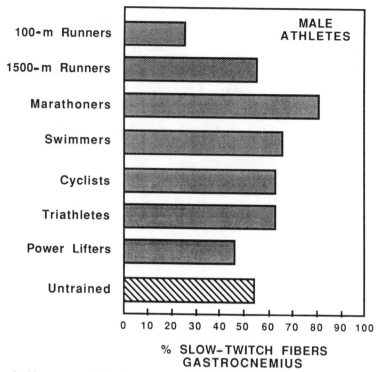

Figure 1-12 Muscle fiber composition (percentage of slow twitch) in the calf muscle (gastrocnemius) of highly trained athletes and untrained men.

will emphasize the use of only the ST fibers, inducing little training effect on the FT_a or FT_b fibers. Thus, long, slow training bouts do not prepare the muscle for the demands of competition, in which greater forces are imposed on the FT fibers. This point will be emphasized more in Chapter 5.

Such information relative to the composition and use of muscle fibers suggests that athletes, who have a high percentage of ST fibers, might have an advantage in long, endurance events, whereas those athletes with a predominance of FT fibers might better be suited for short, explosive activities. Table 1-1 and Figure 1-12 present the muscle fiber make-up of successful athletes from a variety of athletic events. As anticipated, leg muscles of sprinters are composed principally of FT fibers, whereas elite distance runners have a predominance of ST fibers. Although there are tendencies for cyclists and swimmers to have a slightly higher percentage of ST fibers in their

muscles than untrained subjects, this factor does not appear to be a prerequisite for success in these sports.

An average individual has roughly 50 percent ST, 25 percent FT_a, and 25 percent FT_b fibers in his or her leg muscles. Studies of elite male and female distance runners have revealed that some have calf muscles composed of more than 90 percent ST fibers. The calf muscle from a recent world record-holder in the marathon, for example, was found to have 93 percent ST fibers, 7 percent FT_a fibers, and no FT_b fibers. In contrast, muscles of world-class sprinters are composed mostly of FT_a fibers. Although there is a marked difference in the composition of fibers in the muscles of sprinters and distance runners, fiber composition alone is not a reliable predictor of distance success.

Whereas previous studies have shown that training may increase the endurance capacity of muscle, there is little evidence to suggest that the percentage of ST and FT fibers change following only a few months of training. There is some debate as to whether ST and FT fibers can be converted after long-term training. Any changes that might occur in the percentage of ST and FT fibers with training, however, are probably small. That is to say, it would be very unlikely that a sprinter's fiber type could be converted to that of a marathoner's. Most studies have reported that the composition of muscle appears fixed and unaffected by training, suggesting genes and inheritance may be involved. Studies have shown that identical twins, from the same egg, have identical physical characteristics, as well as identical fiber compositions. Fraternal twins, from separate eggs, differ in their physical characteristics as well as fiber composition. The percentage of ST and FT fibers is established soon after birth during the process of natural development and remains relatively unchanged throughout life.

Findings have shown, however, that the subtypes of FT fibers (FT_a and FT_b) may show some modification with training. The FT_a fibers are generally described as being a bit more aerobic (able to use oxygen for energy production) than the FT_b fibers. With endurance training, the FT_b fibers begin to take on the characteristics of the FT_a fibers. This suggests that these fibers are used more during training and gain greater endurance ability. Though the full significance of this change of FT_b fibers to FT_a fibers is not known, it may explain why we find very few, if any, FT_b fibers in the leg muscles of highly-trained distance runners.

The size (diameter) of the muscle fibers varies markedly among elite distance runners, but on the average ST fibers are some 22 percent larger than FT fibers in elite male and female runners' gastrocnemius (see Table 1-1 and Figure 1-12). Experts have proposed that training for endurance or strength may result in selective enlargement (hypertrophy) of the ST and FT fibers, respectively.

Is the percentage of ST and FT fibers the same in all the muscles of the body? Generally, the muscles of the arms and legs have similar fiber compositions, although there are some exceptions. The soleus, a muscle near the bone in the calf area, is almost completely composed of ST fibers in everyone. Studies have shown that an individual with a predominance of ST fibers in the thigh, or gastroc-

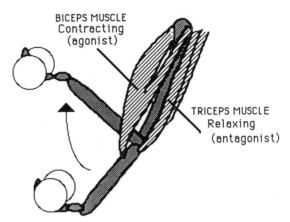

Figure 1-13 Elbow flexion requires the shortening (contraction) of the biceps muscle (antagonist), and the relaxation of the antagonistic muscle (triceps).

nemius, muscles will likely have a high percentage of ST fibers in the arm muscles as well.

How Are Muscles Used?

The more than 215 pairs of muscles in the body vary widely in size, shape, and use. It is important to realize that every coordinated movement requires the application of force by muscles that serve as the prime movers, the **agonistic** muscles, and the relaxation of muscles that might resist that motion, the **antagonistic** muscles. As illustrated in Figure 1-13, the smooth flexion of the elbow requires contracting the biceps muscle (agonist) and the relaxation of the triceps muscle (antagonist).

The principal action of the muscle is to shorten, referred to as **concentric** contraction. There are, however, frequent periods when muscles may contract without reducing their length. Such static contractions are termed **isometric,** and may occur when we attempt to lift an object that is heavier than the force generated by the muscle, or when we hold an object steady with the elbow flexed (see Figure 1-14). When the muscle lengthens during a contraction, as the biceps do when the elbow is extended as in lowering a heavy weight, the con-

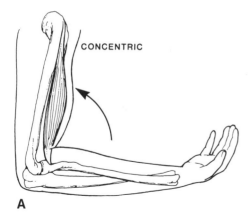

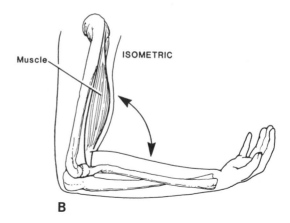

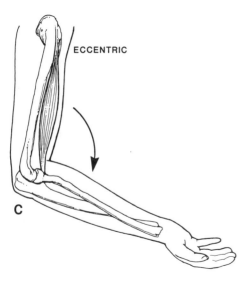

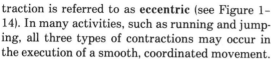

Figure 1-14 Examples of the three types of muscle contractions: (A) concentric contraction, shortening of length, (B) insometric contraction, no change in muscle length, and (C) eccentric contraction, lengthening of muscle during contraction.

traction is referred to as **eccentric** (see Figure 1-14). In many activities, such as running and jumping, all three types of contractions may occur in the execution of a smooth, coordinated movement.

The development of muscle force depends on its initial length and the speed of contraction. If a muscle was not attached to bone, it would assume a relaxed, **equilibrium length.** When attached to the skeleton, a muscle at resting length is normally under slight tension, since it is moderately stretched. Measurements of isometric force are maximal when the length of the muscle at the time of activation is approximately 20 percent greater than the equilibrium length. Increasing or decreasing the muscle length causes a reduction in maximal-force development. When the muscle is elongated to twice its equilibrium length, the force produced by the muscle is nearly zero. This failure to yield force when overstretched is a result of a decrease in the overlap between the actin and myosin filaments. The more they are stretched apart, the fewer cross-bridges are available to bind the filaments and create force.

Muscles and their connective tissues (fascia and tendons) have the properties of **elasticity.** When stretched, this elastic characteristic results in the release of stored energy that creates additional force during a subsequent contraction. In the intact body, muscle length is restricted by the anatomical arrangement and attachment of muscle to bone. When stretched, this anatomical arrangement allows the muscle length to increase 1.2 times the muscle's equilibrium length, the optimal length for maximal force development.

Since the muscles exert their force using skeletal levers, the physical arrangement of these muscle-bone levers are critical to our understanding of

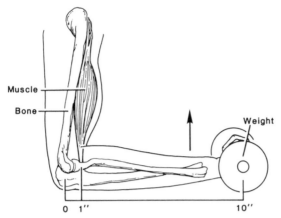

Figure 1–15 The bone-muscle lever system for the application of force.

movement. As shown in Figure 1–15, the tendon attachment for the biceps is only one-tenth the distance from the fulcrum (elbow) to the weighted resistance held in the hand. Thus, in order to hold a ten-pound weight, the muscle must exert ten times (100 lbs.) as much force as the weight. The best joint angle for the application of this force is approximately 100 degrees, since greater or lesser flexion of the elbow will reduce the angle of the force applied to the lever arm.

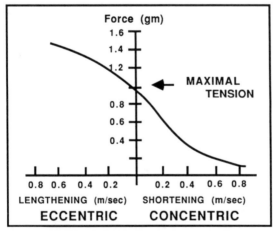

Figure 1–16 The relationship between the rate of movement and the maximal-force development during both eccentric and concentric contractions (modified from Åstrand and Rodahl, 1985).

The ability to develop force also depends on the speed of muscle lengthening or shortening. Figure 1–16 illustrates this relationship, showing that the highest muscle forces occur during fast eccentric contraction. During concentric contractions, on the other hand, maximal force development becomes progressively less at higher speeds. Such measurements are possible only with specialized testing equipment that can control the rate of muscle shortening and/or lengthening.

SUMMARY

It is evident from the preceding discussion that the structural arrangement of the nervous system, bones, connective tissues, and muscles are all essential components of the machinery that allow for human motion. Such movement is achieved by the nervous activation of selected muscle fibers and the transfer of tension to the skeletal levers by the tendons and other connective tissues. The unique ability of muscle to produce just the desired force and speed of motion is accomplished by the selective recruitment of the two major types of fibers—slow and fast twitch. In low-intensity activities it is the slow-twitch fibers that are turned on and carry the major responsibility for force development. As the intensity of the activity is increased, the nervous system recruits more of the slow-twitch fibers and eventually calls into play the fast-twitch fibers. In a maximal effort, both types of fibers are activated in an attempt to involve as many contractile units as possible. Current evidence suggests that one's potential for success in sprint and endurance events may, to some degree, depend on the composition of slow- and fast-twitch fibers in the muscle, a quality that appears to be genetically determined. Although training may alter the endurance and strength of these fiber types, there is some controversy regarding the effect of training on the contractile characteristics of the fibers.

STUDY QUESTIONS

1. How do the bones grow longer and wider?
2. List and define the structure of a muscle fiber.

3. Describe the "sliding filament theory." How do muscle fibers shorten?
4. What are the basic characteristics of slow- and fast-twitch muscle fibers?
5. Describe the relationship between muscle force development and the recruitment of slow- and fast-twitch fibers.
6. What is the pattern of muscle fiber (ST, FT_a, or FT_b) recruitment when high jumping? Running a 10,000 meter race? Running a marathon?
7. List the components of a motor unit.
8. Differentiate between and give examples of (1) concentric, (2) isometric, and (3) eccentric contractions.
9. What is the optimal length of a muscle for maximal force development?
10. What is the relationship between maximal force development and the speed of shortening (concentric) and lengthening (eccentric) contractions?

REFERENCES

Åstrand, P. O., & Rodahl, K. (1985). *Textbook of work physiology* (3rd ed). New York: McGraw-Hill Book Co.

Brobeck, J. R. (Ed) (1979). *Best and Taylor's physiological basis of medical practice* (10th ed.). Baltimore: Williams and Wilkins Co.

Brooke, M. H., & Kaiser, K. K. (1970). Muscle fiber types: How many and what kind? *Archives of Neurology, 23,* 369-379.

Buchthal, F., & Schmalbruch, H. (1970). Contraction times and fiber types in intact muscle. *Acta Physiologica Scandinavica, 79,* 435-452.

Burke, R. E., & Edgerton, V. R. (1975). Motor unit properties and selective involvement in movement. In J. Wilmore & J. Keogh (Eds.), *Exercise and sports sciences reviews* (pp. 31-83). New York: Academic Press.

Costill, D. L. (1986). *Inside running: Basics of sports physiology.* Indianapolis: Benchmark Press.

Crouch, J. E. (1972). *Functional human anatomy* (2nd ed.). Philadelphia: Lea & Febiger.

Edington, D. W., & Edgerton, V. R. (1976). *The biology of physical activity* (pp. 51-72). Boston: Houghton Mifflin Co.

Fox, E. L. (1984). *Sports physiology* (2nd ed.). New York: CBS College Publishers.

Ganong, W. F. (1965). *Review of medical physiology* (2nd ed.). Los Altos, CA: Lange Medical Publications.

Guyton, A. C. (1986). *Physiology of the human body* (7th ed.). Philadelphia: W. B. Saunders Co.

Henneman, E. (1980). Skeletal muscle. The servant of the nervous system. In V. B. Mountcastle (Ed.), *Medical Physiology* (14th ed.): Vol. 1. (pp. 674-702). St. Louis: Mosby Publishing.

Jones, N. L., McCartney, N., & McComas, A. J. (1986). *Human muscle power.* Champaign, IL: Human Kinetics Publishers, Inc.

Katz, B. (1966). *Nerve, muscle and synapse.* New York: McGraw-Hill.

Porter, R., & Whelan, J. (1981). *Human muscle fatigue: Physiological mechanisms* (Ciba Foundation Symposium 82). London : Pitman Medical.

Strauss, R. H. (1979). *Sports medicine and physiology.* Philadelphia: W. B. Saunders Co.

Wickiewicz, T. L., Roy, R. R., Powell, P. L., Perrine, J. J., & Edgerton, V. R. (1984). Muscle architecture and force-velocity relationships in humans. *Journal of Applied Physiology, 57,* 435-443.

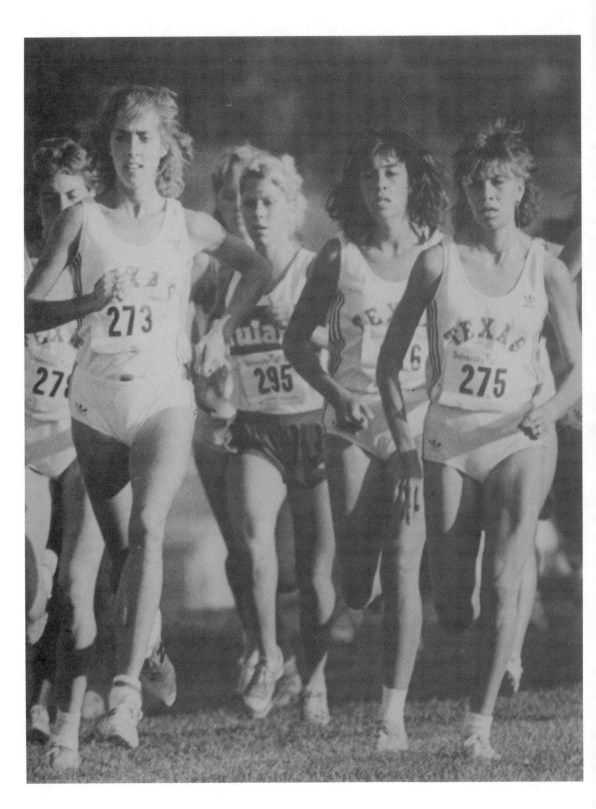

2

Muscle Metabolism: Energy for Exercise

INTRODUCTION

The ability to do work, produce change, and maintain life all require energy. The laws of thermodynamics tell us that all forms of energy, whether chemical, electrical, or mechanical, are interconvertible. Chemical energy, for example, can be used to create electricity, which in turn, can be used to accomplish mechanical work. The first law of thermodynamics states that energy can neither be created nor destroyed.

In order to maintain life and accomplish work, the cells of the body must have a continual supply of chemical energy. The foods we eat provide the **potential energy** to sustain the normal operation of body tissue. The chemical release of energy through metabolism provides the force to activate muscles and to fulfill the functioning requirements of living cells. In active form, it is referred to as **kinetic energy**. Although the foods we eat contain chemical energy, their molecular bonds are relatively weak and provide a low-energy source when the bonds are disassembled. Consequently, the carbohydrates, fats, and proteins we ingest are not used directly for muscular contraction. Rather, the energy that bonds these food molecules together must be chemically released and stored in the form of a "high-energy phosphate," **adenosine triphosphate (ATP)** (see Figure 2–1 on page 20). Assembling and disassembling these energy compounds are facilitated by special proteins, termed enzymes. When acted on by the enzyme **ATP-ase**, the last phosphate group (P_i) is split away from the adenosine triphosphate (ATP) molecule, thereby releasing a great deal more energy (7.6 kcal/mole of ATP) than originally contained in the low-energy foods.

ENERGY PRODUCTION

ATP–PCr System

Another high-energy phosphate molecule, **phosphocreatine (PCr)**, is used to store energy within the cells. Unlike the energy derived from the breakdown of ATP, PCr does not appear to be used directly to accomplish work within the cells. Instead, it is used to rebuild the ATP molecule,

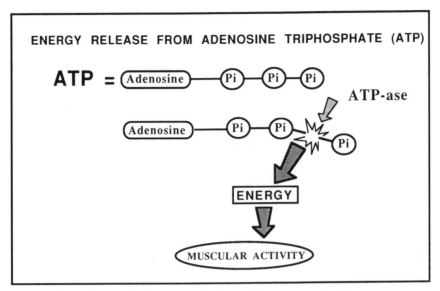

Figure 2–1   Energy release from ATP by the activation of the enzyme ATP-ase.

thereby maintaining a relatively constant supply of this high-energy compound (see Figure 2–2). When energy is released from ATP by the splitting of a phosphate group, the ATP molecule can be reconstructed by reducing PCr to creatine (Cr) and inorganic phosphate (P_i), again providing energy for ATP production.

During the first few seconds of a maximal sprint, the level of ATP remains constant, whereas the level of PCr declines steadily throughout the

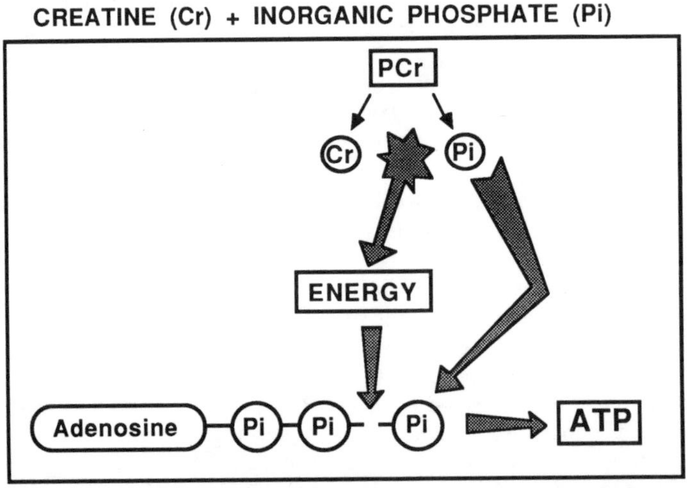

CREATINE (Cr) + INORGANIC PHOSPHATE (Pi)

Figure 2–2   Energy and inorganic phosphate (Pi), derived from splitting creatine phosphate (PCr), are used to bond the third phosphate group to adenosine diphosphate to form adenosine triphosphate (ATP).

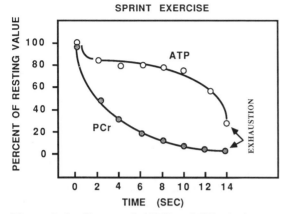

Figure 2-3 Changes in ATP and PCr during exhaustive sprint cycling. Note that ATP declines little during the early seconds of exercise, while PCr drops steadily throughout the activity. Only at exhaustion are both energy sources at low levels.

activity (see Figure 2-3). At exhaustion, both ATP and PCr levels are quite low, unable to provide the energy for further contractions and relaxations.

The capacity to maintain levels of ATP from the energy derived from phosphocreatine is limited. Since the stores of ATP and PCr can only sustain the energy needs of the muscle for a few seconds during an all-out sprint, the muscles must rely on other processes for ATP formation. Aside from the ATP-PCr system, there are two other sources for ATP production: (1) **glycolysis**, ATP production from sugar stored in muscle (glycogen), without the use of oxygen; and (2) **oxidation**, the formation of ATP from carbohydrate, fat, and protein molecules, with the aid of oxygen. Both of these energy systems depend on the availability of fuels commonly consumed in our diets.

Glycolytic System

During the early minutes of exercise, when the intensity of the muscular effort is high, the body is incapable of providing sufficient oxygen to regenerate the needed ATP. To compensate, both the ATP-PCr and glycolytic energy systems generate ATP without the aid of oxygen, a process termed **anaerobic metabolism.** Glycolysis is the breakdown of carbohydrate (starches and sugar) in the absence of oxygen. In this system, **glycogen**, sugar stored within the cells, is broken-down through the action of special **glycolytic enzymes** (see Figure 2-4), resulting in the production and accumulation of lactic acid, producing energy in the form of ATP. Thus, glycolysis generates ATP when there is inadequate oxygen supplied to the system.

Unfortunately, this system of energy production is relatively inefficient, providing only 3 moles of ATP from the anaerobic breakdown of one mole (180 grams) of glycogen. On the other hand, in the presence of oxygen, **aerobic metabolism** can generate 39 moles of ATP from a single mole of glycogen. Thus, the glycolytic system supplements the ATP-PCr system in providing energy for highly-intense muscular effort. Without adequate oxygen, however, the muscles lose their ability to generate tension as their energy reserves dwindle.

The second major limitation of anaerobic glycolysis is that it results in the incomplete breakdown of glycogen, producing lactic acid. In all-out sprint events that last one or two minutes, the demands on the glycolytic system are high, causing muscle lactic acid levels to rise from a resting value of 1 mmol/kg of muscle to over 25 mmol/kg. The high acid content of the muscle fibers inhibits further

GLYCOLYSIS

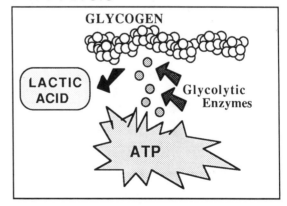

Figure 2-4 Glycolysis—the formation of ATP from the anaerobic breakdown of glycogen.

breakdown of glycogen and may interfere with the muscle's contractile process.

Both the ATP–PCr and glycolytic energy systems serve imporant roles in providing a rapid supply of ATP for intense muscular effort. Since a muscle fiber's rate of energy use during exercise may be 200 times greater than at rest, it is impossible for even these methods of ATP production to supply all the needed energy. Thus, without another more efficient energy system, the maximal duration of exercise may be limited to only a few minutes of activity.

Oxidative Energy System

In order for the muscles to continuously produce the force needed during long-term activity, they must have a steady supply of energy. As noted in Figure 2–5, the energy bound into the ATP molecule is derived from the breakdown of the foods we eat—carbohydrates, fats, and protein. The process of disassembling fuels in the presence of oxygen, is referred to as **aerobic metabolism**. As we have seen, the anaerobic production of ATP, without oxygen, is quite inefficient and inadequate for exercise lasting more than a few minutes. Consequently, aerobic metabolism is the primary method of energy production during endurance

events, placing heavy demands on the athlete's ability to supply oxygen to the exercising muscles.

Within each muscle fiber, there are special powerhouse-like structures called **mitochondria**, which use fuels and oxygen to produce large amounts of ATP. As shown in Figure 2–5, carbohydrate, fat, and protein molecules provide the fuel to drive this system of ATP production. These molecules are disassembled within the fluids (**cytoplasm**) and mitochondria of the cells. To perform this task efficiently and to speed the rate of energy production, mitochondria employ specialized proteins, known as **oxidative enzymes**. In this process, the energy bonding the **carbon** (C), **oxygen** (O_2), and **hydrogen** (H^+) atoms that form the carbohydrate and fat molecules together, is liberated by the action of the oxidative enzymes, resulting in the formation of ATP. If left untended, the hydrogen component of these fuels would be free to disrupt the function of the cells. In the presence of oxygen, however, two hydrogen molecules will bond with oxygen to form water (H_2O), allowing the energy system to flow uninterrupted. Carbon dioxide (CO_2), formed from the combination of carbon and oxygen from the fuels, is another by-product of oxidative metabolism. When carbon dixoide is dissolved in the water of the body it forms, carbonic acid, that upsets the normal cellular homeostasis. Fortunately,

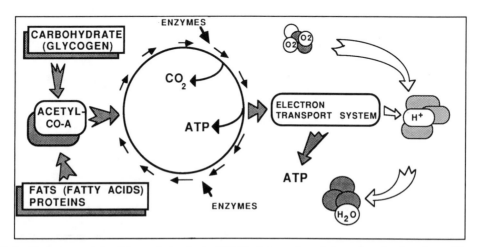

Figure 2-5   Energy contained in carbohydrate (CHO), fat, and protein molecules is released by enzyme actions and used to form ATP for the work of the cells.

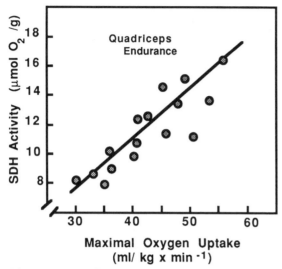

Figure 2-6 Relationship between maximal oxygen uptake and succinate dehydrogenase (SDH) activity of the vastus lateralis (lateral quadriceps) muscle (modified from Ivy, et al., 1980).

CO_2 diffuses easily out of the cells and is transported by the venous blood back to the lungs, where it leaves the body in expired air.

Measurements of oxidative enzyme levels are often used to indicate the capacity of the muscle to do aerobic work. Since these enzymes have rather lengthy names, enzymes such as **succinate dehydrogenase** and **citrate synthase** are often abbreviated to **SDH** and **CS**. Numerous studies have shown a close relationship between the ability of a muscle to perform prolonged exercise and the amount of oxidative enzymes present. Figure 2-6 illustrates that the muscle's endurance is related to enzyme (SDH) activity. Muscles of endurance athletes, for example, have nearly 2 times more oxidative enzymes than untrained men and women.

Although elite distance runners have been reported to possess more slow-twitch (ST) fibers, more mitochondria, and higher oxidative enzyme activities than untrained individuals, little relationship has been found between the percentage of ST fibers and the amount of oxidative enzymes in the muscle. Certainly, endurance training can enhance the oxidative capacity of all fibers, especially the fast-twitch (FT), which naturally have

fewer mitochondria and aerobic enzymes in the untrained state. Thus, even individuals having a small percentage of ST fibers can increase the aerobic capacity of their muscles with endurance training, but it is our general impression that an endurance-trained FT fiber will not develop the same high endurance capacity as a well-trained ST fiber.

Oxygen Delivery. **Oxygen delivery** to the muscle cells is a major factor in maintaining a high rate of aerobic energy production. During mild exercise the blood picks up oxygen as it passes through the lungs, transports it to the muscles where it is exchanged for carbon dioxide (CO_2), then the blood returns to the heart and lungs where it can unload the CO_2 and refill its oxygen supply. The CO_2 is removed from the lungs in exhaled air. As the intensity of the exercise and energy demands increase, the rate of oxidative ATP-production increases. In an effort to satisfy the muscle's need for oxygen, the heart beats faster, pumping more blood and oxygen to the muscles. Since the body stores little oxygen, the amount absorbed by the blood as it passes through the lungs is directly proportional to the amount used for oxidative metabolism. Consequently, an accurate estimate of aerobic metabolism can be made by determining the amount of oxygen being consumed.

In the laboratory we can measure the volume of oxygen consumed ($\dot{V}O_2$) at rest and during moderate exercise to determine the amount of energy being used by the body. Figure 2-7 on page 24 shows some of the equipment used to collect the air that is exhaled from the lungs. As you can see, this measurement equipment is cumbersome and limits the subject's movement. Nevertheless, this technique has been adapted for use under a variety of conditions in the laboratory, on the playing field, and in daily activities.

As the body shifts from rest to exercise, there is an increase in the need for energy. This increase in metabolism is in direct proportion to the increase in the level of work. As with the ATP-PCr and glycolytic energy systems, there is a limit to the amount of energy that can be generated by oxidative metabolism. In the face of increasing energy demands, the body reaches a limit for oxygen delivery ($\dot{V}O_2$ **max**). At this point, there is a leveling

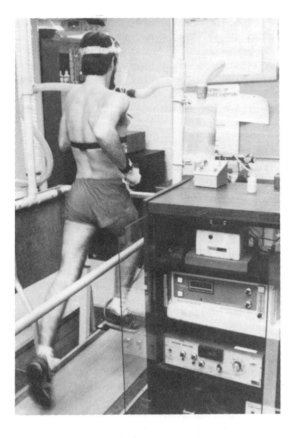

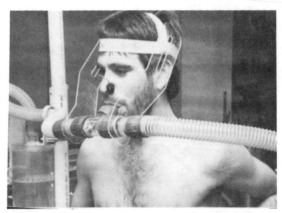

Figure 2-7 The equipment used to measure respiratory exchange during treadmill running.

biological aging and a sedentary life style. In addition, females beyond 10 to 20 years have mean $\dot{V}O_2$ max values considerably lower than their male counterparts. It is questionable whether these represent true differences between the sexes, or whether the female is a victim of her culture, which may impose a sedentary life style once she reaches sexual maturity. This will be discussed in detail in Chapter 17.

of the $\dot{V}O_2$, even though the work level continues to increase (see Figure 2-8). The value at which the $\dot{V}O_2$ plateaus is referred to as the **aerobic capacity** or **maximal oxygen consumption** ($\dot{V}O_2$ **max**). $\dot{V}O_2$ max is regarded as the best single measurement of cardiorespiratory endurance and aerobic fitness.

Since individual needs for energy are influenced by body size, age, and level of fitness, $\dot{V}O_2$ max is frequently expressed relative to body weight—in milliliters of oxygen per kilogram of body weight per minute (ml/kg $\times$ min^{-1}). This allows a more equitable comparison between individuals of different sizes. Normally active 18 to 22 year old college students have been reported to have average $\dot{V}O_2$ max values of 38 to 42 ml/kg $\times$ min^{-1} (women) and 44 to 50 ml/kg $\times$ min^{-1} (men). After the age of 25 to 30 years, inactive individuals have a decrease in $\dot{V}O_2$ max of about one percent per year. This is probably due to a combination of true

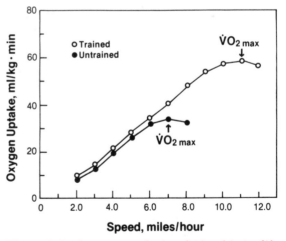

Figure 2-8 Oxygen uptake in relationship to different speeds of walking, jogging, and running for trained and untrained individuals.

Aerobic capacities of 80-84 ml/kg $\times$ min^{-1} have been observed among elite male long-distance runners and cross-country skiers, whereas poorly-conditioned adults may have values below 20 ml/kg $\times$ min^{-1}. The highest value recorded for a champion Norwegian cross-country skier, was 94 ml/kg $\times$ min^{-1}; for a female Russian cross-country skier, was 74 ml/kg $\times$ min^{-1}. A list of $\dot{V}O_2$ max values for athletes in various athletic events is presented in the Appendix.

Oxygen Debt. **Oxygen debt** refers to the volume of oxygen consumed during recovery from exercise that is in excess of the volume normally consumed while at rest. A quick run down the block to catch a departing bus, or a fast climb up several flights of stairs, leaves one with a rapid pulse and an out-of-breath feeling. After several minutes of recovery, the breathing and pulse appear to return to normal. Such post-exercise heavy breathing and oxygen consumption are needed to remove carbon dioxide that has accumulated in the body tissues, and to pay the debt left from the use of the anaerobic energy systems, ATP–PCr and glycolysis.

Most bouts of exercise are performed at levels well below one's aerobic capacity ($\dot{V}O_2$ max). However, it is possible to perform work that requires maximal use of all three systems of energy production, ATP–PCr, glycolysis, and oxidation. As noted earlier in this chapter, when glycolysis is performed with inadequate oxygen delivery to the muscles, there is an accumulation of lactate and hydrogen ions. PCr cannot be conveniently restored to its normal levels during exercise, and must, therefore, be processed during recovery.

There is even an oxygen debt associated with low levels of exercise. This is due to the fact that oxygen consumption requires several minutes to reach the required or steady-state level (see Figure 2-9), even though the requirement to perform the exercise is constant from the very start of the exercise. This initial period, in which the oxygen consumption is below the needed level, is referred to as the period of **oxygen deficit**. This deficit is calculated simply as the difference between the amount of oxygen that is required and that which is actually consumed.

For many years, the oxygen debt curve was mathematically described as having two distinct components: an initial fast, non-lactate component (alactacid portion), and a secondary slow, lactate component (lactacid portion). This classical theory postulated the fast component to be the result of the rebuilding of ATP and PCr. The slow component was theorized to be the result of lactate removal, with 80 percent of the lactate formed during exercise being converted to glycogen, and the remaining 20 percent being oxidized to CO_2 and

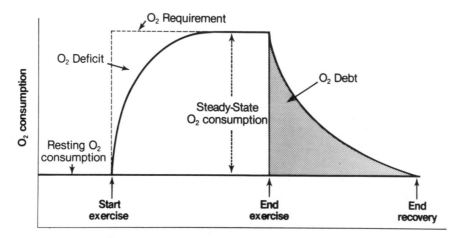

Figure 2-9 Illustration of (A) oxygen deficit, (B) oxygen uptake, and (C) oxygen debt during and after submaximal, steady-state exercise.

H_2O, providing the energy necessary for glycogen repletion. More recent studies have concluded that the classical explanations of oxygen debt are too simplistic, and that the physiological mechanisms responsible for the oxygen debt need to be more clearly defined.

Energy Substrate. The **respiratory exchange ratio (R)** is the ratio between the amount of carbon dioxide produced and the amount of oxygen consumed—R = CO_2 produced divided by the O_2 consumed. In general, the amount of oxygen needed to completely oxidize a molecule of carbohydrate or fat is proportional to the amount of carbon within the fuel. In chemical terms, for example, a glucose molecule can be written as $C_6H_{12}O_6$, containing six units of carbon. Thus, in the combustion of this molecule, six oxygen units would be used with the release of six carbon dioxide units, six water units, and energy. As a result, the ratio between the carbon dioxide produced and the amount of oxygen used, is 1.0.

$$6\ O_2 + C_6H_{12}O_6 = 6\ CO_2 + 6\ H_2O + 39\ ATP$$
$$R = CO_2/O_2 = 6/6 = 1.0$$

As shown in Table 2–1, the R-value (Respiratory Exchange Ratio) will vary with the fuels or substrates being used for energy. Oxidation of fat, for example, results in more oxygen use than carbon dioxide release. In the following equation, for example, the oxidation of the fatty acid, palmitate ($C_{15}H_{31}COOH$), requires 23 moles of oxygen, while producing 16 moles of carbon dioxide, 16 moles of

water, and 129 moles of ATP. It should be noted that it takes significantly more oxygen to combust this molecule of fat than was needed to oxidize a mole of carbohydrate. During carbohydrate oxidation, approximately 6.5 moles of ATP are produced for each mole of oxygen used, compared to 5.6 moles of ATP per mole of oxygen during fatty acid metabolism. Although fat is a more potent source of energy (129 ATP per mole) than carbohydrate (39 ATP per mole), it takes proportionately more oxygen to oxidize fat than carbohydrate. Consequently, the ratio of carbon dioxide production to oxygen use is substantially lower for fat (R = 0.70) than for carbohydrate (R = 1.00).

$$23\ O_2 + C_{15}H_{31}COOH =$$
$$16\ CO_2 + 16\ H_2O + 129\ ATP$$
$$R = CO_2/O_2 = 16/23 = 0.70$$

Since the oxidation of protein is less complete than for fats and carbohydrates, it is impossible to calculate the use of protein from the respiratory exchange. As a result, the R is sometimes referred to as a non-protein R. Traditionally, protein has been thought to contribute little to the energy used during exercise; thus, exercise physiologists have used the non-protein R to calculate energy expenditure and fuel use during physical activity. More recent evidence, however, suggests that in exercise lasting several hours, protein may contribute eight to nine percent of the total energy used. In shorter activities, however, use of the respiratory-exchange ratio to estimate substrate use still seems justifiable.

Table 2–1 Calorie equivalence of the Respiratory Exchange Ratio (R) and fraction (%) of the energy derived from the oxidation of carbohydrates and fats.

Respiratory Exchange Ratio	Calories per Liter of Oxygen	% of Calories from	
		Carbohydrate	Fat
0.71	4.686	0	100
0.75	4.739	15.6	84.4
0.80	4.801	33.4	66.6
0.85	4.862	50.7	49.3
0.90	4.924	67.5	32.5
0.95	4.985	84.0	16.0
1.00	5.047	100.0	0

The R-value may vary from 0.75 to 0.81 at rest, but rises with exercise to reach values in excess of 1.0 as the individual approaches exhaustion. At that point, and during recovery, the R may rise to 1.1 or higher. Such elevations in the R during recovery are associated with an unloading of the excess carbon dioxide that accumulated in the blood during exercise. When R values exceed 1.0 they no longer provide an accurate estimate of the fuel type being oxidized.

The major source of energy, or the fuel for muscular work, was previously thought to be carbohydrates, with fats serving only in a reserve, or secondary, role. It is now evident that fat is a major energy source during exercise. It appears that in aerobic work, where the intensity is below the individual's endurance capacity, 50 to 70 percent of the energy used may be provided by fats; the longer the duration, the higher the contribution of fat.

During intense exercise lasting only a few minutes (anaerobic work), carbohydrate is the primary source of energy. Chapter 12 will discuss how the composition of the diet can have a remarkable influence on athletic performance.

Caloric Expenditure. The standard unit of measure of energy in nutrition is the kilocalorie, or the **kcal.** One kcal is defined as the amount of energy, in the form of heat, necessary to raise the temperature of one kilogram of water 1 degree centigrade, from 15 to 16 degrees centigrade. In nutrition research, a calorimeter is used to measure the absolute amount of heat produced when burning different food materials. When carbohydrate, fat, or protein are burned, each yields a net energy value of 4.10, 9.45, and 4.35 kcal per gram of substance burned, respectively. Large human calorimeters have also been constructed which enable a very accurate analysis of the total heat produced by the body over a 24-hour period. Such information provides an accurate method to calculate the total caloric expenditure, but is too cumbersome and expensive for use in the study by exercise physiologists. Instead, indirect assessments of energy expenditure can be made by measuring the subject's respiratory exchange of oxygen and carbon dioxide. It should be noted that there is a direct relationship between the amount of oxygen consumed, or what is referred to as oxygen uptake, and the number of calories (kcal) expended.

Thus, in addition to estimating the percentage of carbohydrates and fats being oxidized, the R-value can also be used to calculate the rate of heat or caloric production (see Table 2–1). As noted earlier, the system of carbohydrate oxidation is somewhat more efficient than for fat metabolism, since it requires more oxygen to burn fat than to combust carbohydrate. In terms of calories, the oxidation of carbohydrates (R = 1.0) generates 5.047 kcal of energy for every liter of oxygen used. For fats, this value is 4.686 kcal/liter of oxygen consumed, whereas protein generates roughly 4.5 kcal. Combusting a mixture of fuels (R = 0.83) results in a caloric expenditure of 4.838 kcal/liter of oxygen. Under resting conditions the average man will consume about 0.3 liters of oxygen/minute or 18 liters/hour (0.3 l/min × 60 min = 18 liters), which totals 432 liters of oxygen/day (24 hours × 18 liters/hour = 432 liters). If we assume that such a man was burning an even mixture of carbohydrates and fats with an R-value of 0.85 and a caloric equivalence of 4.862 kcal/liter of oxygen, then his daily caloric expenditure could be calculated as follows:

$$
\begin{aligned}
\text{kcal/day} &= (O_2 \text{ consumed}) \times (\text{kcal/liter}) \\
&= (432 \text{ liters/day}) \times (4.862 \text{ kcal/liter}) \\
&= 2100 \text{ kcal/day}
\end{aligned}
$$

This value is in close agreement with the average resting energy expenditure expected for a 154-pound or 70-kilogram man. Of course, it does not include the energy needed for normal daily activity.

Basal metabolic rate (BMR) refers to the rate of energy expenditure for an individual in a totally quiet, supine position, after eight hours of fasting. The BMR will depend on the size of the individual, since the larger the person is, the more total calories expended in a day. While the BMR may vary between 1,500 and 2,000 kcal/day, the average metabolic rate of the individual who is engaged in normal daily activity will range from 1,800 to 2,700 kcal. For athletes engaged in intense daily training, this value can be much higher, approaching 10,000 kcal/day in extremely large individuals.

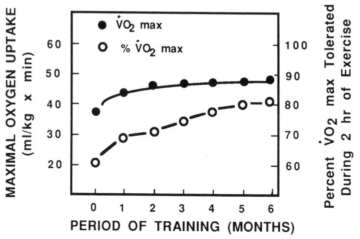

Figure 2-10 Influence of physical training on maximal oxygen uptake ($\dot{V}O_2$ max), and the ability to work at a high percentage of $\dot{V}O_2$ max$_2$ during prolonged exercise.

Lactate Threshold. Although maximal oxygen uptake ($\dot{V}O_2$ max) is often regarded as the best single measurement of one's physiological endurance capacity, it is not a consistently good predictor of success in long distance events. The winner of a marathon race, for example, cannot be predicted from the runner's laboratory measurement of $\dot{V}O_2$ max. Likewise, correlations between endurance-running performance tests (for example, Cooper's 12-minute run or the Balke 1.5-mile run) and $\dot{V}O_2$ max are only moderately high (R = 0.40 to 0.89), indicating that there is more to a good performance than just $\dot{V}O_2$ max. It is also well documented that $\dot{V}O_2$ max will increase with physical training for only 12 to 18 months, at which time it plateaus, even with continued, higher-intensity training. The individuals can still improve their endurance performance, despite the absence of any further gains in aerobic capacity.

Figure 2-10 illustrates one possible explanation for the continued improvement in performance with little change in $\dot{V}O_2$ max—the ability to use a higher percentage of one's $\dot{V}O_2$ max. We have observed that most runners can complete a 26.2-mile race at an average pace corresponding to 75 to 80 percent of their $\dot{V}O_2$ max. Derek Clayton, former world-record holder for the marathon (2 hr, 8 min,

33 sec), had a measured $\dot{V}O_2$ max below that normally expected, based on his world-record performance (69.7 ml/kg × min). Clayton, however, was able to work at 86 percent of his $\dot{V}O_2$ max when running on the treadmill at his racing pace, a value considerably higher than the average world-class marathoner, which probably accounted for his world-record running ability. It would appear that both $\dot{V}O_2$ max and the percentage of $\dot{V}O_2$ max (%$\dot{V}O_2$ max) that the athlete can maintain for a prolonged period of time, are the determining factors in endurance performance. This could explain the lower-than-expected correlations between $\dot{V}O_2$ max and endurance performance tests, and the ability of athletes to improve despite a plateau in their $\dot{V}O_2$ max.

Recently, investigators have introduced a new parameter, the **lactate threshold**, which may be a better indicator of the athletes' endurance potential for prolonged exercise. The lactate threshold has been defined as that point in an exercise of increasing intensity at which the body starts to accumulate blood lactate. Such a definition suggests that we can judge the interaction between the ATP–PCr, glycolytic, and oxidative energy systems. Unfortunately, this is not the case. Rather, the measurements of blood-lactate accumulation

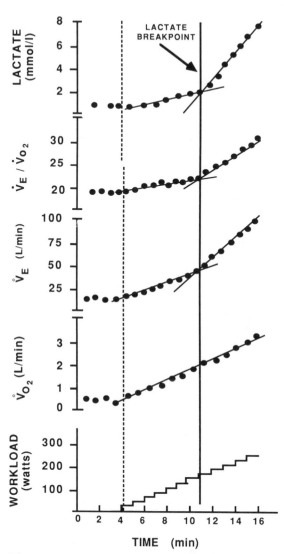

Figure 2–11 Illustration of the changes in blood lactate concentration, oxygen uptake ($\dot{V}O_2$), pulmonary ventilation ($\dot{V}_E$) and the ratio of $\dot{V}_E$ to $\dot{V}O_2$ during varied intensities of exercise. Note that despite a steady increase in oxygen uptake with gradual increments in workload, there is an abrupt increase in respiratory ventilation and carbon dioxide production at an exercise intensity that corresponds to about 75 percent of the subject's $\dot{V}O_2$ max.

simply provide a means of gauging the severity of the exercise relative to the subject's physiological limits. During light physical activity, lactate remains only slightly above the resting level and does not show a significant rise until the subject reaches the lactate threshold. Measurements of respiratory exchange also seem to provide a means of gauging this threshold of exercise intensity. During light activity, ventilation, carbon dioxide production, and ventilatory equivalent (exhaled volume/oxygen uptake) show a steady, linear rise with each increase in the level of effort. This continues to the point of the lactate threshold, at which time there is an increase in the rate of change. This sudden change in blood lactate is disproportionate to the steady rise in oxygen uptake. Figure 2–11 illustrates the relationship between the measurements of ventilatory exchange, exercise intensity, and lactate threshold. The lactate threshold can be expressed in terms of the $\%\dot{V}O_2$ max at which it occurs. A lactate threshold that occurred at 60 $\%\dot{V}O_2$ max would suggest a greater performance potential for the same $\dot{V}O_2$ max than a lactate threshold of 45 $\%\dot{V}O_2$ max. The higher percentage indicates that the individual can work at relatively higher levels of effort before experiencing the physiological stresses associated with the onset of fatigue and ultimate exhaustion.

Recent studies have indicated that the lactate threshold, or the onset of blood lactate accumulation, may well be the reason runners cannot run at a higher perecentage of their $\dot{V}O_2$ max. It has been noted that marathon runners' best pace is one that is just below their lactate threshold. In other words, the experienced, well-trained runner maintains a pace that does not result in the accumulation of blood lactate.

It is generally agreed that there are actually three phases during the progressive transition from low to maximal exercise intensity. These phases are clearly defined by different breakpoints in various physiological parameters during incremental exercise. The transition from Phase I to Phase II has been termed the aerobic threshold, and is characterized by a gradual increase in blood lactate, an increase in the fraction of expired oxygen (FEO$_2$), and a break upward from linearity in ventilation and CO$_2$ production ($\dot{V}CO_2$). The transition from Phase II to Phase III has been termed the lactate threshold, and is characterized by a further increase in blood lactate, a sharp decrease in the fraction of expired CO_2 ($FECO_2$), and an additional break from linearity in ventilation. The aerobic threshold occurs at approximately 40 to 60 percent of $\dot{V}O_2$ max, at a blood lactate level of approximately 2 mmol/liter. The lactate threshold occurs at approximately 65 to 90 percent of $\dot{V}O_2$ max, at a blood lactate level of approximately 4 mmol/liter. The possibility of two thresholds rather than one is intriguing, but still somewhat controversial.

Energy Cost of Various Activities. The amount of energy expended for different activities varies relative to the intensity and mode of exercise. Many activities have been evaluated to determine their energy cost. This is usually accomplished by monitoring oxygen consumption during exercise

Table 2-2 Energy expenditure during various physical activities, based on a 154 lb (70 kg) man.

Activity	Kcal/ min	Kcal/kg × min⁻¹
Sleeping	1.2	0.017
Sitting	1.7	0.024
Standing	1.8	0.026
Walking		
3.5 miles/hr	5.0	0.071
Running		
7.5 miles/hr	14.0	0.20
10 miles/hr	18.2	0.26
Cycling		
7.0 miles/hr	5.0	0.071
10 miles/hr	7.5	0.107
Swimming (Crawl)		
3.0 miles/hr	20.0	0.285
Tennis	7.1	0.101
Weight Lifting	8.2	0.117
Basketball	8.6	0.123
Handball	11.0	0.157
Wrestling	13.1	0.187

to determine an average oxygen uptake per unit of time, which can then be used to calculate the kcal/min. These values typically ignore the anaerobic aspects of exercise, since the oxygen debt is seldom used in these calculations. This is an important point, for an activity that costs a total of 300 kcal to perform, could also cost an additional 100 kcal during the recovery period; thus, the total cost of the activity would be 400, not 300, kcal. The body requires 0.2 to 0.35 liters of oxygen/min to satisfy its resting energy requirements. This would amount to between 1 and 1.8 kcal/min, 60 to 108 kcal/hour, or 1,440 and 2,600 kcal/day. Obviously, any activity above resting levels will add to the projected daily expenditure. The range of values for total daily caloric expenditure are, however, quite varied and will depend on factors such as sex, age, weight, environment, and activity levels.

Sport activities also differ with respect to their energy cost. Some require levels of energy expenditure that are only slightly greater than those at rest. Others have levels so high that they can be maintained for only a matter of seconds, for example, sprinting. With regard to total energy expenditure, the duration of the activity must be considered, in addition to the intensity of the exercise. While approximately 29 kcal/min are expended while running at a speed of 15.5 miles per hour (mph), this level of activity can be endured for only brief periods of time. Jogging at a 7 mph pace (approximately 8.5 min/mile) will, on the other hand, result in an expenditure of 14.5 kcal/min, or only half that expended in running at 15.5 mph, but jogging can be maintained for a considerably longer period of time, resulting in a greater total expenditure of energy.

Table 2-2 provides an estimate of energy expenditure for various activities by average mature men with an approximate body weight of 154 lb (70 kg). Since most activities involve moving the body mass, these figures may vary considerably with the weight, age, sex, and the individual's technical skill (efficiency).

Economy of Exercise. The ability to perform any exercise skillfully results in a reduced demand for energy. This point is illustrated by the data from two distance runners, shown in Figure 2-12.

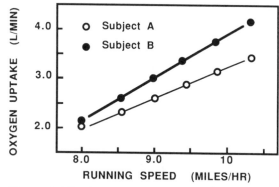

Figure 2-12 Oxygen requirements ($\dot{V}O_2$ liters × min^{-1}) for two distance runners while running at various speeds. Though they had similar $\dot{V}O_2$ max values (*64 to 65* liters × min^{-1}), runner A was the more efficient and, therefore, the faster runner.

At all running speeds faster than eight minutes per mile (200 meters per minute), subject A used significantly less oxygen than subject B. Since these men had similar $\dot{V}O_2$ max values (64 to 65 ml/kg × min), it is apparent that subject A's use of less energy would provide him with a decided advantage during competition.

Since these two men competed on numerous occasions, it is interesting to examine the results of their encounters. We estimated that during marathon races, these men ran at paces requiring them to use 85 percent of their $\dot{V}O_2$ max. Table 2-3 indicates that, on the average, subject A's running efficiency gave him a 13-minute advantage in marathon races. Since these men had similar $\dot{V}O_2$ max values, but markedly different energy needs during distance running, a large part of subject A's advantage in competition can be attributed to his greater running efficiency. Further studies need to be done to explain the underlying causes of these differences in the energy cost of running as exhibited by these men.

Various studies with sprint, middle-distance, and distance runners have shown that marathon runners are more efficient than other trained runners. In general, these ultra-long distance runners tend to use between five and ten percent less energy than middle-distance and sprint runners. Since this economy of effort has only been studied at relatively slow speeds (five to ten min/mile paces), it seems reasonable to assume that distance runners are less efficient at sprinting than those runners who train specifically for the short, faster races.

Table 2-3 Performance data (hr:min:sec) for two middle-aged distance runners.

Mon/yr	Distance	Subject A	Place	Subject B	Place
2/67	42.2 km	2:51:40	8	2:46:21	6
4/67	42.2	2:45:20	81	2:29:55	22
5/67	42.2	2:48:08	11	2:30:06	1
5/67	60.4	4:48:08	4	3:36:52	1
6/67	42.2	3:08:42	14	2:43:42	2
2/68	42.2	2:51:33	8	2:44:40	4
4/68	42.2	2:52:00	43	2:39:34	19
5/68	42.2	2:45:37	6	2:36:35	2
5/68	60.4	4:29:17	3	3:50:11	1
6/68	42.2	3:02:54	10	2:46:51	1
8/68	42.2	2:55:01	8	2:36:36	1
2/69	42.2	2:42:40	9	2:37:25	6
4/69	42.2	2:42:02	56	2:29:07	13
5/69	60.4	3:57:01	2	3:48:11	1
5/69	42.2	2:49:41	5	2:39:34	3 .

Though the difference in energy use between the distance and sprint runners may seem small, it becomes a serious consideration during events lasting several hours. Variations in running form and the specificity of training for sprint versus distance running may account for such differences in running economy. Film analyses reveal that middle-distance and sprint runners have significantly greater vertical movement when running between 7 and 12 miles/hr, than do marathoners. Such speeds, however, are well below those required during middle-distance races, and probably do not represent the running efficiency of competitors in 1,500-m events or less. It is interesting to note that the oxygen consumption at a given running speed is also less for world-class, middle-distance runners than it is for less successful middle-distance runners.

Performance in other athletic events may be affected more by efficiency of movement than running. Energy expended during swimming, for example, is used, in part, to pay the cost to maintain the body on the surface of the water and to generate the force required to overcome the water's resistance to motion. Although the energy needed for swimming is dependent on body size and buoyancy, the efficient application of force against water is the major determinant of economy in this activity. Figure 2–13 illustrates the difference in oxygen requirements of trained, competitive male and female swimmers, and for a group of highly-trained triathletes. Although the triathletes trained daily at swimming, none had a prior background in competitive swimming. It is also interesting to note that many of these triathletes had aerobic capacities that were markedly higher than the competitive swimmers, but few could perform as well as the poorest competitive swimmer. Several female swimmers who possessed $\dot{V}O_2$ max values between 2.1 and 2.3 liters/min were able to swim the 400-meter as fast as triathletes having values above 5.0 liters of oxygen per minute.

Performance in many activities may be limited more by the athlete's skill than by his or her maximal capacity to generate energy. Such information makes it clear that the training time and effort spent improving the mechanical aspects (skill) of the sport may be as important as the time dedicated to improving one's strength and endurance.

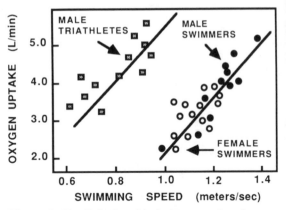

Figure 2–13 Relationship between swimming velocity and oxygen uptake during a 400 yd. front-crawl swim by male (●) and female (○) competitive swimmers, and trained, male triathletes (▨).

FATIGUE

There appear to be multiple definitions and causes for fatigue during exercise. Those who have exercised to exhaustion know that the sensation of fatigue after events lasting 45 to 60 seconds, such as the 400-meter run, is markedly different from fatigue experienced during prolonged, exhaustive muscular effort, such as marathon running. Generally, the term **fatigue** is used to describe the general sensations of tiredness, as well as the decrements in muscular performance. Four basic processes have been suggested as causes of fatigue. It has been proposed that decrements in performance may occur as a consequence of

1. the accumulation of waste products such as lactic acid
2. depletion of substances necessary for activity (for instance, muscle glycogen)
3. changes in the physiochemical state of the muscle (for instance, electrolytes)
4. disturbances in the processes of muscular coordination (for instance, central nervous system).

More recent efforts to describe the underlying causes and sites of fatigue have focused on the energy systems (PCr, glycolysis, and oxidation), the accumulation of metabolic by-products, and the peripheral and central nervous systems. Although the availability of energy may reduce the muscles' capacity to generate tension, the energy systems cannot be held wholly responsible for all forms of fatigue. The sensations of tiredness we often experience at the end of a work-day may, for example, have little or nothing to do with the availability of ATP in the muscles and nerves. Fatigue could also be the result of environmental stresses on the body's homeostasis.

Energy Supply

As noted earlier, ATP provides immediate energy for muscular contraction and is critical in muscle tension development. In sprint activities lasting only a few seconds, muscle ATP levels are maintained at the expense of a breakdown of PCr. As shown in Figure 2–14, PCr declines rapidly during the first minute of an intense, 10-minute exercise bout, which is followed by a more gradual reduc-

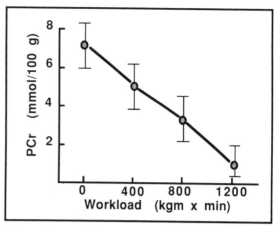

Figure 2–15 Relationship between workload and creatine phosphate levels in the thigh muscle after five minutes of cycling at each work level (modified from Bergstrom, 1967).

tion, until the end of exercise. The rate at which PCr declines during exercise is dependent on the intensity of the muscular effort.

The rate of PCr breakdown increases with higher rates of work, resulting in an earlier onset of fatigue and ultimate exhaustion (see Figure 2–15). Studies of human thigh muscle and isolated muscle preparations have shown that exhaustion during repeated maximal contractions coincides with the depletion of PCr. Although ATP is directly responsible for the energy used during such activities, it declines much less than PCr during muscular effort. At exhaustion, however, both ATP and PCr could be depleted. Thus, to delay the onset of fatigue, the athlete must control the rate of effort through proper pacing, to insure that PCr and ATP are not exhausted prematurely. Selecting a pace that is too rapid at the start of a race will result in a quick decline in the available phosphogens, an early onset of fatigue, and the inability to maintain the pace over the final stage of the event. Training and experience enable the athlete to judge the optimal exercise pace that will result in an even distribution of ATP and PCr use over the entire event, resulting in the best possible performance.

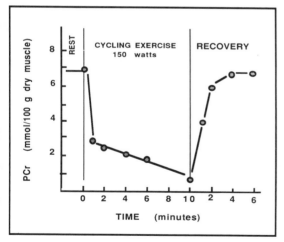

Figure 2–14 Changes in phosphocreatine (PCr) levels during ten minutes of sprint cycling exercise. Note the sudden initial drop in PCr and the more gradual decline to exhaustion. Recovery of PCr is nearly complete within three minutes.

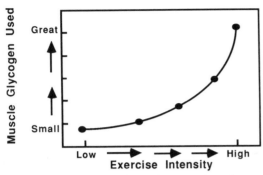

Figure 2-16   Effects of running speed on the rate of muscle glycogen use. The rate of muscle glycogen use may be 40 times faster during sprint running than during walking (modified from Costill, 1986).

In addition to PCr, the levels of muscle ATP are also maintained by the aerobic and anaerobic breakdown of muscle glycogen. In events lasting more than a few seconds, muscle glycogen becomes a primary source of energy for the synthesis of ATP. Unfortunately, the reserves of glycogen are limited and can serve as an energy source for a restricted period. As with PCr use, the depletion rate of muscle glycogen is controlled by the intensity of the activity. As noted in Figure 2-16, an increase in the rate of work causes muscle glycogen to be used at faster rates. It has been estimated that during sprint running, muscle glycogen may be used 35 to 40 times faster than during walking. Even during mild muscular effort, muscle glycogen could become a limiting factor, and the cause for fatigue. Although fat serves as an alternate

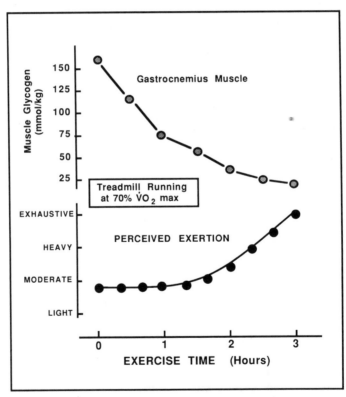

Figure 2-17   Muscle glycogen content and the subject's rating of effort during a three-hour treadmill run. Note that during the first half of the run glycogen was used at a higher rate than during the last 90 minutes of the exercise (modified from Costill, 1986).

source of energy for ATP and PCr resynthesis, the muscle is dependent on a constant supply of glycogen to meet the high energy demands of exercise.

During the first few minutes of exercise, muscle glycogen is used at a higher rate than in the latter stages of activity. This is illustrated by the data in Figure 2–17, showing the change in muscle glycogen content during three hours of treadmill running at 70 percent of the subject's $\dot{V}O_2$ max. Although the test was run at a steady pace, the rate of muscle glycogen metabolized from the calf muscle (gastrocnemius) was greatest during the first 90 minutes of the exercise. Thereafter, the use of glycogen slowed as it approached zero. The subject felt only moderately stressed during the early part of the run, when glycogen stores were still high, though being used at a high rate. It was not until muscle glycogen levels were nearly depleted, that the subject began to experience severe fatigue. Thus, it appears that the sensation of fatigue in long-term exercise could coincide with the lowering of muscle glycogen. Marathon runners commonly refer to the sudden onset of fatigue that they experience between 18 and 22 miles, as "hitting the wall." It is quite possible that at least part of this sensation can be attributed to the depletion of muscle glycogen.

It should be noted, however, that muscle fibers are used and have their energy reserves depleted in selected patterns. That is to say, the muscle fibers most frequently recruited during exercise may become individually depleted of glycogen, thereby reducing the number of fibers available to produce the tension neessary for exercise. This point is demonstrated by the microscopic examination of the glycogen staining in muscle fibers taken from a runner before and after a 30 kilometer run (see Figure 2–18). These biopsy data reveal that the glycogen content of the slow-twitch (ST) fibers is nearly exhausted, while the fast-twitch (FT) fibers still contain considerable quantities. This information suggests that the ST muscle cells are most heavily used when the tension demands of exercise are relatively low.

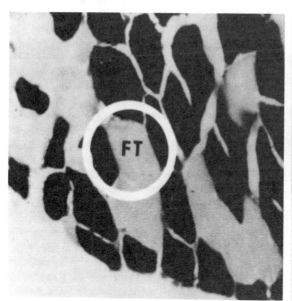 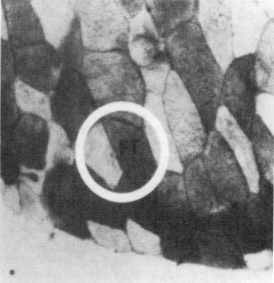

Figure 2–18 Selective muscle glycogen depletion from slow-twitch (ST) and fast-twitch (FT) fibers during a 30-kilometer run. On the left, the FT fibers appear unstained, whereas ST fibers are stained black. The right frame shows the glycogen content of these same fibers. Those fibers with the most glycogen appear darkly stained, whereas the depleted fibers are unstained.

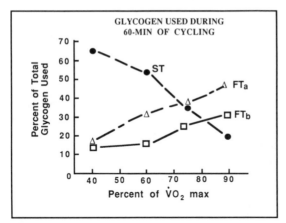

Figure 2–19 Distribution of muscle glycogen used within the slow-twitch (ST) and fast-twitch (FT$_a$ and FT$_b$) fibers of the vastus lateralis during 60 minutes of cycling at varied intensities (modified from P. Blom, Oslo, Norway, unpublished).

The pattern of glycogen depletion from the ST and FT (type a and b) fibers is dependent on the intensity of the exercise. As the tension requirements increase, the FT$_a$ fibers are added to the work force. Finally, during maximal contraction, both slow- and fast-twitch fibers are recruited, even the FT$_b$ fibers. Figure 2–19 illustrates the distribution of glycogen use between the ST, FT$_a$, and FT$_b$ fibers of the vastus lateralis muscle (lateral thigh) during cycling at 40, 60, 75, and 90 percent of the subjects' maximal oxygen uptake. During relatively low-intensity exercise (40 and 60 %$\dot{V}O_2$ max), ST fibers appear more active, whereas the FT$_a$ and FT$_b$ fibers appear relatively inactive. At higher intensities of effort (75 and 90 %$\dot{V}O_2$ max) the FT fibers are recruited more frequently and are depleted of their glycogen at a greater rate than the ST fibers. This should not be interpreted to mean that the ST fibers are used less than the FT fibers during maximal contractions, but simply reflects the greater reliance of FT fibers on glycogen. In reality, all fiber types are recruited during highly-intense, muscular contractions. The ramp-like recruitment of muscle fibers with varied intensities of effort is illustrated in Figure 1–11 on page 12.

When the ST fibers have relinquished their glycogen stores, the FT fibers appear unable to generate enough tension and/or cannot be easily recruited to compensate for the loss in muscle tension. For that reason, it has been theorized that the sensations of muscle fatigue and heaviness that occur during long-term exercise, reflect the inability of some muscle fibers to respond to the demands of exercise.

In addition to selectively depleting glycogen from ST or FT fibers, exercise may place unusually heavy demands on select groups of muscles. During two hours of uphill, downhill, and level treadmill-running, for example, greater amounts of glycogen are used from the gastrocnemius and soleus than from the vastus lateralis muscles (see Figure 2–20). This suggests that the ankle extensor muscles (gastrocnemius and soleus) are more likely to become depleted during distance running than are the thigh muscles, isolating fatigue to the lower leg muscles.

Muscle glycogen alone cannot provide all the carbohydrate necessary for exercise lasting several hours. Glucose delivered to the muscles via the blood has been shown to contribute a sizeable amount of energy during endurance exercise. The liver breaks down glycogen to provide a constant supply of glucose to the blood. In the early stages of exercise, energy production requires relatively little blood glucose, but in the later stages of an endurance event, blood glucose will make a large contribution to the energy needs of the muscles. The longer the exercise period, the greater must be the output of glucose from the liver to keep pace with the glucose uptake by the muscles.

Since the liver has a limited supply of glycogen, and is unable to rapidly produce glucose from other substrates (for instance, gluconeogenesis), blood glucose levels begin to decline when the muscle uptake becomes greater than the liver's output. Unable to obtain sufficient glucose from the blood, the muscles must rely more heavily on their glycogen reserves, resulting in an acceleration of muscle glycogen use and the earlier onset of exhaustion.

In light of the muscle's dependence on glycogen and blood glucose, it is not surprising that endurance performances are improved when the supply of muscle glycogen is elevated at the start of the activity. The importance of nutrition, muscle-gly-

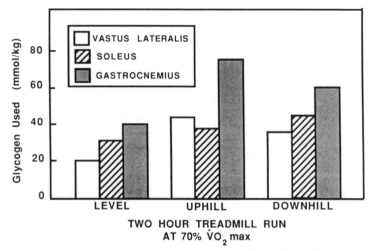

Figure 2-20 Amount of glycogen used from the thigh (vastus lateralis) and calf (soleus and gastrocnemius) muscles during level, uphill, and downhill running for two hours at 70% $\dot{V}O_2$ max.

cogen storage, and endurance performance will be discussed in detail in Chapter 12.

It should be noted that glycogen depletion and hypoglycemia appear to limit performance and cause fatigue in activities lasting 30 to 60 minutes, or longer. Fatigue in shorter events are more likely the result of an accumulation of metabolic by-products, such as lactate and hydrogen ion build-up within the muscles.

Accumulation of Waste Products

The association between fatigue and lactic acid accumulation in the blood has been recognized since the early 1930s. During strenuous exercise, some energy is provided by the formation of lactic acid in the cytosol of the muscle fibers. Since lactic acid is an acid, it dissociates to some degree, resulting in an accumulation of hydrogen ions and a decrease in pH. Although most people believe that lactic acid is responsible for fatigue and exhaustion in all types of exercise, it is only during relatively short-term, highly-intense, muscular effort that lactate accumulates within the muscle fiber and alters its pH. Marathon runners, for example, may have near-resting lactate and pH levels at the end of the race, despite their exhaustion. As noted

in the previous section, the cause for their fatigue is one of inadequate energy supply, not an excess of lactate. Sprint running, cycling, and swimming all result in a large accumulation of lactate, the result of energy production via glycolysis. It should be realized, however, that it is not lactate *per se* that should be blamed for the feeling of fatigue. Hydrogen ion concentration that accompanies lactate and other acid accumulation within the cells may decrease muscle pH from 7.1 at rest to 6.4 at exhaustion, a value that is incompatible with normal cell function (see Figure 2-21 on page 38).

Activities that depend heavily on glycolysis for a sizeable portion of their energy, result in severe acidosis within the muscles and throughout the body. The cells and body fluids possess buffers, such as bicarbonate (HCO^-_3), that function to minimize the disrupting influence of the hydrogen ions (H^+) that dissociate from lactate. If the released H^+ ions were added to an unbuffered solution, the free concentration of H^+ would lower the pH level to about 1.5, effectively killing the cells. Because of the body's buffering capacity, the free H^+ concentration is kept low even in the most severe exercise, allowing the pH to fall to between only 6.6 and 6.4 at exhaustion.

Such changes in pH, however, have a negative effect on energy production and the contraction

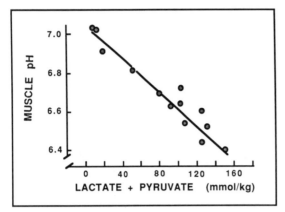

Figure 2-21   Relationship between muscle lactate plus pyruvate and pH during intense exercise. Note that as lactate increases, the pH drops proportionately (modified from Sahlin, 1982).

process within the muscle. A reduction in intracellular pH to less than 6.9 has been shown to inhibit the action of phosphofructokinase (PFK), an important glycolytic enzyme, thereby slowing the rate of glycolysis and ATP production. At pH 6.4, the influence of free H^+ is strong enough to stop any further breakdown of glycogen, resulting in a rapid drop in ATP, inducing exhaustion. In addition, H^+ can act to displace calcium within the fi-

ber, thereby interfering with the coupling of the cross-bridges and a concomitant decline in the muscle's contractile force. It is generally agreed, therefore, that a decrease in pH within the muscle is the major limiting factor and site of fatigue during maximal short-term exercise.

As noted in Figure 2-22, recovery from an exhaustive sprint exercise takes approximately 20 to 30 minutes. At that point, muscle pH has returned to the pre-exercise level, although blood and muscle lactate may still be quite elevated. Experience has shown that athletes can continue to exercise at relatively high intensities even when their muscle pH is below 7.0, with lactate levels above 6 or 7 mmol/liter, which is four to five times the resting value. Currently, coaches and sports physiologists are attempting to use measurements of blood lactate to gauge the intensity and volume of training required to produce optimal training stimulus. Although such measurements provide an index for training intensity, they may not reflect the anaerobic processes or the state of acidosis within the muscles. As lactate and H^+ are generated within the muscles, they diffuse out of the cells, dilute in body fluids, transport to other areas of the body, and are metabolized. Consequently, blood values for lactate are dependent on their rate of production, diffusion, and oxidation. Since there are a variety of factors that can influence this management of lactate and H^+, the validity of their use in evaluating training is questionable.

Neuromuscular and Psychological Fatigue

Thus far we have considered only factors within the muscle that might be responsible for fatigue. There is also evidence to suggest that under some circumstances, fatigue can be the result of an inability to activate the muscle fibers, the nervous system's responsibility. The nerve impulse is transmitted across the motor end plate to activate the muscle fiber's membrane and to release calcium from its sarcoplasmic reticulum, the key to muscle contraction. The calcium, in turn, binds with troponin to initiate muscle contraction. It has been suggested that fatigue may occur at the motor end plate, making it impossible to relay the nerve impulse to the fiber membrane. The failure of impulse transmission from the nerve to the mus-

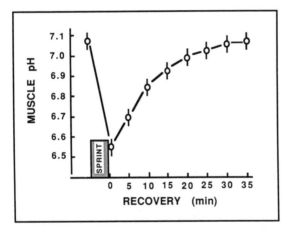

Figure 2-22   Changes in muscle pH during sprint-cycling to exhaustion and during 35 minutes of recovery. Note the slow rate of recovery for pH.

cle fiber in fatigued muscle was clearly established by studies in the early part of this century. This block in the transmission of the impulse to the fiber membrane may involve one or more of the following processes:

1. A reduction in the release or synthesis of **acetylcholine,** the transmitter substance responsible for relaying the nerve impulse from the motor nerve to the muscle membrane.
2. **Cholinesterase**, responsible for destroying acetylcholine, could become hyperactive, preventing acetylcholine from attaining a concentration necessary to initiate an action potential.
3. Cholinesterase activity could become hypoactive, or inhibiting, leading to an accumulation of acetylcholine, thereby paralyzing the fiber.
4. The muscle fiber membrane could develop a higher threshold necessary for activation.
5. The presence of a substance competing with acetylcholine for the receptors on the muscle membrane, without activating the fiber membrane.

Although most of these causes for a transmission block have been associated with muscle disease, for example, myasthenia gravis, they could also be responsible for some forms of neuromuscular fatigue.

There is also some evidence to show that fatigue during exercise may be due to an accumulation of calcium within the T-tubules, with less calcium available for muscle contraction. It has been proposed that depletion of PCr and lactate build-up may simply increase the rate of calcium accumulation within the T-tubules. These theories of fatigue have not been clearly demonstrated and remain speculative.

The central nervous system (CNS) may also be a site of fatigue. Indirectly- or directly-stimulated muscle, *in situ,* is practically indefatigable, whereas voluntary activities of similar loads and frequencies cannot be maintained for a comparable duration. The precise mechanisms underlying such fatigue of the CNS is not fully understood. It is also difficult to determine whether this form of fatigue is isolated to the CNS or linked to peripheral nerve transmission.

Since the recruitment of muscle depends, in part, on conscious control, the psychological trauma of exhaustive exercise may consciously or subconsciously inhibit the athlete's willingness to tolerate further pain. Slowing the exercise pace to a tolerable level may, therefore, be the result of limited central nervous system control, rather than local fatigue in the muscle. It is generally agreed that the perceived discomfort of fatigue precedes the onset of a physiological limitation within the muscles. Unless they are highly motivated, most individuals will terminate the exercise before their muscles are physiologically exhausted. In order to achieve a peak performance, athletes train to learn proper pacing and must be willing to tolerate the discomfort of fatigue.

Heat Stress and Fatigue

The influence of environmental conditions on exercise performance will be discussed in greater detail in Chapter 14, but for the moment let us consider the impact of warm environmental conditions on fatigue. Heat produced by the muscles during exercise is dissipated from the body principally through sweat evaporation. The evaporation of each liter of sweat from the skin takes away approximately 560 kcal of heat. Anything that blocks this evaporation, such as excess humidity, will limit the removal of metabolically produced heat and increase body heat storage. High air temperatures, humidity, and bright sunlight can reduce heat dissipation, thereby inducing a rise in the internal temperature of the body and blood. It is not uncommon to observe internal (rectal) temperatures in excess of 40° centigrade (104° F) among distance runners at the end of a ten kilometer race when the environmental temperature is only 21° centigrade (70° F), with bright sun and a relative humidity of 60 to 70 percent. While sprint performances under these conditions are unaffected, endurance capacity for longer periods is markedly reduced.

One of the responsibilities of the circulatory system is to transport heat from the muscles to the surface of the body where it can be transferred to the environment. Since the volume of blood in the body is limited, exercise poses a complex problem for the circulatory system. During exercise, a large

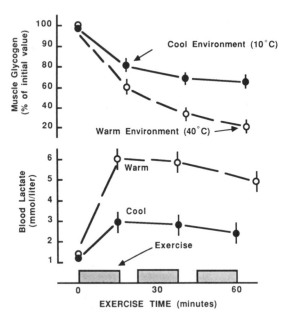

Figure 2-23   Effects of air temperature on muscle glycogen use and blood lactate accumulation during one hour of cycling at 70% V̇O₂ max.

part of the cardiac output must be shared by the skin and working muscles. An increase in the demand for blood flow to either the skin or muscles will automatically decrease flow to the other. During exercise in a warm climate, more blood must be diverted to the skin, thereby reducing blood flow and oxygen delivery to the muscles. Consequently, the athlete perceives the effort as more difficult. There is also evidence to indicate that muscle glycogen is used at a greater rate during exercise in warm environments as compared to cooler conditions, thus, leading to an earlier onset of fatigue (see Figure 2-23).

The volume of sweat lost during warm-weather exercise leads to a reduction in plasma and blood volume. Consequently, the already compromised circulatory capacity is further weakened, thereby reducing the capacity of the blood to deliver oxygen and nutrients to the muscle, and limiting heat transfer to the skin. The build-up of internal body heat (hyperthermia) elevates the temperature of the brain, blood, and muscles. Since these tissues are normally maintained and function best within a narrow temperature range (36 to 40° C), exercise

hyperthermia offers another possible cause for the subject's sense of fatigue. Heat stress is a major limitation to endurance peformance, inducing early fatigue by impairing the function of the circulatory system, altering muscle metabolism, and stressing the body's systems for temperature regulation.

SUMMARY

The ability of muscles to produce movement depend on the availability of the high-energy phosphate compound ATP. In short, the energy for intense effort lasting only a few seconds, is provided by the breakdown of ATP stored within the muscle fiber, and the resynthesis of ATP from the energy in PCr. Exhaustive exercise bouts lasting more than a few seconds require that energy be derived from the breakdown of sugar stored within the muscle fibers (glycogen). In the absence of adequate oxygen, the muscles can only partially metabolize glycogen, resulting in a limited supply of energy and the accumulation of lactic acid. The most efficient system for energy production during exercise is oxidative metabolism (the combustion of carbohydrates and fats with the aid of oxygen). This system, however, depends on the circulatory system to provide a continual supply of oxygen to the working muscles, and to remove metabolically-produced carbon dioxide and heat.

Energy expenditure during exercise is calculated in terms of calories (kcal). Measurements of respiratory exchange provide an effective method for determining the rate of energy expenditure and to estimate the fuel type being combusted during aerobic activities. Exercise poses a strong stimulus to the energy systems within the muscle fibers, increasing the rate of energy production from rest to maximal effort by nearly 200-fold. The limits of aerobic exercise, however, are determined by the transport of oxygen and its use within the muscles. If all energy was produced by aerobic means, the muscles would only be able to increase their rate of energy production by 20 to 25 times the resting level. Thus, in most athletic events, peak performances depend on the combined contributions of all energy sytems.

Efficiency of movement is a key factor in sports performance. The ability to expend a minimal amount of energy in performing a given skill, allows athletes to gain the most from the energy expended in the activity. Such efficient use of their energy systems allows the athlete greater functional endurance and greater potential for success.

The sites of fatigue are multiple and, at present, only partly identified. It is generally agreed, however, that the causes of fatigue and exhaustion are dependent on the availability of energy, the accumulation of metabolic waste products, environmental conditions, and/or limitations within the peripheral and central nervous systems. Despite research efforts since the late 1800s, the precise mechanisms underlying fatigue are not completely understood. Like many questions facing exercise physiologists, there is no single factor responsible for fatigue. Rather, there are a multitude of conditions and causes underlying the sensation and discomforts associated with exercise fatigue and exhaustion.

STUDY QUESTIONS

1. Why are the ATP-PCr and glycolytic energy systems considered anaerobic?
2. What role does oxygen play in the process of aerobic metabolism?
3. What is the role of PCr?
4. Describe the relationship between muscle ATP and PCr during sprint exercise.
5. Describe the by-products of energy production from ATP-PCr, glycolysis, and oxidation.
6. What is the primary function of muscle enzymes?
7. What is the relationship between oxygen consumption and energy production?
8. Why is oxygen consumption often computed as milliliter of oxygen per kilogram of body weight (ml/kg $\times$ min^{-1})?
9. Define and distinguish between oxygen debt and oxygen deficit.
10. What is the respiratory exchange ratio (R)? Explain how it is used to determine the oxidation of carbohydrate and fat.
11. What is the lactate threshold?
12. How can we use measurements of caloric expenditure to estimate one's exercise efficiency?
13. Describe the possible causes of fatigue during exercise bouts lasting between 15 and 30 seconds; two and four hours.
14. What is $\dot{V}O_2$ max? Discuss its importance in endurance activities.

REFERENCES

Armstrong, R. B. (1979). Biochemistry: Energy liberation and use. In R. H. Strauss (Ed.) *Sports medicine and physiology*. Philadelphia: W. B. Saunders Co.

Åsmussen, E. (1979). Muscle fatigue. *Medicine and Science in Sports, 11,* 313-321.

Åstrand, P. O., & Rodahl, K. (1986). *Textbook of work physiology.* New York: McGraw-Hill.

Bergstrom, J. (1967). Local changes of ATP and phosphorylcreatine in human muscle tissue in connection with exercise. In *Physiology of muscular exercise,* monograph no. 15 (pp. 191-196). New York: American Heart Association.

Bigland-Richie, B., Jones, D. A., Hosking, G. P., & Edwards, R. H. T. (1978). Central and peripheral fatigue in sustained maximum voluntary contractions of human quadriceps muscle. *Clinical Science of Molecular Medicine, 541,* 609-614.

Brooks, G. A., Brauner, K. E., & Cassens, R. G. (1973). Glycogen synthesis and metabolism of lactic acid after exercise. *American Journal of Physiology, 224,* 1162-1166.

Costill, D. L., Gollnick, P. D., Jansson, E. D., Saltin, B., & Stein, E. M. (1973). Glycogen depletion pattern in human muscle fibers during distance running. *Acta Physiologica Scandinavica, 89,* 374-383.

Costill, D. L., Jansson, E., Gollnick, P. D., & Saltin, B. (1974). Glycogen utilization in leg muscles of men during level and uphill running. *Acta Physiologica Scandinavica, 91,* 474-481.

Farrell, P. A., Wilmore, J. H., Coyle, E. F., Billing, J. E., & Costill, D. L. (1979). Plasma lactate accumulation and distance running performance. *Medicine and Science in Sports, 11,* 338-344.

Ivy, J. L., Costill, D. L., & Maxwell, B. D. (1980). Skeletal muscle determinants of maximum aerobic power in man. *European Journal of Applied Physiology, 44,* 1-8.

Lamb, D. R. (1978). *Physiology of exercise: Responses and adaptations.* New York: Macmillan Publishing Co.

Pernow, B., & Saltin, B. (1971). *Muscle metabolism during exercise.* New York: Plenum Press.

Sahlin, K. (1982). Effect of exercise on intracellular acid-base balance in the skeletal muscle of man. In P. Komi (Ed.) *Basic metabolism and exercise.* (pp. 3-14). Champaign, IL: Human Kinetics Publishers.

Simonson, E. (1971). *Physiology of work capacity and fatigue.* Springfield, IL.: C. C. Thomas.

Skinner, J. S., & McLellan, T. H. (1980). The transition from aerobic to anaerobic metabolism. *Research Quarterly for Exercise and Sport, 51,* 234-248.

Wasserman, K., & McIlroy, M. B. (1964). Detecting the threshold of anaerobic metabolism. *American Journal of Cardiology, 14,* 844-852.

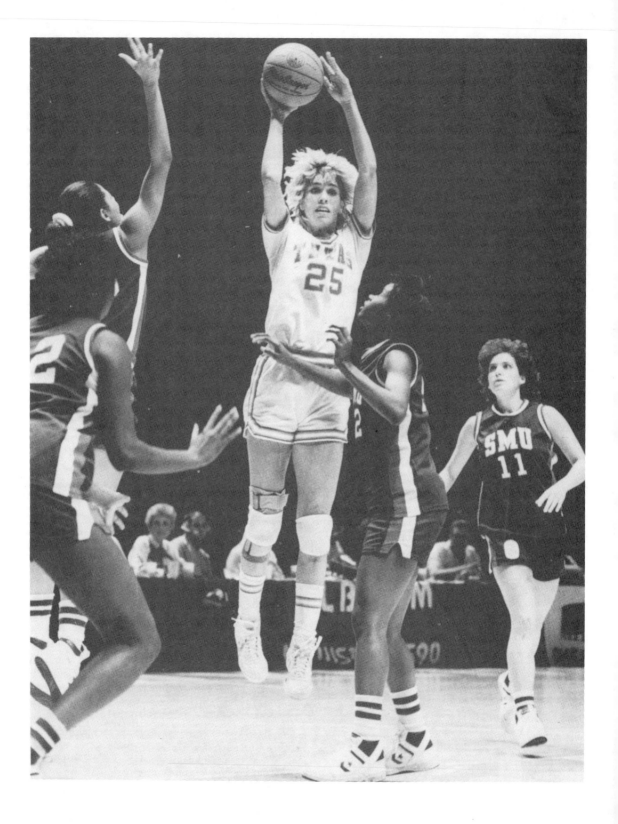

3

Respiration and Acid-Base Balance

INTRODUCTION

Respiration is the process in which carbon dioxide is removed from and oxygen is delivered to the body tissues. This process can be differentiated in two separate phases: external and internal respiration. **External respiration** is the process of moving air into and out of the lungs, and the subsequent exchange of gases between the gas in the lungs and the blood as it flows through the capillaries of the lung tissue. **Internal respiration** refers to the process of oxygen and carbon dioxide exchange between the blood and the body tissues. Thus, external respiration identifies the process of gas exchange in the lung, whereas internal respiration defines the process of gas exchange at the level of the muscles and other body tissues. The process of external respiration is commonly referred to as **pulmonary ventilation.**

STRUCTURES OF RESPIRATION

The anatomy of the respiratory system is illustrated in Figure 3-1 on page 44. Air comes into the lungs through the nose; the mouth is also used when the demand for air exceeds levels comfortably provided through the nose. There are certain advantages to inhaling air through the nose that are lost with mouth breathing. First, the air is warmed and humidified as it swirls through the irregular surfaces (**turbinates**) inside the nose. Cold air or dry air can be irritating to the lungs and the associated air passages, so this heating and humidifying process is very important. Of equal importance, the turbinates cause agitation in the air flowing into the lungs, causing dust and other particulate matter to adhere to the nasal surfaces. This is a very efficient system that filters out almost all but the very smallest particles, reducing irritation and discomfort to a minimum. From either, or both the nose and mouth, the air travels through the **pharynx, larynx, trachea, bronchi,** and **bronchioles,** until it finally reaches the smallest units, the **alveoli.** The throat is commonly referred to as the **pharynx,** and separates into the **trachea** for the passage of air and the **esophagus** for the passage of food. The ability of the body to differentiate between food and air is the result of nerve reflexes. Whenever food touches the surface of the pharynx, the vocal cords and the **epiglottis** close by reflex action, allowing food to slide only into the esophagus. With certain accidents, injuries, or disease states, it becomes necessary to insert a tube into the trachea, usually at the **larynx,** to allow for continued breathing or provide assisted breathing.

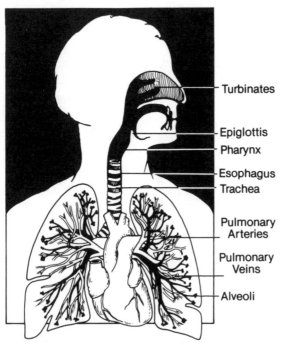

Figure 3-1 Anatomy of the respiratory system.

Turbinates

Epiglottis
Pharynx

Esophagus
Trachea

Pulmonary
Arteries

Pulmonary
Veins

Alveoli

Gas exchange takes place in the alveoli. Blood returning to the right side of the heart via the venous system is low in oxygen and high in carbon dioxide. From the right ventricle this blood is pumped to the lungs, where it enters the pulmonary capillaries, forming a dense network around the **alveolar sacs.** The distance between the air in the alveoli and the blood in the pulmonary capillaries is quite small (approximately 0.00016 inch). The space is filled with the epithelial cells of the alveoli and the endothelial cells of the capillaries. The red cells pass through the pulmonary capillaries in single file, thus each cell is exposed to the surrounding lung tissue. The close proximity of the alveoli to the capillary blood allows for the relatively rapid exchange of gases between the alveolar air and the blood gases.

Mechanics of Breathing

Inspiration is an active process involving the diaphragm, which is the primary muscle of respiration, and the muscles responsible for enlarging the thoracic or chest cavity, referred to as the **second-**

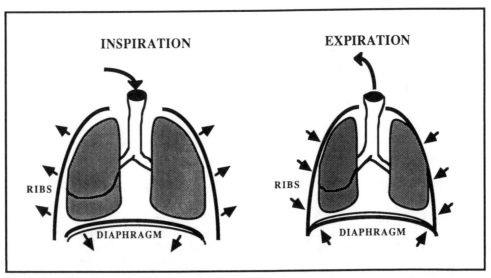

Figure 3-2 In mechanical aspects of breathing, movement of the rib cage and diaphragm increase and decrease the volume of the thoracic cavity, creating positive and negative pressures within the lungs.

ary muscles of respiration. As noted in Figure 3–2, the ribs and sternum assist with breathing by changing the size of the **thoracic cavity.** The muscles between the ribs, the intercostals, rotate and lift the rib cage, contributing to the expansion of the thoracic cavity. When the diaphragm contracts, it moves away from the lungs toward the abdominal cavity. These actions decrease the pressure within the thoracic cavity, creating a reduced pressure or vacuum within the lungs, allowing outside air to flow into the lungs. Expiration is usually a passive process involving the relaxation of the diaphragm and a dropping of the rib cage, increasing the pressure within the thoracic cavity, and forcing air out of the lungs. In forced or labored breathing, such as in exercise, the secondary muscles of respiration play a major role in inspiration, whereas the abdominal muscles play a major role in forced expiration. Contracting the abdominal muscles increases the intra-abdominal and intra-thoracic pressures and reduces the size of the thoracic cavity by pulling the rib cage down and inward.

These changes in intra-abdominal and intra-thoracic pressure assist not only in forced breathing, but also in the return of blood back to the heart. As the pressure increases, this pressure is transmitted to the veins that are transporting blood back to the heart through the abdominal and thoracic areas, and assists the blood returning to the heart through a squeezing-like action. When the pressure decreases, the veins return to their original size and fill with blood. A potentially dangerous respiratory procedure, frequently performed in certain types of exercise, is known as the **Valsalva maneuver.** This occurs when an individual holds his or her breath, and increases the pressure in the intra-abdominal cavity by a forceful contraction of the abdominal muscles, and in the intra-thoracic cavity by a forceful contraction of the diaphragm and the secondary muscles of respiration, with the glottis closed so the air will be trapped in the lungs. This maneuver is typically performed in lifting heavy weights. The high intra-abdominal and intra-thoracic pressures restrict venous return by collapsing the great veins. This maneuver, if held for an extended period of time, can greatly reduce the volume of blood returning to the heart, a situation that can initiate a fatal chain of events. A similar maneuver may occur when one is attempting to defecate when constipated. While very helpful in certain circumstances, it is important to realize that this maneuver can be dangerous and should be avoided if one has hypertension or known heart disease.

MEASUREMENTS OF PULMONARY VENTILATION

Lung function can be divided into several anatomical and functional fractions, as illustrated in Figure 3–3 on page 46. The **tidal volume (TV)** is that volume of air that goes into or out of the lungs with each breath. It can vary from approximately 0.5 liters at rest to 2.5 to 3.0 liters during heavy exercise. The **respiratory rate** refers to the number of times one breathes in a minute, and will vary from twelve breaths per minute at rest to from 40 to 50 breaths per minute, or higher, during heavy exercise. **Pulmonary ventilation,** abbreviated V_l, is the product of the tidal volume and respiratory rate, also referred to as the **minute respiratory volume.** At rest, pulmonary ventilation values are in the range of five to seven liters per minute. During exercise, pulmonary ventilation increases to levels in excess of 100 liters per minute, and can exceed 200 liters per minute in very large, well-conditioned athletes. The control of ventilation is mediated through the respiratory centers of the medulla oblongata and pons of the brain stem.

Vital capacity is the largest volume of air that can be forcibly expired following a maximal inspiration. Normal values range from approximately three liters for small females, to over seven liters for large, well-conditioned athletes. **Residual volume** represents that volume of air that remains in the lungs following a maximal expiration, for instance, at the end of the vital capacity maneuver. No matter how forcibly or how long you expire, the lungs will never completely empty or collapse. Normally, the residual volume is relatively small, varying between 0.8 and 1.6 liters, depending on the size of the individual. As a percentage of total lung volume, the residual volume should not exceed 30 percent. (Example: If the vital capacity is 4.0 liters, the residual volume is 2.0 liters, then total lung volume is 6.0 liters; the ratio of residual

Ventilation

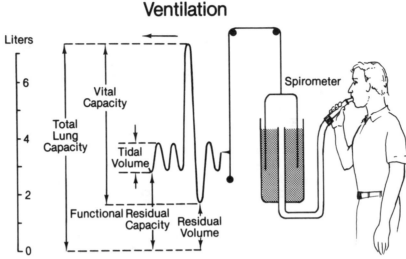

Figure 3-3   Measurements of lung volumes.

volume to total lung volume equals 2.0/6.0, which equals 0.33, or 33 percent.) This ratio, in addition to the vital capacity measure and other tests to determine the speed with which you can empty your lungs, are valuable screening tests for the detection of chronic obstructive lung disease. It is important to recognize that lung volumes are a function of body size, especially height, age, and sex.

Physics of Breathing

Gas exchange in the lungs involves the removal of carbon dioxide from the venous blood returning from various parts of the body, and the replenishment of oxygen which has been removed at the tissue level. The process of gas exchange is a function of pressure gradients between the lungs and the blood. Concentrations of various gases are typically described either relative to their percentage concentration, or their partial pressure (see Table 3-1). In percentage concentration, the air we breathe is composed of 79.03 percent nitrogen, 20.93 percent oxygen, and 0.03 percent carbon dioxide. At sea level, the atmospheric pressure is approximately 760 millimeters of mercury (mmHg). This is considered the total pressure, or 100 percent. Each gas exerts pressure in direct proportion

Table 3-1   Composition of atmospheric air and the corresponding partial pressures of respiratory gases at sea level.

| Gas | Percent in dry | Dry air | Partial pressure (mm Hg) | | Diffusion gradient |
			Alveolar air	Venous blood	
Total	100	760	760	760	
H_2O	0	0	47	47	
O_2	20.93	159	104	40	60
CO_2	0.03	0.2	40	47	5
N_2	79.04	600.8	573	573	

From H. A. DeVries, *Physiology of exercise for physical education and athletics*, 2nd ed. (Dubuque, Iowa: William C. Brown Co., Publisher, 1974), p. 172. Reproduced by permission of the publisher.

to its concentration. Thus, if the total pressure was 760 mmHg, then the partial pressure of nitrogen in air would be 600.6 mmHg (0.7903 x 760). Oxygen would be 159.1 mmHg (0.2093 x 760), and carbon dioxide would be 0.2 mmHg (0.0003 x 760). As we ascend from sea level to the higher elevations, the total atmospheric pressure decreases, the decrease being in direct proportion to the increase in elevation. As an example, at an elevation of 10,000 feet, the total atmospheric pressure is 523 mmHg, thus the partial pressure of oxygen in air would be reduced to 109.5 mmHg (0.2093 x 523). A gas will dissolve in a liquid in direct proportion to its partial pressure, assuming temperature remains constant. Thus, the gases and their movement from one part of the body to another are controlled by their partial pressures. The exchange of gases, for example, between the alveoli and blood or between blood and the tissues, is influenced most by the pressure gradient between two areas or tissues.

The partial pressure of oxygen in dry air is 159 mmHg, dropping to a level of 100 to 105 mmHg in the alveoli. Part of the reason for this drop in pressure is that considerable quantities of water vapor and carbon dioxide are found in the alveoli, with partial pressures of approximately 47 and 40 mmHg, respectively. The alveolar gas concentrations remain relatively stable. The venous blood coming into the pulmonary capillaries from the right side of the heart has a partial pressure of oxygen that is typically 40 to 45 mmHg. The pressure gradient for oxygen between the alveoli and blood would then be typically between 55 and 65 mmHg. It is this pressure gradient that drives the oxygen from the alveoli into the blood. By the time the blood exits the lungs on its return to the heart, the partial pressure for oxygen will have nearly equilibrated with that in the alveoli. The greater the pressure or diffusion gradient, the more rapidly the gases will diffuse across the membrane. Carbon dioxide reacts in a similar manner; however, diffusion gradients aren't as important for carbon dioxide since it diffuses at a rate approximately twenty times faster than oxygen. At the tissue level, the same gas laws apply to the unloading of oxygen and the loading of carbon dioxide from the blood to the tissue, and vice versa (see Figure 3–4).

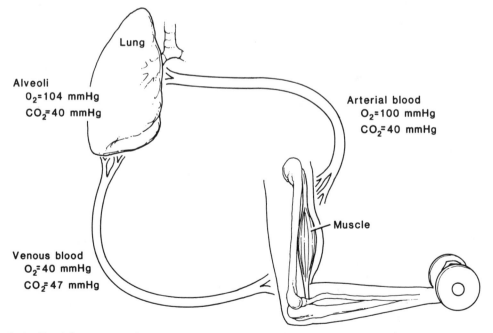

Figure 3-4 Partial pressure of oxygen and carbon dioxide levels in the body during rest.

The influence of altitude on the transport of oxygen to the tissues can be better understood in light of the preceding discussion. At a 10,000-foot altitude or elevation, the partial pressure of oxygen in air is reduced to 109 mmHg, and in the alveoli to 69 mmHg. If the partial pressure of oxygen in the mixed venous blood remains at 40 mmHg, the diffusion gradient would drop from approximately 60 mmHg at sea level to 29 mmHg at this altitude, which is more than a 50-percent reduction. This will have relatively little influence on the loading of oxygen at the level of the lungs, since the gradient is sufficient to almost totally saturate the blood with oxygen. At the tissue level, however, the reduced pressure gradient will reduce the amount of oxygen released from the blood to the tissues. Thus, altitude presents a significant challenge to the body, particularly during exercise. This topic will be discussed in greater detail in Chapter 14.

Transport of Oxygen and Carbon Dioxide

Oxygen is carried by the red blood cells in combination with **hemoglobin (Hb)**, and in plasma. Only about three milliliters (ml) of oxygen is dissolved in each liter of plasma. This means that approximately 10 to 15 ml of oxygen can be carried in the dissolved state, assuming a plasma volume of 3 to 5 liters. Such a supply of oxygen is wholly inadequate to even meet the needs of the tissues of the resting body, which requires more than 250 ml of oxygen per minute.

Hemoglobin in the four to six billion red blood cells of the body makes it possible for the blood to transport nearly 70 times more oxygen than can be dissolved in plasma. Each molecule of hemoglobin can carry four molecules of oxygen. The binding of oxygen to hemoglobin is a relatively loose, reversible reaction, that depends on the partial pressure of oxygen in solution.

$$Hb_4 + 4\ O_2 \rightarrow Hb_4\ O_8$$

The oxygen-carrying capacity also depends on the blood's hemoglobin content. Each 100 ml of blood contains an average of 14 to 16 grams of hemoglobin in men, and approximately 12 to 14 grams in women. Since each gram of hemoglobin can combine with about 1.34 ml of oxygen, the blood's oxygen-carrying capacity is approximately 20 ml per 100 ml of blood, when fully saturated with oxygen. As the blood passes through the lungs, it is in contact with the alveolar air for approximately 0.75 seconds, sufficient time for hemoglobin to pick up nearly all the oxygen it can hold, resulting in a 98 percent saturation. Individuals who have a low hemoglobin content, which occurs in **iron-deficiency anemia,** have a reduced capacity to transport oxygen, since the blood's carrying capacity is reduced. At rest these people may feel little effect of being anemic, since their cardiovascular systems can compensate for the lower oxygen content by increasing the flow of blood. During activities where oxygen delivery may become a limitation, the reduced oxygen content of the blood limits oxidative energy production and performance.

At rest, the oxygen content of arterialized blood is about 20 ml per 100 ml, which drops to 15 to 16 ml per 100 ml as it passes through the capillaries into the venous system. This arterial-venous difference in oxygen content (**a-vO$_2$ diff**) reflects a four to five ml of oxygen per 100 ml of blood uptake by the tissues. The amount of oxygen used by the tissues is proportional to its use for energy production. As the rate of oxygen usage increases, the a-vO$_2$ diff widens. During intense exercise the a-vO$_2$ diff of contracting muscles may increase to 15 ml per 100 ml of blood. The unloading of oxygen from the blood to the muscles is facilitated by the low partial-pressure of oxygen in the tissue, and increase in tissue acidity, temperature, or carbon dioxide concentration, factors all known to occur during muscular activity.

The increasing demand for oxygen during exercise can also be met by an increase in the volume of blood-flow through the muscle, thereby requiring less removal of oxygen from each 100 ml of blood. Consequently, oxygen delivery and uptake depends on the oxygen content of blood, blood flow, and the local conditions within the muscle. During maximal exercise, several of these factors may contribute to limit oxygen delivery, thereby restricting the muscle's ability to meet the oxidative demands of the effort.

Carbon dioxide exits the cells by diffusion in response to the partial pressure gradient between the tissue and the capillary blood. Whereas a small amount of carbon dioxide is dissolved in plasma, it is chiefly transported to the lungs in combination with hemoglobin and water (**carbonic acid**). The latter form provides the largest avenue for carbon dioxide transport. With the aid of the enzyme **carbonic anhydrase (c.a.)**, the carbon dioxide and water molecules combine in the tissue capillaries to form carbonic acid (H_2CO_3). After leaving the capillaries, carbonic acid dissociates a hydrogen ion (H^+), thereby forming a bicarbonate ion (HCO_3^-).

Tissue
$$CO_2 + H_2O \rightarrow (c.a.) \rightarrow H_2CO_3 \rightarrow H^+ + HCO_3^-$$

The hydrogen (H^+) is subsequently buffered by hemoglobin, which maintains the relatively normal acidity (pH) of the blood. As a consequence of this reaction, nearly 70 percent of the carbon dioxide is carried in the form of bicarbonate (HCO_3^-).

In the lungs, the partial pressure of carbon dioxide is lowered, resulting in the reformation of carbonic acid. At this stage, carbon dioxide and water are reformed, allowing the carbon dioxide to leave the blood, entering the alveoli to be exhaled during pulmonary ventilation.

Lung
$$H^+ + HCO_3^- \rightarrow H_2CO_3 \rightarrow (c.a.) \rightarrow CO_2 + H_2O$$

Controls of Breathing

The involuntary regulation of the rate and depth of breathing is not fully understood, although many of the intricate neural controls have been identified. The maintenance of arterial oxygen, carbon dioxide, and pH within very narrow limits, depends on a high level of coordination between pulmonary ventilation and circulation. As illustrated in Figures 3–5A and 3–5B, these systems

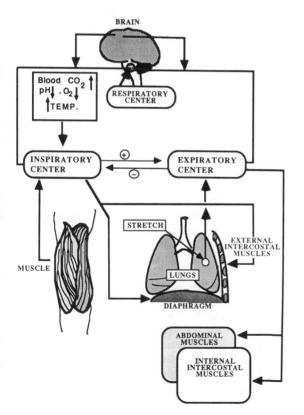

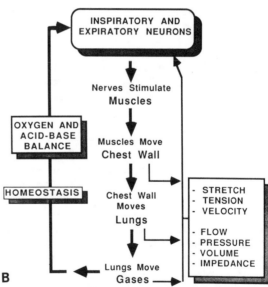

Figure 3–5A and 3–5B The controls of pulmonary ventilation during exercise. Note that a number of inputs to the respiratory center—motor centers of the brain, changes in pH, CO_2, and O_2, skeletal and respiratory muscles, and stretch receptors in the lung—are responsible for the control of breathing.

are closely monitored and regulated by both peripheral and central nervous receptors. The control center for pulmonary ventilation (**respiratory center**) is located in the medial portion of the medulla, although other areas of the brain—cerebral hemispheres and pons—contribute to fine regulation of breathing. At rest, changes in the Pco_2, Po_2, pH, and temperature of arterial blood activate neurons within the medulla and the arterial system. Signals are then relayed to the inspiratory and expiratory centers which control the rate and depth of breathing (see Figures 3–5A and 3–5B).

A decrease in arterial Po_2 activates the chemical receptors (**chemoreceptors**) in the aortic and carotid bodies. These same receptors are also responsible for sensing a rise in carbon dioxide (Pco_2), blood temperature, blood pressure, and a drop in pH. Under resting conditions, the partial pressure of carbon dioxide is the strongest stimulus for the regulation of breathing. As noted in the preceding section, small changes in carbonic acid, formed from carbon dioxide and water, result in an increase in hydrogen ion concentrations, the result of a dissociation of carbonic acid to bicarbonate and hydrogen ions. This increase in blood hydrogen-ion concentration stimulates breathing, thereby eliminating carbon dioxide, which lowers the hydrogen ion concentration as water is formed. This sequence of reactions regulates the acidity of the blood, while controlling the mechanism for inspiration and expiration.

The sensation of **dyspnea**, shortness of breath during exercise, is most common among individuals who are in poor physical condition, who attempt to exercise at levels that produce a sudden increase in arterial carbon dioxide and a drop in pH. As noted earlier, both of these stimuli send strong signals to the respiratory center, resulting in an increased demand on ventilation. Although exercise-induced dyspnea is sensed as an inability to breath, the underlying cause is an increase in blood hydrogen and carbon dioxide levels.

VENTILATION DURING EXERCISE

It has been suggested that the motor cortex is the principal site for stimulating the respiratory center to the high ventilatory rates observed during

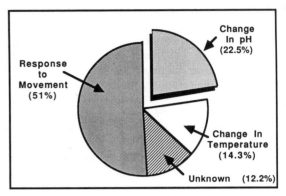

Figure 3–6   Factors responsible for the rise in pulmonary ventilation during exercise.

voluntary breathing and exercise. As shown in Figure 3–6, the response of movement appears to provide the greatest stimulus to breathing during exercise, although changes in blood acidity (pH) and temperature have a strong influence on ventilation. The anticipation of exercise results in a sudden increase in respiration, above the metabolic needs. Such over-breathing is termed **hyperventilation,** which may result in an excessive unloading of carbon dioxide, and a rise in pH above normal levels. Such voluntary, deep, rapid breathing can lead to light-headedness and even unconsciousness when performed for only a few seconds, revealing the sensitivity of the respiratory system's regulation of carbon dioxide and acid-base balance.

At the onset of activity there is a two-phase increase in ventilation: there is an almost immediate increase in ventilation, followed by a continued, more gradual rise in the depth and rate of breathing (see Figure 3–7). This two-phase adjustment suggests that the initial rise in ventilation is produced by the mechanical aspects of movement, whereas the more gradual increase is produced by changes in the temperature and chemical status of the arterial blood. At the end of mild exercise, the energy demands of the muscles drop almost immediately to resting levels, whereas pulmonary ventilation returns to normal at a relatively slow rate. If the rate of breathing was perfectly matched to the metabolic demands of the tissues, respiration would drop to the resting level within seconds after exercise. The fact that recovery of breathing

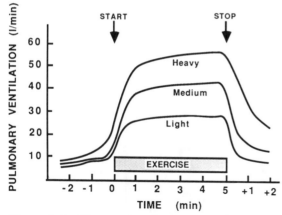

Figure 3-7 Changes in pulmonary ventilation before, during, and after five minutes of exercise at three levels of effort.

takes several minutes to return to the resting level, suggests that post-exercise breathing is regulated by acid–base balance and temperature of the blood.

During long periods of mild, steady-state activity, respiration appears to match the rate of energy metabolism. Although the partial pressure of oxygen and carbon dioxide remains relatively constant in the alveoli and arterial blood, ventilation tends to be more in proportion to the volume of oxygen consumed and the carbon dioxide produced by the body. The ratio between the amount of oxygen consumed (liters/minute) and the volume of pulmonary ventilation, provides an indicator of breathing economy referred to as the **ventilatory efficiency** ($\dot{V}E$).

$$\dot{V}E = \text{ventilation / oxygen consumption}$$
$$or$$
$$\dot{V}E = \dot{V}_e / \dot{V}o_2$$

At rest the $\dot{V}E$ may range from 23 to 28 liters of air per liter of oxygen consumed, which changes very little during mild exercise, such as walking. When the work intensity is increased to near maximum, the $\dot{V}E$ may be greater than 30, reflecting a rise in ventilation that is disproportionate to the uptake of oxygen. In general, however, the $\dot{V}E$ re-

mains relatively constant over a wide range of exercise levels, indicating that the control systems for breathing are properly matched to the body's need for oxygen. Even in activities such as swimming, where breathing must be synchronized with the arm-stroke cycle, the $\dot{V}E$ does not differ from other, free-breathing activities.

As the intensity of exercise is increased toward maximum, there is a disproportionate increase in ventilation in relation to oxygen consumption. When the workload exceeds 55 to 70 percent of maximal oxygen uptake, the delivery of oxygen to the muscles is insufficient to support the required energy needs via oxidation. To compensate, more energy is derived from glycolysis, resulting in an increase in the production and accumulation of lactic acid. This lactic acid combines with sodium bicarbonate to form sodium lactate, water, and carbon dioxide. The increase in carbon dioxide stimulates the chemoreceptors, amplifying the signals to the respiratory center to increase ventilation. Since this occurs without an equal increase in oxygen consumption, there is a disproportionate increase in the R-value, carbon dioxide production, and ventilation (see Figure 3–8). The workload at which these changes occur is termed the **lactate threshold,** or the **onset of blood lactate accumulation** (OBLA). Although such measurements of blood lactate are often used as indicators of anaerobic metabolism, this may be an oversimplification. Lactate accumulation occurs when the production and diffusion of lactate exceeds the rate of its removal. Admittedly, both the lactate threshold and OBLA reflect the level of stress imposed by the exercise, and may provide an objective tool for monitoring the stresses and adaptations to training (see Chapter 8).

Energy for Respiration

Like all aspects of tissue activity, lung ventilation and gas transport within the body require energy. At rest, only about two percent of the total energy used by the body is for breathing. As the rate and depth of ventilation increases, so does its energy cost. More than 15 percent of the oxygen consumed during heavy exercise may be used by the muscles of the chest wall (external and internal intercostal muscles), diaphragm, and abdomen, to

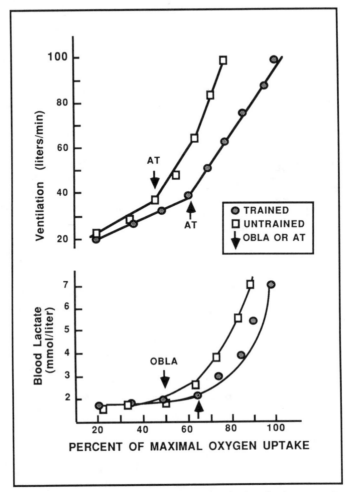

Figure 3-8 Blood lactate concentration and pulmonary ventilation during exercise of varied intensities (percent of maximal oxygen uptake) in untrained and endurance-trained men. The sharp increase in lactate accumulation and ventilation is identified as the onset of blood lactate accumulation (OBLA), and the anaerobic threshold (AT). The AT has been used to identify the sudden, disproportionate rise in respiration that occurs at about the same time as OBLA.

ventilate the lungs. During recovery from exercise, the work of breathing continues to demand a sizeable amount of energy, using 9 to 12 percent of the total oxygen being consumed.

Although it is clear that the muscles of respiration are heavily taxed during exercise, there is sufficient ventilatory reserve to prevent a rise in al-

veolar carbon dioxide or a decline in alveolar oxygen tension during activities that last for only a few minutes. During maximal effort, ventilation is usually less than the individual's capacity to voluntarily move air in and out of the lungs **maximal voluntary volume (MVV)**. In addition, most athletes can voluntarily increase their ventilation at the end of exercise. Nevertheless, recent evidence suggests that pulmonary ventilation may be a limiting factor in highly-trained subjects during maximal, exhaustive exercise (Dempsey, et al., 1986).

It has been suggested that heavy breathing for several hours may result in glycogen depletion and fatigue of the respiratory muscles. There are, however, few studies to support this theory. One experiment using untrained rats during exercise, found a smaller depletion of respiratory muscle glycogen as compared with the limb muscles. Such data are not available for humans.

It should be noted that the respiratory muscles are better designed for long-term activity than are the muscles of the arms and legs. Diaphragm muscle, for example, has two to three times the oxidative capacity (oxidative enzymes and mitochondria) and capillary density of skeletal muscle. Consequently, a larger part of the energy production for respiration can be derived from fat and lactate oxidation than in skeletal muscles.

In the normally healthy individual, the airway resistance and gas diffusion within the lungs is not a limiting factor for exercise. Despite marked reductions in mixed venous oxygen content, and a four- to fivefold increase in pulmonary blood flow, blood leaving the lungs is nearly saturated with oxygen, even near maximal effort. Although the volume of air passing through the trachae, bronchioles, etc., may increase 10- to 20-fold with exercise, airway resistance is maintained near the resting levels by dilation of the airway (increase in laryngeal aperature). Thus, the respiratory system is well-designed to accommodate the demands of heavy breathing during short- and long-term physical effort, and may only be a limiting factor in individuals with unusually large capacities to consume oxygen during exhaustive exercise.

Constriction of the bronchial tubes or a swelling of their mucous membranes causes considerable resistance to ventilation and shortness of breath. This ailment, termed **asthma,** is triggered by a wide variety of allergenic substances, such as pollen, mold spores, animal dander, or dust. Exercise is also known to have an adverse affect on subjects with asthma. The mechanism or mechanisms through which exercise causes airway obstruction in asthmatic subjects is unknown, despite exten-

sive study. A thorough review of this topic has been presented by Sly (1986) and Eggleston (1986).

Voluntary Regulation of Breathing

The conscious control of breathing enables us to alter the balance in our blood pH and carbon dioxide level, but has little influence on its oxygen content. At rest, voluntary hyperventilation results in a decrease in alveolar and arterial carbon dioxide from 40 to 15 mmHg, with a concomitant rise in blood pH. This reduction in circulating carbon dioxide and hydrogen reduces the ventilatory drive. Since the blood leaving the lungs is nearly always 98 percent saturated with oxygen, an increase in the partial pressure of oxygen in the alveoli does not increase the oxygen content of the blood. Consequently, the reduced desire to breathe and the increased ability to hold one's breath after hyperventilation, is due to an unloading of carbon dioxide rather than an increase in blood oxygen.

In an attempt to reduce the respiratory distress of exercise, swimmers often hyperventilate before competition. Since holding one's breath during swimming offers some advantages to stroke mechanics, most swimmers hyperventilate in the seconds before the start of most sprint events. Although they may feel little desire to breathe during the first eight to ten seconds of the race, their alveolar and arterial oxygen content may decline to critically low levels, impairing muscle oxidation and oxygen delivery to the central nervous system. In events lasting more than 20 to 30 seconds, this practice of hyperventilation may impair performance rather than improve it.

This practice is also common among individuals who attempt to perform long, underwater swims. By hyperventilating for several seconds before the dive they again decrease the drive to breathe, but do not increase their body oxygen stores. Breath-holding usually becomes intolerable when the partial pressure of carbon dioxide in arterial blood reaches 50 mmHg. During a dive that is preceded by hyperventilation, the oxygen content of the blood may reach critically low levels long before carbon dioxide signals the swimmer to surface and begin breathing. These events may cause the diver to lose consciousness before experiencing a desire to breathe.

ACID–BASE BALANCE IN EXERCISE

As noted earlier, intense muscular activity often results in the production and accumulation of lactate and H^+ that can impair energy metabolism and reduce the contractile force of the muscles. **Acids,** such as lactic acid and carbonic acid, are those substances that release **hydrogen ions (H^+).** The metabolism of carbohydrates, fats, and proteins all produce inorganic acids that dissociate to increase the H^+ concentration of body fluids. In order to minimize the presence of free H^+, the blood and muscles contain **base** substances, such as bicarbonate and proteins, that combine with or **buffer** H^+:

$$H^+ + buffer \rightarrow (H\text{-}buffer)$$

An increase in H^+ concentration is referred to as **acidosis,** whereas a decrease in H^+ below the normal level is termed **alkalosis.** The level of acid and base in the blood and muscles is measured in **pH** units, with a neutral pH balance at 7.0. Values above pH 7.0 indicate the presence of more base than H^+, whereas values below 7.0 reflect an excess of H^+, or an acid condition. Under resting conditions body fluids have more base—bicarbonate, phosphates, and proteins—than acid, resulting in a tissue pH that ranges from 7.1 in muscle to 7.4 in arterial blood. The tolerable limits for arterial pH extend from 6.9 to 7.5, although such extremes can only be tolerated for a few minutes (see Figure 3–9).

The pH of intra- and extracellular body fluids is kept within a relatively narrow range by (1) chemical buffers, (2) pulmonary ventilation, and (3) kidney function. The three major chemical buffers in the body are bicarbonate (HCO_3^-), phosphates (P_i), and proteins. In the blood, the most important buffers are the hemoglobin in the red blood cells, sodium bicarbonate ($NaHCO_3$), plasma protein, and phosphate. Table 3–2 illustrates the relative contributions of these buffers in handling acids. The relatively large contribution of bicarbonate to the buffer capacity of blood depends on the amount of bicarbonate present and upon the fact that when it combines with H^+, it converts to carbonic acid and disappears. The carbon dioxide formed from the carbonic acid is removed by the lungs, and only water is left. The amount of acid buffered is equal to the amount of bicarbonate that disappears. More than 60 percent of the bicarbonate initially present in the blood is used when lactic acid reduces the pH from 7.4 to 7.0. Even under resting conditions, the acid produced by the end-products of metabolism would eliminate a major portion of the bicarbonate from the blood if there was no other avenue of H^+ removal from the body. Fortunately, the blood and its buffers are required to carry the metabolic acids from the muscles to

Arterial Blood pH

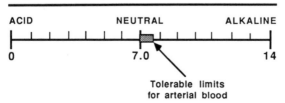

Tolerable limits
for arterial blood

Muscle pH

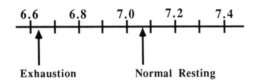

Figure 3-9 The range of pH from acid to alkaline for arterial blood and muscle, pH 7.0 being neutral. Note the small range of physiological tolerance for blood pH (6.9 to 7.5).

Table 3-2 Buffering capacity of bicarbonate, hemoglobin, plasma protein, and phosphate. Units in the "Slykes" column represent the milliquivalents of hydrogen ions consumed by the acid buffers of each liter of blood, from pH 7.4 to 7.0.

Buffer	Slykes
Bicarbonate	18
Hemoglobin	8
Plasma Protein	1.7
Phosphate	0.3
Total	28

the kidneys or other tissues where they can be eliminated.

Within the muscle fibers and kidney tubules, H^+ is buffered by phosphates, such as phosphoric acid and sodium phosphate. Unfortunately, less is known about the capacity of the buffers that are housed within cells, although it is known that cells contain more protein and phosphates, and less bicarbonate than exist in extracellular fluids.

As noted earlier, any increase in free H^+ in the blood stimulates the respiratory center to increase alveolar ventilation. This facilitates the combining of H^+ and bicarbonate (HCO_3^-) and the removal of carbon dioxide. The end result is a lowering of free H^+ and a rise in blood pH. Both the chemical buffers and the respiratory system provide a temporary means of neutralizing the acute effects of exercise acidosis. In order to establish a more stable buffer reserve, the accumulated H^+ is removed from the body via the kidneys and urinary system. Hydrogen ions (H^+) are removed from the blood along with other waste products during glomerular filtration, which occurs in the renal tubules. This process provides a means of eliminating H^+ from the body while raising the concentration of extracellular bicarbonate.

During a sprint exercise, the muscles generate a large amount of lactate and H^+, which lowers the muscle pH from a resting level of 7.08 to less than 6.70. As shown in Table 3-3, an all-out, 400-meter

sprint results in a drop in leg muscle pH from 7.08 to 6.63 with a concomitant rise in muscle lactate from a resting value of 1.2 mmol/kg to 19.7 mmol/kg of muscle. As noted earlier, such disturbances in acid–base balance impair muscle contractility and its capacity to generate ATP. Lactate and H^+ accumulate within the muscle, in part, because it does not freely diffuse across the fiber membranes. Despite the large production of lactate and H^+ during the 60 seconds required to run the 400 meters, diffusion and equilibrium of these by-products within the body fluids takes five to ten minutes of recovery. Five minutes after the exercise, the runners in Table 3-3 were found to have blood pH and lactate values of 7.10 and 12.3 mmol/liter, respectively, compared to resting values of 7.40 and 1.5 mmol/liter.

Returning the blood and muscle lactate levels to normal after such an exhaustive exercise bout is a relatively slow process, often requiring one or two hours. As shown in Figure 3-10, recovery of blood lactate to the resting level is facilitated by continued, lower-intensity exercise (**active recovery**). After a series of exhaustive sprint bouts, the

Table 3-3 Blood and muscle pH and lactate concentration (LA) after a 400-meter run for each of four men (Ss).

Ss	400 m Run Time (sec)	Muscle		Blood	
		pH_m	LA_m	pH_b	LA_b
1	61.0	6.68	19.7	7.12	12.6
2	57.1	6.59	20.5	7.14	13.4
3	65.0	6.59	20.2	7.02	13.1
4	58.5	6.68	18.2	7.10	10.1
Average	60.4	6.63	19.7	7.10	12.3

*Note that blood lactate is measured in mmol/liter and muscle lactate is in mmol/kg muscle; blood and muscle pH are in mmol/liter ($\times 10^{-8}$), and mmol/kg ($\times 10^{-8}$), respectively.

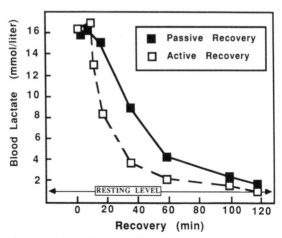

Figure 3-10 Effects of active and inactive (passive) recovery of blood lactate to the resting level after a series of exhaustive sprint bouts. Note the faster rate of recovery when the subjects performed mild exercise (50 percent of their maximal oxygen uptake). The subjects sat quietly during the passive recovery.

subjects in this study either sat quietly (**passive recovery**) or exercised at a work level that required them to use 50 percent of their maximal oxygen uptake (active recovery). The faster removal of blood lactate with active recovery occurs as a consequence of a higher rate of blood flow through the active muscle, increased lactate diffusion out of the muscles, and an increase in the rate of lactate oxidation.

Although blood lactate remains elevated for one to two hours after a highly anaerobic exercise bout, blood H^+ concentration is readjusted to normal within 30 to 40 minutes of recovery. Chemical buffering, principally bicarbonate, and respiratory removal of excess carbon dioxide are responsible for this relatively rapid return to a normal acid–base homeostasis.

It has been suggested that performance in highly anaerobic events can be improved by first elevating blood and muscle bicarbonate concentrations, thereby enhancing their buffering capacity. Although the oral intake of sodium bicarbonate

does elevate the plasma bicarbonate, it has little effect on the intracellular concentration of bicarbonate. Consequently, dietary manipulation of blood bicarbonate has little or no influence on muscle fatigue in activities that produce exhaustion in less than two minutes. These events are too brief to allow much H^+ diffusion out of the muscle fibers or to benefit from the enhanced extracellular buffering provided by the ingested bicarbonate.

The level of blood bicarbonate does appear important for performance levels in anaerobic events lasting two to five minutes, or during repeated sprint bouts. As shown in Figures 3–11 and 3–12, when the blood bicarbonate concentrate was artificially elevated before and during five, one-minute sprint-cycling bouts, performance on the final trial was improved 42 percent. This elevation in bicarbonate reduced the concentration of free H^+ both during and after the exercise, thereby elevating blood pH. As a result of the sprints, muscle pH fell to only 6.85 after the third sprint, compared to a muscle pH of 6.70 when blood bicarbonate was

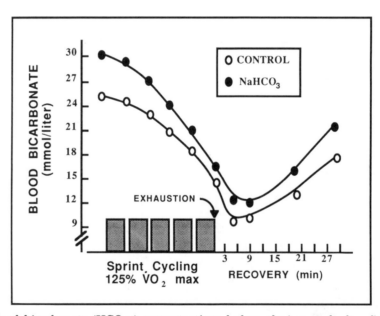

Figure 3–11 Blood bicarbonate (HCO_3^-) concentrations before, during, and after five sprint cycling bouts with and without sodium bicarbonate ($NaHCO_3$) ingestion. The fifth sprint was performed to exhaustion. The higher blood HCO_3^- levels resulted in a significant improvement in performance (modified from Costill, et al., 1984).

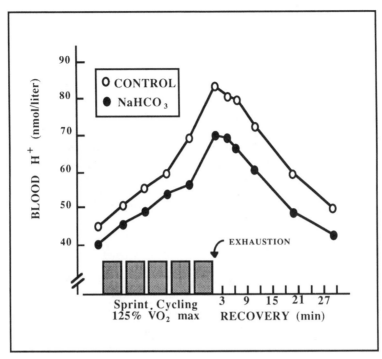

Figure 3-12 Blood hydrogen (H$^+$) concentrations before, during, and after the five sprint bouts described in Figure 3-11. The elevated blood HCO$_3^-$ concentrations resulted in an elevation of blood H$^+$, a smaller drop of blood pH, and a faster recovery after the sprint bouts (modified from Costill, et al., 1984).

normal. Thus, in addition to its improved buffering capacity, the extra bicarbonate appears to speed the removal of H$^+$ from the muscle fibers, thereby lessening the drop in intracellular pH.

Although bicarbonate plays an important role in controlling acid-base balance during exercise, neither sprint nor endurance training have an effect on its concentration. At rest, there is no difference in blood H$^+$, lactate, or bicarbonate concentrations between trained and untrained individuals. However, there is evidence that muscle buffer capacity is increased 37 percent with sprint training. Endurance training, on the other hand, appears to have no influence on the muscle's buffer capacity. Although there is no direct evidence to explain the adaptation to sprint training, it has been theorized that this improved buffer capacity is the result of an increase in muscle phosphates and/or proteins.

The role of training adaptations to anaerobic training will be presented in greater detail in Chapter 8.

SUMMARY

Pulmonary ventilation plays an important role in the homeostasis of oxygen delivery and removal of carbon dioxide from the body. The structural design of the lungs and pulmonary vasculature provides a protected interface between respiratory air and blood. Inspiration and expiration of air is accomplished by the contractile force of the diaphragm, intercostal, and abdominal muscles.

Gas exchange between the tissues, blood, and alveolar air is dependent on the difference in partial pressure between the gases in each compartment.

Gases will diffuse across the membranes more rapidly when there is a greater difference in partial pressure or diffusion gradient between the tissues. During passage through the lungs, there is sufficient time for the blood and alveolar air to reach a carbon dioxide and oxygen equilibrium. Consequently, even during heavy exercise, arterial blood is nearly saturated with oxygen (98 percent saturated). During passage through the working muscle, the blood's partial pressure of oxygen declines from 100 mmHg to 40 mmHg, whereas carbon dioxide rises from 40 to 47 mmHg. The synchronization of such gas exchange is critical to the processes of energy metabolism and acid–base balance.

The rate and depth of breathing is controlled by a combination of neural, thermal, and chemical factors. At rest, the hydrogen ion and carbon dioxide concentrations of the blood are the most important mechanisms for respiratory regulation. During exercise, however, actions of the muscles and joints, and neural inputs from the motor centers of the brain, account for more than 50 percent of the drive and regulation for breathing.

By eliminating carbon dioxide, the respiratory system maintains a balance between blood and tissue pH. Since these tissues can only survive within a narrow range of pH, the body's buffering capacity and ability to remove free hydrogen ions is critical for the function and life of the cells. Although lactic acid is buffered during highly anaerobic activities, blood and muscle pH can be markedly distorted, requiring 30 to 120 minutes of recovery time before returning to normal. This process is influenced by blood bicarbonate concentration and the level of activity during the recovery period.

Thus, the interaction between pulmonary respiration and the regulation of acid–base balance are critical to exercise performance. Any impairment in the body's capacity to exchange gases, to buffer the metabolically produced acids, or to eliminate free-hydrogen ions will lead to a reduction in exercise performance. Although the lungs, *per se*, do not appear trainable, the mechanisms that control the function of ventilation and acid–base regulation are enhanced with regular physical activity.

STUDY QUESTIONS

1. Describe the structural mechanisms that are responsible for external respiration.
2. Identify the muscles and their function in pulmonary ventilation.
3. What effect does exercise have on tidal and minute respiratory volumes?
4. What are the partial pressures of oxygen and carbon dioxide in inspired air, alveoli gas, and arterial and mixed venous blood? How are they affected by altitude?
5. In what forms are oxygen and carbon dioxide transported in the blood?
6. Define acids and bases. What role does the respiratory system play in acid–base balance?
7. What are the chemical stimuli that control the depth and rate of breathing? How do they control respiration during exercise? How are they affected during voluntary hyperventilation?
8. What other stimuli control ventilation during exercise?
9. What is "ventilatory efficiency"?
10. Define "OBLA" and the "anaerobic threshold." How do they differ in trained and untrained subjects?
11. What risks are associated with voluntary hyperventilation prior to underwater swimming? Describe the physiological mechanisms that cause this risk.
12. What is the "normal" resting pH for arterial blood? Muscle? How are these values changed as a result of exhaustive sprint exercise?
13. What are the primary buffers in the blood? Muscles?
14. How long does it take blood pH and lactate levels to return to normal after an all-out sprint? How is recovery affected by the oral administration of sodium bicarbonate?

REFERENCES

Brooks, G. A. & Fahey, T. D. (1984). *Exercise physiology: Human bioenergetics and its applications.* New York: John Wiley & Sons, pp. 221–278.

Comroe, J. H. (1974). *Physiology of respiration* (2nd ed). Chicago: Year Book Medical Pub.

Costill, D. L. (1970). Metabolic responses during distance running. *Journal of Applied Physiology*, 251–255.

Costill, D. L., Barnett, A., Sharp, R., Fink, W. J., & Katz, A. (1983). Leg muscle pH following sprint running. *Medicine and Science in Sports and Exercise, 15*, 325–329.

Costill, D. L., Verstappen, F., Kuipers, H., Janssen, E., & Fink, W. (1984). Acid-base balance during repeated bouts of exercise: Influence of HCO_3. *International Journal of Sports Medicine, 5.* 228–231.

Costill, D. L., Kovaleski, J., Porter, D., Kirwan, J., Fielding, R., & King, D. (1985). Energy expenditure during front crawl swimming: Predicting success in middle-distance events. *International Journal of Sports Medicine, 5*, 266–270.

Craig, A. B., Jr. (1980). Principles and problems of underwater diving. *Physician and Sportsmedicine, 8*, 72.

Dempsey, J. A., Vidruk, E. H., & Mastenbrook, S. M. (1980). Pulmonary control systems in exercise. *Federation Proceedings, 39*, 1498–1505.

Dempsey, J. A. (1985). Pulmonary control systems in exercise: Update. *Federation Proceedings, 44*, 2260–2270.

Dempsey, J. A. & Fregosi, R. F. (1985). Adaptability of the pulmonary system to changing metabolic requirements. *American Journal of Cardiology, 55*, 59D–67D.

Dempsey, J. A., Vidruk, E. H., & Mitchell, G. S. (1986). Is the lung built for exercise? *Medicine and Science in Sports and Exercise, 18*, 143–155.

Eggleston, P. A. (1986). Pathophysiology of exercise-induced asthma. *Medicine and Science in Sports and Exercise, 18*, 318–321.

Hermansen, L. (1981). Effect of metabolic changes on force generation in skeletal muscle during maximal exercise. In *Human muscle fatigue: Physiological mechanisms.* London: Pitman Medical.

McArdle, W. D., Katch, F. I., & Katch, V. L. (1986). *Exercise physiology: Energy, nutrition, and human performance.* Philadelphia: Lea and Febiger.

Sharp, R. L., Costill, D. L., Fink, W. J., & King, D. S. (1986). Effects of eight weeks of bicycle ergometer sprint training on human muscle buffer capacity. *International Journal of Sports Medicine, 7*, 13–17.

Sly, R. M. (1986). History of exercise-induced asthma. *Medicine and Science in Sports and Exercise, 18*, 314–317.

Sutton, J. R., & Jones, N. L. (1979). Control of pulmonary ventilation during exercise and mediators in the blood: CO2 and hydrogen ion. *Medicine and Science in Sports and Exercise, 11*, 198.

Sutton, J. R., Jones, N. L., & Toews, C. J. (1981). Effect of pH on muscle glycolysis during exercise. *Clinical Science, 61*, 331–338.

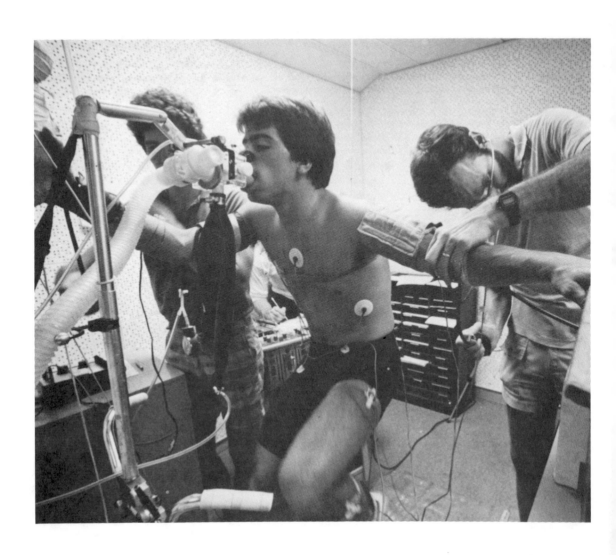

4

Cardiovascular Regulation

INTRODUCTION

As you progressively move from a lying position to sitting, from sitting to standing, from standing to walking, from walking to jogging, and from jogging to running, the body continuously adjusts physiologically, allowing a progressive increase in the rate of work. As just one example, if your heart rate is 50 beats/minute while lying down, it will increase to about 55 beats/minute while sitting, and to 60 beats/minute while standing. The major reason your heart rate increases is to compensate for the decrease in the volume of blood the heart can pump with each beat, the **stroke volume.** This decrease in stroke volume as you go from a lying to a standing position, is a result of a reduction in the amount of blood returned to the heart, an effect of gravity. In fact, blood tends to pool in the lower extremities as you stand quietly at rest.

Thus, the increase in heart rate with a change in position from lying, to sitting, to standing, maintains the volume of blood pumped per minute, or the **cardiac output** (cardiac output = heart rate x stroke volume, or $\dot{Q}$ = HR x SV). As you move from a standing position to jogging, the heart will increase from about 60 to 120 beats/minute, and as you progress to a fast run the heart rate could reach 180 beats/minute, or more. While the increase in heart rate from a lying position to standing was for the purpose of maintaining cardiac output, the increases with jogging and running are to facilitate increases in cardiac output, enabling delivery of substantially more blood to your working muscles to meet the requirements of that activity. These relationships are illustrated in Figure 4–1 on page 62.

The cardiovascular system serves a number of functions in the body, functions that are essential for survival. The body depends on the cardiovascular system to deliver nutrients to and remove waste products from every cell in the body; to provide a means of cooling the body as it produces heat during exercise, or as it gains heat during hot and humid weather; to control the degree of acidity and alkalinity of your body; and to promote resistance to disease organisms. The cardiovascular system serves many other functions, but these are of lesser importance to our understanding of the physiological bases of sport and physical activity.

Any system of circulation requires three essential components: a pump, a system of channels or vessels, and a fluid medium. The heart, blood vessels, and blood, respectively, comprise these essential components.

THE HEART

The heart is a four-chambered organ that serves as a primary pump for circulating blood throughout the entire cardiovascular system. Figure 4–2 on page 62 illustrates the heart, showing the flow of

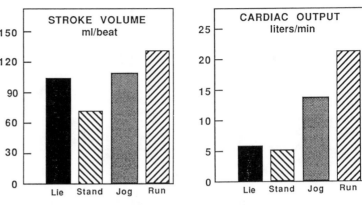

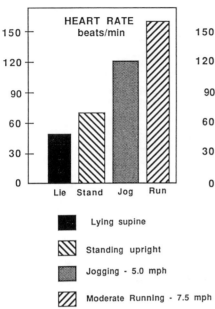

Figure 4-1 Changes in heart rate, stroke volume, and cardiac output with changes in posture and exercise.

blood through the pulmonary and systemic circulatory systems. The circulation from the right ventricle through the lungs and back to the left atrium is referred to as the lesser, or **pulmonary circulation**, while circulation from the left ventricle through the remainder of the body and back to the right atrium is referred to as the greater, or **systemic circulation**. Blood enters the right side of the heart, from the great veins (**superior and inferior vena cava**) into the **right atrium**. From the

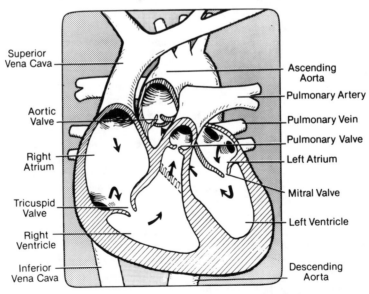

Figure 4-2 The heart, illustrating the pulmonary and systemic circulation.

right atrium, the blood is pumped through the **tricuspid valve** into the **right ventricle.** The right ventricle pumps the blood through the **pulmonary valve** into the **pulmonary artery** which transports the blood directly into the lungs. The blood exits the lungs through the **pulmonary vein** into the **left atrium.** From the left atrium, the blood is pumped through the **mitral valve** and into the **left ventricle.** The left ventricle is the most powerful of the four chambers of the heart, since it must pump the blood through the **aortic valve,** into the **aorta,** and through the entire systemic circulation.

The four valves (pulmonary, tricuspid, mitral, and aortic) function to prevent backflow or regurgitation of blood into the chamber from which it has been pumped. A **heart murmur** describes a condition in which abnormal heart sounds are detected by listening to the chest through a stethoscope. These abnormal sounds reflect the turbulent flow of blood through narrowed or leaky valves, or through a hole in one of the walls separating the chambers of the heart. Heart murmurs are quite common in the growing child and adolescent. During periods of growth, the growth of the valves often fails to keep up with the growth of the openings or **orifices** of the heart. Heart murmurs also reflect diseased valves, such as **aortic stenosis** (narrowed aortic valve) and **mitral stenosis** (narrowed mitral valve).

The blood travels through the major arteries to minor arteries, and then to the arterioles before it reaches the capillary bed. From the capillaries, the blood returns via venules to the lesser veins, and then to the greater veins back to the right atrium. Figure 4–3 illustrates the transport of blood through this system of vessels, the vascular system.

The Myocardium

The heart is a muscle, but it is distinctly different from both skeletal and smooth muscle (see Chapter 1). The heart muscle is called the **myocardium.** The inner lining is referred to as the **endocardium** and the outer lining is the **epicardium.** The thickness of the myocardium varies in direct relationship to the stress placed on the walls of each chamber. The left ventricle has the thickest walls since it must pump blood throughout the entire body, with the

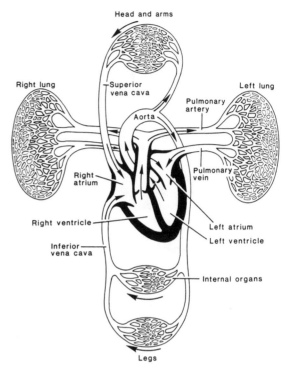

Figure 4–3 The vascular system.

exception of the lungs, and faces a much greater resistance than that encountered by any of the other three chambers of the heart.

Athletes in training, as well as non-athletes who train for health-related benefits, typically have enlarged hearts. For those who have trained through endurance-types of activities, this enlargement is thought to be the result of an increase in size of the left ventricular chamber, allowing more blood to be pumped per beat. Resistance-types of training, such as weight lifting, are thought to result in an increased left ventricular muscle mass, allowing a more forceful contraction of the heart. The reasons for this differential response to training, such as endurance training versus resistance training, will be discussed in Chapter 9.

The myocardium differs from skeletal muscle in one very important way. Cardiac muscle fibers or cells are anatomically interconnected end-to-end by intercalated discs. This feature allows the heart to act as one large muscle fiber—when one fiber contracts, all fibers contract. In fact, the atria and ventricles form two independent units, referred to as **functional syncytia**, allowing the atria and then the ventricles to contract as functional units.

Control of Heart Rate

Heart muscle is striated like skeletal muscle, but has the unique feature of being able to contract rhythmically on its own in the absence of nervous stimulation. Without either neural or hormonal stimulation, the intrinsic rate of the heart is approximately 100 beats per minute in the untrained individual, but can drop to levels of 80 beats per minute or lower in endurance-trained individuals. Under normal conditions, the heart rate is controlled by both the sympathetic and parasympathetic nervous systems, and by certain hormones (see Chapters 5 and 6). The parasympathetic system, through the vagus nerve, has a depressant effect on the heart, slowing the rate of the heart, decreasing the force of atrial contraction, and delaying atrioventricular conduction. Maximal vagal stimulation can lower the heart rate between 20 and 30 beats per minute. The sympathetic system has just the opposite effect, increasing both the rate of contraction and the force of contraction. Maximum sympathetic stimulation will allow the heart rate to reach values up to 250 beats per minute. **Chronotropic** and **inotropic factors** are terms used to describe those factors that influence either or both rate (chronotropic) and strength of contraction (inotropic).

Under resting conditions the parasympathetic system predominates. The normal resting heart rate typically varies between 60 and 85 beats per minute. With extended periods of endurance training, for instance, months to years, the resting heart rate can decrease to 35 beats per minute or lower. We have observed a resting heart rate of 28 beats per minute in a world-class long-distance runner. It is postulated that these lower resting rates are the result of increased parasympathetic stimulation, or tone, through the vagus nerve, with the reduction in sympathetic activity serving a lesser role.

As was stated earlier, the myocardium has its own rate of contraction independent of nervous stimulation. In fact, various areas within the myocardium have their own rates of contraction. The sinoatrial, **S–A node,** is a small group of specialized cardiac muscle fibers located on the posterior wall of the right atrium. Without nervous or hormonal stimulation, it will contract at a rate of approximately 80 to 95 times per minute. Similarly, the atrium and the ventricle will contract at 60 and 20 times per minute, respectively. Since the S–A node has the faster rate compared to other parts of the heart, the impulses generated by the S–A node spread into the atria and ventricles at a rate that exceeds their natural slower rate of contraction. Thus, the S–A node establishes the rate and rhythm for the entire heart, and for this reason it is referred to as the **pacemaker** of the heart. Occasionally, chronic problems develop within the S–A node that result in its inability to maintain an appropriate sinus rhythm. In such cases, it has become quite common to surgically install an artificial pacemaker, a small battery-operated electrical stimulator implanted under the skin, with electrodes attached to the right ventricle. The artificial pacemaker takes over the control of the ventricles. The batteries need to be replaced about once every five years.

Once the impulse is initiated at the S–A node, it spreads by special pathways to the atrioventricular, or **A–V node,** located toward the center of the heart on the right atrial wall. From the A–V node the impulses spread rapidly through the A–V bundle (Bundle of His), out to specialized conduction fibers, the **Purkinje fibers.** The Purkinje fibers transmit the impulses to the right and left ventricles at a velocity approximately six times faster than normal heart muscle. The A–V bundle divides into right and left bundle branches shortly after entering the ventricles. After reaching the walls of the ventricles, each branch divides into many small Purkinje fiber branches that make direct contact with the cardiac muscle. The high speed of conduction of the impulses along the Purkinje fibers is an important aspect of ventricular contraction, as this allows all parts of the ventricle to contract at the same time, not one segment at a time.

The sequence of contraction is as follows: First, the impulse travels relatively slowly from the S–A node to the A–V node, where the A–V node delays the impulse about 1/10th of a second before sending it on to the ventricles. Since the impulse travels through the atria on its way from the S–A node to the A–V node, contraction of the atria occurs at this time. The delay of the impulse at the A–V node allows the atria to complete contraction, pumping the blood into the ventricles, prior to activation of the ventricles.

Occasionally, disturbances occur in this normal sequence of events leading to an irregular heart rhythm, dysrhythmia. These disturbances vary in the degree of seriousness. **Premature ventricular contractions** that result in the feeling of either skipped beats or extra beats are relatively common and result from impulses outside the S–A node. **Atrial flutter** or **atrial fibrillation** are more serious dysrhythmias, in which the atria contract at rates of 200 to 400 times per minute, but pump little or no blood. **Ventricular tachycardia,** defined as four or more consecutive premature ventricular beats, is a very serious dysrhythmia and can lead directly to **ventricular fibrillation,** where large masses of the myocardium contract simultaneously. During ventricular fibrillation, the heart is unable to pump blood. Most cardiac deaths occur

as a result of ventricular fibrillation. Use of a defibrillator to shock the heart back into normal sinus rhythm must occur within several minutes if the person is to survive. Cardiopulmonary resuscitation will take over the function of the heart and maintain life for up to several hours, but the sooner emergency treatment, including defibrillation, is started, the better the chances of survival.

The electrical activity of the heart, as just described, can be recorded for purposes of diagnosing potential cardiac problems. Electrodes are placed in specific locations on the arms, legs, and multiple locations on the chest. A permanent recording of the electrical activity between any two or more electrodes is made using an electrocardiograph (see Figure 4–4). The resulting tracing is referred to as an electrocardiogram (see Figure 4–5 on page 66). Heart defects, disease, and electrical conduction abnormalities can be identified from a detailed interpretation of the electrocardiogram. Often, electrocardiograms will be obtained during exercise (see Figure 4–6 on page 66). As the intensity of exercise is increased, the heart is called on to beat faster and work harder to deliver more

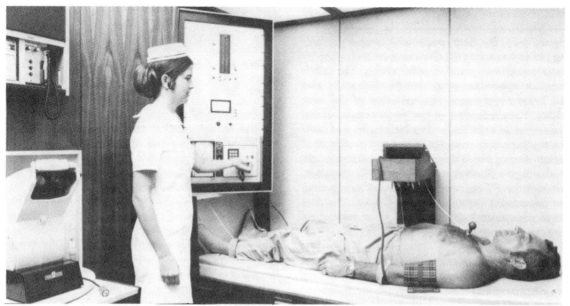

Figure 4-4 Obtaining a resting electrocardiogram.

A. Resting electrocardiogram   Heart rate: 75 beats/min

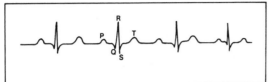

B. Exercise electrocardiogram   Heart rate: 150 beats/min

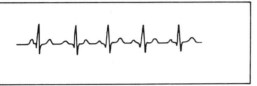

C. Ischemic response during exercise

ST segment depression

D. Premature ventricular contraction

Figure 4-5 The first two graphs compare a resting (A) and exercise (B) electrocardiogram. The P-wave represents atrial depolarization, the QRS-complex represents ventricular depolarization, and the T-wave represents repolarization of the ventricles. Repolarization of the atria occurs at the same time as ventricular depolarization, and thus the repolarization complex is not observable as it occurs during the QRS-complex. The third graph of this figure illustrates an ischemic (C) response, in which the ST-segment is depressed, suggesting the presence of coronary artery disease. The last graph illustrates a dysrhythmia, as in premature ventricular contraction (D).

blood to the active muscles. If the heart is diseased, evidence of the disease becomes evident on the electrocardiogram as the heart increases its rate of work (see graphs C and D in Figure 4-5). The electrocardiogram provides information only

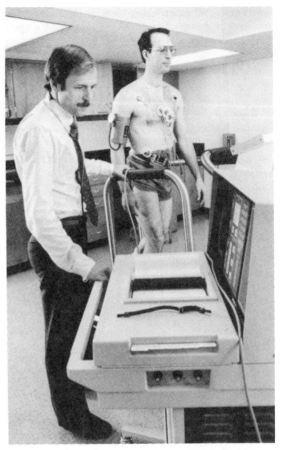

Figure 4-6 Obtaining the exercise electrocardiogram.

on the electrical activity of the heart and not on the mechanical aspects, such as valve function or the filling and emptying of the four chambers of the heart. Heart murmurs, or the leakage of blood through an imperfectly closed valve, will not be evident on the electrocardiogram.

The contraction phase for either the atria or ventricles, during which time they expel most of the blood from their chambers, is referred to as the period of systole. The relaxation phase, during which time the atrium or ventricle fill with blood, is referred to as the period of diastole. At a heart rate of 74 beats per minute, diastole accounts for 0.50 seconds and systole for 0.31 seconds, for a total of 0.81 seconds for the entire cardiac cycle. As the heart rate increases, these absolute time intervals are proportionately shortened. During systole, a certain volume is ejected from the left ventricle, referred to as the **stroke volume (SV)** of the heart, or the volume of blood pumped per stroke. The volume of blood in the ventricle at the end of diastole (**end-diastolic volume** or **EDV**) minus the volume of blood in the ventricle at the end of systole (**end-systolic volume** or **ESV**) is equal to the stroke volume (EDV − ESV = SV). The proportion of blood pumped out of the left ventricle with each beat is referred to as the **ejection fraction,** and is determined by dividing the stroke volume by the end-diastolic volume (EF = SV ÷ EDV). This value, generally expressed as a percentage, averages 60 percent at rest. As an example, 60 percent of the blood in the ventricle at the end of the diastole will be ejected with the next contraction of the heart.

As was defined earlier, cardiac output ($\dot{Q}$) is the volume of blood pumped per minute, or simply the product of heart rate (HR) and stroke volume ($\dot{Q}$ = HR · SV). The stroke volume at rest in the standing position will average between 60 and 80 milliliters in an average-sized adult. Thus, at a resting heart rate of 80 beats per minute, the resting cardiac output will vary between 4,800 and 6,400 milliliters per minute, or between 4.8 and 6.4 liters per minute.

THE VASCULAR SYSTEM

The vascular system is composed of a series of vessels that transport blood from the heart to the tissues and back to the heart. In addition, the heart, as an active muscle, has its own vascular system to provide it with necessary nutrients and to rid it of waste products. The coronary arteries, which supply the heart muscle or myocardium, originate from the base of the aorta as it leaves the heart. The coronary arteries are very susceptible to atherosclerosis, or narrowing, which can lead to coronary artery disease. This will be discussed in much greater detail in Chapter 18.

The system of arteries, arterioles, capillaries, venules, and veins was described earlier and is illustrated in Figure 4–2. Since we spend so much of our time in an upright position—sitting, standing,

or actively walking or running—it is necessary to provide assistance in returning the blood from the lower part of the body back to the heart. This is accomplished by two basic mechanisms, breathing and the muscle pump. With breathing, each time you breathe in and out the resulting changes in pressure within the abdominal and thoracic cavities work to assist the return of blood to the heart. The muscles, as they contract, also assist the return of blood to the heart. This is accomplished by a series of valves located in the veins that allow blood to flow in only one direction—back to the heart. Thus, backward flow is prevented. Each time the surrounding muscles contract, the veins in the immediate vicinity are compressed and the blood is pushed up towards the heart. When an individual stands for an extended period of time with minimal contraction of the leg muscles, there will be a pooling of blood in the leg veins as they become distended three to five times their normal size. As the valves undergo progressive destruction, the distention continues, even in the presence of muscle contractions, leading to the condition of **varicose veins.**

Blood flow to all parts of the body is controlled largely by the autonomic nervous system. Under normal resting conditions, the total blood flow is distributed as follows: brain (14%), heart (4%), kidneys (22%), liver (27%), muscle (15%), bone (5%), skin (6%), and other tissues (7%). Under the stress of exercise, following a big meal, or after exposure to cold temperatures, there is a general redistribution of blood flow to those areas where it is needed most. With heavy endurance exercise, as an example, muscles receive 75 percent or more of available blood. This allows, in combination with increases in cardiac output, up to a 25 times greater flow of blood to the active muscle (see Figure 4–7 on page 68).

Arteries, arterioles, and the splanchnic (visceral or internal abdominal organs), and cutaneous (skin) veins of the systemic circulation, are richly supplied with nerves from the sympathetic nervous system. Sympathetic stimulation results in constriction of these vessels. In order to maintain adequate blood pressure under normal conditions, the blood vessels continuously receive impulses from the sympathetic nerves, maintaining the vessels in a constant state of moderate constriction.

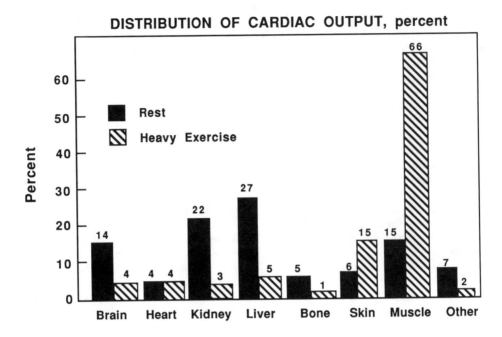

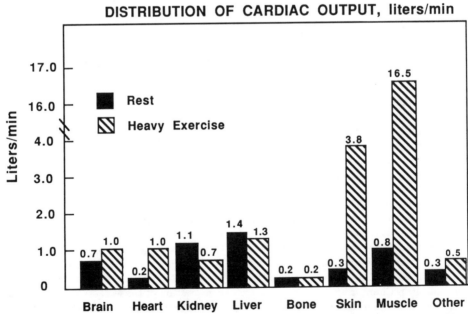

Figure 4–7   The redistribution of the cardiac output as one moves from a resting state to maximal levels of exercise.

This is referred to as **vasomotor tone.** Increasing stimulation further constricts the blood vessels in a specific area. Decreasing the intensity of stimulation below base levels allows the vessels in that immediate area to dilate. There is also a sympathetic vasodilator system in which sympathetic vasodilator fibers accompany the constrictor fibers to skeletal muscle. Activation of the vasodilator fibers results in a generalized dilation of the blood vessels in the immediate area.

When it becomes necessary to redistribute blood to areas where there is an increased need, such as the muscles during exercise, this is accomplished by a generalized sympathetic stimulation of those areas from which blood flow is to be reduced. Constriction of these vessels will divert blood flow to those areas where increased flow is needed. In contrast, to those areas needing an increased blood supply, sympathetic stimulation to the constrictor fibers is reduced, sympathetic stimulation to the vasodilator fibers is increased, the local vessels dilate, and additional blood is supplied. In the example of exercise, the metabolic waste products begin to accumulate as exercise continues, attenuating the local release of norepinephrine, which allows further dilation in the immediate area.

Regulation of body temperature is controlled in much the same way. During heavy exercise, or even at rest in a hot environment, blood is shunted to the skin through reduced sympathetic stimulation, leading to dilation of the superficial vessels supplying the skin. This promotes heat loss and allows for the maintenance of a constant body temperature. When faced with a cold environment, body heat is conserved by increasing sympathetic stimulation to the skin, thus constricting the superficial vessels and diverting blood away from the surface of the skin. The bright red color of the skin in the heat and the white color of the skin in the cold provide visual evidence of this effective shunting of blood.

The rate of blood flow through the various areas or regions of the body is controlled primarily by the arterioles. This is due to the following:

1. The arterioles control approximately 50 percent of the total resistance to blood flow in the systemic circulation.

2. The arterioles have a strong muscular wall that allows the diameter of the vessel to be altered three to five times.
3. The arterioles respond to autoregulation in addition to direct sympathetic stimulation.

Autoregulation is the ability of the vessel to self-regulate, based on the needs of the tissues which are supplied by those vessels.

Oxygen demand appears to be the single most important factor in this local self-regulation. As the tissue increases its use of available oxygen, the local vessels dilate to allow more blood, and thus more oxygen to perfuse that area. The capillary bed also has a system by which blood can be shunted away from the primary capillary network. As it enters the capillary bed, the arteriole reduces in size, becoming a metarteriole. True capillaries arise from the metarteriole, but small muscular precapillary sphincters surround the initial portion of these true capillaries. These sphincters have the ability to open and close the flow of blood into the associated capillaries, and are controlled primarily by the local tissue needs, such as a lack of oxygen. This system of control is illustrated in Figure 4–8 on page 70.

Alterations in blood pressure are largely controlled by the specific changes in arteries, arterioles, and veins. Generalized constriction of blood vessels leads to an increase in blood pressure; generalized dilation results in reduced blood pressure. **Hypertension** is the medical term for blood pressure chronically elevated above normal, healthy values. While the cause of hypertension is generally unknown in approximately 90 percent of diagnosed cases, it can be effectively controlled with appropriate medication. Diuretics and adrenergic or beta-blocking drugs are prescribed singly, or in combination, as the first line of medication. Diuretics promote urine flow by inhibiting the renal tubular reabsorption of sodium, thus reducing blood volume. Adrenergic-blocking agents act to block the beta receptors, attenuating the response to sympathetic stimulation. The exact manner in which they work to control blood pressure is not clearly understood at this time. If these are unsuccessful, the next line of medication involves the

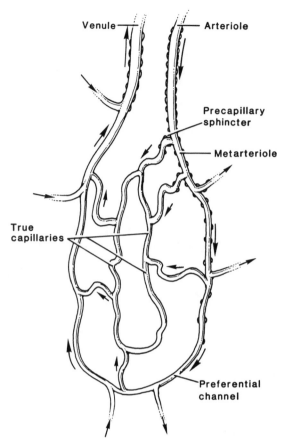

Figure 4-8 Illustration of arterioles, metarterioles, precapillary sphincters, and true capillaries.

use of direct vasodilators to achieve a reduction in blood pressure.

BLOOD

Any system of circulation must have a circulating medium. Blood and lymph serve this important function, as they are responsible for transporting various materials between the different cells or tissues of the body. The lymphatic system is extremely important to general health and coordinated physiological function, but it has little known relevance to the major focus of this book, so it will not be discussed.

Blood serves many useful purposes in the regulation of normal body function. Three functions of primary importance here are transportation, temperature regulation, and acid-base balance. With respect to the blood's transportation function, it carries nutrients and oxygen to the cell and transports carbon dioxide, lactate, and other metabolic waste products from the cell to the lungs, liver, and kidneys. The blood also transports hormones from endocrine glands, or their storage depots, to their respective target organs (that tissue or organ that reacts specifically to a particular hormone). Blood is critical in temperature regulation as it picks up heat from the core of the body, or from areas of increased metabolic activity, to deliver it throughout the body during normal environmental conditions, and to the periphery or skin when the body becomes overheated. With regard to acid-base balance, the blood has the ability to buffer, or neutralize, the acids produced with anaerobic metabolism.

The composition of blood is highly variable from one individual to the next, and can even vary considerably within the same individual over time, with alterations in plasma volume. Generally, however, the **plasma volume** constitutes approximately 55 percent of the total blood volume, with the red blood cells, white blood cells, and platelets constituting the remaining 45 percent. Approximately 90 percent of the blood plasma content is water, seven percent is comprised of blood proteins (serum albumin, serum globulin, and fibrinogen), and the remaining three percent is comprised of cellular nutrients (salts, enzymes, hormones, antibodies, and wastes). The ratio of total blood cell mass to the total blood volume is referred to as the **hematocrit,** and typically varies between 40 and 50 percent. Total blood volume varies considerably on the basis of both the size and the state of training of the individual, with larger blood volumes being associated with increased size and high levels of endurance training. Values will range from 5 to 6 liters in men and four to four and a half liters in women of average size and level of physical training. Since high levels of endurance training are typically reflected by increases in plasma volume, the resulting hematocrit could lead one to assume that the individual is anemic. Instead, there has been an expansion of the plasma volume with only

Table 4–1　Differences in total blood volume (TBV), plasma volume (PV), blood cell volume (BCV), and hematocrit (HCT) between a highly-trained athlete and an untrained individual.

Subjects	Age, yr	Ht, cm	Wt, kg	TBV ℓ	PV ℓ	BCV ℓ	HCT %
Highly-trained male athlete	25	180	80.1	7.4	4.8	2.6	35.1
Untrained male	24	178	80.8	5.6	3.2	2.4	42.9

Note: TBV = total blood volume; PV = plasma volume; BCV = blood cell volume; HCT = hematocrit [{blood cell volume ÷ total blood volume}·100]; yr = years; cm = centimeters; kg = kilograms; and ℓ = liters

a slight increase or no change in the cellular mass. Thus, the number of red blood cells is normal, or maybe even slightly above normal, but they are diluted in a much larger plasma volume. Table 4–1 and Figure 4–9 illustrate this apparent paradox, comparing two individuals of exactly the same size. The hematocrit of the endurance-trained athlete would lead one to suspect that he has a low red blood cell count, and is possibly anemic, when in fact, he has a high blood cell volume which has been diluted by a very high plasma volume.

The presence of a low hematocrit with a high plasma volume appears to have certain beneficial effects with respect to the transportation function of blood. Viscosity is that property of a fluid that resists internal flow. The more viscous a fluid, the more resistant that fluid is to flow. The viscosity of blood is normally about twice that of water. The higher the hematocrit, the greater the viscosity and the greater the resistance to flow. While an increase in red blood cells would appear to be highly desirable to increase the transportation of oxygen, this increase in red blood cells, assuming no increase in plasma volume, would greatly increase the viscosity of the blood, and restrict the flow of blood. Thus, a low hematocrit in the presence of a normal or slightly elevated number of red cells would actually facilitate the transportation of oxygen.

With respect to oxygen transport, the red blood cell plays a vital role. The red blood cell contains approximately 34 grams of hemoglobin per 100 milliliters of cells, or 15 grams per 100 milliliters of whole blood. Each gram of hemoglobin is capable of combining with 1.33 milliliters of oxygen, or 20 milliliters of oxygen per 100 milliliters of whole blood (1.3 ml/gram · 15 grams/100 ml of whole blood). **Hemoglobin** is composed of a protein (globin) and a pigment (hematin). Hematin contains iron which binds with oxygen. Hematin also has a high affinity for carbon monoxide, approximately 250 times stronger than its affinity for oxygen. For this reason, it is important not to breathe gas mixtures that contain moderate to high levels of carbon monoxide. Those who exercise out of doors are warned to avoid exercising on days when the carbon monoxide levels are high. The oxygen-carrying capacity of the blood is greatly compromised under these polluted conditions.

Red blood cells are continuously undergoing production and destruction, with the normal life span

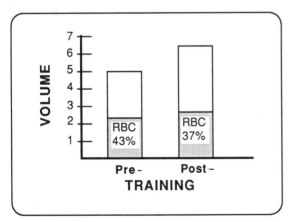

Figure 4–9　The total plasma volume increases in response to training. While the hematocrit is lowered, there is actually an increase in the number of red blood cells.

of a red blood cell approximately four months. The rate of red blood cell production in the bone marrow is approximately equal to the rate of red blood cell destruction. In **anemia,** there is a marked deficiency of either total red blood cells and/or hemoglobin in the total blood volume. Obviously, oxygen transport capabilities would be greatly limited by anemia. General weakness, chronic fatigue, and decreased performance are typical side effects or symptoms of anemia. Anemia can result from excessive blood loss, red cell destruction, or a decrease in the rate of red cell production. When donating blood, the removal of one unit, or nearly 500 milliliters, will represent approximately an eight- to ten-percent reduction in the total blood volume and in the circulating red blood cells. It will take approximately six weeks or more to reconstitute the red blood cells, while plasma volume returns to normal within 24 to 48 hours. Red blood cells can also undergo destruction during exercise. The membrane of the red blood cell appears to be disrupted by both the wear and tear associated with increased rates of circulation as well as by increased body temperature. Studies have demonstrated that the constant pounding of the bottom of the foot (shoe) during distance running can lead to increased fragility and destruction of red blood cells. Finally, a decreased rate of red blood cell production is a relatively common cause of anemia, and is most often associated with inadequate intake of iron, or the inability to assimilate sufficient iron from that taken in with the diet. This area of anemia will be discussed in much greater detail in Chapter 12.

White blood cells are represented by only one out of every 500 blood cells. White blood cells function to protect the body against invasion by disease organisms. The body is continuously exposed to bacteria, many of which could cause serious disease if they invaded the deeper tissues. The white blood cells play an extremely important function in combating any infectious agent that tries to invade the body. The white blood cells either directly destroy invading agents through the process of **phagocytosis** or form antibodies to destroy the invading agent. The adult human has approximately 7,000 white blood cells per cubic millimeter of blood, including polymorphonuclear eosinophils (2.3%), polymorphonuclear neutrophils (62.0%),

polymorphonuclear basophils (0.4%), monocytes (5.3%), and lymphocytes (30.0%). In addition, blood platelets are fragments of a sixth type of white blood cell. Platelets are small, round, or oval discs that are extremely important in the mechanisms of blood clot formation to prevent bleeding.

CARDIOVASCULAR RESPONSES TO EXERCISE

The major function of the cardiovascular system during exercise is to deliver blood to the active tissues. This includes the delivery of oxygen and nutrients and the removal of the metabolic waste products. If the exercise bout is prolonged, the cardiovascular system also assists in maintaining body temperature to prevent overheating. A series of complex interactions allows these cardiovascular adaptations to occur in a smooth and integrated manner.

Heart Rate

The heart rate (HR) is the simplest and one of the most informative of the cardiovascular parameters that can be measured. At rest, the heart beats at a rate of 60 to 80 beats/minute. This is easily determined by locating the radial (thumb-side of the wrist) or the carotid (junction of the head and neck) artery pulses, counting for 15 seconds, and multiplying the result by four [HR = (beats/15 sec) x 4]. The technique for monitoring pulse rate is illustrated in Figure 4–10. In very sedentary, unconditioned individuals, the resting heart rate can exceed 100 beats/minute, while in highly-conditioned, endurance athletes, resting heart rates in the range of 28 to 40 beats have been reported.

The lowest heart rate is found at rest in the supine position. As discussed in the introduction to this chapter, it will be elevated slightly upon sitting, and increase even further with standing. This is the result of the influence of gravity, which reduces the amount of blood returning to the heart when one shifts from a supine to an upright posture, thus reducing the stroke volume (SV). For cardiac output ($\dot{Q}$) to remain the same, the heart

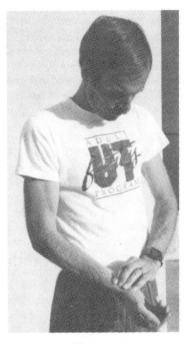 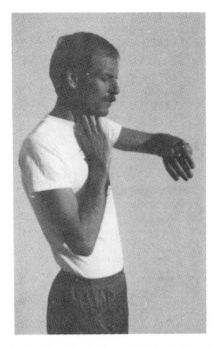

Figure 4-10 Illustration of the correct procedure for taking both the radial (wrist) and carotid (neck) pulse rate.

rate must increase, since $\dot{Q}$ = HR · SV. Resting heart rate is also influenced by age and the environment. It typically decreases with age and increases with extremes in temperature and altitude. Prior to the start of exercise, the pre-exercise heart rate will normally be increased well above normal resting values. This is referred to as an **anticipatory response** and is mediated through catecholamine secretion from both the sympathetic nervous system and the adrenal medulla. Reliable estimates of actual resting heart rate should be made only under conditions of total relaxation, such as early in the morning, prior to arising from a restful night's sleep. Pre-exercise heart rates should not be used as estimates of resting heart rate.

When exercise begins, the heart rate will increase rapidly to a rate that is directly proportional to the intensity of the exercise. This is illustrated in Figure 4-11 on page 74. In this figure, the intensity of exercise is represented by the oxygen uptake, for there is a direct linear relationship between the rate of work and the corresponding oxygen uptake. When exercise is performed on a cycle ergometer, where the rate of work can be accurately controlled and measured, the oxygen uptake for any given level of work is very predictable, varying little from one individual to another. Thus, expressing the level of work or the intensity of exercise in terms of the oxygen uptake is not only accurate, but appropriate for comparing different individuals, or the same individual under different circumstances. From Figure 4-11, it is apparent that the heart rate increases in a direct or linear manner with increases in the intensity of exercise, until near the point of exhaustion. As exhaustion is approached, there is a leveling off of the heart rate response, indicating that you are approaching your maximal value. The maximal heart rate is a highly reliable value which remains constant from day-to-day and changes only slightly from year-to-year.

Estimates of your maximal heart rate can be made on the basis of your age, as there is a slight but steady decrease in maximal heart rate with aging. This is illustrated in Figure 4-12 on page 74.

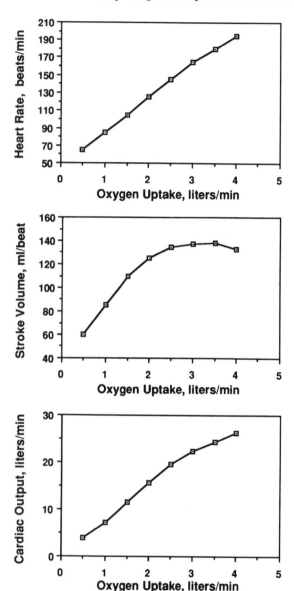

Figure 4-11 Changes in heart rate, stroke volume, and cardiac output with increasing rates of work.

Subtracting your age from the figure 220 provides an approximation of the maximal heart rate average for your particular age group. However, individual values vary considerably around this mean, or average, value. To illustrate, for a 40-year-old, maximal heart rate would be estimated 180 beats/

minute (HR max = 220 − 40 years). For all 40-year-olds, however, 68 percent of them will have actual maximal heart rate values between 168 and 192 beats/minute (mean ± 1 S.D.), and 95 percent will fall between 156 and 204 beats/minute (mean ± 2 S.D.). This example illustrates the tremendous potential for error when attempting to estimate or predict maximal heart rate for any one individual.

At submaximal levels of exercise, when the rate of work is held constant, the heart rate increases fairly rapidly until it reaches a plateau. This plateau is called the **steady state heart rate**. For each subsequent level of exercise, from very low to moderately high intensities, the heart rate will reach a steady state value within one to two minutes. However, the more intense the exercise, the longer it takes to achieve this steady state value. The concept of steady state heart rate is important as it forms the basis of several tests that have been developed to measure physical fitness. Individuals are placed on an exercise device, such as a cycle ergometer, and are exercised at two or three standardized rates of work. Those who are in better physical condition on the basis of their cardiorespiratory endurance capacity will have lower heart rates for the same level of work, thus indicating a more efficient heart. When a constant rate of exercise is performed over a prolonged period of time, particularly under heat-stress conditions, the heart rate tends to drift upward, not maintaining a steady state value. This phenomenon is referred to as **cardiovascular drift** and will be discussed later in this chapter.

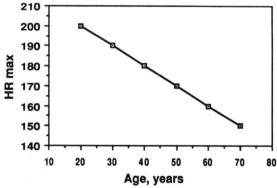

Figure 4-12 Decrease in maximal heart rate with aging.

Stroke Volume

Stroke volume, defined as the quantity of blood pumped per heart beat, is determined by four factors:

1. return of venous blood to the heart
2. ventricular distensibility
3. ventricular contractility
4. aortic or pulmonary artery pressure

The first two factors influence the filling capacity of the ventricle—how much blood is available for filling the ventricle and the ease with which the ventricle is filled at the available pressure. The last two factors influence the ability of the ventricle to empty—the force with which the blood is ejected and the pressure against which it must flow in the arteries. These factors control the alterations in stroke volume in response to increasing intensities of exercise.

Stroke volume increases with increasing rates of work, up to exercise intensities between 40 and 60 percent of maximal capacity. At this point, stroke volume appears to plateau, remaining essentially unchanged up to and including the point of exhaustion (see Figure 4–11). Recent evidence has challenged this classic concept. Data from trained athletes exercising on a treadmill suggests that the stroke volume continues to increase up to the point of exhaustion. This apparent disagreement may be the result of the type of testing device used, or the state of training of the subject population. Where studies have shown plateaus in stroke volume at intensities between 40 and 60 percent of maximal capacity, cycle ergometers have typically been used. Previous studies have shown that blood is trapped in the legs during cycle ergometer exercise, thus the plateau in stroke volume may be unique to cycle ergometer exercise, resulting from a decreasing return of blood from the lower extremities. It is also possible that the more highly-trained athlete can continue to increase stroke volume above this 40 to 60 percent of maximal level—a possible adaptation to training. In the upright position, stroke volume approximately doubles from resting to maximal values—from 60 to 120 ml in the untrained and from 110 to 200 ml in the highly endurance-trained individual. During supine exercise, such as swimming, stroke volume can increase from 20 to 40 percent above resting values. Table 4–2 illustrates the expected changes in heart rate (HR), stroke volume (SV) and cardiac output ($\dot{Q}$) at rest, during steady state submaximal exercise, and at maximal levels of exercise in the activities of running, cycling, and swimming.

When the body shifts from a reclining to a standing position, there is an immediate drop in stroke volume and a compensatory increase in the heart rate to maintain a constant cardiac output. This decrease in stroke volume is due primarily to a pooling of the blood in the legs, which reduces the volume of blood returning to the heart. This pooling of blood in the lower extremities is the result of what has been termed the **hydrostatic pressure effect.** Gravity exerts a dramatic effect on any fluid column. The pressure of the fluid in the

Table 4–2 Changes in heart rate (HR), stroke volume (SV), and cardiac output ($\dot{Q}$) from rest to maximal levels of exercise when running, cycling, and swimming.

Activity	*Condition*	*HR* beats/min	*SV* ml/beat	$\dot{Q}$ liters/min
Running	Resting	60	70	4.2
	Max Exercise	190	130	24.7
Cycling	Resting	60	70	4.2
	Max Exercise	180	120	21.6
Swimming	Resting*	55	95	5.2
	Max Exercise	170	120	20.4

*Measurements taken in the supine position

column is a direct result of where that pressure is measured, with the pressure being essentially zero at the top of the column and reaching its highest value at the bottom of the column. In the standing position, the blood pressure is highest at the level of the feet and lowest at the level of the head. This increased pressure in the lower extremities presents a barrier to the return of blood to the heart, resulting in the pooling of blood in the legs and a reduced stroke volume. In the supine position, blood does not pool in the lower extremities. Thus, the increase in stroke volume in response to maximal levels of exercise in the supine position is not as great, since resting stroke volume values are much higher in the supine position. Of particular interest, the highest stroke volume attainable in upright exercise is only slightly greater than the resting value observed in the supine position. Thus, the increases seen in stroke volume during low to moderate levels of work appear to be only compensating for or overcoming the hydrostatic pressure effect.

Resting stroke volume varies from 60 to 100 ml at rest and can increase to values in excess of 200 ml. The actual values will depend, however, almost entirely on both the size and state of conditioning of the individual, with the larger, better-trained person having the higher values. Also, it has been speculated that stroke volume may, in fact, decrease at very high heart rates, 180 beats/minute or higher, since the time available to fill the ventricle is greatly reduced. There is, however, little scientific evidence for this theory since it is difficult to obtain accurate estimates of stroke volume at maximal levels of exercise.

Cardiac Output

Cardiac output, the product of both heart rate and stroke volume, follows a rather predictable course with increasing levels of work (see Figure 4-11). From a resting value of approximately 5.0 liters/minute, the cardiac output increases as a direct function of the level or intensity of the exercise to a maximal value of 20 to 40 liters/minute, or higher, with the absolute value again reflecting the individual's size and state of conditioning. During the initial stages of exercise, the increased cardiac output is due to an increase in both heart rate and

stroke volume. As the level of exercise exceeds 50 to 60 percent of the individual's capacity, further increases are theoretically the result of increases in heart rate, since stroke volume is presumed to have plateaued.

Blood Flow

Blood flow patterns change rather markedly as the individual moves from rest to exercise. Blood is redirected away from areas where it is not essential, to those areas that are active during the exercise bout. Only 15 to 20 percent of the resting cardiac output goes to muscle, while in exhaustive exercise, the muscles receive 80 to 85 percent of the cardiac output. This shift in blood flow to the muscles is accomplished primarily by a decrease in blood flow to the kidneys, liver, stomach, and intestines, as was demonstrated in Figure 4-7. As the body starts to overheat, either as a direct result of the exercise, or because of high environmental temperatures, an increasing amount of blood is redirected to the skin for the specific purpose of conducting heat away from the body core to its periphery, where the heat is transferred to the environment not only by sweat, but by conduction and convection. This increase in skin blood flow reduces the amount of blood available to supply the muscles, and explains why most athletic performances in the heat are well below average.

An additional problem with prolonged exercise or exercise in the heat, is a reduction in blood volume due to a loss of water in the form of sweat, and a generalized shifting of fluid out of the blood into the tissues, a condition referred to as **edema.** With the total blood volume gradually decreasing as the duration of exercise increases, and with a shunting of more blood to the periphery for cooling, the cardiac filling pressure is reduced, leading to a decreased venous return to the right side of the heart. This leads to a reduction in stroke volume and a compensatory increase in heart rate to maintain stroke volume. These alterations, described earlier in this chapter as cardiovascular drift, allow the continuation of exercise at low to moderate intensities. However, the body is unable to fully compensate for the decreased stroke volume at high intensities as heart rate attains its peak value at a much lower exercise intensity, limiting maximal performance capabilities.

The shift in blood flow from inactive to active tissues during exercise is the result of constriction of vessels in the inactive areas and dilation of vessels in the active areas. These changes in vascular tone are controlled through the autonomic nervous system and through the local effects of increased metabolism at the site of muscular contraction. Increased metabolism causes an increase in the acidity, CO_2, and temperature of the local tissue, and this can have a direct effect on dilating the local arterioles and increasing blood flow through the local capillaries. This local regulation is referred to as **autoregulation.** Local regulation is also affected by low partial pressure of oxygen in the tissue (pO_2), muscle contraction directly, and possibly other vasoactive substances released as a result of muscle contraction.

Blood Pressure

Systolic blood pressure increases in direct proportion to increases in exercise intensity, with values ranging from approximately 120 mmHg at rest to 200 mmHg or greater at the point of exhaustion. Systolic pressures of 240 to 250 mmHg have been reported in healthy, highly-trained athletes at maximal levels of exercise. This increase in systolic blood pressure is a direct reflection of the increase in cardiac output ($\dot{Q}$) with increasing rates of work, without an equivalent decrease in total peripheral resistance (TPR), $P = \dot{Q} \cdot TPR$. Diastolic blood pressure changes little, if any, during exercise, irrespective of the intensity. In fact, increases in diastolic pressure of 10 mmHg or more are considered to be abnormal responses to exercise and are considered as one of several criteria for stopping the exercise test prematurely. Figure 4–13 illustrates a typical blood pressure response to increasing rates of work.

The Blood

The oxygen content of blood at rest varies from 20 ml of oxygen for every 100 ml of arterial blood to 14 ml of oxygen for every 100 ml of venous blood. The difference between these two values, 20 ml − 14 ml = 6 ml, is referred to as the **arterial-venous**

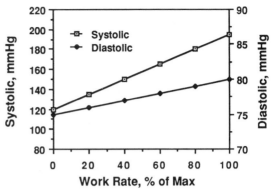

Figure 4–13   Blood pressure response to exercise.

oxygen difference (a - $\bar{v}$ O_2 diff), and reflects the extent to which oxygen is extracted or removed from the blood as it passes through the body. With exercise, there is a progressive increase in the a-$\bar{v}$ O_2 diff, reflecting a decreasing venous oxygen content, with the arterial oxygen content remaining essentially unchanged. There have been reports of a decreased arterial oxygen content in highly-trained athletes at maximal levels of exercise. The venous oxygen content drops to values approaching zero in the active muscles, but the mixed venous blood in the right atrium of the heart rarely drops below 2 ml per 100 ml of blood, since the blood returning from the active tissues is mixed with blood from inactive areas as it returns to the heart. The a-$\bar{v}$ O_2 diff can increase approximately threefold from rest to maximal levels of exercise.

The composition of the blood changes as the individual moves from resting to an exercising state. The red blood cell may actually undergo a decrease in size as exercise continues for a prolonged period of time with substantial losses in body fluid. Proteins may also be lost from the plasma volume, although the results of studies investigating this area are not in agreement.

There is a substantial fluid loss in prolonged exercise due to sweating which leads to a reduction in plasma volume. This results in a **hemoconcentration** of red blood cells and plasma proteins. Since the fluid portion of the blood volume is reduced, the cellular and protein portions represent

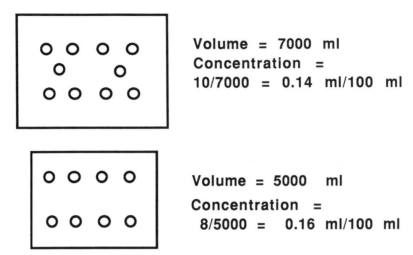

Volume = 7000 ml
Concentration =
10/7000 = 0.14 ml/100 ml

Volume = 5000 ml
Concentration =
8/5000 = 0.16 ml/100 ml

Figure 4-14 Any substance in the blood will appear in a higher concentration as plasma volume decreases.

a larger fraction of the total blood volume (see Figure 4-14). This hemoconcentration results in a substantial rise of up to 20 to 25 percent in the red blood cell concentration. At one time it was thought that red blood cells were added to the circulation to facilitate oxygen transport. Many animals have the capacity to increase the actual number of circulating red blood cells by dumping out red blood cells stored in their spleen. The spleen does not serve this function in the human. It is now recognized that the plasma volume is reduced with fluid loss causing an increase in the relative number of red blood cells, not in the absolute number. Plasma volume loss is a result of a shift of fluid from the plasma to the interstitial fluid—the fluid between the cells.

As the length of the exercise period increases, body fluid changes and temperature regulation become important to the efficient performance of the athlete. In activities lasting several minutes or less, body fluid changes and temperature regulation are of little or no practical importance. For the football player or the marathon runner, however, these processes are critically important, even to the point of being necessary for survival. Deaths have occurred during or following various sport activities as a result of dehydration and hyperthermia.

With the onset of exercise, there is an almost immediate loss of the non-protein fluid from the plasma volume to the interstitial and intracellular fluid spaces, which is probably the result of increased hydrostatic pressure within the vascular system. The increase in blood pressure forces water from the vascular compartment to the nonvascular compartment. A 10 to 20 percent or greater reduction in plasma volume can occur with prolonged work. If the exercise intensity or the environmental conditions promote sweating, additional fluid loss can be expected from the plasma volume, although the major source of fluid for sweating is from the interstitial and intracellular spaces. This reduction in plasma volume is likely to be detrimental to performance. For longer-duration activities, in which heat loss is a problem, an increasingly higher percentage of blood must be diverted to the skin to reduce body heat. Reduced plasma volume will also result in an increased viscosity of the blood as a result of the hemoconcentration of the red blood cells. An increased blood viscosity can limit the oxygen transporting capacity of the blood.

As sweating continues, there will be a loss of interstitial and intracellular fluid. This will create an increased osmotic pressure (a higher concentration of solids) in the interstitial fluid, causing even more fluid from the plasma volume to diffuse into the interstitial space. Although intracellular fluid volume is impossible to measure directly and, therefore, accurately, research suggests that there is also fluid loss from the intracellular fluid and even from the red blood cells, which may shrink.

Finally, the blood pH can experience considerable change with moderate to high intensity exercise. At rest, the blood pH remains constant at a value slightly below 7.4. A pH of 7.0 is considered neutral, greater than 7.0 is alkaline or basic, and less than 7.0 is acidic (see Chapter 3). Thus, normal blood at rest is slightly alkaline. There is little change in blood pH from rest up to an intensity of about 50 percent of maximal aerobic capacity. As the intensity increases above 50 percent, the pH starts to decrease, the blood becoming more acidic. This drop will be gradual at first, but it will become more rapid as the individual approaches exhaustion. Blood pH values of 7.0 or lower have been reported following maximal exercise. Tissue pH reaches levels even lower than 6.5. The lowering of the blood pH is primarily the result of an increased reliance on anaerobic metabolism and corresponds to the increases in blood lactate observed with increasing intensity of exercise.

SUMMARY

During exercise, the cardiovascular system's major responsibilities include supplying all parts of the body with necessary oxygen and nutrients, removing metabolic waste products, maintaining an appropriate pH, and serving as the body's cooling system for the regulation of body temperature. The heart, blood vessels, and the blood comprise the essential components of the cardiovascular system. The heart is a four-chambered organ that serves as the primary pump for circulating blood throughout the entire cardiovascular system. Blood returning to the heart from all parts of the body enters the right side of the heart into the right atrium, to the right ventricle, and then out into the pulmonary circulation where the blood becomes oxygenated. It returns to the left side of the heart into the left atrium, to the left ventricle, and then is pumped into the systemic circulation of the body.

The heart muscle is striated like skeletal muscle, but it has the unique ability to contract rhythmically on its own without neural or hormonal stimulation, and the fibers contract synchronously as two units, the atria and the ventricles. Heart rate is controlled by both parasympathetic (decreasing) and sympathetic (increasing) nervous activity, and hormonal activity. Rates can vary from a low of 30 to 40 beats/minute in the highly-trained endurance athlete at rest, to over 200 beats/minute during maximal levels of exercise. As the intensity of the exercise increases, the heart rate and stroke volume increase proportionally, although stroke volume theoretically reaches its peak value at approximately 40 to 60 percent of capacity. Increases in heart rate and stroke volume result in large increases in cardiac output, allowing an increased blood flow to the active muscle mass. This ability of the heart rate to increase by a factor of four to five, coupled with the ability of the stroke volume to double from rest to exercise, allows the cardiac output to increase by a factor of eight to ten. Combining this with the ability of the vascular system to redirect the majority of the cardiac output to the active muscle enables local muscle blood flow to increase up to 25-fold.

The arterial-venous oxygen difference widens with increasing exercise intensity, indicating a greater extraction of oxygen at the tissue level. Plasma volume is reduced and the blood becomes hemoconcentrated. Blood pH decreases after exercise exceeds 50 percent of the individual's capacity, a change that is related to the appearance of lactate in the blood. As exercise is prolonged, plasma volume may decrease from 10 to 20 percent or more as sweating reduces both plasma volume and interstitial fluid. The body depends on convection, radiation, conduction, and evaporation for heat loss to maintain the body's core temperature. With a relative high intensity of exercise, or with exercise in hot and/or humid environments, the body begins to rely almost exclusively on evaporation for heat loss. Thus, adequate fluid replacement during the activity is essential for both fluid balance and temperature regulation.

STUDY QUESTIONS

1. What events take place that allow the heart to contract? How is heart rate controlled?
2. Describe the structure of the heart, the pattern of blood flow through the valves and chambers of the heart, and how the heart as a muscle is supplied with blood. What happens when the resting heart must suddenly supply an exercising body?
3. What is the difference between systole and diastole, and how does this relate to systolic blood pressure and diastolic blood pressure?
4. What are inotropic and chronotropic factors with respect to the control of cardiac output with increasing rates of work?
5. How is blood flow to the various regions of the body controlled? How does this vary with exercise?
6. Describe the primary functions of blood.
7. Describe two important mechanisms for returning blood back to the heart when you are exercising in an upright position.
8. What are the major determinants of maximal heart rate and maximal stroke volume?
9. Describe how heart rate, stroke volume, and cardiac output respond to increasing rates of work.
10. What changes occur in plasma volume with increasing levels of exercise? With prolonged exercise in the heat?
11. What is anemia? What are its causes? How might this affect athletic performance?
12. How do you determine your maximal heart rate? What are alternative methods using indirect estimates? What are the major limitations to indirect estimates?
13. What is cardiovascular drift? Why might this be a problem with prolonged exercise?
14. What are the major cardiovascular adjustments made by your body when you are overheated during exercise?

REFERENCES

Åstrand, P. O., & Rodahl, K. (1986). *Textbook of work physiology* (3rd ed.). New York: McGraw-Hill Book Co.

Åstrand, P. O., Cuddy, T. E., Saltin, B., & Stenberg, J. (1964). Cardiac output during submaximal and maximal work. *Journal of Applied Physiology, 19,* 268–274.

Brooks, G. A., & Fahey, T. D. (1984). *Exercise physiology: Human bioenergetics and its applications.* New York: John Wiley & Sons.

Carlsten, A., & Grimby, G. *The circulatory response to muscular exercise in man* (1966). Springfield, IL: Charles C. Thomas.

Clausen, J. P. (1977). Effect of physical training on cardiovascular adjustments to exercise in man. *Physiological Reviews, 57,* 779–815.

Costill, D. L., Branam, G., Eddy, D., & Fink, W. (1974). Alterations in red cell volume following exercise and dehydration. *Journal of Applied Physiology, 37,* 912–916.

Costill, D. L., & Fink, W. (1974). Plasma volume changes following exercise and thermal dehydration. *Journal of Applied Physiology, 37,* 521–525.

Dowell, R. T. (1983). Cardiac adaptations to exercise. *Exercise and Sport Sciences Reviews, 11,* 99–117.

Edington, D. W., & Edgerton, V. R. (1976). *The biology of physical activity.* Boston: Houghton Mifflin Company.

Ekblom, B., & Hermansen, L. (1968). Cardiac output in athletes. *Journal of Applied Physiology, 25,* 619–625.

Fox, E. L. & Mathews, D. K. (1981). *The physiological basis of physical education and athletics* (3rd ed.). Philadelphia: Saunders College Publishing.

Guyton, A. C. (1986). *Textbook of medical physiology* (7th ed.). Philadelphia: W. B. Saunders Company.

Hammand, H. K., & Froelicher, V. F. (1985). Normal and abnormal heart rate response to exercise. *Progress in Cardiovascular Diseases, 27,* 271–296.

Hermansen, L., Ekblom, B., & Saltin, B. (1970). Cardiac output during submaximal and maximal treadmill and bicycle exercise. *Journal of Applied Physiology, 29,* 82–86.

Hossack, K. F., Kusumi, F., & Bruce, R. A. (1981). Approximate normal standards of maximal cardiac output during upright exercise in women. *American Journal of Cardiology, 47,* 1080–1086.

Laughlin, M. H., & Armstrong, R. B. (1985). Muscle blood flow during locomotory exercise. *Exercise and Sport Sciences Reviews, 13,* 95–136.

McArdle, W. D., Katch, F. I., & Katch, V. L. (1986). *Exercise physiology: Energy, nutrition, and human performance* (2nd ed.). Philadelphia: Lea & Febiger.

Miyamura, M., & Honda, Y. (1973). Maximum cardiac output related to sex and age. *Japanese Journal of Physiology, 23,* 645–656.

Poliner, L. R., Dehmer, G. J., Lewis, S. E., Parkey, R. W., Blomqvist, C. G., & Willerson, J. T. (1980). Left ventricular performance in normal subjects: A comparison of the responses to exercise in the upright and supine positions. *Circulation, 62,* 528–534.

Rowell, L. B. (1974). Human cardiovascular adjustments to exercise and thermal stress. *Physiological Reviews, 54,* 75–159.

Rowell, L. B. (1986). *Human circulation regulation during physical stress.* New York: Oxford University Press.

Saltin, B. (1985). Hemodynamic adaptations to exercise. *American Journal of Cardiology, 55,* 42D–47D.

Saltin, B., & Rowell, L. B. (1980). Functional adaptations to physical activity and inactivity. *Federation Proceedings, 39,* 1506–1513.

Senay, L. C., Jr., & Pivarnik, J. M. (1985). Fluid shifts during exercise. *Exercise and Sport Sciences Reviews, 13,* 335–387.

Shepherd, J. T. (1982). Reflex control of arterial blood pressure. *Cardiovascular Research, 16,* 357–383.

Shepherd, J. T., & Vanhoutte, P. M. (1979). *The human cardiovascular system: Facts and concepts.* New York: Raven Press.

Smith, E. E., Guyton, A. C., Manning, R. D., & White, R. J. (1976). Integrated mechanisms of cardiovascular response and control during exercise in the normal human. *Progress in Cardiovascular Diseases, 18,* 421–443.

Steingart, R. M., Wexler, J., Slagle, S., & Scheuer, J. (1984). Radionuclide ventriculographic responses to graded supine and upright exercise: Critical role of the Frank-Starling mechanism at submaximal exercise. *American Journal of Cardiology, 53,* 1671–1677.

Stone, H. L., Dormer, K. J., Foreman, R. D., Thies, R., & Blair, R. W. (1985). Neural regulation of the cardiovascular system during exercise. *Federation Proceedings, 44,* 2271–2278.

Vander, A. J., Sherman, J. H., & Luciano, D. S. (1980). *Human physiology: The mechanisms of body function* (3rd ed.). New York: McGraw-Hill Book Company.

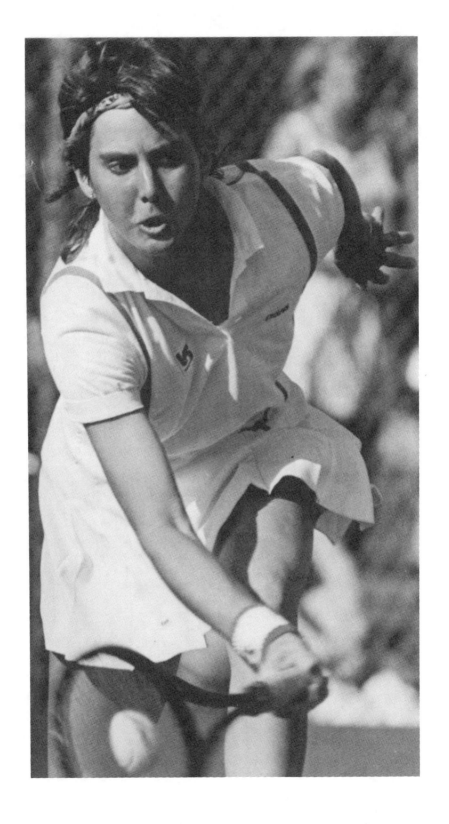

5

Neural Control of Physical Activity

INTRODUCTION

The various physiological functions of the body discussed in the previous four chapters are regulated by two major control systems, the nervous system and the endocrine system. The nervous system is able to exert its control in fractions of a second, and its effect is relatively short-lived. The endocrine system takes much longer to initiate change, from several seconds to days, months, or even years, and its effect is relatively long-lived. The two systems are intricately interrelated. This chapter provides an overview as to how the human body is able to efficiently integrate its various physiological systems through neural control. This discussion will be limited to those specific aspects of neural control that directly relate to the performance of sport and activity. Hormonal control will be the topic of the next chapter (Chapter 6).

The muscular system provides the force that causes movement of the skeletal system. The nervous system acts to initiate this movement. Just as the skeleton is motionless without the force production of the supporting muscles, the muscle is unable to move without activation by the nervous system. The nervous system is probably the most complex of the body's systems. The master control center is located in the brain, although simple movement patterns that originate from reflexes, such as the "knee-jerk" reflex, do not depend on the brain for initiating or controlling the resulting movement. In addition to the brain, intricate networks of nerve cells emanate to all parts of the body from the brain and spinal cord, providing intricate instructions to the target areas. Other nerve cells originate in such areas as vessels, organs, muscles, and skin, and end in the spinal cord or brain, where they continuously convey information regarding the body's physical status.

The nervous system can be divided into its various components according to the following classification:

A. Central Nervous System
   1. Brain
   2. Spinal Cord
B. Peripheral Nervous System
   1. Afferent Division
   2. Efferent Division
      a. Somatic nervous system
      b. Autonomic nervous system
         1) Sympathetic division
         2) Parasympathetic division

Anatomically, the nervous system has a central and a peripheral component. The **central nervous system** is comprised of the brain and the spinal cord, while the **peripheral nervous system** consists of the nerves, which have the brain and spinal cord as either their origin or destination. Prior to discussing in some detail the central and peripheral nervous systems, it is first appropriate to focus on the basic functional unit of the nervous system, the nerve cell or **neuron.**

THE NEURON

A typical neuron is composed of three parts: the **soma** or cell body of the neuron, the **dendrites,** and the **axon.** A motor neuron and its attachment to a muscle fiber are illustrated in Figure 5-1. A nerve impulse can be transmitted only in one direction.

It proceeds from the dendrite to the cell body and then out along the axon to either the end organ, such as a muscle fiber, or to another neuron. Each neuron contains many dendrites which function to transmit impulses from adjacent neurons to the cell body for that neuron. There is, however, only one axon for each neuron, and the impulses travel from the cell body along the length of the axon to the point where it branches into many terminal fibrils.

The small terminal fibrils from the axon of a single motor neuron either connect to a muscle fiber, forming a **neuromuscular junction,** or to adjacent neurons forming a **synapse.** The neuromuscular junction is composed of the terminal fibrils of the neuron, which end in sole feet, and the muscle fiber, which is invaginated at that point forming a cavity to accommodate the sole feet of the terminal fibrils. The cavity is referred to as a **synaptic**

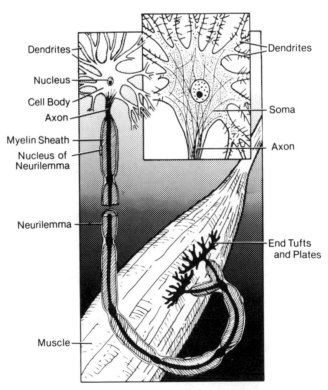

Figure 5-1   The motor neuron and its connection with a muscle fiber.

gutter, and the small space between the sole feet and the muscle fiber is referred to as the **synaptic cleft.** When one neuron connects with an adjacent neuron to form a synapse, the terminal fibrils end in synaptic knobs, which lie on the surface of the cell body and the dendrites of the adjacent neuron. The synapse is the actual junction between each synaptic knob and the adjacent dendrite or soma. Branches on terminal fibrils from many different axons of other neurons can all converge on the dendrites and cell body of a single neuron.

There are two basic types of synapses, electrical and chemical. Almost all synapses used for signal transmission in the central nervous system are of the chemical type. Once a single neuron is stimulated, the impulse is transmitted the length of that neuron to the terminal fibrils. Once the impulse reaches the synaptic knobs or sole feet a chemical substance, referred to as a **neurotransmitter,** transmits the impulse across the synaptic cleft to the muscle fiber, dendrites, or soma of the adjacent neuron. When this transmission occurs between adjacent neurons, the neurotransmitter can either excite or inhibit the adjacent neuron, or modify its sensitivity. Over 30 different transmitter substances have been identified and categorized into four basic classes:

Class I—Acetylcholine
Class II—The Amine
        (norepinephrine, epinephrine,
        dopamine, and serotonin)
Class III—Amino Acids
Class IV—Peptides

Acetylcholine is the major neurotransmitter for the motor neurons of the skeletal muscle system, for the postganglionic neurons of the parasympathetic nervous system, and for some of the postganglionic neurons of the sympathetic nervous system. Norepinephrine is the major neurotransmitter for most of the postganglionic neurons of the sympathetic nervous system.

The cell membrane of the neuron has a resting electrical potential of −70 millivolts (mV). This negative charge results from the fact that the cell membrane has a higher concentration of potassium ions on the inside, a higher concentration of sodium ions on the outside, and a greater permeability to potassium ions than to sodium ions. Further, there is an active transport of sodium ions out of the cell and potassium ions into the cell by a sodium-potassium pump.

When a neural impulse reaches the dendrites, or soma, of the neuron, the impulse is propagated along the length of the neuron through the process of depolarization. The impulse is referred to as an **action potential.** During an action potential, the permeability of the membrane to sodium and potassium ions is markedly altered. Initially, the membrane permeability to sodium ions undergoes an increase by several hundredfold and sodium ions rush into the cell. During this initial phase, more sodium ions are entering the cell than potassium ions leaving the cell, and the inside of the cell membrane becomes positively charged in comparison to the outside, for instance, from a −70 mV to a +30 mV. This is immediately followed by a period in which sodium permeability is reduced and there is an increase in potassium permeability, which quickly brings the cell membrane back to its original resting charge of −70 mV.

The actual number of ions that cross the membrane during an action potential are surprisingly small, and the sodium-potassium pumps maintain the proper balance of sodium and potassium inside and outside the cell. The action potential lasts only about one thousandth of one second (one millisecond) and will occur only when the membrane is depolarized to the point where the entry of sodium exceeds the departure of potassium. Further, there is a period of time immediately following an action potential where the membrane is unable to respond to a second stimulus. This is referred to as the **absolute refractory period.** The absolute refractory period is followed by a period of time during which only a stimulus well above the normal threshold level will elicit an action potential. This is referred to as the **relative refractory period.** The absolute and relative refractory periods represent those periods of time where the membrane is returning to its original resting state with respect to sodium and potassium permeability.

There are several additional aspects of neural impulse transmission that are important to understand. Referring back to Figure 5-1, the axon of most neurons is covered with a **myelin sheath.** Myelin, a fatty substance, acts to insulate the cell

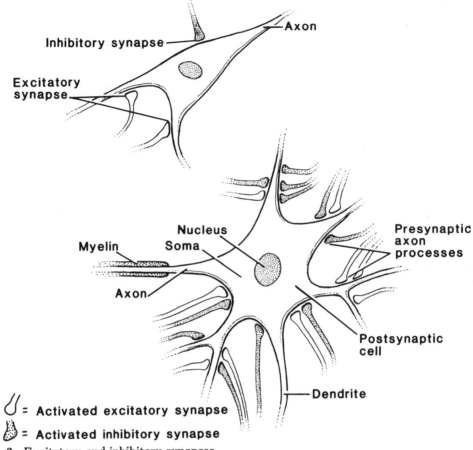

Inhibitory synapse

Excitatory synapse

Axon

Nucleus

Myelin

Soma

Axon

Presynaptic axon processes

Postsynaptic cell

Dendrite

⟨ = Activated excitatory synapse

⟨ = Activated inhibitory synapse

Figure 5-2   Excitatory and inhibitory synapses.

membrane, reducing the flow of current between fluid compartments. As shown in this figure, the myelin sheath is not continuous as it courses the length of the axon, but exhibits periodic breaks or interruptions. These interruptions are referred to as **nodes of Ranvier**. The action potential appears to jump from one node to the next as it traverses along a myelinated fiber. This is referred to as **saltatory conduction**, and results in a much faster rate of conduction. Further, the velocity of nerve impulses is determined by the size of the neuron. The larger the fiber diameter, the faster the velocity of conduction since the larger fiber offers less resistance to the flow of local current. The velocity of nerve impulse transmission in large myelinated fibers can approach 120 meters/second or 250 miles/hour, where nonmyelinated fibers of the same size conduct impulses at only ¹⁄₁₀th of that velocity.

Finally, once an impulse has traversed the length of the neuron, it has the potential to be either excitatory or inhibitory to the adjacent neuron, depending on how it was originally programmed (see Figure 5-2). The excitatory or inhibitory nature of a specific impulse is determined by the interaction of the neurotransmitter and the postsynaptic cell of the adjacent neuron. Further, the triggering of an action potential at the adjacent neuron is dependent on the combined effects of all of the synapses activated, as a single excitatory synaptic

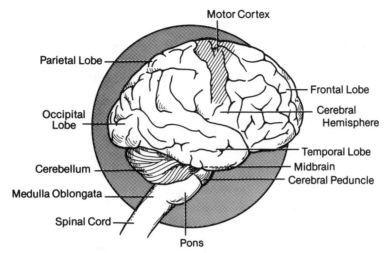

Figure 5-3 The brain and its functional areas.

event is not sufficient to elicit a threshold stimulus. Thus, a number of action potentials converging from different neurons to one specific neuron will be necessary to initiate an action potential, providing the excitatory impulses predominate.

THE CENTRAL NERVOUS SYSTEM

The brain and its various functional areas are illustrated in Figure 5-3. Information coming into the brain from various regions of the body is transmitted by the **afferent** or **sensory division** of the peripheral nervous system. The sensory division conducts impulses from the various sensory organs or receptors to the brain by **afferent** or **sensory nerves**. Vision, hearing, touch, smell, pressure, and pain illustrate some of the various sources of sensory information that allow the brain to be aware of its immediate surrounding environment.

Once the brain has processed the information it receives through the sensory nerves, a decision is made, and the action is initiated by impulses traveling from the brain to that area of the body where movement is to occur. The brain transmits information out to various regions of the body through the **efferent** or **motor division** of the peripheral nervous system. The motor division controls the contraction of skeletal muscle, the con-

traction of smooth muscle in hollow organs and tubes, for example the stomach and blood vessels, and the secretion of the exocrine and endocrine glands. Skeletal muscles are controlled by impulses conducted by **efferent** or **motor nerves** originating from any one of three levels—the motor area of the cerebral cortex, the basal regions of the brain, and the spinal cord. As the level of control moves from the spinal cord to the **motor cortex**, the degree of movement complexity increases from simple reflex control to complicated movements requiring basic thought processes.

The Brain

The brain is composed of six subdivisions—the cerebrum, the diencephalon, the mesencephalon or midbrain, the pons, the medulla, and the cerebellum. The **brainstem** is the stalk of the brain through which all sensory and motor nerves pass as they relay information between the brain and the spinal cord. It is comprised of the midbrain, pons, and medulla. A specialized collection of neurons running the entire length of the brainstem is referred to as the **reticular formation**. The neurons comprising the reticular formation are affected by yet influence nearly all areas of the central nervous system. The reticular formation helps to coordinate skeletal muscle function, contains primary cardiovascular and respiratory control centers, and determines our state of consciousness through three neuronal systems, one causing arousal and two causing sleep.

The **cerebellum** is critical to the control of rapid and complex muscular activities. It helps coordinate the motor activities by monitoring and making corrective adjustments in the motor activities elicited by other parts of the brain. It is thought to act as an integration system, comparing the programmed or intended activity with the actual changes occurring in the body, and then initiating corrective adjustments through the motor system.

The **forebrain** consists of the central core (the **diencephalon**) and the cerebral hemispheres, which together are referred to as the **cerebrum**. The right and left cerebral hemispheres are connected to each other by fiber bundles referred to as the **corpus callosum**. The **cerebral cortex** forms the outer portion of the cerebral hemispheres and has been referred to as the site of the mind and intellect. It is also referred to as the gray matter, which simply reflects the distinctive color of the many cell bodies located in this area. The cortex is comprised of four lobes, the frontal, temporal, parietal and occipital, as illustrated in Figure 5–3. The frontal lobe is associated with general intellect and motor control, the temporal lobe is associated with auditory (hearing) sensory input and its interpretation, the parietal lobe is associated with general sensory input and its interpretation, and the occipital lobe is associated with visual input and its interpretation. The diencephalon contains the **thalamus**, which is an important integration center for all sensory input, except smell. The **hypothalamus**, which lies directly below the thalamus, is responsible for the integration of most of the activity that controls the body's internal environment. Centers for the regulation of body temperature, heart rate and blood pressure, fluid balance, neuroendocrine control, emotions, thirst, and the control of food intake are believed to be located within the hypothalamus.

The Spinal Cord

The **spinal cord** is composed of tracts of nerve fibers which allow the flow of signals from the sensory receptors to the upper levels of the spinal cord and to the brain, as well as from the brain and upper spinal cord to the motor end-organs. It is encased within the vertebral canal, which provides protection and support. Small notches on the pedicles of each vertebra form the intervertebral foramen, through which spinal nerves pass. Sensory, or afferent, fibers combine to form the **dorsal roots** and enter the spinal cord on the dorsal or back side. Their cell bodies form the **dorsal root ganglia** just prior to entering the spinal cord. Motor, or efferent, fibers leave the spinal cord via the **ventral roots**.

THE PERIPHERAL NERVOUS SYSTEM

The **peripheral nervous system** is comprised of the afferent, or sensory, division and the efferent, or motor, division. The autonomic nervous system, which is technically a part of the efferent division, will be discussed separately.

Sensory Division

The sensory division of the nervous system receives information concerning the body from four primary sources—exteroceptive sensors, proprioceptive sensors, visceral sensors, and the special senses. **Exteroceptive sensations** are those that arise from the skin, including touch, pressure, heat, cold, and pain. **Proprioceptive sensations** arise from special sensory organs that sense muscle tension, tendon tension, joint angle, and deep pressure. **Visceral sensations** are received from the internal organs, and include the sensations of pain, fullness, and heat. The **special senses** include vision, hearing, taste, and smell.

Sensations are detected by special nerve endings in the skin, muscles, tendons, or deeper areas of the body. The impulses are transmitted via the sensory nerves to the spinal cord, at which point they can form a local reflex at that level of the spinal cord, or they can travel up to the upper regions of the spinal cord and brain. Sensory pathways to the brain terminate either in the sensory areas of the brain stem, the cerebellum, the thalamus, or the cerebral cortex. Impulses that terminate in the spinal cord initiate cord reflexes. As an example, if one was to accidentally touch a hot stove, his or her hand would be withdrawn quickly to avoid further pain and discomfort—a reaction that would not require conscious effort. In this example, the sensory impulses from heat and pain traveled to the spinal cord, terminated at that level of entry, connected with a motor nerve, which then activated the muscles necessary to withdraw the individual's hand.

Sensory signals that terminate in the lower brain stem result in subconscious motor reactions of a higher and more complex nature than those resulting in simple spinal-cord reflexes. Postural control would be an example of this level of sensory input. Sensory signals that terminate at the level of the cerebellum also result in subconscious control of movement. This appears to be the center of coordination, smoothing out movements by coordinating the actions of the various muscle groups that are contracting to perform the desired movement. Both fine and gross motor movements appear to be coordinated by the cerebellum. Without the control exerted by the cerebellum, all movement would be uncontrolled and obviously uncoordinated. Sensory signals that terminate at the thalamus begin to enter the level of consciousness, and you begin to distinguish between the various types of sensation. Only when the sensory signals enter the cortex is one able to discreetly localize the nature of the signal.

Sensory receptors are basically of two types— **free nerve endings** and **special end-organs.** Free nerve endings detect the sensations of crude touch, pressure, pain, heat, and cold. Special end-organs are of several types and have several different functions. Each type of end-organ is sensitive to a specific stimulus. The end-organs of most significance to human movement are the proprioceptive receptors. The joint kinesthetic receptor is located in the joint capsule, and is sensitive to joint angles and rates of change in joint angles. **Muscle spindles** and **Golgi tendon organs** are specialized receptors that provide information on the status of muscle. Muscle spindles provide information regarding the degree to which a muscle is stretched, and Golgi tendon organs detect the resulting tension applied to the tendon, providing information relative to the strength of muscle contraction.

Motor Division

Once a sensory impulse is received, this typically evokes a response through a motor neuron, irrespective of the level at which the sensory impulse stops. In a simple reflex, such as the example used earlier of touching a hot stove, the sensory receptors detect heat and pain and transmit this information by impulses to the spinal cord through sensory nerve fibers. At this point, the impulses continue to the brain, informing the brain of what has transpired. More importantly, the impulses are transmitted by an interneuron, at that same level in the spinal cord at which the sensory input entered, to a motor neuron, which then activates the appropriate muscle group to withdraw your hand. The motor response to the more complex movement patterns typically originates in the motor cortex of the brain.

Once an electrical impulse reaches a motor neuron, the impulse travels the length of the neuron to the neuromuscular junction or **motor endplate,** and from here the impulse is propagated to the muscle fibers innervated by that particular motor neuron. The motor neuron and the muscle fibers it innervates is referred to as a **motor unit.** Each muscle fiber is innervated by only one motor neuron, but each motor neuron innervates from several fibers to several hundred fibers, depending on the function of that particular muscle. Muscles that exert control over fine movements, such as movement of the eye, are characterized by a small number of muscle fibers for each motor neuron. Those muscles that have more general functions, such as the gluteal muscles that form the buttocks, have a very high number of muscle fibers for each motor neuron. The muscle fibers comprising a specific motor unit are homogeneous with respect to their fiber type. In fact, there is general support for the theory that the characteristics of the motor neuron actually determine the fiber types of the muscle fibers innervated by that motor neuron.

It is now accepted that motor units are generally recruited on the basis of a fixed order, referred to as the phenomenon of orderly recruitment. It appears that for a given muscle, there is a rank ordering of motor units. Using the biceps brachii as an example, if there were a total of 200 motor units, they would be ranked on a scale of 1 to 200. For an extremely fine contraction requiring very little force production, the motor unit ranked number one would be recruited. As the requirements for force production increase, numbers two, three, four, etc. are recruited, up to a maximal contraction which would require activation of all 200 motor units. For a given force production, the same motor units are recruited each time.

A mechanism which may partially explain the principle of orderly recruitment is the **size principle.** The size principle states that the recruitment of a motor unit is directly related to the size of the soma or cell body of the motor neuron. Those motor units with the smaller cell bodies will be recruited first. Since the slow twitch motor units have the smaller cell bodies, they are typically recruited first in graded movement, with the fast twitch motor units recruited as the force needed to perform the movement is increased. There is still some question as to how this size principle relates to most athletic movements, as it has only been studied in graded movements that represent relative intensities of contraction of 25 percent and below.

Sensory-Motor Integration

Skeletal muscle function is precisely controlled by a complex series of events that transpire within the muscle, and between the muscle and its sensory and motor activation. Muscle spindles and Golgi tendon organs play a vital role in controlling muscle contraction and the resulting tension developed by the muscle. Surrounding muscle spindles (see Figure 5-4) are ordinary muscle cells referred to as **extrafusal fibers.** Muscle spindles are composed of several small specialized muscle fibers called **intrafusal fibers,** and the nerve endings which attach to these fibers. The endings of the intrafusal fibers are attached to the sheaths of the surrounding skeletal muscle fibers. These specialized muscle fibers, the intrafusal fibers, are controlled by specialized motor nerve fibers, **gamma motorneurons.** Extrafusal muscle fibers are controlled by **alpha motorneurons.** The middle portion of the intrafusal fiber does not have the ability to contract, thus when the ends of these fibers contract they stretch or elongate the central portion. Sensory nerve endings are wrapped around this middle portion of the intrafusal fibers and transmit information back to the central nervous system, informing the higher centers of the state of contraction or relaxation of that portion of the muscle.

When a muscle is suddenly stretched, such as when a heavy weight is placed in the palm of an extended arm, the middle of the muscle spindle becomes stretched or elongated, sending impulses to

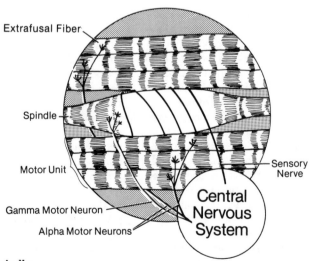

Figure 5-4 The muscle spindle.

the spinal cord. These impulses then excite the alpha motorneurons, causing the muscle to contract, overcoming the stretch. The gamma motorneurons function to excite the intrafusal fibers, placing them into a slightly prestretched position, making the central portion of each fiber more sensitive to even small degrees of stretch.

The muscle spindle also assists in normal muscle contraction. It appears that when the alpha motorneurons are stimulated to excite contraction of the extrafusal muscle fibers, the gamma system is activated at the same time, causing contraction of the ends of the intrafusal fibers. This elongates the middle portion of the muscle spindle which stimulates impulses to travel back through the sensory nerves to the spinal cord and immediately back to the muscle to facilitate the original impulses. Thus, the contraction and final force or tension development is a result of both direct stimulation through the alpha motorneurons and indirect stimulation through the muscle spindle.

Golgi tendon organs are encapsulated sensory receptors through which muscle tendons pass just prior to their attachment to muscle fibers. These tendon organs are sensitive to tension in the muscle-tendon complex. The sensory receptors perform a protective function by reducing the potential for injury. When stimulated, these receptors inhibit the contracting or agonist muscles and excite the antagonist muscles, thus diminishing the strength of contraction before it causes damage. It is speculated that reducing the influence of Golgi tendon organs results in **disinhibition**, allowing a more forceful muscle contraction, a factor which could explain at least part of the gains in strength that accompany strength training.

There are a number of reflexes that enable the body to function under a variety of conditions. Each of these reflex patterns has an intricate control system. Current texts in physiology, neurophysiology, or motor control are available for additional information on this topic.

Most movements used in sport activities involve control and coordination through the higher brain centers, specifically the motor cortex, the basal ganglia, and the cerebellum. The motor cortex is a part of the cerebral cortex in the higher brain centers and is responsible for the control of fine and discreet muscle movements. The basal ganglia are located deep in the cerebral hemispheres, and are composed of separate large pools of neurons that control complex, semi-voluntary movements such as walking and running. The cerebellum is located behind the lower brain stem, and it assists both the motor cortex and the basal ganglia in the performance of their functions. It facilitates movement patterns by smoothing out the movement, which would normally be jerky and uncontrolled in the absence of the cerebellum.

When a new motor skill is learned, the initial periods of practice require intense concentration. As the new motor skill becomes increasingly familiar, less concentration is needed. Finally, once the skill has been perfected it can be recalled with little or no conscious effort. Specific learned motor patterns appear to be stored in the brain to be replayed on call. These memorized motor patterns are referred to as motor programs, or **engrams**. Engrams are apparently stored in both the sensory and motor portions of the brain. Those in the sensory portion of the brain are for slower motor patterns, and those in the motor portion are for rapid movements.

THE AUTONOMIC NERVOUS SYSTEM

The preceding discussion of neural control was based solely on the sensory and motor aspects of body movement. The **autonomic nervous system** controls the internal functions of the body which are typically not subject to voluntary control, such as blood pressure, heart rate, and respiration. The autonomic nervous system has two major divisions: the **sympathetic nervous system** and the **parasympathetic nervous system**. These two divisions originate from different sections of the spinal cord and base of the brain. The effects of the two systems are often antagonistic to one another and they usually secrete different neurotransmitter substances.

The sympathetic division originates from the thoracic and upper lumbar regions of the spinal cord, while the parasympathetic division originates from the cranial nerves and the sacral region of the spinal cord. Approximately 90 percent of the parasympathetic fibers originate from the tenth cranial nerve, the **vagus nerve**. The primary neurotransmitter for the sympathetic division is norepinephrine or noradrenalin, and the neurons are referred to as adrenergic neurons. The primary neurotransmitter for the parasympathetic division is acetylcholine, and the neurons are referred to as cholinergic neurons. A few of the neurons originating from the sympathetic division secrete acetylcholine. Acetylcholine and norepinephrine both have the ability to excite some end-organs and inhibit others, although they usually act in opposition.

The functions of the two divisions are typically opposing. As an example, sympathetic stimulation of the heart increases heart rate, while parasympathetic stimulation decreases heart rate. The sympathetic nervous system is responsible for constricting most of the blood vessels, which provides control over blood pressure and cardiac output. Sympathetic stimulation, however, results in dilation of the coronary blood vessels that supply the myocardium or heart muscle. Thus, during exercise, sympathetic stimulation is very important since it increases heart rate, which, in turn, increases the work of the heart. Further, it causes dilation of the coronary blood vessels, allowing more blood to perfuse the heart muscle in order to provide necessary nutrients and remove waste products associated with an increased rate of work. Finally, sympathetic stimulation elevates the blood pressure to allow sufficient blood to return to the heart to maintain an adequate cardiac output. If all of the blood vessels in the body were to dilate simultaneously, there would be no return of blood to the heart, since the capacity of the blood vessels to hold blood far exceeds the total volume of blood in the body. When an individual goes into a state of shock, referred to as neurogenic shock, this is essentially what happens: there is a sudden cessation of sympathetic impulses, the blood vessels dilate, the blood pressure drops, and blood pools in the veins, greatly reducing the return of blood to the heart. This would be a typical series of events when one faints following an acute emotional stress. The parasympathetic nervous system plays a very minor role in controlling the systemic blood vessels.

Closely related to the example of sympathetic nervous system control during exercise, the sympathetic nervous centers in the brain, when excited, produce a mass discharge throughout the body, preparing the body for action. A sudden loud noise, a life-threatening situation, or those last few seconds prior to starting a race or game, are examples of times when one experiences this mass sympathetic discharge. Heart rate and blood pressure increase, the rate of metabolism increases, the degree of mental activity is increased and facilitated, glucose is released into the blood from the liver as an energy source, kidney function decreases, and sweating is initiated. These basic alterations in body function facilitate action, demonstrating the importance of the autonomic nervous system in preparing an individual for acute stress.

SUMMARY

The nervous and hormonal systems work in concert to initiate and control movement, and provide direction to the various physiological systems, allowing them to meet the demands of the sport or activity. There is a great deal of similarity between the nervous and endocrine systems relative to the way in which they integrate and control movement. There are also important ways in which they differ. The nervous system functions quickly and its effects are rather short-lived and localized, where the endocrine system functions more slowly, and its effects are longer lasting and more general.

The nervous system is comprised of the central nervous system, which includes the brain and spinal cord, and the peripheral nervous system, which is comprised of an efferent, or motor, division and an afferent, or sensory, division. The efferent division can further be divided into the somatic and autonomic nervous systems. The neuron is the basic functional unit of the nervous system and is comprised of a soma or cell body, dendrites which act as receivers for incoming signals from adjacent neurons, and an axon which is the fiber-like extension of the nerve cell. Nerve impulses or action potentials pass from the dendrites through the cell body and along the length of the axon to the terminal fibrils of the axon. From here, a neurotransmitter is released which allows the impulse to be passed along to adjacent neurons or to an end-organ such as a muscle fiber. Sensory impulses are sent to the spinal cord and brain from the various receptors in the periphery, including proprioceptors such as muscle spindles and Golgi tendon organs; exteroceptive receptors for touch, heat, cold, and pain; visceral receptors; and the special sensory receptors for vision, hearing, taste, and smell.

Information comes into the spinal cord and brain from these sensory receptors and when corrective action is required, signals to initiate action or movement are relayed back to the periphery via efferent, or motor, neurons. The more complex the action or movement, the higher the signals travel in the spinal cord or brain. When an impulse reaches a specific motor neuron it will be passed along to each of the muscle fibers innervated by that motor neuron. The motor neuron and the muscle fibers it innervates is referred to as a motor unit. Neuromuscular activity is graded on the basis of a fixed order of recruitment from the available pool of motor units. The more force needed to execute a certain movement, the more motor units recruited.

STUDY QUESTIONS

1. What are the major divisions and subdivisions of the nervous system? What are their functions?
2. Explain how movement occurs in response to a local trauma, such as touching a hot object.
3. Explain how movement occurs when you make the decision to bend down to pick up a ball.
4. Describe those parts of the brain which are critical to coordinating your movement as you dribble down the basketball floor preparing to slam-dunk your opponent.
5. What is a neuromuscular junction? Explain how impulses cross this junction.
6. What is disinhibition, and how might this be important for an athlete in training for high-level competition?
7. Describe the role of the muscle spindle in muscle contraction.
8. Describe the role of the Golgi tendon organ in controlling muscle contraction.
9. What is a motor unit? How are motor units recruited?
10. What is a neuron? How are action potentials generated?
11. Explain the importance of the autonomic nervous system during physical activity.
12. How do the sympathetic and parasympathetic nervous systems differ in their functions during exercise?
13. Describe the concept of excitatory and inhibitory impulses and its importance for controlling human movement.
14. What are engrams? How would they be important for someone learning a new sports skill such as the serve in tennis?

REFERENCES

Åstrand, P. O. & Rodahl, K. (1986). *Textbook of work physiology* (3rd ed.). New York: McGraw-Hill Book Co.

Brooks, G. A. & Fahey, T. D. (1984). *Exercise physiology: Human bioenergetics and its applications.* New York: John Wiley & Sons.

Edington, D. W. & Edgerton, V. R. (1976). *The biology of physical activity.* Boston: Houghton Mifflin Company.

Fox, E. L. & Mathews, D. K. (1981). *The physiological basis of physical education and athletics* (3rd ed.). Philadelphia: Saunders College Publishing.

Ginzel, K. H. (1977). Interaction of somatic and autonomic functions in muscular exercise. *Exercise and Sport Sciences Reviews, 4,* 35–86.

Goodwin, G. M. (1977). The sense of limb position and movement. *Exercise and Sport Sciences Reviews, 4,* 87-124.

Guyton, A. C. (1986). *Textbook of medical physiology* (7th ed.). Philadelphia: W.B. Saunders Company.

Hasan, Z., Enoka, R. M., & Stuart, D. G. (1985). The interface between biomechanics and neurophysiology in the study of movement: Some recent approaches. *Exercise and Sport Sciences Reviews, 13,* 169-234.

McArdle, W. D., Katch, F. I., & Katch, V. L. (1986). *Exercise physiology: Energy, nutrition, and human performance* (2nd. ed.). Philadelphia: Lea & Febiger.

Vander, A. J., Sherman, J. H., & Luciano, D. S. (1980). *Human physiology: The mechanisms of body function* (3rd ed.). New York: McGraw-Hill Book Company.

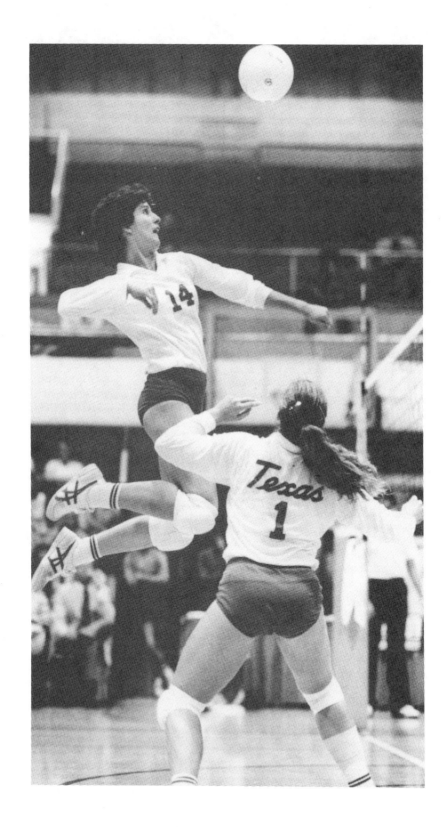

6

Endocrine Control
of Physical Activity

INTRODUCTION

Muscular activity can only be accomplished by the coordinated interaction of many physiological and biochemical systems, requiring a strong communicative link between the various bodily functions. Although the nervous system is responsible for much of this communication, the fine-tuning is accomplished by the **endocrine system.** During endurance exercise, for example, the supply of energy for muscle contraction depends on the hormonal regulation of blood glucose. As noted in Chapter 2, blood glucose is maintained relatively constant, both at rest and during several hours of exercise, by the continued release of glucose from the liver in proportion to the glucose uptake by the muscles. Without some way to sense the level of blood glucose and a means of regulating the breakdown of liver glycogen to form glucose, blood levels would drop to critically low values within a few minutes. As illustrated in Figure 6-1 on page 96, the **pancreas** is sensitive to changes in blood glucose, and is capable of releasing hormones, such as insulin, that can increase the levels of blood glucose.

This is but one example of the important role played by the endocrine system in maintaining ho-

meostasis. This chapter will describe the important general contributions of hormonal regulation to exercise performance. The details of more specific hormone functions related to the regulation and control of the exercise response will be included in the appropriate chapters throughout this book.

The endocrine system is composed of a series of glands referred to collectively as endocrine glands. **Endocrine glands** are defined as ductless glands, or glands that secrete their products directly into the blood stream. **Exocrine glands** secrete their products into ducts leading to specific compartments or surfaces. The sweat gland is an example of an exocrine gland, as ducts allow for the direct passage of sweat to the skin surface for purposes of evaporation and cooling. The pancreas is an example of a gland that has both endocrine and exocrine functions. Digestive enzymes secreted by the acini of the pancreas flow to the duodenum of the small intestine via the pancreatic duct (exocrine function). Insulin and glucagon are derived from the islets of Langerhans in the pancreas, and are secreted directly into the blood stream (endocrine function). Only those glands that secrete hormones into the blood are considered to be a part of the endocrine system. This chapter will present a

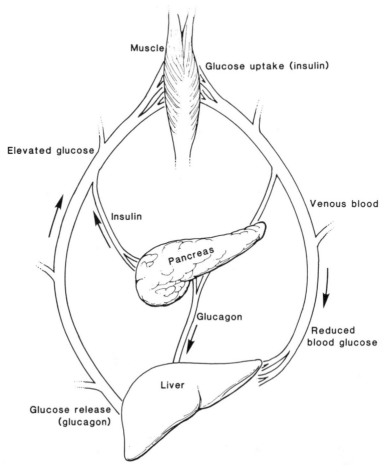

Figure 6-1   Communicative controls of the pancreas in regulating blood glucose levels during prolonged muscular activity. The removal of glucose from the blood results in the release of glucagon from the pancreas, which stimulates the breakdown of liver glycogen and an increase in the release of glucose.

general overview of those hormones responsible for regulating exercise performance.

HORMONES AND HORMONE RECEPTORS

Hormones are the chemical messengers of the endocrine system. Hormones can also be secreted by non-endocrine tissue. Acetylcholine, as discussed in Chapter 5, is a hormone neurotransmitter secreted by the parasympathetic and somatic nerve endings. Within the endocrine system, a hormone is a specific chemical substance that is synthesized by an endocrine gland, secreted into the blood on demand, and has its effects on specific tissues of the body. There are three basic types: steroid hormones, protein or peptide hormones, and amino acid derivative hormones. Hormones are considered to be either local or general in their effects. Acetylcholine has a very specific local effect, while epinephrine and norepinephrine secreted from the adrenal medulla, are much more general in their effects.

Hormones travel in the blood, which places them in contact with virtually all tissues of the body. How, then, are they able to limit their effects to specific organs or cells, called target organs or target cells? It is now known that each cell has between 2,000 and 10,000 receptors which are located within the membrane of the cell, for instance, receptors for epinephrine and norepinephrine; in the cytoplasm, for instance, receptors for steroid hormones; or in the nucleus, for instance, receptors for thyroxine and triiodothyronine. Each receptor is usually highly specific for a single hormone. Therefore, any single hormone will bind only with receptors which are specific to that hormone, and thus to tissues that contain those specific receptors. This specialization of target cell receptors explains the specificity of hormone action.

Once the hormone molecule attaches to its receptor site, it can have a direct effect on that site, such as the effects of epinephrine and norepinephrine on their target cells. More common, however, hormones either activate the cyclic AMP system of the cell, which then activates other intracellular functions, or they can activate the genes of the cell, causing the formation of intracellular proteins that activate specific cellular functions.

Blood levels of specific hormones tend to fluctuate both over short time periods of one hour or less, as well as over longer time periods such as the 24-hour diurnal cyclic variations. Hormones appear to be released in bursts lasting relatively short periods of time, with little or no activity between bursts. Blood levels of each of the specific hormones are controlled by a system of negative feedback. Once the target organ reaches the appropriate or desired level of activity, signals are sent back to the endocrine gland responsible for that specific hormone, causing the gland to reduce or stop secretion of that hormone.

Actual blood levels of specific hormones are not always the best indicators of actual hormone activity, as the number of receptors on a cell can be altered to increase or reduce that cell's sensitivity to a certain quantity of hormone. In obese individuals, for example, there appears to be a reduction in the number of insulin receptors on each cell. The body responds by increasing the release of insulin from the pancreas. This leads to an increase in blood levels of insulin. Thus, to obtain the same degree of blood sugar control as the normal, healthy individual, the obese individual needs to release more insulin to maintain blood insulin at higher levels.

THE ENDOCRINE GLANDS AND THEIR HORMONES

The endocrine glands and their respective hormones are illustrated in Figure 6-2, and further amplified in Table 6-1 on pages 98-99. It must be emphasized that the figure and table are greatly oversimplified to focus on those hormones of greatest importance to sport and physical activity.

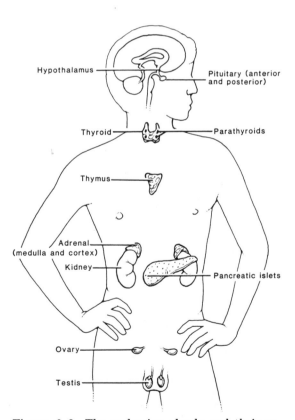

Figure 6-2 The endocrine glands and their respective hormones.

Table 6-1 The Endocrine Glands, their Hormones, their Target Organs, and Major Functions of the Hormones.

Endocrine Gland	Hormone	Target Organ	Major Functions
Pituitary Anterior Segment	Growth Hormone (GH)	All cells in the body	Promotes development and enlargement of all body tissues up through maturation; increases rate of protein synthesis; increases mobilization of fats and uses fat as an energy source; decreases rate of carbohydrate utilization
	Thyrotropin or Thyroid-stimulating Hormone (TSH)	Thyroid Gland	Controls the amount of thyroxin and triiodothyronine produced and released by the thyroid gland
	Adrenocortico-tropin (ACTH)	Adrenal cortex	Controls the secretion of hormones from the adrenal cortex
	Prolactin	Breasts	Stimulates breast development and milk secretion
	Follicle-stimulating hormone (FSH)	Ovaries, testes	Initiates growth of follicles in the ovaries and promotes secretion of estrogen from the ovaries; promotes development of sperm in testes
	Luteinizing hormone (LH)	Ovaries, testes	Promotes secretion of estrogen and progesterone, and causes the follicle to rupture, releasing the ovum; causes testes to secrete testosterone
Posterior Segment (Hypothalamus)	Antidiuretic hormone (ADH or vasopressin)	Kidneys	Assists in controlling water excretion by the kidneys; elevates blood pressure by constricting blood vessels
	Oxytocin	Uterus, breasts	Stimulates contraction of uterine muscles; milk secretion
Thyroid	Thyroxine and Triiodothyronine	All cells in the body	Increases the rate of cellular metabolism; increases rate and contractility of the heart
	Calcitonin	Bones	Controls calcium-ion concentration in the blood
Parathyroid	Parathormone or Parathyroid Hormone	Bones, intestine, and kidneys	Controls calcium-ion concentration in extracellular fluid through its influence on bone, intestine, and kidneys
Adrenal Medulla	Epinephrine	Most cells in the body	Mobilizes glycogen; increases skeletal muscle blood flow; increases heart rate and contractility; oxygen consumption

Table 6-1   (Continued)

Endocrine Gland	Hormone	Target Organ	Major Functions
	Norepinephrine	Most cells in the body	Constricts arterioles and venules thereby elevating blood pressure
Cortex	Minerocorticoids (Aldosterone)	Kidneys	Increases sodium retention and potassium excretion through the kidneys
	Glucocorticoids (Cortisol)	Most cells in the body	Controls metabolism of carbohydrates, fats, and proteins; anti-inflammatory action
	Androgens and Estrogens	Ovaries, breasts, and testes	Assists in the development of the female and male sex characteristics
Pancreas	Insulin	All cells in the body	Controls blood glucose levels by lowering glucose levels; increases the utilization of glucose and the synthesis of fat
	Glucagon	All cells in the body	Increases blood glucose; stimulates the breakdown of protein and fat
	Somatostatin	Islets of Langerhans and gastrointestinal tract	Depresses the secretion of both insulin and glucagon
Gonads			
Testes	Testosterone	Sex organs, muscle	Promotes development of male sex characteristics, including growth of testes, scrotum and penis; facial hair and change in voice; promotes muscle growth
Ovaries	Estrogen	Sex organs, adipose tissue	Promotes development of female sex organs and characteristics; provides increased storage of fat; assists in regulating the menstrual cycle
	Progesterone	Sex organs	Assists in regulating the menstrual cycle
Kidneys	Renin	Adrenal cortex	Assists in blood pressure control
	Erythropoietin	Bone marrow	Erythrocyte production

Note: These represent the *major* endocrine glands and hormones. Others of lesser importance to sport and physical activity have not been included.

Pituitary Gland

The **pituitary gland,** also referred to as the hypophysis, is a very small, marble-sized gland that lies in a bony cavity beneath the base of the brain. It was at one time considered to be the "master gland" of the human body. However, subsequent research has demonstrated that the hypothalamus, which lies directly above the pituitary, is the major area of production of several of the pituitary hormones and controls the secretion of all the pituitary hormones.

The pituitary gland is composed of three lobes: anterior, intermediate, and posterior. The intermediate lobe is very small and has little or no function in the human body. The posterior lobe is actually an outgrowth or continuation of neural tissue from the hypothalamus. The two hormones of the posterior pituitary, **antidiuretic hormone (ADH or vasopressin)** and **oxytocin,** are synthesized in the hypothalamus. They travel down the neural tissue and accumulate at the nerve endings in the posterior lobe where they are released into the capillaries.

Although little is known about the effects of exercise on these secretions from the posterior lobe of the pituitary gland, it is well-known that a reduction in blood flow and oxygen to the kidneys results in an increase in the level of blood ADH. Since this hormone acts to reduce urine production, it plays an important role in conserving body water, thereby minimizing the risk of dehydration during periods of heavy sweating and hard exercise. As shown in Figure 6–3, exercise results in a

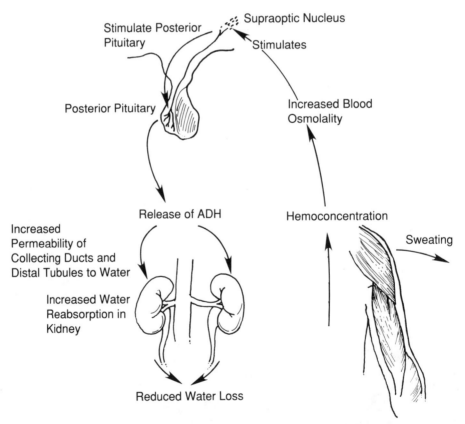

Figure 6–3　Sequence of events that result in an antidiuretic hormone release from the posterior lobe of the hypothalamus and a subsequent reduction in water excretion by the kidney.

decrease in blood flow and oxygen to the kidneys, causing the release of renin. **Renin** is a protein formed in the kidney which acts as an enzyme to convert alpha globulin, a blood protein, to **angiotensin,** a strong blood vessel constrictor. This renin-angiotensin system serves as a messenger to the posterior pituitary gland causing the release of ADH, thereby blocking water loss via the kidney.

The six anterior pituitary hormones are released into the blood in response to hypothalamic releasing and inhibiting factors. Specific releasing and inhibiting factors control the release or secretion of each of these hormones. Exercise appears to be a strong stimulant for these hormones, causing an increase in all six of these hormones. **Adrenocorticotropin (ACTH)** is controlled by **corticotropin-releasing hormone (CRH).** ACTH controls the release of the adrenocortical hormones from the adrenal cortex. **Thyrotropin** or **thyroid-stimulating hormone (TSH)** is controlled by **thyrotropin releasing hormone (TRH).** TSH controls the release of thyroxine and triiodothyronine from the thyroid gland. **Growth hormone (GH)** is controlled by both **growth hormone releasing hormone,** which stimulates the secretion of GH, and **somatostatin** or **growth hormone release inhibiting hormone (GIH),** which inhibits the secretion of GH.

Gonadotropin-releasing hormone (GnRH) stimulates the secretion of **luteinizing hormone (LH)** and **follicle-stimulating hormone (FSH).** LH is involved in ovulation and causes secretion of female sex hormones by the ovaries and testosterone by the testes. FSH causes growth of follicles in the ovaries prior to ovulation and promotes formation of sperm in the testes. Finally, the secretion of **prolactin,** which promotes development of the breasts and secretion of milk, is controlled by both **prolactin-releasing hormone (PRH)** and **prolactine-release inhibiting hormone (PIH).**

Communication between the hypothalamus and the anterior pituitary occurs through a specialized circulatory system that allows passage of the releasing hormones through the stalk connecting the hypothalamus and pituitary.

Thyroid Gland

The **thyroid gland** (see Figure 6–2) is located immediately beneath the larynx on both sides of the tra-

chea. It secretes two important hormones for regulating cellular and general body metabolism, **thyroxine** and **triiodothyronine,** and an additional hormone, **calcitonin,** which assists in the regulation of calcium metabolism. Thyroxine and triiodothyronine increase the metabolic rate of almost all tissues, and can increase the basal metabolic rate by as much as 60 to 100 percent above normal values. These hormones can also increase protein synthesis, increase the synthesis of enzymes, and increase the size and number of mitochondria in most cells of the body. They also promote rapid uptake of glucose by the cells, enhance glycolysis and gluconeogenesis, and enhance lipid mobilization, thus increasing free fatty-acid concentration and oxidation.

During exercise, the thyroid-stimulating hormone (TSH) increases progressively with work loads above 50 percent of $\dot{V}O_2$ max. The concentration of TSH appears to reach a steady-state level after 40 minutes of exercise. TSH controls the release of the thyroid hormones, thyroxine (T_4) and triiodothyronine (T_3). It is generally agreed that exercise produces an increase in blood thyroxine. However, a delay seems to exist between the rise in TSH during exercise and the associated increase in the blood thyroxine level.

Parathyroid Glands

The **parathyroid glands** are located on the dorsal surface of the thyroid glands (refer back to Figure 6–2) and they secrete parathyroid hormone or **parathormone.** Parathormone acts upon bone, causing it to increase its release of calcium into the blood in response to low blood concentrations of calcium. It also acts on the kidneys to increase the reabsorption of calcium at the renal tubules and decrease the reabsorption of phosphate, thus allowing a greater urinary loss of phosphate. Calcitonin, secreted by the thyroid glands, lowers plasma calcium primarily by inhibiting bone reabsorption, but the overall role of calcitonin on calcium balance is much less important than that of parathormone.

Adrenal Glands

The **adrenal glands** are situated directly on top of each kidney and are composed of two parts, the

adrenal medulla and the **adrenal cortex.** The adrenal medulla produces and releases two hormones, **epinephrine** and **norepinephrine,** which are collectively referred to as the **catecholamines.** When the adrenal medulla is stimulated, approximately 80 percent of the secretion is epinephrine and 20 percent is norepinephrine, although these percentages will vary with different physiological conditions. The catecholamines have a powerful effect on the cardiovascular and nervous systems, smooth and skeletal muscles, and metabolism. This effect is similar to that of the sympathetic nervous system, but the duration of the effect is sustained due to the fact that these hormones are removed from the blood at a relatively slow rate. These two hormones prepare an individual for immediate action, "fight or flight," when suddenly aroused.

The major function of epinephrine is to increase the rate and force of contraction of the heart, resulting in an increase in cardiac output. Epinephrine also causes increases in the following: metabolic rate, glycogenolysis in the liver and muscle, and release of glucose and free fatty acid into the blood. It has a small effect on the blood vessels, slightly increasing the systolic and mean arterial pressure, with little or no effect on diastolic pressure and total peripheral resistance. Norepinephrine has less of an effect on the heart and metabolism, but exerts a very strong effect on blood vessels, causing generalized constriction of all of the body's blood vessels. This leads to substantial increases in systolic, diastolic, and mean arterial pressure, and in total peripheral resistance.

The release of epinephrine and norepinephrine is affected by a wide variety of factors, including changes in body position, psychological stress, and exercise. As shown in Figure 6-4, the concentration of norepinephrine increases at work rates above 50 percent of $\dot{V}O_2$ max, whereas the blood concentration of epinephrine does not show a significant increase until the exercise intensity is above 75 percent of $\dot{V}O_2$ max. Figure 6-5 illustrates the rise in both hormones throughout steady-state activity lasting more than three hours at 60 percent of $\dot{V}O_2$ max. Epinephrine levels will return to the resting level within only a few minutes of recovery, while norepinephrine may remain elevated for several hours after the activity.

The adrenal cortex secretes over 30 different steroid hormones, referred to as **corticosteroids.**

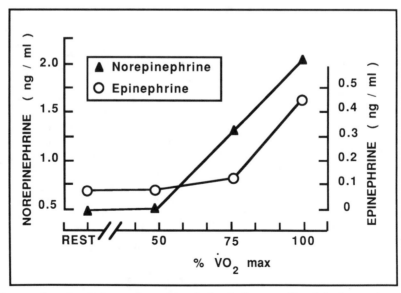

Figure 6-4 Changes in epinephrine and norepinephrine in forearm blood during rest and treadmill running.

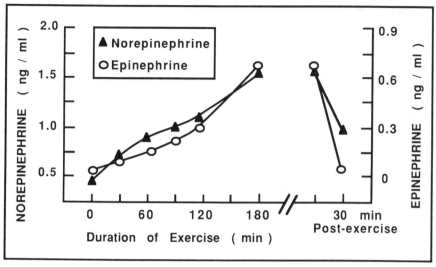

Figure 6-5   Changes in the concentration of epinephrine and norepinephrine in blood during prolonged treadmill running at 60 percent of the $\dot{V}O_2$ max and during recovery.

These are generally classified into three major types, mineralocorticoids, glucocorticoids, and androgens. The two major corticosteroids are **aldosterone,** the principal mineralocorticoid, and **cortisol,** the principal glucocorticoid. Aldosterone exerts at least 95 percent of the mineralocorticoid activity. Its major function is to promote the transport of sodium and potassium through the renal tubular walls of the kidney in an attempt to maintain an appropriate fluid balance within the body. Cortisol exerts at least 95 percent of the glucocorticoid activity within the body. Known also as hydrocortisone, cortisol stimulates gluconeogenesis in the liver by a factor of six to tenfold, decreases the rate of glucose utilization by the cells, increases the mobilization of free fatty acids, and acts as an anti-inflammatory agent. The adrenal cortex also synthesizes and releases androgens, estrogens, and progesterone in relatively small quantities, although their specific role has not been well-defined.

Pancreas

The **pancreas** is located behind and slightly below the stomach. As noted earlier in this chapter, the pancreas secretes two major hormones directly from its islets of Langerhans, **insulin** and **glucagon,** that are responsible for controlling blood glucose levels. The beta cells of the islets secrete insulin and the alpha cells secrete glucagon. A third type of cell found in the islets, delta cells, secrete the hormone **somatostatin.** Somatostatin, a recently discovered hormone, appears to function locally within the islets, acting to inhibit the secretion of both insulin and glucagon. **Hyperglycemia** refers to elevated blood glucose levels and **hypoglycemia** refers to blood glucose levels that are below normal.

Insulin promotes the rapid uptake, storage, and use of glucose from the blood into various tissues of the body. When blood glucose levels are elevated, the pancreas receives signals to release insulin into the blood. Insulin facilitates the transport of glucose from the blood into the cell, particularly in the liver and skeletal muscle. Insulin also promotes fat synthesis and storage in fat cells (adipocytes).

Diabetes mellitus, a disease in which blood sugar levels remain elevated, is the result of either or both a diminished rate of secretion of insulin by the beta cells of the islets, or a reduced sensitivity

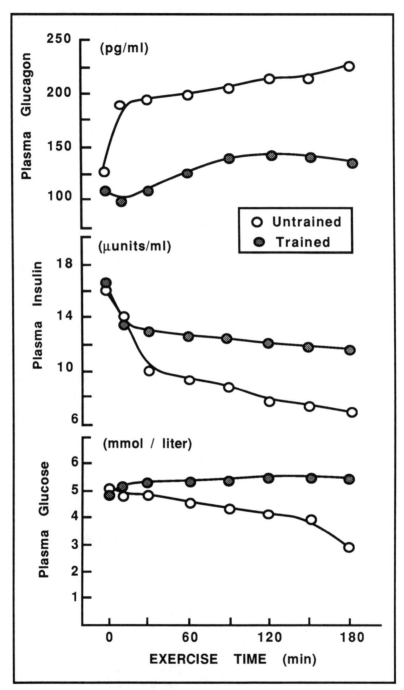

Figure 6–6 Changes in the concentration of plasma glucagon, plasma insulin, and plasma glucose during prolonged cycle ergometry at 60 percent of the VO_2 max in trained and untrained individuals.

of the body's cells to insulin. Type I, or juvenile diabetes, usually begins early in life and is associated with disruption of beta cell function leading to the inability to produce sufficient quantities of insulin. Type II, or maturity-onset diabetes, results from degeneration or suppression of the beta cells, a reduced responsiveness of the beta cells to stimulation by increased blood glucose levels, or a reduction in the number of insulin receptors on the cell. Type II diabetes is often associated with obesity. This will be discussed in Chapter 18.

Glucagon is secreted by the alpha cells of the islets when blood glucose falls below normal levels, and its effects are largely in opposition to those of insulin. Glucagon leads to an increased breakdown of liver glycogen (glycogenolysis) and increases gluconeogenesis in the liver, in an attempt to increase blood sugar levels.

During exercise lasting thirty minutes or longer, plasma insulin levels tend to decline, although blood glucose may remain relatively constant (see Figure 6-6). This appears to compensate for an increase in the muscle membrane's sensitivity to insulin as exercise duration increases. Consequently, less insulin is needed to aid in transporting glucose from the blood to the interior of the muscle fiber. Plasma glucagon, on the other hand, shows a gradual rise throughout the period of exercise, thereby stimulating liver glycogen breakdown and the maintenance of blood glucose (see Figure 6-6). Thus, the decline in insulin and concomitant increase in plasma glucagon function together to maintain a constant glucose supply for all body tissues.

Gonads

The **gonads** are the reproductive glands of the endocrine system and they include the testes in the male and the ovaries in the female. The testes secrete three hormones, referred to as androgens, which include **testosterone, dihydrotestosterone, and androstenedione.** Testosterone is the most important of the three, and is responsible for the development of the primary and secondary sexual characteristics, and the promotion of growth in skeletal muscle and bone. A major problem in athletics today involves the use of synthetic steroid hormones by male and female athletes to mimic

the anabolic or tissue-building characteristics of testosterone. This will be discussed in much greater detail in Chapter 13.

The ovaries secrete two types of hormones, the **estrogens** and **progestins. Estradiol** is the most important of the estrogen hormones and **progesterone** is the most important progestin. The estrogens promote proliferation and growth of specialized cells in the body and facilitate development of the secondary sex characteristics. The progestins prepare the uterus for pregnancy and the breasts for lactation.

Kidneys

The **kidneys** secrete two hormones which serve major roles in maintaining homeostasis during acute bouts of exercise and during training. **Renin** is synthesized and secreted by juxtaglomerular cells, specialized cells lining the arterioles in the kidneys. In response to a decrease in blood volume, the arterial pressure in the renal arteries decreases. This decrease in renal arterial pressure, and a concomitant increase in the activity of the renal sympathetic nerves, leads to renin release. Renin cleaves the polypeptide **angiotensin I** from the larger plasma protein **angiotensinogen.** After several transformations, angiotensin acts as a potent stimulator of aldosterone secretion, which promotes water conservation at the kidneys in an attempt to re-establish blood volume. Angiotensin is also a potent constrictor of the arterioles, which increases peripheral resistance to increase mean arterial pressure.

Erythropoietin is another hormone secreted by the kidneys. **Erythropoietin** is responsible for regulating the production of erythrocytes or red blood cells by stimulating the bone marrow. This is an extremely important mechanism for increasing red blood cell production in response to training, altitude, and blood loss.

GENERAL RESPONSE TO ACUTE AND CHRONIC EXERCISE

The hormonal responses to an acute bout of exercise are summarized in Table 6-2. This table focuses only on those hormones of major importance

Table 6-2 Hormonal Changes during Exercise and with Training.

Hormone	Changes during Exercise	Changes with Training	Significance
Growth Hormone	Increases with increasing rates of work	Less of a response in trained subjects	May increase FFA mobilization and gluconeogenesis
Thyrotropin	Increases with increasing rates of work	Unknown	Of no known significance
Thyroxine	Little or no change	Increase in thyroxine turnover without toxic effects	Of no known significance
LH and FSH	No changes have been observed	Unknown	Unknown
Adreno-corticotropin	Increases with increasing rates of work	Unknown	Increases availability of glucocorticoids
Glucocorticoids (cortisol)	Increases with higher relative rates of work	Increases less for the same workrate, may increase more at exhaustion	Increased glycogen deposition, increased liver gluconeogenesis, increased lipoloysis, and anti-inflammatory agent
Mineralocorticoids (aldosterone)[a]	Increases with increasing rates of work	May increase less for the same absolute rate of work	Maintenance of plasma volume
Parathormone and Calcitonin	Unclear at this time	Unknown	Important for normal bone development and bone health
Epinephrine	Little change at low rates of work over short duration, but increases with increased rates of work and with longer duration work	Increases less for the same absolute rate of work	Increased blood glucose, muscle blood flow, and heart rate and contractility
Norepinephrine	Relative marked increases with increases in the rate of work, difficult to isolate adrenal vs. sympathetic source	Increases less for the same absolute rate of work	Blood pressure control
Insulin	Decreases with increasing rates of work	Decreases less after training	Reduces the stimulus to utilize blood glucose

Table 6-2   (Continued)

Hormone	Changes during Exercise	Changes with Training	Significance
Glucagon	Increases with duration of activity, but decreases from an elevated level with high intensity, short duration activity	Increases less following training	Increased blood glucose by glycogenolysis and gluconeogenesis
Testosterone	Increases with higher rates of work	Unknown	Unknown
Estrogen and Progesterone	Increases with higher rates of work	Unknown	Unknown
Erythropoietin	Unknown, but postulated to increase with exercise	Unknown	Increased production of red blood cells

*Antidiuretic hormone (ADH) and renin are thought to respond in a similar manner.

Note: The information for this table was taken from Galbo, H. (1983) *Hormonal and Metabolic Adaptation to Exercise.* New York: Thieme-Stratton, Inc., and Terjung, R. (1980) Endocrine response to exercise. *Exercise and Sport Sciences Reviews, 7,* 153–180.

to sport and physical activity, and for which substantial information is available. The majority of these hormonal responses are discussed in detail in those chapters where their application is most relevant. Table 6-2 also summarizes the responses of these hormones following a period of training.

INTERPRETIVE FACTORS

As discussed in the previous section, during a single bout of exercise many of these hormones will undergo significant changes in their blood levels. These changes are dependent on such factors as the intensity of the exercise, the duration of the exercise bout, and the level of training. It should also be noted that plasma volume undergoes considerable change with exercise, decreasing by as much as ten percent or more with high-intensity, short-term exercise, or with low-intensity, long-duration exercise. Since hormones are typically expressed relative to their concentration in the blood, it is important to consider changes in

plasma volume when tracking hormonal changes with an acute bout of exercise. What appears to be an increase in the release of a specific hormone with exercise may only be a reflection of a reduction in the plasma volume. A reduction in plasma volume leads to **hemoconcentration** where the constituents of the blood are more tightly packed together. When hemoconcentration occurs, there will be an increase in the concentration of a specific blood constituent even when the absolute amount of that constituent has not changed. In some instances, this has been incorrectly interpreted as an increase in the release of a particular hormone, enzyme, or other blood constituent.

When interpreting the significance of specific levels of hormones in the plasma, it is also important to appreciate that the plasma level is the net result of the interaction of increases or decreases in hormone release and in hormone clearance or removal. Increased levels of a particular hormone, without a change in plasma volume, could be reflecting either an increase in the rate of production of that hormone, a decrease in its rate of clearance or removal, or a combination of increased rate of production and decreased rate of clearance. Similar consideration must be given when interpreting low levels of a particular hormone.

SUMMARY

This chapter has reviewed the mechanisms by which the endocrine system initiates, controls, and integrates physical activity. The endocrine and nervous systems work in concert to initiate and control movement, and to provide direction to the various physiological systems, allowing these systems to meet the demands of the sport or activity. There is a great deal of similarity between the nervous and endocrine systems relative to the way in which they integrate and control movement. There are also important ways in which they differ. The nervous system functions quickly and its effects are rather short-lived and localized, while the endocrine system functions much more slowly, and its effects are much longer-lasting and more general.

The endocrine system is composed of a series of glands referred to collectively as endocrine glands. Endocrine glands secrete hormones, which are potent chemical substances usually carried in the blood from the glands to other parts of the body where they assist in the control of specific body functions. The pituitary gland and the hypothalamus work in concert to release a number of the major hormones responsible for controlling body function. These include vasopressin (ADH) for controlling water balance and blood pressure; growth hormone; thyrotropin for controlling the release of the two major thyroid hormones; adrenocorticotropin for controlling the release of the hormones of the adrenal cortex; and several of the hormones that control secondary sex characteristics and reproductive functions.

The thyroid gland controls metabolic rate through its two major hormones, thyroxine and triiodothyronine, and blood calcium levels through calcitonin. The parathyroid glands secrete parathormone, which also control blood calcium levels. The adrenal glands are composed of two parts: the adrenal medulla secretes the potent catecholamines, epinephrine and norepinephrine, which

have a powerful effect on the nervous and cardiovascular systems, smooth and skeletal muscle, and metabolism; the adrenal cortex secretes mineralocorticoids such as aldosterone to control sodium and potassium excretion, glucocorticoids such as cortisol to control the metabolism of proteins, carbohydrates, and fats, and androgens and estrogens. The pancreas regulates glucose levels in the blood through its two hormones, insulin and glucagon. Finally, the gonads, which include the ovaries and testes, control the development of the female and male sex characteristics through the progestins, estrogens, and androgens, with testosterone being the major androgen.

The responses of these hormones to acute and chronic exercise were discussed. Much more extensive discussions of specific hormones and hormonal responses to exercise are included in the appropriate sections of various chapters throughout this book.

STUDY QUESTIONS

1. What is an endocrine gland? What are the functions of hormones?
2. Explain the difference between an endocrine and an exocrine gland.
3. Explain the similarities and differences between neural control and hormonal control of basic bodily functions.
4. Explain how hormones are able to limit their effects to specific functions when these hormones reach nearly all parts of the body through the blood.
5. How are blood levels of specific hormones controlled?
6. Are blood levels of specific hormones accurate indicators of actual hormone activity? Explain why or why not.
7. Explain the rather complex relationship between the hypothalamus and the pituitary gland.
8. Briefly outline the major endocrine glands, their hormones, and the specific action of these hormones.
9. Which of the hormones outlined in the previous question would be of major significance during exercise? During training?

10. Explain how hemoconcentration might influence your interpretation of blood levels of specific hormones.
11. Discuss the concept of hormone production and hormone clearance in interpreting hormone levels in the blood.

REFERENCES

Åstrand, P. O., & Rodahl, K. (1986). *Textbook of work physiology.* (3rd ed.). New York: McGraw-Hill Book Co.

Brooks, G. A., & Fahey, T. D. (1984). *Exercise physiology: Human bioenergetics and its applications.* New York: John Wiley & Sons.

Edington, D. W., & Edgerton, V. R. (1976). *The biology of physical activity.* Boston: Houghton Mifflin Company.

Fox, E. L., & Mathews, D. K. (1981). *The physiological basis of physical education and athletics.* (3rd ed.). Philadelphia: Saunders College Publishing.

Galbo, H. (1983). *Hormonal and metabolic adaptation to exercise.* New York: Thieme-Stratton Inc.

Ginzel, K. H. (1977). Interaction of somatic and autonomic functions in muscular exercise. *Exercise and Sport Sciences Reviews, 4,* 35–86.

Guyton, A. C. (1986). *Textbook of medical physiology,* (7th ed.). Philadelphia: W. B. Saunders Company.

McArdle, W. D., Katch, F. I., & Katch, V. L. (1986). *Exercise physiology: Energy, nutrition, and human performance.* (2nd ed.). Philadelphia: Lea & Febiger.

Shangold, M. M. (1984). Exercise and the adult female: Hormonal and endocrine effects. *Exercise and Sport Sciences Reviews, 12,* 53–79.

Shephard, R. J., & Sidney, K. H. (1975). Effects of physical exercise on plasma growth hormone and cortisol levels in human subjects. *Exercise and Sport Sciences Reviews, 3,* 1–30.

Svedenhag, J. (1985). *The sympathoadrenal system in physical conditioning.* (Report). Stockholm, Sweden: Karolinska Institute.

Terjung, R. (1979). Endocrine response to exercise. *Exercise and Sport Sciences Reviews, 7,* 153–180.

Turner, C. D., & Bagnara, J. T. (1976). *General endocrinology.* (6th ed.). Philadelphia: W. B. Saunders Company.

Vander, A. J., Sherman, J. H., & Luciano, D. S. (1980). *Human physiology: The mechanisms of body function.* (3rd ed.). New York: McGraw-Hill Book Company.

Wade, C. E. (1984). Response, regulation, and actions of vasopressin during exercise: A review. *Medicine and Science in Sports and Exercise, 16,* 506–511.

Winder, W. W. (1985). Regulation of hepatic glucose production during exercise. *Exercise and Sport Sciences Reviews, 13,* 1–31.

SECTION B

Physiological Adaptations to Physical Training

The skilled performance of an athlete is the final result of many long hours of physical training and practice. The end product does not happen by chance, but requires an intense dedication on the part of the athlete and exceptional insight by both coach and athlete as to what constitutes the best training program for that athlete in that particular sport or event. Just as each sport is different and requires its own unique training program, each athlete is also unique and requires an individualized training program to maximize his or her potential. To individualize training programs requires a basic knowledge of those physiological components that constitute the foundation of physical training. This section is devoted to a discussion of these individual components, with one chapter devoted to each of the following: muscular strength and power; muscular endurance and anaerobic power; cardiorespiratory endurance and aerobic power; and body build and composition. Each component will be defined, followed by a discussion of those adaptations that occur with training specifically related to that component, training procedures to best develop that component, and finally, an integrative assessment of the importance of that component to general athletic performance. The final chapter of this section will integrate these components into a working model through a discussion of their interrelationships during periods of deconditioning or undertraining, periods of overtraining, and periods of peaking for optimal performance.

This section is intended to apply to all sports and activities. Much of the research to date has been conducted on a limited number of sports. As a result, the individual chapters may appear to be biased toward one or two specific sports or activities. The basic principles introduced in these chapters are presented so that they can be applied to any sport. In addition, while the term athlete *is used throughout this section, the information is, in most cases, equally applicable to the nonathlete, or noncompetitive athlete, who pursues exercise for health-related benefits.*

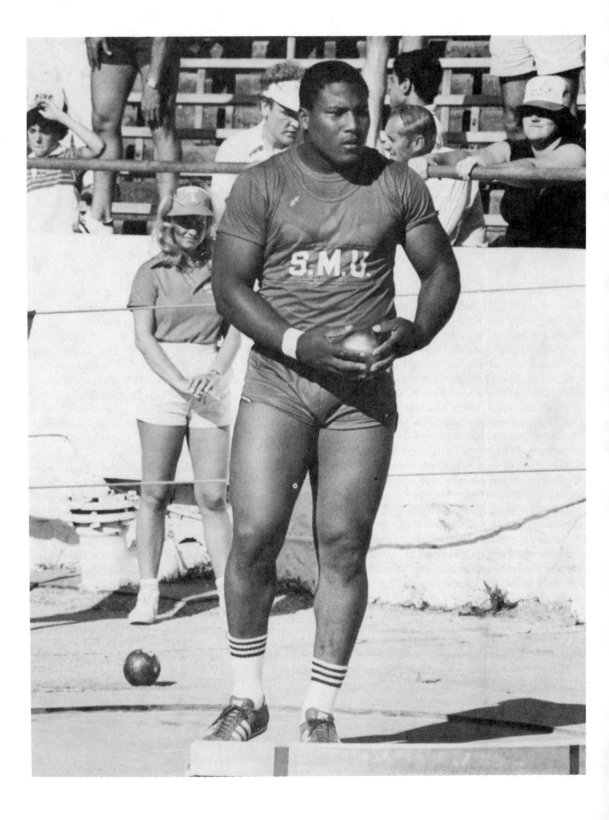

7

Muscular Strength and Power

INTRODUCTION

As the shot putter crouches low at the back of the circle in preparation for the next put, it is obvious that great muscular strength and power will be necessary for a successful performance. Likewise, muscular strength and power are needed to throw a ball, jump to the rim of a basket, and run a 100-meter dash. Are strength and power also important in activities such as golf, tennis, and distance running? The answer, while not as obvious, is indeed, yes! Virtually all activities depend on the ability of the muscles to generate force. Research has shown that success in many sports is closely related to the athlete's ability to develop strength and power.

Training to improve strength and power was, at one time, considered taboo for all athletes other than those in competitive weight lifting, weight events in track and field, and, on a limited basis, for football players, wrestlers, and boxers. It is now recognized that strength training is important to successful performance in almost all sports and activities. This change in attitude or philosophy has been largely the result of innovations in strength-training procedures that have taken place over the last few years.

How do we define the terms strength, power, and endurance? Are they synonymous, and can they be used interchangeably? Although the terms are interrelated, each has its own meaning. **Strength** can be defined as the maximum ability to apply or to resist force. The individual who can press 200 pounds of weight over his head has twice the strength of the individual who can only press 100 pounds. **Power** is simply the product of strength and speed, or more appropriately, power = force × velocity. If two individuals can each bench press 250 pounds, but one is able to do it in one-half the time of the other, the faster individual would have twice the power of the slower individual, providing the distance the weights moved was the same. While absolute strength is an important component of performance, power is probably even more important for most activities.

Although this chapter focuses on strength and power development, many sporting activities depend on the ability of muscle to repeatedly develop near maximal force, an ability termed **muscular endurance** (see Chapter 8). This capacity of muscle to sustain repeated contractions is what allows you to perform sit-ups, push-ups, and to sustain a fixed or static contraction for an extended period of time, such as in hanging from a bar. While stength appears to be a pure component, independent of power and muscular endurance, both muscular endurance and power are dependent on your level of strength.

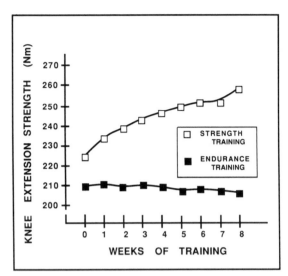

Figure 7-1 Specificity of training. Note that leg muscle strength improved throughout the ten-week training period when the subject strength-trained, whereas endurance training had no effect on knee extension strength.

STRENGTH: ADAPTATIONS IN MUSCLE

With chronic exercise, there are a number of adaptations that occur in the neuromuscular system. First, the extent of these adaptations will depend on the type of training program followed. If training is of a cardiorespiratory endurance nature, as in jogging or swimming, then little or no gains in strength will occur. This point is illustrated in Figure 7-1, where knee extension strength did not improve following a ten-week endurance training program. Likewise, a program of stretching to increase flexibility, combined with light calisthenics, will produce only small-to-moderate gains in muscular strength.

Strength training programs, where increased strength is a primary goal, will produce substantial gains in strength, ranging from 25 to 100 percent improvement, or greater, within a period of three to six months. When strength training is stopped, however, the strength that was gained is gradually lost over time, thus a basic maintenance program must be established once desired goals

for strength development have been achieved. Maintenance programs are designed to provide sufficient stress to the muscles in order to maintain the existing levels of strength, while allowing a reduction in the intensity and/or the duration, as well as the frequency, of the program. Preliminary research indicates that one or two exercise sessions per week is sufficient to maintain strength, but is probably not adequate to stimulate further increases in strength.

How does an individual become stronger? What physiological adaptations take place that allow one to exert greater levels of strength? For many years it was assumed that strength gains were a direct result of increases in muscle size. This increase in the size of the muscle with training is referred to as **hypertrophy**. This was a logical assumption, since those individuals who trained regularly with free weights or other strength-training modes, developed large, bulky muscles. In addition, when a broken limb is placed in a cast and immobilized for weeks or months, it is only a matter of a few days before the muscles start to decrease in size and lose strength, a process referred to as **atrophy**. Gains in muscle size are paralleled by gains in strength, whereas losses in the size of a muscle correlate highly with losses in strength when the muscles become immobilized. Thus, it is tempting to conclude that a cause-effect relationship exists, such as gains in strength are the result of increases in the size of the muscle. However, recent research suggests that there is more involved in understanding the basic mechanisms of strength gains than a simple relationship to the size of the muscle.

First, there have been numerous stories in newspapers and magazines in which individuals have performed superhuman feats of strength at times of great psychological stress. As noted by the newspaper headline in Figure 7-2, even a child can exhibit exceptional levels of strength when exposed to a highly-charged emotional situation. Straitjackets were specifically designed to control patients in mental hospitals who would suddenly go berserk and become impossible to restrain. Even in the world of sport, there have been isolated examples of superhuman athletic performances, such as Bob Beamon's long jump of 29 feet, 2½ inches at the 1968 Olympic Games held in

Boy, 9, lifts 4,100-pound car off chest of trapped father

Jamestown, N.D. (UPI) — Nine-year-old Jeremy Schill weighs just 65 pounds. But that didn't stop him from lifting a 4,100-pound car to help his father, who was trapped underneath.

Jeremy said he "just knew what to do" when the family's Ford LTD fell off a jack and onto his father. He lifted the car, easing the pressure on his father's chest so he could breathe.

Rique Schill, 31, told the *Jamestown Sun* he was working on his car Sunday when it slipped off the jack, pinning him under the rear axle.

"I WAS slowly suffocating. It was getting harder to breathe. But the boy pretty much kept his head together."

Jeremy, a third-grader who weighs 65 pounds, said, "I thought he was dead. But then I heard Daddy screaming.

"I never panicked, but I was pretty scared," he said.

Schill said his son lifted the car enough to ease his breathing, but could not give Schill enough room to slip out from under it.

The boy had to let the car go and ran to the family's farmhouse screaming, "Mommy, Mommy, the car fell on Daddy,'" said Schill's wife, Vicky, 25.

JEREMY SAID he "just knew what to do. My brain told me to get another jack."

He said he remembered another jack was buried in the snow under the front steps. He and his mother used the jack to free Schill, who was taken to the hospital.

He was released Tuesday. Nurse Donna Gullickson said he had a bruised chest and ribs.

Mrs. Schill said her husband's first words were, "'Oh no. Now I'm going to have to watch the Super Bowl from a hospital room.'"

Figure 7-2 Newspaper clipping illustrating the exceptional strength potential in man. Such feats of strength appear to be feasible only under unusual emotional conditions.

Mexico City—a jump which exceeded the previous world record by nearly two feet! World records are usually broken by inches, or more often, by fractions of inches.

An additional fact also casts doubt on the simplistic view that strength gains are solely the result of increases in the size of the muscle. Studies of strength training have shown that women experience gains in strength similar to men who perform the same training program, but the women do not experience the same degree of hypertrophy (Wilmore, 1974). In fact, several subjects in these studies doubled their levels of strength in the absence of any observable change in the size of the muscle. Thus, strength gains can occur in the absence of hypertrophy!

How, then, do you explain gains in strength? The preceding examples should not be taken to imply that muscle size is not an important factor in the ultimate strength potential of the muscle. All other things being equal, size is extremely important, as is illustrated by the world and Olympic records for competitive weight lifting. From the lightest to the heaviest weight classification, there is a progressive increase of total weight lifted. However, these examples indicate that the mechanisms responsible for gains in strength are very complex, and at this time not well understood. There is accumulating evidence to indicate that motor unit recruitment is important in explaining gains in muscular strength, particularly those gains in strength that occur in the absence of hypertrophy, as well as those episodic superhuman feats of strength (McDonagh & Davies, 1984).

There is evidence that motor units are controlled by a number of different neurons, or interneurons, which have the ability to produce both excitatory as well as inhibitory impulses. It has been suggested that inhibitory mechanisms in the neuromuscular system are necessary to prevent the muscles from exerting more force than can be tolerated by the bones and connective tissues. **Autogenic inhibition** is a reflex inhibition of the lower motor-neuron discharge, directed to a specific muscle when the tension on that muscle's tendons and internal connective tissue structures exceeds the threshold of the imbedded Golgi tendon organs. At higher levels in the nervous system, the reticular formation in the brain stem and the cerebral cortex both have the ability to initiate and propagate inhibitory impulses. It is quite possible that these inhibitory impulses are gradually overcome or counteracted with training, enabling the muscle to reach greater levels of strength, as would typically occur following a strength-training program. It is possible that strength gains may be achieved by releasing the neurological inhibitors that control muscle-force development.

The final decision as to whether an individual motor unit will fire and contribute to the contractile force, or remain in the relaxed state, depends on the summation of the many impulses it receives at any one time. If the inhibitory impulses equal or exceed the excitatory impulses, that particular motor unit will not be activated and will not contribute to the overall contraction of the muscle. If the excitatory impulses exceed the inhibitory impulses, the unit will then be activated and contribute to the force production capabilities of that muscle. Gains in strength may well be the result of a gain in the ability to recruit additional motor units and to synchronize their firing to facilitate the contraction. The improvement in recruitment patterns could be the result of a blocking of, or reduction in, the number of inhibitory impulses, thereby allowing more motor units to be activated simultaneously. In any case, McDonagh and Davies (1984) have concluded that there is a neurogenic component to the adaptive responses to strength training, particularly during the initial stages of training.

When hypertrophy does occur with strength training, what basic adaptations are taking place that lead to an increase in the size of the muscle? As compared to females, males experience a significantly greater increase in muscle size for the same strength-training program, even with equivalent gains in strength. Therefore, it is hypothesized that the male androgen, **testosterone,** is responsible, at least in part, for muscular hypertrophy. In Chapter 6, it was noted that one of the functions ascribed to testosterone was its promotion of muscle growth. It is also known that massive doses of anabolic steroids will lead to rather marked increases in muscle mass. This will be discussed in detail in Chapter 13.

Although testosterone appears to play a key role in the process of hypertrophy, it alone does not determine the growth in muscle size with strength training. There is, for example, a poor correlation between blood testosterone concentrations and the degree of muscle hypertrophy experienced during strength training. Some women will experience considerable hypertrophy with strength gains, while others experience essentially no change in muscle girth. It is speculated that the testosterone/estrogen ratio is higher in the former group which results in a greater increase in muscle mass.

What actual changes occur within the muscle? When the size of the whole muscle increases, how is this accomplished? First, there are two types of hypertrophy: transient and chronic. **Transient hypertrophy** is that "pumping-up" of the muscle that takes place during a single exercise bout. This is largely the result of fluid accumulation, or edema, in the muscle caused by water accumulation in the interstitial and intracellular spaces of the muscle. Transient hypertrophy, as its name implies, lasts only for a short period of time, since the fluid eventually returns to the blood within hours after exercise. **Chronic hypertrophy** refers to the increase in muscle size that results from strength training. Chronic hypertrophy is the result of structural changes in the muscle and can be explained either as an increase in the number of muscle fibers (**hyperplasia**), or an increase in the size of existing fibers. Controversy surrounds the several theories that attempt to explain the underlying cause for chronic muscle hypertrophy.

Early research demonstrated that the number of muscle fibers is established by birth, or shortly thereafter, and that this number remains fixed throughout life. If this is true, then chronic hypertrophy would be the result of muscle fiber enlargement, which could be explained by an increase in the number of myofibrils and/or filaments, an increase in the sarcoplasm, and/or an increase in the connective tissue. As noted in the microscopic photographs in Figure 7–3, a significant increase in the cross-sectional area of muscle fibers occurs as

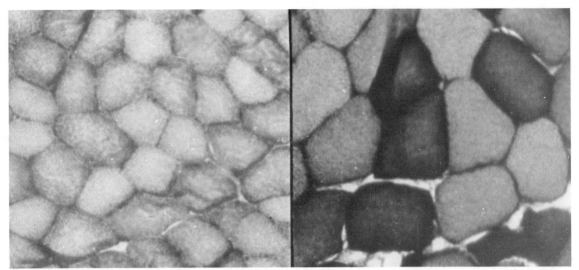

Figure 7-3   Microscopic view of a muscle cross-section from the leg muscles of a man before (left) and after (right) six months of isotonic strength training. This subject was a body builder who had not trained for two years prior to these measurements. Note the significantly larger fibers (hypertrophy) after training.

a result of intense strength training. This dramatic enlargement of the muscle fibers does not, however, appear to occur in all cases of muscle hypertrophy. Some weight lifters and body builders, for example, have developed an unusually large muscle mass but have normal fiber cross-sectional areas. Tesch and Larsson (1982) reported that mean muscle fiber areas of the vastus lateralis and the deltoids in three high-caliber body builders were smaller than a reference group of competitive power/weight lifters, and nearly identical to physical education students and non-strength trained individuals. A subsequent study by Larsson and Tesch (1986) confirmed these original findings. Nevertheless, an increase in myofibrils and filaments has been demonstrated in many research studies, and this would provide more cross bridges to produce force during a maximal contraction.

Recent research has pointed to the possibility that hyperplasia may be a factor in total muscle hypertrophy. Studies on cats have provided fairly clear evidence that with extremely heavy weight training, a splitting of fibers actually takes place (Gonyea, 1980). Cats were trained to use their fore-

paw to move a heavy weight a fixed distance in order to get their food. As a result, these cats learned to generate considerable amounts of force. With this intense strength training, selected muscle fibers appeared to actually split in half, with each half then increasing in size to that of the parent fiber. These series of events is illustrated in Figure 7-4 on page 118.

Subsequent studies by Gollnick, et al. (1981, 1983) and by Timson, et al. (1985), have disputed the concept of muscle hyperplasia, and have demonstrated that hypertrophy of the rat soleus, plantaris, and extensor digitorum longus muscles, the chicken anterior latissimus dorsi muscle, and the mouse soleus muscle, resulting from a chronic exercise overload, is due solely to a hypertrophy of existing fibers. In these studies by Gollnick and Timson, each fiber in the whole muscle was actually counted in order to provide an absolute count of the total fiber population in the muscles being studied. They felt the histological sectioning method used by Gonyea (1980) was producing artifacts that had led him to conclude that his cats were experiencing hyperplasia, when, in fact, the

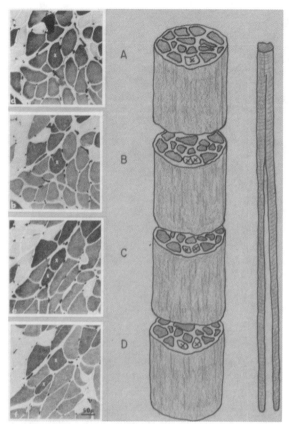

Figure 7-4 Muscle fiber splitting. The model of fiber splitting in the center and right of the figure have been assumed from the series of microscopic slides shown on the left (modified from Gonyea, et al., 1977).

size increases were more likely due to fiber enlargement. Their results using direct fiber counts showed no change in fiber number with training.

This led Gonyea and his colleagues (1986) to repeat their strength training study with cats, using actual fiber counts to determine if total muscle hypertrophy was the result of hyperplasia or single muscle fiber hypertrophy. They found a nine percent increase in the number of actual fibers consequent to their training program, confirming their original conclusions of muscle fiber hyperplasia. The difference in results between the studies of Gonyea and those of Gollnick, Timson, and

their colleagues is quite possibly due to both methodological differences and, more likely, to differences in the mode of training. Gonyea used a pure form of strength training—high resistance, low-repetition training, whereas Gollnick and Timson used more endurance-type activity—low resistance, high-repetition training.

The possible role of fiber hyperplasia and hypertrophy in human muscle in response to strength training is unclear, but the evidence appears to support the concept that individual fiber hypertrophy accounts for most, if not all, of the hypertrophy seen in the whole muscle. The results of the study by Tesch and Larsson (1982, 1986) on body builders, however, would suggest that hyperplasia is possibly a factor in humans as well. Taylor and Wilkinson (1986) recently conducted an extensive review of the hypertrophy versus hyperplasia issue with similar findings.

The ability to change one muscle fiber type to another with physical conditioning is an additional topic for debate. Based on the simple classification system of slow-twitch and fast-twitch fibers (see Chapter 1), the early studies indicated that neither strength nor endurance (aerobic) training altered the basic fiber types (Costill, 1979; Gollnick, 1973). As an example, an individual who possesses 75 percent slow-twitch fibers and 25 percent fast-twitch fibers would have these same fiber-type proportions even after intensive strength training, which theoretically would promote an increase in fast-twitch fibers, if fibers could change characteristics. These early studies did show that fibers begin to take on certain characteristics of the opposite fiber type if the training is of the opposite kind; although actual conversion from one fiber type to the other, as Type I to Type II or Type II to Type I, was not observed.

More recent research with animals has shown that fiber type conversion is possible under conditions of cross-innervation, where a fast-twitch motor unit is innervated by a slow-twitch motor neuron, and vice versa. Further, chronic stimulation of fast-twitch motor units with low-frequency nerve stimulation transforms fast-twitch into slow-twitch motor units within a matter of weeks (Pette, 1984). Several recent studies in both rats (Green, et al., 1984) and humans (Simoneau, et al., 1985) have indicated a shift in fiber type as a result

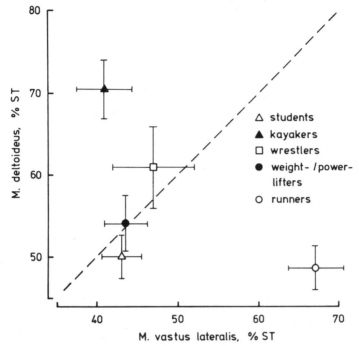

Figure 7-5 Relationship between muscle fiber type distribution in vastus lateralis and deltoids in athletes trained for different sports (from Tesch & Karlsson, 1985).

of long-term, high-intensity training, with an increase in Type I and a decrease in Type IIb fibers. Further, Tesch and Karlsson (1985) found what could be long-term training adaptations of muscle fiber type in highly-trained athletes. Using the vastus lateralis muscle to represent the leg and the deltoid to represent the arm, they found kayakers to have a higher percentage of slow-twitch fibers in the deltoid as compared to their vastus lateralis, while the reverse pattern was seen in long-distance runners. This is illustrated in Figure 7-5.

Power (P) is simply the product of muscle force (F) and velocity (V) of movement (P = F × V). Thus, any increase in power must be the result of improvements in either strength or speed, or both. Since muscle training substantially increases muscle strength and can also increase speed of movement, the increase in power with muscle training is often substantial. Unlike strength, the mechanisms responsible for these increases in power are obvious.

It is generally accepted that muscular endurance is best increased through muscle training that emphasizes high repetitions and relatively low resistance. Yet, there is also a high correlation between strength and absolute muscular endurance. This would tend to suggest that even programs designed to produce optimal gains in strength, for instance, low repetitions and high resistance, provide some improvements in muscular endurance. As noted in Figure 7-6 on page 120, strength training increased the total work that could be performed during a maximal, 60-second exercise bout (isokinetic knee extension), but had little influence on the rate of muscle fatigue, as there was no improvement once the subject exceeded twenty to twenty-five seconds. It appears, therefore, that strength is one of the major determinants of muscle endurance in explosive, sprint events. Other factors important to endurance in these events, include local patterns of circulation, the availability of fuels such as glycogen, and the removal of waste

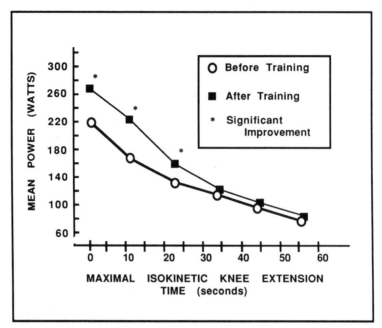

Figure 7-6 Effects of training on muscle strength and endurance. The subjects performed a series of repeated, maximal knee extensions for 60 seconds. Note that the greatest improvements in force development occurred during the first half of the endurance test.

products such as lactate and hydrogen ions. The more efficient the circulation and the greater the development of circulatory capacity within that local area, the greater the potential for muscular endurance. Numerous research studies have indicated that muscle training between 20 and 30 repetitions per minute is the most efficient way to increase muscular endurance. This routine, however, will have little effect on muscle strength and bulk. Thus, factors other than strength are important in the development of endurance.

MUSCLE SORENESS

Muscle soreness may be present during the latter stages of an exercise and/or immediate recovery, between twelve and forty-eight hours after a strenuous bout of exercise, or at both times. Pain that is felt during and immediately after exercise may be due to the accumulation of the end-products of

exercise and tissue edema caused by the high hydrostatic pressures that force fluid to shift from the blood plasma into the tissues. This is the "pumped-up" feeling that the athlete is conscious of following heavy endurance or strength training. This pain and soreness is usually of short duration, disappearing within minutes or hours after the exercise.

The muscle soreness that is felt a day or two following a heavy bout of exercise is not clearly understood. There are several theories that have been presented to explain this form of muscle soreness, but they do not have universal support or agreement. Abraham (1979) has provided data supporting Hough's torn tissue hypothesis, which was originally formulated in 1902. He found muscle soreness to correlate with the appearance of myoglobin in the urine, myoglobin being a marker of muscle fiber trauma. Since myoglobinuria is associated with all strenuous work, independent of muscle soreness, he also looked at hydroxyproline excretion, which is indicative of connective tissue breakdown. He found a significant correlation between the day of maximum hydroxyproline excretion and the day when the subjects experienced their greatest soreness.

The presence of muscle enzymes in the blood after intense exercise suggests that some structural damage may occur in the muscle membranes. Following bouts of *heavy* training, these enzymes have been reported to increase between two and ten times their normal levels. Recent studies tend to support the idea that these changes in blood enzymes may reflect varied degrees of muscle tissue breakdown. Examination of tissue from the leg muscles of marathon runners has revealed that there is remarkable damage to the muscle fibers after training and marathon competition. The onset and time course of these muscle changes seemed to parallel the degree of muscle soreness experienced by the runners.

The electronmicrograph presented in Figure 7-7 shows a sample of the damage done to some muscle fibers as a result of marathon running. In this case the cell membrane or sarcolemma has been totally ruptured, with its contents floating freely between the other normal fibers. Not all of the damage done to the muscle cells is as severe as that shown in Figure 7-7. Other examples of disruptions within the fibers are illustrated in Figures 7-8A on page 122 and 7-8B on page 123.

Figures 7-8A and 7-8B illustrate changes in the contractile filaments, or Z-lines, which are the points of contact and support for the contractile proteins, before (A) and after (B) a marathon race. They provide structural support for the transmission of force when the muscle fibers are activated

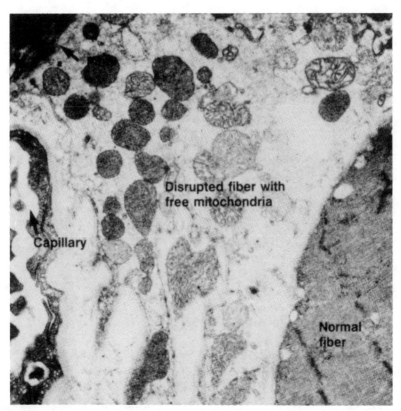

Figure 7-7 An electronmicrograph of a muscle sample taken immediately after a marathon, showing the disruption of the cell membrane in one muscle fiber (from Hagerman, et al., 1984).

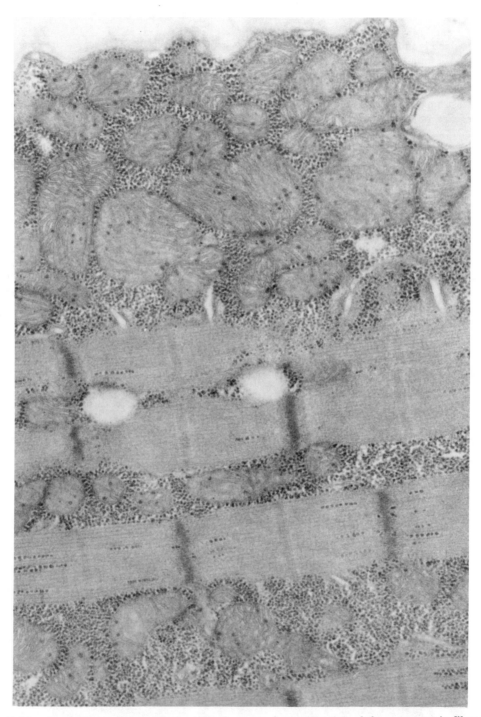

Figure 7–8A An electronmicrograph showing the normal arrangement of the actomyosin filaments and Z-line configuration in the muscle of a runner before a marathon race (from Hagerman, et al., 1984).

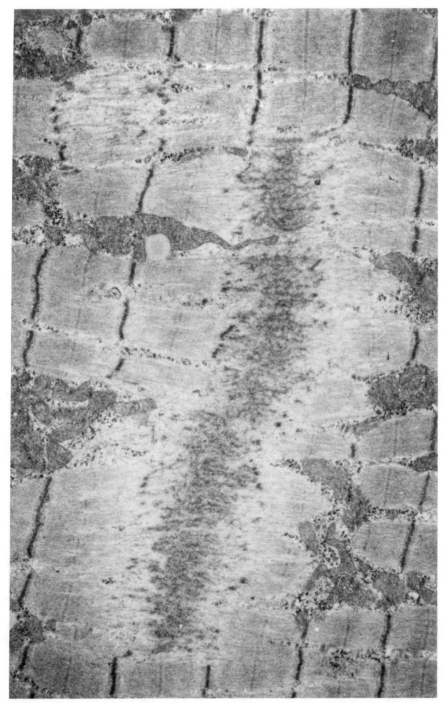

Figure 7–8B   An example of Z-line streaming caused by the eccentric contractions of running. This sample of muscle was taken immediately after a marathon race (from Hagerman, et al., 1984).

to shorten. Figure 7–8A shows the normal ultrastructure of the muscle fiber before the marathon race, with the Z-lines intact. Figure 7–8B shows the Z-lines after the marathon, pulled apart as a result of the force of eccentric contractions or the stretching of tightened muscle fibers.

Although the effects of muscle damage on performance are not fully understood, experts generally agree that it may be, in part, responsible for the localized muscle pain, tenderness, and swelling associated with muscle soreness. There is, however, no evidence that this condition is directly linked to the symptoms of muscle soreness. It is possible that blood enzyme levels rise and muscle fibers are damaged frequently during exercise, without symptoms of muscle soreness.

White blood cells, or eosinophils, serve as a defense against foreign materials that enter the body or conditions that threaten the normal function of its tissues. Since the white blood cell count tends to rise following activities that induce muscle soreness, some investigators have suggested that soreness is the result of an inflammatory reaction within the muscle. However, the link between these reactions and muscle soreness is not clearly established. Efforts to block the inflammatory reaction in muscle with drugs have been unsuccessful in reducing either the amount of muscle soreness or the degree of inflammation (Kuipers et al. 1985). Thus, no link can be made between muscle soreness and these observed inflammatory reactions.

While actual structural damage is a possible outcome of certain types of explosive or violent exercise, it is suspected that this would not account for all cases of muscle soreness. The "spasm theory" is a theory for muscle soreness suggested by de Vries (1974). According to de Vries, exercise brings about localized muscle ischemia (deficiency of blood), the ischemia causes pain, the pain generates increased reflex motor activity, greater motor activity creates even greater local muscle tension, resulting in even greater degrees of ischemia. His research supports this theory, and he has also found that static stretching exercises help to prevent soreness, as well as to relieve soreness when it is present.

This is an attractive theory to explain the basic cause of muscle soreness. The theory fails, however, to explain two phenomena. First, muscle soreness will usually haunt the athlete only during the initial stages of training—the first week or two. Following this period, the athlete has relatively little trouble with soreness, even though he or she may be working at substantially higher absolute and relative work loads. The spasm theory does not seem to explain this phenomenon.

Second, isokinetic strength training has produced an interesting and an unexpected outcome. Little or no muscle soreness has been found following exhaustive bouts of isokinetic exercise. Talag (1973) investigated the relationship between muscle soreness and eccentric, concentric, and isometric contractions. She found that a group training solely with eccentric contractions experienced extreme muscle soreness, while the isometric- and concentric-contraction groups experienced little soreness with their training. The fact that isokinetic procedures use only concentric contractions with a passive recovery, combined with the results from the preceding study, suggest that muscle soreness is unique to those activities that have a component of eccentric contraction. This has been further explored by Schwane, et al. (1983a and b), who had their subjects run on a treadmill for 45 minutes, both on a ten percent downhill grade at 57 percent of their maximal oxygen uptake, and on a level grade at 78 percent of their maximal oxygen uptake. There was no muscle soreness associated with the level running, but considerable soreness within 24 to 48 hours following the downhill running, even though the blood lactate levels were higher with level running.

In 1984, Armstrong conducted a review of the possible mechanisms for exercise-induced delayed-onset muscular soreness (DOMS). He concluded that DOMS is associated with elevations in plasma enzymes, myoglobinemia, and abnormal muscle histology and ultrastructure. He developed a model of DOMS which proposed that: a) high tensions in the contractile/elastic system of muscle result in structural damage; b) this cell membrane damage leads to a disruption of calcium-ion homeostasis in the injured fibers, resulting in necrosis, which peaks about 48 hours after exercise; and c) the products of macrophage activity and intracellular contents accumulate in the interstitium, which, in turn, stimulate the free nerve endings of the group IV sensory neurons in the muscle. This process appears to be accentuated in eccentric exercise, where large forces are distributed over relatively small, cross-sectional areas of the muscle.

MUSCULAR TRAINING PROCEDURES

Improvement in strength, power, and muscular endurance will result from muscle training programs. There are two basic types of muscle training: static or isometric training, and dynamic training. Dynamic training can be broken down further into the categories of isotonic, isokinetic, and variable-resistance training. Each will result in substantial increases in strength and power, but only isotonic, isokinetic, and variable resistance procedures increase muscular endurance. Additionally, a muscle can contract **concentrically,** where the muscle shortens, and **eccentrically,** where the muscle lengthens. Using the two-arm curl with a barbell as an example, lifting the weight from the arms fully extended to the fully-flexed position would be an example of a concentric contraction of the elbow flexor muscles. Lowering the weight from the fully-flexed to the fully-extended position would be an example of an eccentric contraction of the same elbow flexor muscles. It is often incorrectly assumed that the elbow extensors are responsible for lowering the weight, since the elbow is moving from a flexed to an extended position. The elbow flexors perform a controlled lengthening, or eccentric contraction, to slow the lowering of the weight, overcoming the effects of gravity.

Isometric Training Procedures

Isometric training procedures follow the theory that strength can be efficiently gained by training the muscle, or muscle group, against a fixed, immovable resistance. This concept evolved in the early twentieth century, but gained greater popularity and support in the mid-1950s as a result of the work of Hettinger and Müller (1953) in Germany. Their initial studies indicated that tremendous gains in strength would result from isometric training procedures, and, in fact, these gains would exceed those resulting from the more traditional isotonic procedures. This caused a consider-

able change in the training patterns during this era; most athletes switched exclusively to isometric training or combined isometric training with isotonic training. Hettinger and Müller claimed increases by five percent of the original strength value per week as a result of one, six-second contraction per day at only 67 percent of maximum contraction strength. Supposedly, little difference in improvement resulted when the tension was increased to 100 percent of maximum contraction strength, or when repeated exercises totaling 45 seconds were completed.

Subsequent research was unable to confirm the original work by Hettinger and Müller. Most of the later studies demonstrated sizeable strength increases with isometric exercises, but not increases of the five percent per week magnitude reported in the original studies. However, it is difficult to use the percentage improvement as an objective evaluation of the value of any program. This is due to the widely-accepted belief that the closer one is to his or her theoretical maximum strength, the more difficult it is to show a high percentage improvement in strength. The further one is from his or her theoretical maximum, the easier it is to demonstrate substantial improvement. Thus, the same procedure or program may result in a five percent increase in a group of highly-trained athletes and a 20 percent increase in a group of sedentary, unconditioned individuals.

Those early studies, which followed the original work by Hettinger and Müller, appeared to support their contention that it does not require a contraction of 100 percent of maximum contraction strength or more than one, six-second contraction to attain significant gains in strength (Clarke, 1973). One study compared two groups, one group exercising at 67 percent of maximum contraction strength one, six-second contraction per day, and the other at 80 percent of maximum contraction strength with five, six-second contractions per day (Rarick and Larsen, 1958). Both groups made significant gains in strength, but there were no differences between the groups in their increases in strength. However, studies by Müller and Rohmert (1963) suggest that, while the 67-percent of maximum contraction held for six seconds once a day will increase strength, the more demanding routine of six-second contractions at 100 percent of maximum contraction strength, repeated five to ten times, gives substantially greater strength gains. Obviously, additional research is necessary to gain an understanding of which is the best routine for maximizing strength gains. Until then, it appears the best results can be obtained by using maximum, or near-maximum contractions, held for a period of six seconds, or until all muscle fibers can be recruited, and repeated several times per day (Atha, 1982).

Several studies have indicated that the gains in strength with isometric training are specific to the joint angle trained (Clarke, 1974a). As an example, performing isometric training at a 90-degree angle in the biceps curl will lead to substantial strength gains at that particular angle, but will result in only small increases at 45 degrees and 135 degrees in that same range of motion. While other studies have not supported this finding, in order to optimize training, it seems justified to suggest that the athlete perform a series of five to ten, six-second maximal contractions, at each of three angles in the full range of motion. Otherwise, strength gains will be limited to a rather small portion of the total range of motion.

Specific isometric exercises will not be reviewed in this book, since they can easily be designed to fit the specific needs of the athlete. Also, since there are no equipment needs, simple props, such as chairs and doorways, can be improvised to provide suitable resistance. An isometric power rack can be constructed inexpensively and used for a wide variety of exercises. Two four × four-inch stationary posts with holes drilled every two to three inches along the length of the post, and several bars to insert into the holes to provide the static resistance to the exercise, are all that is needed.

An interesting concept in the area of isometrics, introduced in the early 1960s, is referred to as functional isometric training. O'Shea (1969) has devoted an entire chapter to this concept in his book, *Scientific Principles and Methods of Strength Fitness*. A power rack is used. The barbell is placed on the bars of the power rack and additional bars, or pins, are placed two to four inches above the bars, supporting the barbell. The athlete gets into the starting position, executes a fast isotonic movement through the two to four

inches, and then holds the barbell isometrically against the upper bars or pins for three to five seconds. Thus, functional isometric training is a combination of both isometrics and a short, explosive period of isotonics. In performing this system of training, it is important to isolate that muscle group that is to be trained. As an example, it is better to perform an overhead press in a sitting position in order to isolate the upper-body muscles and eliminate unwanted assistance from the legs. Little, if any, research has been conducted to date on the advantages of functional isometric training over the more traditional procedures.

Isotonic Training Procedures

Traditionally, **isotonic training procedures** have involved the use of weights in the form of barbells, dumbbells, and pulleys. Weight training procedures using the isotonic concept date back as far as recorded history and are even mentioned in Greek mythology. According to mythology, Milo of Crotona desired to become the strongest man in the world. When he was a young boy, he began lifting a young bull once a day and continued lifting it daily until the bull was fully grown. Milo eventually developed enough strength to lift the full-grown bull and to carry it around on his shoulders.

This story, although mythical, does illustrate two important, basic concepts in isotonic muscle training: the concept of overload and the concept of progressive resistance exercise. The concept of **overload** refers to the fact that in order to gain strength through muscle training procedures, it is necessary to load the muscles beyond that point to which they are normally loaded. Consider the example of an assembly line worker who must transfer a seventy-five-pound object from a conveyor belt into a packing carton. For his first few days on the job, this is a considerable stress and his muscles are taxed to near-capacity. As a result, the strength of his muscles increases to the point where he can handle this task with ease, a process that may take several months. At this point, however, his muscle strength levels off and does not continue to increase. If the factory suddenly shifted to ninety-pound objects, this would constitute an overload and he would then continue to gain in strength. Thus, the muscles must be taxed beyond so-called "normal" levels of work in order for significant increases in strength to occur.

The concept of **progressive resistance exercise** was illustrated earlier by Milo—as the muscles become stronger, they must work against a proportionately greater resistance to gain further increases in strength. In essence, this is the systematic application of the overload principle. As an example, a young man who initially performs only ten repetitions of a bench press using 150 pounds of weight, will, within a week or two of weight-training, be able to increase his repetitions for the same weight to fourteen or fifteen. If he then adds five pounds of weight to the bar, giving him a total of 155 pounds, his repetitions will drop to between eight and ten. As he continues to train, the repetitions continue to increase, and within another week or two, he is ready to add an additional five pounds of weight. Thus, there is a progressive increase in the amount of weight, or resistance, lifted.

DeLorme (1945), and later DeLorme and Watkins (1948), have been credited with the initial efforts to systemize isotonic training procedures. Their primary interests were in the areas of physical medicine and rehabilitation. The DeLorme and Watkins system emphasized the use of low resistance and high repetitions to develop muscular endurance. Initially, it was suggested that the subject do 70 to 100 repetitions divided into ten sets of ten repetitions per set. Later, this was modified to the traditional DeLorme system, in which three sets of ten repetitions were performed. The ten-repetition maximum (10-RM) was thus established. This represents the greatest resistance that can be lifted ten, but not more than ten, consecutive times. The first set was then performed at a resistance equal to 50 percent of the 10-RM, the second set at 75 percent of the 10-RM, and the third at 100 percent of the 10-RM. The amount of weight used was adjusted, periodically, as strength increased. This was determined by the individual's success in the third set, when lifting one 10-RM. If he or she could lift this weight fourteen to fifteen times, it no longer represented the 10-RM, and a new, heavier weight, or resistance, was used.

Zinovieff (1951) proposed an alternate technique, since he felt the DeLorme technique had inherent weaknesses. He felt that it was difficult to maintain the quality of contraction in the last set at a full resistance of 10-RM, because of the impaired range of motion and painful joints with maximal contraction. He proposed the Oxford technique, which consisted of a total of one hundred contractions, divided into ten sets of ten repetitions each, the first being performed at 10-RM. Subsequent sets were performed at a lowered resistance to match the decrease in strength that accompanies fatigue. Theoretically, this allowed the individual to do all ten sets at 10-RM, since the decrease in resistance (theoretically) matched the decrease in strength.

Over the years, research has attempted to identify the best possible combination of sets, repetitions, and resistance to maximize strength gains resulting from isotonic training. From these findings, it would appear that isotonic training should be performed at 5- to 7-RM, with three sets being executed per training session, in order to maximize strength gains. Training frequency should be three times per week, although this can be increased to five times per week if the muscles have been preconditioned to take this additional stress.

A new form of isotonic training, **plyometrics,** became popular during the late 1970s and early 1980s. Proposed to bridge the gap between speed and strength, plyometrics uses the stretch reflex to facilitate the recruitment of additional motor units and loads both the elastic and contractile components of muscle. Plyometrics has been referred to as bounce loading or rebounding jumping. As an example, to develop knee extensor muscle strength, the athlete jumps from a 24-inch high box to the ground, lands with the knees in a state of partial flexion, for instance at 90 degrees, then rebounds with an explosive upward movement by forceful maximal contraction of the knee extensor muscles. There are a number of variations that can be performed, including repetitive jumping on and off of a 12-inch box, and jumping with weight belts attached to the body. There is little research available to allow an objective evaluation of the benefits of plyometrics at this time.

Another popular form of isotonic training involves an emphasis on the eccentric phase of muscle contraction. Since eccentric strength is some 32 percent greater than concentric strength (Atha,

1982), one can load any given muscle more in the eccentric than in the concentric mode. Subjecting the muscle to this greater stimulus theoretically would produce greater gains in strength with training. While this is theoretically sound, the research to date has not been able to show any clear advantage of eccentric training over either concentric or isometric training (Atha, 1982).

Isokinetic and Variable Resistance Training Procedures

The concept of isokinetic muscle contraction was introduced by Perrine in 1968. It is a totally different form of muscle contraction when compared to the more traditional forms of isometric and isotonic contractions. First, in an isometric contraction, the contraction can always be performed at 100 percent of maximum contraction strength, but the strength that is gained is localized to the specific joint angle that is trained. In isotonic exercise, the resistance is constant throughout the full range of the movement, for instance, a loaded barbell. Since the maximum strength will vary according to the angle of pull and the length of the muscle throughout the entire range of motion, the contraction must be defined as submaximal during most of the range of motion, even if the resistance can be lifted only once. The lift would be maximal only at the weakest points in the range of motion. This is illustrated in Figure 7-9. Isokinetic exercise attempts to utilize the advantages and eliminate the disadvantages of both isometric and isotonic exercises.

In true **isokinetic exercise**, the resistance varies so that it is exactly matched to the force applied by the muscles. Thus, if one is able to motivate himself or herself to apply maximum force throughout the entire range of the lift, the resistance will vary directly with the force applied to allow a maximum contraction throughout this range. This is accomplished by having one exert force against a resistance that has a fixed speed of movement. No matter how much force is applied, the resistance will only move at a pre-set speed and no faster. As an example of this principle, if a car was placed on a hoist in a service station and raised to chest level, no matter how hard one pushed on the hoist, the car would not move upward. If, however, the hoist was moved further up-

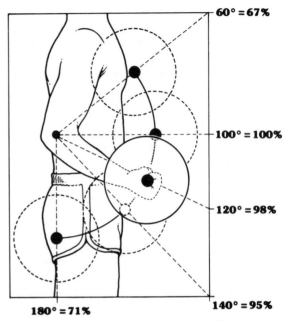

Figure 7-9 Variation in strength relative to the angle of contraction, with 100 percent representing the angle at which strength is optimal.

ward at a slow speed by its normal hydraulic operation, one could then push upward with maximal force from chest level to full extension, as in an overhead press. The car and hoist would move upward, but no faster than the hoist was set to go. Isokinetic training equipment works on the same principle.

The ability to vary the speed of contraction is another interesting aspect of the isokinetic concept. Traditionally, strength training has been performed either at zero velocity (isometric contraction) or at very low velocities (traditional isotonic 6-RM to 10-RM sets). Athletic performances, however, are typically performed at very high velocities. The question must then be raised: would muscle training at high velocities have a more favorable influence on the athlete's performance than the traditional, slow-training procedures of isometric and isokinetic exercise? It would appear that high-velocity strength training would develop substantial muscle power. Unfortunately, the few

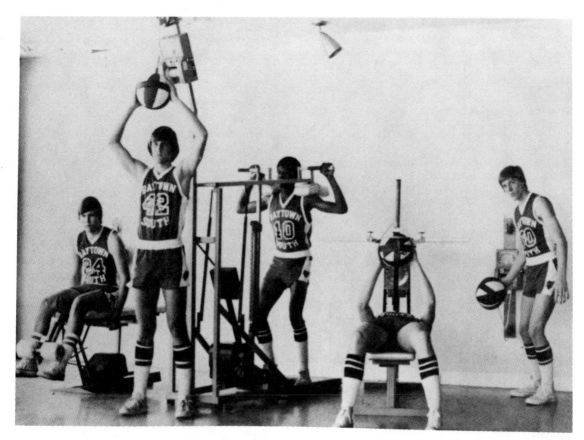

Figure 7–10 Mini-Gym specialized circuit for basketball (photo courtesy of Glen Hensen, Mini-Gym, Inc. Independence, MO 64051).

studies that have been conducted on various aspects of isokinetic exercise have not clearly demonstrated its potential in this area due to a lack (until recently) of pure measures of muscle power. Several studies have investigated the ability of isokinetic exercise to facilitate increases in muscle strength. Unfortunately, however, most of the limited work completed has been of a clinical nature.

Variable resistance training is a form of training where the resistance is systematically varied in an attempt to match the change in force-producing capabilities of the muscles as they act on a specific joint through its range of movement. Accommodating resistance training, a form of variable resistance training, attempts to match the resist-

ance precisely to the strength curve for that specific joint movement.

During the past ten years, a number of new training devices have been designed which have attempted to provide either direct isokinetic training or variable resistance training. Figure 7–10 illustrates the Mini-Gym device, which utilizes a rope that, when pulled, is released at a pre-set speed. The speed of the rope is controlled internally and is essentially independent of the force exerted during the exercise movement. As illustrated, this device can be used in a number of different configurations to simulate basic sports activities. Models are available which allow one to vary the speed of contraction. Nautilus strength-training machines (see

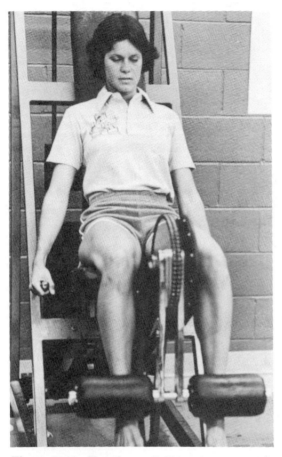

Figure 7-11 Nautilus variable resistance weight training machine.

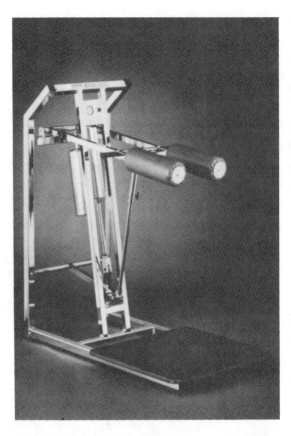

Figure 7-13 The CAM II pneumatic variable resistance machine (photo courtesy of Randy Keiser, Keiser Sports Health Equipment, Fresno, CA 93706).

Figure 7-12 Universal Gym, multiple station variable resistance training system (photo courtesy of Norman Barnes, Universal Gym, Cedar Rapids, IA 52406).

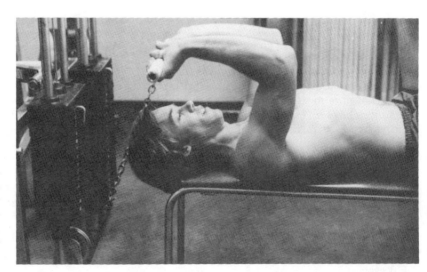

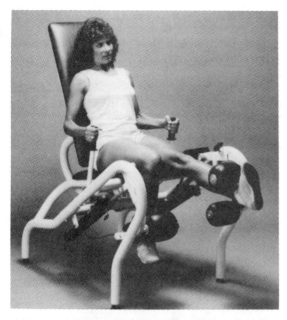

Figure 7-14 Hydra-Fitness hydraulic variable resistance machines (photo courtesy of Jerry Brentham, Hydra-Gym, Belton, TX 76513).

Figure 7-11) are very popular for the training of athletes. Special cams have been designed which attempt to duplicate the variations in force-producing capabilities of the muscle group as it contracts through the range of motion, providing a form of accommodating resistance. Universal Gym and Paramount have developed variable resistance systems which allow the use of their traditional weight stacks (see Figure 7-12). The CAM II system utilizes pneumatic or air resistance which is achieved with compressed air and pneumatic cylinders. Rather than "pumping iron," the athlete is pumping air! This system is illustrated in Figure 7-13. HydraFitness is another accommodating resistance device which controls the speed of movement by restricting the speed of movement of hydraulic fluid through a hydraulic cylinder. The speed of movement can be varied with this device (see Figure 7-14). A new strength training system was introduced in 1987 which is computerized and utilizes artificial intelligence. The Powercise equipment illustrated in Figure 7-15 actually

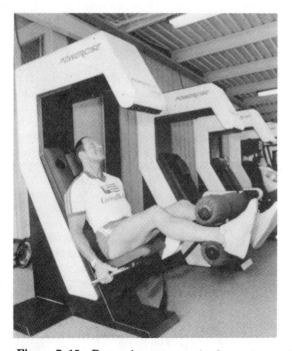
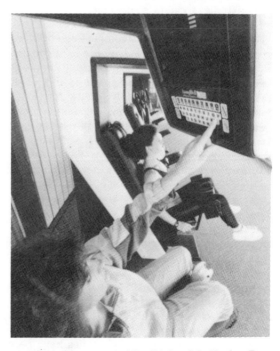

Figure 7-15 Powercise computerized exercise equipment (photos courtesy of Dr. Richard O. Keelor, Powercise, Houston, TX 77024).

coaches the individual through his or her workout, giving verbal encouragement, and stating when an increase in resistance is needed.

Comparison of Strength Training Procedures

From the discussion in the preceding sections, it is obvious that substantial strength gains can be obtained from each of the different muscle training procedures. Does any one of them offer a distinct advantage over the others? Does each provide equal gains in strength, power, and muscular endurance as compared to others, for an equal quantity of time and effort invested? These are questions that should be asked by the coach and the athlete, since they are both interested in obtaining the greatest benefit in the shortest time possible.

The majority of research that has been conducted to date in evaluating these different types of muscle training have dealt with isometric and isotonic training. This is to be expected, however, since isokinetic and variable resistance training are relatively new concepts and have not been explored in depth. However, there are sufficient numbers of studies to allow some general conclusions to be made.

The problem with making comparisons between types or systems of muscle training is in equalizing the intensity of training by equating work rates. Because of the principle of isometric or static contraction, to accurately equate work loads is nearly impossible. Irrespective of this problem, many studies have had reasonable success in their attempts to equate the training stimulus for purposes of accurate comparison. These studies have been summarized by both Clarke (1973) and Atha (1982). Isometric, isotonic, isokinetic, and variable resistance procedures produce substantial gains in muscular strength. While some studies indicate little or no difference between these procedures, most have demonstrated that isometric exercise provides smaller gains. Among isotonic, isokinetic, and variable resistance procedures, there appears to be no consistent difference in the magnitudes of the strength gains, when the appropriate controls have been used. Further, no one system or product has been found to be superior to any of the others when the studies have been well-controlled. Muscular endurance is more effec-

tively developed through isotonic, isokinetic, and variable resistance procedures, and recovery from muscular fatigue is faster in muscles that have been trained by these procedures. Isometric procedures appear to develop strength in only a limited portion of the total range of motion, therefore, isotonic, isokinetic, and variable resistance procedures will produce a more uniform development of strength throughout that range of motion. Isometric procedures can be used during a period of convalescence from injury. Normally, the athlete with a joint or bone injury is completely immobilized, and the lack of exercise will result in a reduction in both muscle size (atrophy) and strength. Isometric contractions involve no joint movement and can be safely and effectively used during the period of recovery from most injuries, to prevent substantial loss of muscle function.

In addition to such research findings, there are several practical considerations. Isometric exercises can be performed with little or no supportive apparatus, eliminating the need for expensive equipment. They can also be performed anywhere, at anytime, and the time requirement for completing a workout is considerably less than that for isotonic exercises. This would allow the coach the incentive to assign strength-conditioning exercises for athletes to perform at home, both in-season and off-season. On the negative side, isometric exercises present motivational problems. Unless the exercise is performed with elaborate testing equipment, it is impossible to quantify the amount of strength that is applied during the contraction. Furthermore, with training, it is difficult to demonstrate improvement. This lack of positive feedback has led many athletes to abandon their isometric programs.

Isometric exercises are potentially dangerous for older individuals and individuals who have diagnosed cardiovascular disease, such as coronary artery disease (heart disease), hypertension, or stroke. When performing isometric exercises, the individual typically closes the glottis, creating a very high pressure within the thoracic, or chest cavity. This is similar to taking in a full breath of air and then trying to exhale it as forcefully as possible with the mouth and nose closed. The resulting high pressure in the thoracic cavity makes it difficult, if not impossible, for the blood to return from the lower extremities, since the intrathoracic pressure will exceed the pressure in the inferior vena cava. This results in increased blood pressure and a reduced availability of blood for the heart and brain.

One advantage of isokinetic exercises over other forms of training is related to the problem of muscle soreness. While extreme soreness is present a day or two following muscle training with isometric, isotonic, and variable resistance exercise, little or no soreness has been noted with isokinetic exercises. The possible reason for this was discussed in one of the earlier sections in this chapter and is thought to result from the lack of an eccentric component with isokinetic exercise.

Circuit Training

Circuit training, developed in England in 1953, was designed as an all-purpose type of training program for the development of strength, power, muscular endurance, speed, agility, flexibility, and cardiovascular endurance (Morgan & Adamson, 1961). The concept has a built-in versatility, which allows the program to be varied to meet the needs of the individual, or the group. Logically, circuit training should be one of the most popular of the many training programs. Unfortunately, it has not been widely accepted in the United States.

Circuit training is a formal type of training in which one goes through a series of selected exercises or activities that are performed in sequence or in a circuit. Circuits can be set up inside gymnasia, exercise rooms, hallways, or outside on courts, fields, or on roof tops. There are usually six to ten stations in a circuit. An individual will perform a specific exercise at each station and then proceed to the next station. The idea is to progress through the circuit as rapidly as possible. Improvement is accomplished by decreasing the total time it takes to complete the circuit, increasing the amount of work accomplished at each station, or both. The stations are distributed throughout the area assigned to circuit training. The greater the distance between stations, the greater the degree of cardiovascular conditioning as one runs from one station to the next. An example of a circuit training program is illustrated in Table 7-1.

Various levels are established, depending on the skill level and ability of the group or individual. A group of highly-skilled and well-conditioned athletes would have higher levels of accomplishment than a group of sedentary college students who were attempting to get into condition. Start at the lowest level, level Red-1 from the example in Table 7-1. Go through the circuit a total of three times without stopping. The total time it takes to complete three repetitions at level Red-1 is recorded.

Table 7-1 Example of a Circuit Training Circuit.*

Target Times		Red—23 minutes				Blue—25 minutes			
Station Number	Exercise	Weight, lbs	Red Circuit Repetitions			Weight, lbs	Blue Circuit Repetitions		
			1	2	3		1	2	3
1	Bench press	60	8	10	12	80	8	10	12
2	Squat thrust		10	13	16		19	22	25
3	Chins		1	3	5		7	9	10
4	Stair climb		4	6	8		10	12	14
5	Two-arm curl	45	8	10	12	55	8	10	12
6	Half-squat	75	9	12	15	100	12	14	16
7	Sit-ups		10	14	18		20	25	30
8	Running lap		1	1	2		2	3	3

*Adapted from R. P. Sorani, *Circuit Training*. Dubuque, Iowa: William C. Brown Co., 1966. Reproduced by permission of the publisher.

If Red-1 is finished under the target time of 23 minutes, move to the next level, Red-2.

Circuit training offers a number of unique advantages. It combines a number of different components of training, thus **total fitness** is emphasized. It provides an interesting training environment for the athlete, and there are established times and levels to motivate the athlete to continue improving. The circuit can be modified to fit the needs of any one group or individual, it can be adapted within the time constraints of the individual, and it can accommodate large groups of individuals at a relatively low expense. Progression in all activities is a likely result of circuit training.

In designing a circuit, first establish the training needs of the athletes who will be using the circuit. Adapt the circuit to fit the specific needs of the individuals, if possible. Identify an area that can be used for the circuit, ideally where permanent stations can be accommodated in the space allotted. Arrange the stations in such an order that exercises for similar body areas do not follow one another sequentially. Alternate exercises with an upper-body strength exercise, flexibility exercise, muscular endurance exercise, lower-body strength exercise, and cardiovascular endurance exercise, in sequence. Place the station number and the specific instructions at each station. This information should also include a list of the various levels and the required weights and repetitions.

As mentioned, the trainer or coach who has a basic knowledge of the principles behind circuit training will find that it is one of the easiest training programs to implement. Once established, it requires little or no supervision, and can be an excellent adjunct to any regular training program, or it can function as a complete off-season training program in itself.

In 1976, Allen et al. investigated a new concept in training that has a great deal of application for off-season conditioning. They merged the circuit training concept with traditional weight training into a form of training now referred to as circuit weight training. Traditional weight training is usually performed in a slow, methodical manner, with very short work intervals and very long rest intervals. With circuit weight training, the individual works at 40 to 60 percent of his or her maximum strength, as determined by the one repetition maximum (1-RM), for periods of approximately 30 seconds, with 15-second rest intervals interspersed between work periods. The program begins at the first station, completing as many repetitions as possible in 30 seconds, take a 15-second rest to move to the next station, and then start the second 30-second work period. This continues until the six to eight stations in the circuit have been completed. This form of training has been demonstrated to provide modest increases in $\dot{V}O_2$ max; major increases in strength, muscular endurance, and flexibility; and substantial alterations in body composition, as increased lean weight, and decreased fat weight.

Gettman and Pollock (1981) have conducted an extensive review of the research that has been conducted in the area of circuit weight training through 1980. According to their summary, the major advantages of circuit weight training include: (1) it is an activity that attends to the major components of athletic fitness; (2) it can be conducted in a very small area (small room with a multi-station weight training machine); and (3) the complete workout (three sets) can be completed in less than 30 minutes. Further, the workout can be highly motivating!

MUSCULAR TRAINING AND ATHLETIC PERFORMANCE

Gaining strength, power, or muscular endurance simply for the sake of becoming stronger, more powerful, or possessing greater muscular endurance, is of relatively little importance to athletes, unless it will also translate into improvements in their athletic performance. The use of strength training by field-event athletes in track and competitive weight lifters intuitively makes a great deal of sense. What about the gymnast, distance runner, baseball player, high jumper, swimmer, or ballerina? Will muscular training assist them in preparation for their events, activities, or sport? Since training is costly in terms of time, athletes cannot afford to waste time on activities that will not result in better athletic performances. What do research findings indicate?

With regard to specific sports, muscular training appears to be a highly-desirable supplement to the general training program for almost any athlete. In three studies involving baseball, muscle training as a supplement to regular baseball practice resulted in significant improvements in throwing speed and in the speed for sprinting 90 feet. In a single study of softball, underhand throwing ability for distance was improved with functional, isometric exercises, as well as the endurance to maintain maximum distance for 80 underhand throws. In all of these studies, the improvements noted were significantly greater in the muscular training groups than in other groups who did not supplement their practice with muscular training.

Strength training programs have been a part of the conditioning programs for competitive swimmers for the past 50 years. This is in spite of the fact that lifting weights (isotonic, free-weights) does not produce significant improvements in swimming performance. Recent studies have shown that sprint swimming produces the same performance benefits as most other forms of strength training. This should not be interpreted to mean that strength is unimportant to swimming performance. To the contrary, there is a close relationship between upper body strength and sprint swimming performance. This simply means that the gains in strength needed for performance are achieved during regular swimming training, which often includes explosive, short sprints. Thus, specialized equipment is not needed to strength train for this sport.

In football, the influence of both isometric and isotonic strength training on the speed and force of the offensive football charge was investigated in a single study. The isometric group and the isotonic group improved significantly in both speed and the force of the offensive charge, while the control group did not improve on either test.

A number of studies have observed the influence of muscular training on the speed of movement. At one time, it was felt that muscular training would result in a muscle-bound, inflexible athlete and that speed would actually be decreased. Most subsequent studies have shown that speed can be improved with muscular training, although there are several studies with conflicting results. One study using isokinetic exercises found a substantial improvement in 40-yard dash speed, from 5.3 to 5.1 seconds, following eight weeks of training.

Many studies have investigated the influence of muscular training on the performance of general motor tasks. Most studies have found that isotonic training substantially improves vertical jumping ability, while isometric training does not. The standing long jump has also been found to improve with isotonic training. Campbell (1962) observed the effects of systematic isotonic exercise on the motor fitness of college football, basketball, and track and field squads during their competitive seasons. Motor fitness was assessed from a composite score consisting of performances for right grip, vertical jump, squat thrusts, pull-ups, sit-ups, 300-yard shuttle run, and 50-yard dash. Each team was divided into two groups: one group supplemented their training for the first half of the season with isotonic exercises, while the other group used only normal training procedures. At the midpoint of the season, the groups switched procedures. Isotonic training resulted in large gains in motor fitness, but the group that stopped weight training midseason had actually decreased in motor fitness when tested at the end of the season.

From such findings, muscle training does appear to have a great deal to offer athletes who wish to improve their performances. A word of caution must be inserted, however—only a handful of activities or sports have been studied. It is possible, but not too likely on the basis of the information presently available, that muscle training will not be beneficial for every athlete, event, activity, or sport. At this time, the best advice appears to be to proceed with caution, and if the results prove beneficial, a more aggressive approach can be taken. This is particularly true of skill sports (such as golf), or positions (such as baseball pitcher). Further, the concept of specificity of training must be considered. Is it better to strength train by simulating the movements used in the sport or activity, or will general strength training provide the same results? Research has not adequately addressed this issue. Refer to Table 7–2 on page 136 for suggested strength-training activities for selected sports.

Table 7-2 Strength Training Activities for Various Sports or Events.*

Column groups: Columns *Backstroke–Freestyle* fall under **Swimming**; columns *Sprinting–Discus and Shot Put* fall under **Track and Field**. All columns fall under **Sport, Activity, or Event**.

Movement	Baseball	Basketball	Golf	Gymnastics	Football	Soccer	Rowing	Tennis	Wrestling	Skiing	Hockey	Backstroke	Breaststroke	Butterfly	Freestyle	Sprinting	Hurdling	Javelin	Long jump	Distance running	Pole vault	High jump	Discus and Shot Put
Neck flexion and extension					X	X			X		X												
Shoulder shrug					X			X	X	X						X					X		
Military or overhead press			X	X				X	X					X		X							X
Behind the neck press												X	X										
Upright rowing	X	X	X	X			X	X			X	X	X	X		X					X	X	
Bent rowing				X				X						X			X						
Lat machine		X		X	X		X		X	X	X	X	X	X		X							
Triceps extension	X			X				X	X	X	X	X	X	X				X	X	X			X
Lateral arm raise	X	X			X						X										X		
Bent-arm pull-over	X	X					X	X				X	X	X				X	X		X	X	
Biceps curl		X					X																X
Dumbbell curl	X	X	X	X	X	X	X	X	X							X					X	X	X
Bench press		X			X			X		X		X	X	X		X			X	X	X	X	
Incline press	X		X	X	X		X					X	X	X				X	X	X	X	X	X
Parallel bar dip		X	X		X	X			X	X	X				X								
Back hyperextension				X	X			X			X	X			X	X							
Trunk extension	X							X		X	X	X				X							X
Weighted sit-ups	X	X	X		X	X	X	X	X	X	X							X	X	X	X	X	X
Hip flexion												X	X	X	X				X				
Stiff leg dead lift		X	X	X		X								X							X		
Knee flexion													X	X		X	X	X					
Knee extension	X			X	X				X	X	X	X				X	X	X	X			X	X
Squat	X	X	X		X	X	X		X														X
Hack squat			X	X				X	X	X	X	X	X	X	X	X	X	X	X	X	X	X	
Toe raise	X									X						X	X	X			X	X	

*Adapted from J. P. O'Shea, *Scientific Principles and Methods of Strength Fitness.* 2nd ed. Reading, MA.: Addison-Wesley Publishing Co., 1976. Reproduced by permission of the publisher.

SUMMARY

The athlete's performance can be separated into a number of individual components. The components of strength, power, and muscular endurance appear to be extremely important for most athletic performances. Strength is defined as the maximum ability to apply or to resist force. Power is the functional application of both strength and speed—power = force × velocity. Muscular endurance refers to the ability of a muscle, or group of muscles, to sustain either repeated or static contractions for an extended period of time.

Strength can be expressed either statically (isometric contraction) or dynamically (isotonic, isokinetic, or variable resistance contraction), and muscular contractions can either be concentric (shortening) or eccentric (lengthening). With muscle training programs, there are generally increases in strength, power, and muscular endurance. Static and dynamic training procedures result in marked gains in strength, but dynamic training appears to produce somewhat greater gains in strength and substantially greater gains in muscular endurance.

Maximum gains in isometric strength appear to come from five to ten, six-second isometric contractions at 100 percent of maximal strength, repeated at three different points in the full range of motion. Isotonic training is apparently maximized by performing three sets per day of each exercise at 5- to 7-RM. Research is too limited at this point to make recommendations relative to an optimal training procedure for isokinetic or variable resistance exercise. High-speed contraction does appear to be important, but it is too early to tell at this time. Training three to five days per week appears to be optimal for all strength-training procedures.

Circuit training is a unique concept, as it incorporates strength, power, muscular endurance, speed, agility, flexibility, and cardiovascular endurance training into the same workout. A circuit usually consists of six to ten stations, each focusing on one exercise, so that all areas of the body are covered in a complete circuit. The entire circuit should be completed as rapidly as possible, repeating the circuit three times. A specific amount of work is preassigned at each station. As one becomes better-conditioned, the amount of time it takes to complete the circuit is reduced and the amount of work accomplished at each station is increased. In addition, the circuit is designed for different levels of competence so that, with improvement, one moves up to the next highest level. Each successive level requires a greater amount of work at each station. Circuit weight training is a variation of general circuit training, applying the same principles in a weight training mode.

Strength gains result from changes occurring within the central nervous system as well as changes within the muscle itself. Facilitation of motor unit recruitment through reducing autogenic inhibition and/or increasing general neural traffic, as well as increased synchronization of motor unit firing, are possible neurogenic explanations for increased strength with training, particularly during the early stages of training. Possible myogenic factors include hypertrophy of individual muscle fibers through increases in myofibrils and filaments, and hyperplasia. Power is increased by gains in either or both strength and speed. Muscular endurance is increased through gains in muscular strength and probably through changes in local circulatory patterns as well.

Muscle soreness is a phenomenon that is now much better understood. One theory explains soreness on the basis of small tears in the muscle or its connective tissue. A second theory attributed soreness to localized muscle spasms. Neither theory appears to hold under all conditions. Recent findings suggest that soreness results predominantly from eccentric contraction types of exercises, or from activities or exercises that use eccentric contractions. It appears to be associated with major damage within the muscle cell which leads to disruptions of calcium-ion homeostasis in the injured fibers, resulting in necrosis, increased macrophage activity, and a stimulation of the free nerve endings.

Finally, muscle training has been shown to significantly improve performance in sport and in a number of motor activities. It seems obvious at this time that almost all athletes, no matter what their sport, can gain substantial benefits from muscle training. For many sports, however, strength training programs can be developed using the specific activities of the sport (sprint running and sprint swimming) rather than specialized equipment. Regardless of the approach to developing muscle strength, the transfer of strength gains to athletic performance appears to depend on the specificity of the training program.

STUDY QUESTIONS

1. Define and differentiate between strength, power, and muscular endurance. How do each of these components relate to athletic performance?
2. What is the difference between eccentric contraction and concentric contraction?
3. What is the importance of power in specific sports or events?
4. Define isometric, isotonic, isokinetic, and variable resistance training.
5. What is the optimal routine for isometric strength training?
6. Define the overload principle and the principle of progressive resistance exercise.
7. Describe two distinct advantages of isokinetic or variable resistance training over isometric and isotonic training.
8. How does a muscle increase in size?
9. Discuss the different theories which have attempted to explain how muscles gain strength with training. What are the potential myogenic and neurogenic components?
10. What is the physiological explanation for muscle soreness?
11. Should all athletes strength train? If your answer is no, what criteria should be used to determine who should strength train?
12. What is circuit training? How does this differ from circuit weight training?
13. What advantages might circuit training, or circuit weight training, have over other training procedures used for developing strength, power, and muscular endurance?

REFERENCES

Abraham, W. M. (1979). Exercise-induced muscle soreness. *Physician and Sportsmedicine, 7*, 57–60.

Allen, T. E., Byrd, R. J., & Smith, D. P. (1976). Hemodynamic consequences of circuit weight training. *Research Quarterly, 47*, 299–306.

Armstrong, R. B. (1984). Mechanisms of exercise-induced delayed-onset muscular soreness: A brief review. *Medicine and Science in Sports and Exercise, 6*, 529–538.

Atha, J. (1982). Strengthening muscle. *Exercise and Sport Sciences Reviews, 9*, 1–73.

Berger, R. A. (1962). Effects of varied weight training programs on strength. *Research Quarterly, 33*, 168–181.

Berger, R. A. (1962). Comparison of static and dynamic strength increases. *Research Quarterly, 33*, 329–333.

Campbell, R. L. (1962). Effects of supplemental weight training on the physical fitness of athletic squads. *Research Quarterly, 33*, 343–348.

Clarke, D. H. (1973). Adaptations in strength and muscular endurance resulting from exercise. *Exercise and Sport Sciences Reviews, 1*, 73–102.

Clarke, H. H. (1973, January). Toward a better understanding of muscular strength. *Physical Fitness Research Digest.* President's Council on Physical Fitness and Sports. Washington, D.C.: U.S. Government Printing Office.

Clarke, H. H. (1974a, January). Development of muscular strength and endurance. *Physical Fitness Research Digest.* President's Council on Physical Fitness and Sports. Washington, D.C.: U.S. Government Printing Office.

Clarke, H. H. (1974b, October). Strength development and motor-sports improvement. *Physical Fitness Research Digest.* President's Council on Physical Fitness and Sports. Washington, D.C.: U.S. Government Printing Office.

Costill, D. L., Coyle, E. F., Fink, W. F., Lesmes, G. R., & Witzmann, F. A. (1979). Adaptations in skeletal muscle following strength training. *Journal of Applied Physiology, 46*, 96–99.

DeLorme, T. L. (1945). Restoration of muscle power by heavy resistance exercise. *Journal of Bone and Joint Surgery, 27*, 645–667.

DeLorme, T. L., & Watkins, A. L. (1948). Technics of progressive resistance exercise. *Archives of Physical Medicine, 29*, 263–273.

deVries, H. A. (1986). *Physiology of exercise for physical education and athletics* (3rd ed.). Dubuque, Iowa: William C. Brown.

Edgerton, V. R. (1976). Neuromuscular adaptations to power and endurance work. *Canadian Journal of Applied Sports Sciences, 1*, 49–58.

Gettman, L. R., & Pollock, M. L. (1981). Circuit weight training: A critical review of its physiological benefits. *Physician and Sportsmedicine, 9*, 44–60.

Goldberg, A. L., Etlinger, J. D., Goldspink, D. F., & Jablecki, C. (1975). Mechanisms of work-induced hypertrophy of skeletal muscle. *Medicine and Science in Sports, 7*, 248–261.

Gollnick, P. D., Armstrong, R. B., Saltin, B., Saubert IV, C. W., Sembrowich, W. L., & Shepherd, R. E. (1973). Effect of training on enzyme activity and fiber composition of human skeletal muscle. *Journal of Applied Physiology, 34*, 107–111.

Gollnick, P. D., Parsons, D., Riedy, M., & Moore, R. L. (1983). Fiber number and size in overloaded chicken anterior latissimus dorsi muscle. *Journal of Applied Physiology, 54*, 1292–1297.

Gollnick, P. D., Timson, B. F., Moore, R. L., & Riedy, M. (1981). Muscular enlargement and number of fibers in skeletal muscles of rats. *Journal of Applied Physiology, 50*, 936–943.

Gonyea, W. J. (1980). Role of exercise in inducing increases in skeletal muscle fiber number. *Journal of Applied Physiology, 48,* 421–426.

Gonyea, W. J., Ericson, G. C., & Bonde-Petersen, F. (1977). Skeletal muscle, fiber splitting induced by weightlifting exercise in cats. *Acta Physiologica Scandinavica, 19,* 105–109.

Gonyea, W. J., Sale, D. G., Gonyea, F. B., & Mikesky, A. (1986). Exercise induced increases in muscle fiber number. *European Journal of Applied Physiology, 55,* 137–141.

Green, H. J., Klug, G. A., Reichmann, H., Seedorf, U., Wiehrer, W., & Pette, D. (1984). Exercise-induced fibre type transitions with regard to myosin, parvalbumin, and sarcoplasmic reticulum in muscles of the rat. *Pflugers Archives, 400,* 432–438.

Hagerman, F.C., Hikida, R. S., Staron, R. S., Sherman, W. M., & Costill, D. L. (1984). Muscle damage in marathon runners. *Physician and Sportsmedicine, 12,* 39–48.

Hettinger, T. (1961). *Physiology of strength.* Springfield, IL: Charles C. Thomas.

Hettinger, T., Müller, E. A., (1953). Muskelleistung and muskel training. *Arbeitsphysiology, 15,* 111–126.

Ikai, M., & Fukunaga, T. (1968). Calculation of muscle strength per unit cross sectional area of human muscle by means of ultrasonic measurements. *Internationale Zeitschrift Angewandte Physiology, 26,* 26–32.

Jensen, C. R. & Fisher, A. G. (1979). *Scientific basis of athletic conditioning* (2nd ed.). Philadelphia: Lea and Febiger.

Jesse, J. P. (1979). Misuse of strength development programs in athletic training. *Physician and Sportsmedicine, 7,* 46–52.

Kuiper, H., Keizer, H. A., Verstappen, F. T. J., & Costill, D. L. (1985). Influence of a prostaglandin-inhibiting drug on muscle soreness after eccentric work. *International Journal of Sports Medicine, 6,* 336–339.

Lamb, D. R. (1984). *Physiology of exercise: Responses and adaptations* (2nd ed.) New York: MacMillan Publishing Co.

Larsson, L., & Ansved, T. (1985). Effects of long-term physical training and detraining on enzyme histochemical and functional skeletal muscle characteristics in man. *Muscle Nerve, 8,* 714–722.

Larsson, L., & Tesch, P. A. (1986). Motor unit fibre density in extremely hypertrophied skeletal muscles in man. *European Journal of Applied Physiology, 55,* 130–136.

Lesmes, G. R., Costill, D. L., Coyle, E. F., & Fink, W. J. (1978). Muscle strength and power changes during maximal isokinetic training. *Medicine and Science in Sports, 10,* 266–269.

McDonagh, M. J. N., & Davies, C. T. M. (1984). Adaptive response of mammalian skeletal muscle to exercise with high loads. *European Journal of Applied Physiology, 52,* 139–155.

Morgan, R. E., & Adamson, G. T. (1961). *Circuit weight training.* London: G. Bell and Sons.

Müller, E. A., & Rohmert, W. (1963). Die geschwindigkeit der muskelkraft zunahme bei isometrischen training. *Internationale Zeitschrift Angewandte Physiology, 19,* 403–419.

O'Shea, J. P. (1969). *Scientific principles and methods of strength fitness.* Reading, MA: Addison-Wesley Pub. Co.

Perrine, J. J. (1968). Isokinetic exercise and the mechanical energy potentials of muscle. *Journal of Health, Physical Education, and Recreation, 39 (No. 5),* 40–44.

Pette, D. (1984). Activity-induced fast to slow transitions in mammalian muscle. *Medicine and Science in Sports and Exercise, 16,* 517–528.

Rarick, G. L., & Larsen, G. L. (1958). Observations on frequency and intensity of isometric muscular effort in developing strength in post-pubescent males. *Research Quarterly, 29,* 333–341.

Rasch, P. J., & Morehouse, L. E. (1957). Effect of static and dynamic exercise on muscular strength and hypertrophy. *Journal of Applied Physiology, 11,* 29–34.

Salmons, S. & Henriksson, J. (1981). The adaptive response of skeletal muscle to increased use. *Muscle Nerve, 4,* 95–105.

Schwane, J. A., Johnson, S. R., Vandenakker, C. B., & Armstrong, R. B. (1983). Delayed-onset muscular soreness and plasma CPK and LDH activities after downhill running. *Medicine and Science in Sports and Exercise, 15,* 51–56.

Schwane, J. A., Watrous, B. G., Johnson, S. R., & Armstrong, R. B. (1983). Is lactic acid related to delayed-onset muscle soreness? *Physician and Sportsmedicine, 11* (No. 3), 124–131.

Simoneau, J. A., Lortie, G., Boulay, M. R., Marcotte, M., Thibault, M. C., & Bouchard, C. (1985). Human skeletal muscle fiber type alteration with high-intensity intermittent training. *European Journal of Applied Physiology, 54,* 250–253.

Sorani, R. P. (1966). *Circuit training.* Dubuque, IA: William C. Brown Co.

Steinhaus, A. H. (1968, May). Inhibitory mechanisms operative in the expression of human strength. Paper presented at the Annual Meeting, American College of Sports Medicine, Pennsylvania State University.

Talag, T. S. (1973). Residual muscular soreness as influenced by concentric, eccentric and static contractions. *Research Quarterly, 44,* 458–469.

Taylor, N. A. S., & Wilkinson, J. G. (1986). Exercise-induced skeletal muscle growth: Hypertrophy or hyperplasia? *Sports Medicine, 3,* 190–200.

Tesch, P. A., & Karlsson, J. (1985). Muscle fiber types and size in trained and untrained muscles of elite athletes. *Journal of Applied Physiology, 59,* 1716–1720.

Tesch, P. A., & Larsson, L. (1982). Muscle hypertrophy in bodybuilders. *European Journal of Applied Physiology, 49,* 301–306.

Timson, B. F., Bowlin, B. K., Dudenhoeffer, G. A., & George, J. B. (1985). Fiber number, area, and composition of mouse soleus muscle following enlargement. *Journal of Applied Physiology, 58,* 619–624.

Withers, R. T. (1970). Effect of varied weight-training loads on the strength of university freshman. *Research Quarterly, 41,* 110–114.

Zinovieff, A. N. (1951). Heavy resistance exercises: The Oxford technique. *British Journal of Physical Medicine, 14,* 129–132.

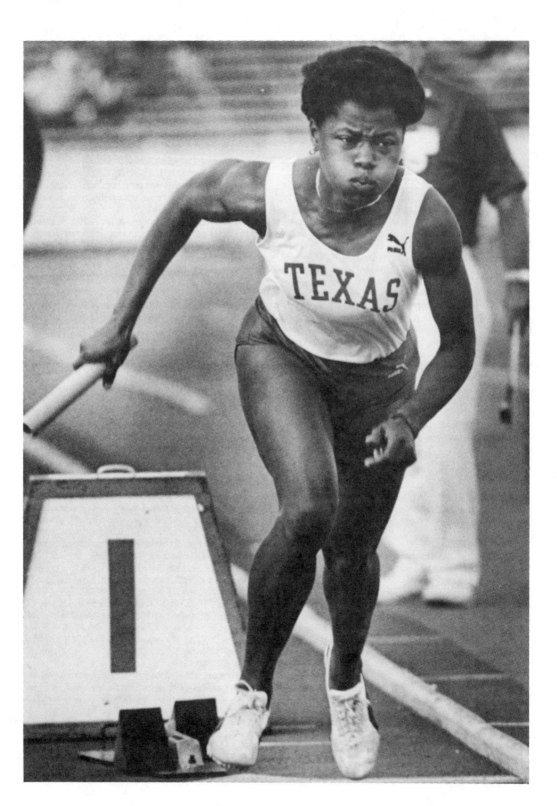

8

Muscular Adaptations to Anaerobic and Aerobic Training

INTRODUCTION

Both sprint and endurance events depend to a large extent on the muscle's ability to generate force and to maintain a constant energy supply. The stress of chronic exercise results in adaptations within and around the muscle fibers that make them more tolerant of strenuous effort. In the following discussion we will describe the changes that occur with training, which give the muscles greater endurance capacity. The peripheral changes result in greater energy production and more efficient metabolic waste removal, thereby reducing factors considered responsible for fatigue.

In general, physical training imposes stress on the body tissues, in particular, the muscles. Chronic muscular activity, which occurs during training, can be considered a positive form of stress because it stimulates growth and improves muscular performance. Most of the changes that occur in the muscle as a result of training are gradual and occur over several weeks or months. The magnitude of these muscular adaptations is somewhat proportional to the amount of exercise performed during training. Unfortunately, this fact has led many coaches and athletes to overwork the muscles by imposing unrealistic training demands on the athlete. This results in a breakdown in the

processes of adaptation (overtraining, see Chapter 11). The key concept to remember is that the muscles will adapt optimally to exercise that moderately exceeds its capacity, necessitating a gradual progression in training load in order to maximize performance. At the same time it must be realized that there is a limit to the body's ability to adapt to physical training. In other words, there is a limit to the physiological and anatomical development that can be achieved with training, a factor that is probably determined by genetics. We were not *all* created with the same adaptive potential for exercise. Consequently, the factors that control the improvements with training differ from individual to individual, explaining why athletes who exercise under the same training regimen often show different levels of improvement.

AEROBIC TRAINING

The improvements in endurance that occur with daily aerobic training appear to be the result of changes in both central and peripheral circulation (such as cardiac output, muscle blood flow) and muscle metabolism (such as muscle respiratory capacity). Chapter 9 will detail the important changes that take place in the circulatory system with endurance training. Training adaptations within the muscles range from an improvement in blood flow around the fibers to dramatic changes in oxidative metabolism.

Fiber Composition

Despite the extensive reliance on the slow-twitch (ST) fibers during distance running, these fibers do not appear to grow any larger than the fast-twitch (FT) fibers. There is, however, considerable variability in the size of these muscle fibers among different athletes. Some individuals have unusually large ST fibers, while others have large FT fibers. This observation may be of only academic importance since the endurance athlete's muscle size seems to have little relationship to either aerobic capacity or performance. The size of the fibers may be more critical in events that demand greater power and strength, such as sprinting and weight lifting.

There is some question as to whether endurance training can increase the number of ST fibers. In a few cases, athletes who have undergone knee surgery followed by several weeks of immobilization, have shown a remarkable decrease in the percentage of ST fibers. Most studies, however, have shown that the percentage of ST and FT fibers does not change with endurance training. Although few studies have examined young children over many years of training, current evidence tends to support the concept that fiber types are not interconvertible; that is, endurance training will not convert FT fibers to ST fibers. Some subtle changes among the subtypes of fast-twitch fibers (type FT_a and FT_b) have been determined. Many years of endurance training seem to convert the FT_b fibers to FT_a fibers. Neither the cause nor the effect for this change is known. Various studies have suggested that the FT_b fibers are used less frequently than the FT_a fibers, and for that reason have a lower aerobic capacity. It seems that long duration exercise may recruit the FT_b fibers into action, demanding output in a manner normally expected of the FT_a fibers. As a result, the FT_b fibers begin to take on some of the characteristics of the FT_a fibers. This subtle conversion of FT_b to FT_a fibers may simply reflect the greater use of the fast-twitch fibers during long, exhaustive training runs.

It is unlikely that endurance exercise will convert FT fibers to ST fibers, since such a change would require a structural modification of the size and function of the motor nerve that controls the muscle cell. As noted in Chapter 1, fiber type is determined by the type and size of the neurons (nerve cell) that innervate each muscle fiber. The only methods known to change the muscle fiber type are: (1) surgical change of the nerve input to the muscle fiber, giving an FT fiber a slow-twitch nerve, or (2) chronic, electrical stimulation, sending false signals to the muscle fibers.

Oxygen Delivery

One of the most important changes that occurs during training is an increase in the number of capillaries surrounding each muscle fiber (see Figure 8-1). As shown in Figure 8-2, endurance-trained men may have 50 percent more capillaries in their leg muscles than sedentary individuals. With eight weeks of conditioning, the number of capillaries increased 15 percent. An increase in the number of capillaries allows greater exchange of gases, heat, and fuels between the blood and the working muscle fibers. This increased exchange maintains an environment conducive to energy production and repeated muscle contractions. It appears that most of the increase in muscle capillary density occurs within the first few months of training. Little research has been performed to determine what changes occur with longer periods of training.

Once oxygen has entered the muscle fiber, it is transported within the cell by myoglobin, a compound similar to hemoglobin. Myoglobin's main function is to deliver oxygen from the cell membrane to the mitochondria. It has been postulated that myoglobin also acts as a storage compartment for oxygen, and supports aerobic metabolism by releasing oxygen to the mitochondria when oxygen becomes limited during muscle contraction. Other researchers have suggested that myoglobin is of little importance in endurance exercise, since this form of exercise does not deplete the intracellular oxygen content. Nevertheless, aerobic training increases the myoglobin content of the muscles to the same extent as other biochemical adaptations.

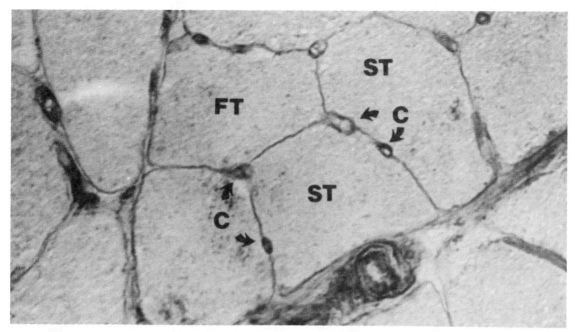

Figure 8-1 A microscopic view of a cross-section of muscle from the gastrocnemius muscle of an elite female marathon runner. Note the abundance of capillaries which surround each fiber, facilitating gas and nutrient exchange between the blood and the muscle.

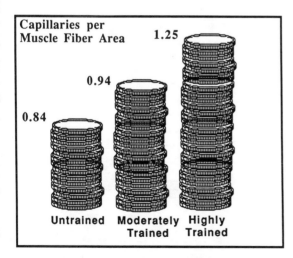

Status of Training

Figure 8-2 Average number of capillaries per 1000 μm^2 of muscle in sedentary (A), moderately active (B), and endurance trained (C) men (modified from Saltin, 1980).

Energy Production

As noted in Chapter 2, aerobic energy production is the exclusive responsibility of the mitochondria. Endurance training induces changes in the mitochondria, which will improve the capacity of the muscle fibers to produce ATP. In the laboratory it is possible to measure the aerobic capacity of a specimen of muscle tissue obtained by needle biopsy. By grinding the muscle sample in a solution containing other essential items, the mitochondria are stimulated to use oxygen and to produce ATP. As a result, it is possible to measure the maximal rate at which the muscle homogenate uses oxygen, referred to as the muscle's **respiratory capacity** or Qo_2. In effect, this procedure measures the maximal oxygen uptake of a piece of muscle. In the untrained state, muscles have a Qo_2 of 1,500 microliters per hour per gram of muscle ($\mu l/hr^{-1} \times g^{-1}$). Individuals who expend 1,500 to 2,500 kcal per week during training (such as joggers) have a muscle Qo_2 approximately 1.8 times greater than the

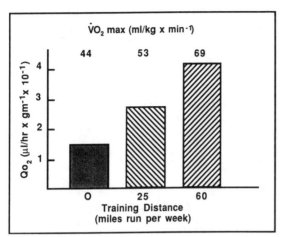

Figure 8–3 Respiratory capacity (Qo_2) in the gastrocnemius muscle of untrained, moderately-trained (joggers), and highly-trained (marathon) men. Note that the Qo_2 is somewhat proportional to the individual's training volume (from Costill, 1986).

untrained person (see Figure 8–3). Highly-trained marathon runners, who use more than 5000 kcal per week in training, have been reported to have Qo_2 values in excess of 4000 $\mu l/hr^{-1} \times g^{-1}$, a value nearly 2.7 times greater than the untrained muscle.

Although it appears that the respiratory capacity of the muscle is proportional to the athlete's training volume, training in excess of 5000 or 6000 kcal per week (for instance, running fifty to sixty miles per week) does not increase the Qo_2. The highest average values reported in human muscle (5174 $\mu l/hr^{-1} \times g^{-1}$) is in swimmers who expended more than 10,000 kcal per week during training (Costill, 1985). Thus, it appears that there is a limit to the muscle's capacity to adapt to aerobic training, and near-maximal adaptations occur at a training energy expenditure of about 6,000 to 8,000 kcal per week. This means that training in excess of these levels may do little to improve the aerobic capacity of the muscles.

How does training increase the respiratory capacity of the muscle? The ability to use oxygen and to produce ATP oxidatively depends on the number, size, and efficiency of the mitochondria.

It has been demonstrated that endurance training produces a weekly increase of approximately five percent in the number of mitochondria over a 27-week period. At the same time, the average size of the mitochondria increases by about 35 percent. These gradual changes suggest that improvements in the muscle's energy systems may take months and perhaps years to fully develop.

Chapter 2 explained that the oxidative breakdown and ultimate production of ATP depends on the action of special protein molecules called enzymes, which speed the chemical reactions of energy metabolism. As a result of aerobic training, there is a dramatic increase in the amount of these enzymes. Figure 8–4 illustrates the changes in the muscle's oxidative enzymes during 12 weeks of gradually increased training. It is interesting to

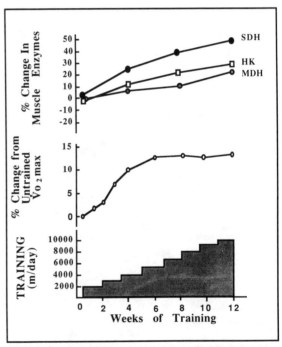

Figure 8–4 Changes in muscle enzymes and maximal oxygen uptake during 12 weeks of swim training. Note the gradual increase in the oxidative enzymes SDH (succinate dehydrogenase), HK (hexokinase), and MDH (malate dehydrogenase) during the gradual increase in the training load.

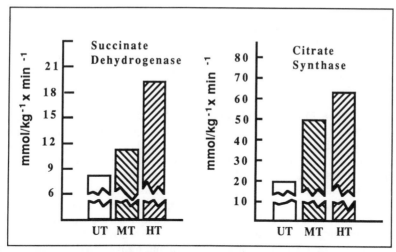

Figure 8-5 Leg muscle (gastrocnemius) enzyme activities of untrained (UT), moderately-trained joggers (MT), and highly-trained marathon runners (HT). The enzyme levels shown in this figure are succinate dehydrogenase (SDH) and citrate synthase (CS), two of the many enzymes that participate in the oxidative production of ATP (from Costill, et al., 1979, and unpublished data).

note that these enzymes continue to rise throughout the period of training, but little change in whole body maximal oxygen uptake occurred during the final six weeks of training. It is also interesting to observe that during this same period the enzymes of glycolysis remained unchanged, or tended to decline slightly.

The concentrations of such muscle enzymes as SDH (succinate dehydrogenase) and CS (citrate synthase) are dramatically influenced by endurance training. Even moderate amounts of daily activity will increase the muscle's aerobic capacity and the activity of these enzymes (see Figure 8-5). For example, jogging and cycling for as little as 20 minutes per day has been shown to increase the leg muscle's SDH activity by more than 25 percent above the levels in sedentary individuals. Training more vigorously (60 to 90 minutes per day), on the other hand, produces a 2.6-fold increase in muscle SDH activity.

As in the case of the Q_{O_2} measurements, the incremental increase in these oxidative enzymes with endurance training reflects an increase in the number and size of the muscle's mitochondria and an improved capacity for ATP production. These improvements in muscle aerobic capacity coincide

with improvements in the individual's maximal oxygen uptake (see Figure 8-6). There is, however, some question as to whether this is a cause-and-effect relationship. There are some researchers who argue that $\dot{V}O_2$ max is controlled by the oxygen transport system (circulation), whereas others

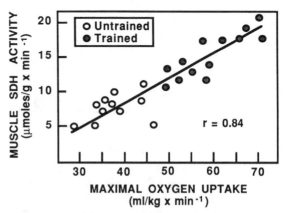

Figure 8-6 The relationship between maximal oxygen uptake ($\dot{V}O_2$ max) and the SDH activities in the leg muscles of untrained and trained men.

believe that it is the oxidative capacity of the muscle that dictates aerobic capacity. This debate over which system is more important for physiological endurance may be purely academic, since it is impossible to separate the contributions of these central and peripheral factors, and both improve with training.

Adjustments in the action of the aerobic enzymes make it possible for the endurance-trained muscle to burn fat more effectively, thereby lessening the demands placed on the muscle's limited supply of glycogen. Samples of muscle taken from the thigh of men before and after cycle training have shown a 30 percent increase in their ability to burn free fatty acids (see Figure 8-7). Other studies have reported that endurance training also increases the release of free fatty acids from the fat cells during exercise, thereby making them

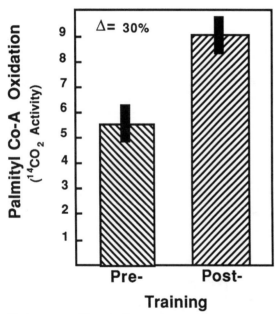

Figure 8-7 The effect of endurance training on the capacity of skeletal muscle to oxidize fats. These experiments tested the ability of skeletal muscle to metabolize a radioactive form of palmityl Co-A to carbon dioxide ($^{14}CO_2$) before and after eight weeks of endurance training (from Costill, et al., 1979).

available for the muscle's use. Thus, improvements in the muscle's aerobic energy system result in a greater capacity to produce energy, and a shift toward a greater reliance on fat for ATP production.

Fuel Storage

Endurance training places repeated demands on the muscle's energy supplies of glycogen and fat. Muscle glycogen, in particular, may be drastically reduced with each training session. As a result, the mechanisms responsible for the resynthesis of glycogen stimulate greater storage when the athlete has adequate rest and sufficient dietary carbohydrate. When distance runners, for example, stop training for several days and eat a diet rich in carbohydrates (400 to 550 grams/day) their muscle glycogen levels will increase to nearly twice the levels seen in sedentary individuals who follow the same regimen.

In addition to its greater glycogen stores, endurance-trained muscle has substantially more fat (triglyceride) than can be found in untrained fibers. Although there is only limited information regarding this improved fuel storage with endurance training, a 1.8 percent increase in muscle triglyceride content has been found to occur after only eight weeks of endurance running. In general, the droplets of triglyceride are distributed throughout the muscle fiber, but are in close proximity to the mitochondria, making them readily available as a fuel source during exercise. In addition, many of the muscle enzymes (such as lipoprotein lipase and carnitine palmityl transferase) responsible for the oxidation of fat are increased with endurance training.

Concomitant with other adaptations to aerobic training, muscles improve their capacity for oxidative ATP production by shifting to the use of more fat with less reliance on carbohydrate as a source of fuel. In athletic events that last for several hours, these adaptations prevent early depletion of muscle fuels, thereby improving performance.

Training for Aerobic Endurance

Improvements in aerobic capacity are determined, in part, by the number of calories expended during

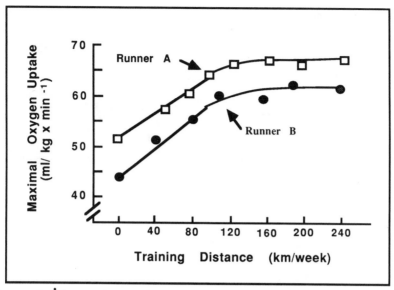

Figure 8-8 Changes in $\dot{V}O_2$ max for two distance runners training at various distances. Note that training 40 to 80 kilometers per week resulted in improvement in their aerobic capacities, whereas greater training distances produced no greater increase (modified from Costill, 1986).

each training bout and the total amount of work performed each week. This has been interpreted by many athletes and coaches to mean that gains in aerobic endurance will be proportional to the volume of training. If this were the single most important stimulus for muscular adaptations, then those individuals who expend the most energy during training should have the highest $\dot{V}O_2$ max values. As pointed out in Chapter 2 and to be discussed later in Chapter 14, this is not the case. The degree of adaptation to endurance training depends on genetic qualities, as well as the intensity of exercise during training.

Not all individuals have the same potential for adaptation to training. Men or women who perform a given training regimen will experience varied levels of muscular and circulatory improvements—some will show tremendous adjustment, while others may experience little or no change in their aerobic capacity. In addition, there seems to be an upper limit to the amount of adaptation that can be achieved with endurance training. Athletes who train with progressively greater workloads

will eventually reach a maximal level of improvement; additional increments in the training volume will not improve endurance. This point is illustrated by the data in Figure 8-8, which shows the changes in $\dot{V}O_2$ max for two distance runners before and at various levels of training. The runners' $\dot{V}O_2$ max increased dramatically with the initiation of training at 40 km per week and continued to improve when their training was increased to 80 km per week. Beyond that level of training, however, no additional gains in endurance were observed. During a one-month period, these same runners increased their training to over 350 km per week, with no improvement in endurance.

Thus, it seems that in all forms of endurance training there is an optimal amount of physical work that will produce maximal improvements in one's aerobic capacity and endurance performance. Although this optimal training load probably differs from one individual to another, observations with distance runners suggests that, on the average, the ideal training regimen may be equivalent to an energy expenditure of between 6,000 and

10,000 kcal per week, which translates to between 60 and 100 miles of running per week. The swimmer, on the other hand, would need to swim between 14 and 26 miles per week to achieve the same benefits. Of course, these are only estimates of the stimulus required for muscular conditioning, and some athletes may show greater improvements with more training, while others may show the best results with substantially less training.

Although the amount, rather than the intensity, of work performed during training, seems to be the most important determinant for developing aerobic endurance, peak performance also depends on the quality, or speed, of training. The major fault with long distance, low-intensity training is that it fails to develop the neurological patterns of muscle fiber recruitment and the high rate of energy production required for peak athletic competition. Muscular adaptations are specific to both the speed and duration of effort performed during training. Runners, cyclists, and swimmers who incorporate intermittent, high-intensity bouts of exercise into their training regimen show significant improvements in performance over those who perform only long, slow, training bouts.

High-intensity, speed training may include either intermittent exercise (intervals) or continuous exercise at a near-competition pace. Although interval training has been used for many years, most athletes consider this form of training to be highly anaerobic. While some interval training can be performed at speeds that produce a large amount of lactate, it is also possible to use this training format as a means to develop the aerobic system. Although long, continuous exercise will develop the aerobic system, repeated bouts at a faster pace, over shorter time periods, with brief rest intervals will achieve the same benefits. This form of **aerobic interval** training has become the framework for aerobic swimming conditioning. It involves repeated short swims (50 to 200 meters) at slightly slower than race pace, but with very brief rest intervals (5 to 15 second rest).

Table 8-1 offers an example of some aerobic intervals for runners who are preparing to compete in a 10 km race. Since volume is the key to successful aerobic training, the runner must perform a large number of these repeated runs. In this example, 20 repetitions of 400 meters results in a total

Table 8-1   Example of aerobic intervals for runners training to run a 10-km race.

Best 10 km min:sec	Reps	Interval Set Distance (meters)	Rest (sec)	Pace (min:sec)
46:00	20	400	10–15	2:00
43:00	20	400	10–15	1:52
40:00	20	400	10–15	1:45
37:00	20	400	10–15	1:37
34:00	20	400	10–15	1:30

of 8,000 meters (roughly five miles) at a pace that is slightly slower (5 to 6 sec/400 m) than that used during the 10 km race, but generally faster than can be sustained easily during a straight five-mile run. The hard part of this interval set is that the prescribed rest between repetitions is relatively brief, 10 to 15 seconds. Such short rest intervals allow little time for the muscles to recover, but it gives the athlete a brief period of escape from the muscular stress of the faster running.

It can be argued that a single, continuous bout of exercise can give the same aerobic benefits as a set of aerobic intervals, but there are some athletes who find continuous, endurance exercise to be boring. When it comes to the aerobic aspects of training, personal preference may be the deciding factor. At present, there is no direct evidence to show that aerobic interval training will produce greater muscular adaptations than continuous training bouts. Whether the training is performed as one long bout of continuous exercise, or in a series of shorter intervals, the aerobic muscular benefits seem to be the same.

ANAEROBIC TRAINING

Some of the muscular adaptations that occur during anaerobic training were detailed in Chapter 7. As mentioned earlier, most of the energy for such exercise is derived from the anaerobic breakdown of muscle glycogen and the muscle's ATP and PCr stores. In competitive events lasting only a few seconds, most of the energy demands are met by the breakdown of ATP and PCr (as discussed in Chapter 2). This anaerobic system is controlled by several enzymes, namely myokinase (MK) and creatine phosphokinase (CPK), though neither of these enzymes limits the rate of ATP resynthesis. Maximal efforts lasting more than four to five seconds rely on the glycolytic resynthesis of ATP and CP. In this system there are two enzymes that limit the rate of ATP formation: phosphorylase and phosphofructokinase (PFK).

In an effort to assess the effects of anaerobic training on muscular adaptations, a group of men trained one leg with repeated 6-second, maximal, exercise bouts. The subject's other leg was trained with an equal volume of work performed in 30-second interval bouts, four days per week for seven weeks. These repeated bouts of 6- and 30-second intervals were selected to stress the ATP–PCr and glycolytic systems, respectively. Measurements of muscle and blood lactate after the 6-second training bouts revealed little, if any accumulation, whereas the 30-second maximal efforts, caused a 10- to 15-fold increase in muscle lactate. The elevation in muscle lactate demonstrates the reliance on glycolysis for energy production in the short, intense exercise bouts.

These two training regimens produced similar gains in thigh strength and endurance performance during a 60-second sprint test. The muscle enzymes of the ATP–PCr system, namely CPK and MK, showed significant increases in activity as a result of the 30-second training bouts, but were unchanged in the leg trained with repeated 6-second maximal efforts (see Figure 8–9). Other investigators, however, have shown improvements in these enzymes with training bouts lasting only five seconds (Thorstensson, et al., 1975). In any event, these studies provide evidence that the mechanisms responsible for ATP resynthesis are adaptable with anaerobic training. Whether these changes enable the muscle to perform more anaerobic work remains unanswered. The 60-second sprint-fatigue test suggests that anaerobic training does not enhance anaerobic endurance.

The results of the 6- and 30-second training regimens on the enzymes of glycolysis are shown in Figure 8–10 on page 150. Again, only the 30-second training bouts produced an increase in the glycolytic enzymes. This difference in response to training appears to be the result of the greater glycolytic demands of the longer, 30-second efforts. Since both PFK and phosphorylase are key links in the anaerobic yield of ATP, it might be theorized that such training will enhance the glycolytic capacity and enable the muscle to develop greater tension for a longer period of time. This conclusion was not, however, supported by the results of a 60-

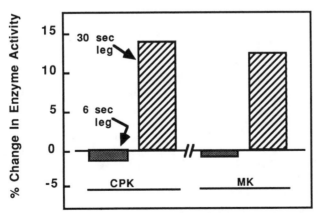

Figure 8–9   Changes in muscle myokinase (MK) and creatine phosphokinase (CPK) activities as a result of 6-second and 30-second bouts of maximal anaerobic training.

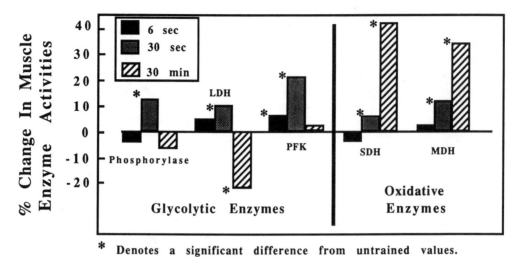

* Denotes a significant difference from untrained values.

Figure 8–10   Changes in muscle enzymes as a result of anaerobic (6- and 30-second) and aerobic (30-minute) training.

minute performance test carried out by these same individuals (see Figure 8–11). As might have been expected, the maximal power generated during the early seconds (1 to 25 seconds) of the test was improved in both legs after training. Since both legs achieved about the same power output and demonstrated a similar rate of fatigue, it appears that the performance gains achieved with training are the result of improvements in strength rather than an

improvement in the anaerobic yield of ATP. Despite the fact that the leg that had been trained with repeated 30-second bouts had greater glycolytic and ATP–CP enzymes, this leg demonstrated no greater resistance to fatigue or improvement in anaerobic power.

How then does anaerobic sprint-training improve performance? In addition to enhancing muscle strength, sprint training has been shown to improve the muscle's buffering capacity. Since the accumulation of lactate and free hydrogen ions within the muscle are considered to be responsible for fatigue during sprint exercise, an increase in muscle buffering capacity would delay the onset of fatigue during anaerobic exercise. It is interesting to note that the calculated buffer capacity increased 12 to 50 percent as a result of eight weeks of sprint training, but was not changed with endurance training (see Figure 8–12). As with other muscular adaptations (enzymes) to training, changes in buffer capacity are specific to the intensity of exercise performed during training.

As a result of this increase in muscle buffer capacity, sprint-trained subjects accumulate more blood and muscle lactate during and following an all-out sprint test. It appears that with an enhanced buffer capacity, the subjects' muscles can

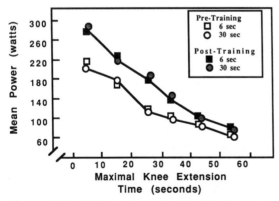

Figure 8–11   Effects of maximal isokinetic training on power development during a maximal 60-second work bout.

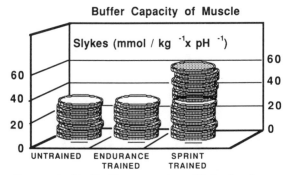

Figure 8-12 Buffer capacity (Slykes) of untrained (Pre-training), sprint-trained (Post-training), and endurance-trained (ET) muscle. Slykes were calculated from changes in muscle lactate and pH ratios.

continue to generate energy for a longer period before a critically high concentration of hydrogen develops and inhibits the contractile process. It is interesting to note that under similar circumstances, such as sprinting to exhaustion, endurance trained subjects do not accumulate as much muscle lac-

Table 8-2 Selected muscle enzyme activities ($\mu mol/g^{-1} \times min^{-1}$) for untrained, sprint-trained and endurance-trained men.

	Untrained	*Sprint*	*Endurance*
Aerobic Enzymes			
SDH	8.1	8.0	20.8*
MDH	45.5	46.0	65.5*
CPT	1.5	1.5	2.3*
Anaerobic Enzymes			
CPK	609	702*	589
MK	309	350*	297
Phosph	5.3	5.8	3.7*
PFK	19.9	29.2*	18.9
LDH	766	811	621*

*Denotes a significant difference from the untrained value. SDH = succinate dehydrogenase; MDH = malate dehydrogenase; CPT = carnitine palmityl transferase; CPK = creatine phosphokinase; MK = myokinase; Phosph = phosphorylase; PFK = phosphofructokinase; LDH = lactate dehydrogenase.

tate or experience the unusually low pH values seen in sprint-trained men. Although it is difficult to explain this difference between sprint- and endurance-trained subjects, it is tempting to speculate that muscle pH is not a limiting factor in this type of exercise for endurance-trained subjects. Since aerobically-trained muscles have significantly lower glycolytic enzymes, it may be that they have a lower capacity for anaerobic metabolism (see Table 8-2). More research is needed to explain the implications of the muscular changes that accompany both anaerobic and aerobic training.

MONITORING TRAINING CHANGES

The ability to judge the optimal training load is not an easy task. Some investigators have proposed that central, circulatory and peripheral muscular adaptations, which accompany training, are best judged by measuring the athlete's $\dot{V}O_2$ max, a test that requires the sophisticated equipment of an exercise physiology laboratory. Although this test may be sensitive to the changes in one's aerobic capacity, it is not available to most coaches and athletes. Also, it does not measure the muscular adaptations that are associated with anaerobic and aerobic training. In recent years, sports physiologists have proposed that measuring the level of blood lactate during training might provide a gauge of training stress and serve to monitor the muscle's adaptations to training.

It has been proposed that the sudden accumulation of blood lactate that occurs during incremental exercise represents a shift from aerobic to anaerobic metabolism, thereby providing a means to judge the intensity of the exercise. As illustrated in Figure 8-13 on page 152, endurance training raises the threshold for the onset of lactate accumulation. Endurance-trained men are able to exercise at a higher percentage of their maximal oxygen uptake before blood lactate begins to accumulate. Although this phenomenon has been interpreted in different ways and has been given several names (such as anaerobic lactate threshold; OBLA), it is generally felt to be a good predictor of endurance performance, and is more sensitive to training than $\dot{V}O_2$ max.

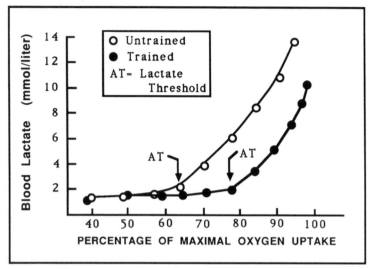

Figure 8-13 Effects of endurance training on blood lactate accumulation.

In an effort to detect the onset of anaerobic metabolism (anaerobic threshold) by noninvasive means, changes in selected respiratory parameters measured during incremental exercise have been correlated with the changes in blood pH and lactate. Additional details relative to the anaerobic threshold are presented in Chapter 3. Under laboratory conditions these measurements are good indicators of the cardiorespiratory adjustments to training. Davis et al. (1979), for example, studied nine middle-aged men before and after nine weeks of endurance training. They observed an increase in $\dot{V}O_2$ max of 25 percent; whereas the anaerobic threshold increased 44 percent.

Although these laboratory tests offer sensitive methods to monitor both the intensity of exercise and the adaptations to training, they are impractical for athletic training. Consequently, blood lactate measurements have been adapted for use with various sports, namely running and swimming. These athletes are asked to perform a series of standard exercise bouts at varied intensities, and with 30 to 60 minutes of rest between efforts. Blood taken from a forearm vein or fingertip is used to measure lactate after each bout. These values are then graphed against the athlete's running or swimming velocity. As illustrated in Figure 8-

14, it is possible to identify the lactate threshold by examining the relationship between blood lactate concentration and swimming velocity. After training, the onset of lactate accumulation occurs at a higher swimming velocity.

The need for repeated blood samples and the time required for these measurements, do not justify the value of such testing. A simpler protocol has been used to monitor training—the measurement of blood lactate accumulation after a single, standard exercise bout. Since the slope of the blood lactate-swimming velocity curve remains relatively unchanged with training, it is possible to judge the effect of training on muscle metabolism by having the swimmer or runner perform a single exercise trial at a controlled speed. Costill et al. (1985) have used a 200-meter swim, in which the swimmer's pace is controlled with a computer-operated series of lights positioned along the length of the swimming pool. Most athletes do not need this aid to control their pace. As shown in Figure 8-15, blood lactate accumulation following this standard swim declined steadily over a five-month period of training.

Other attempts to monitor training appear to be less sensitive or reliable, more expensive, and too time-consuming for use with athletes. Even this

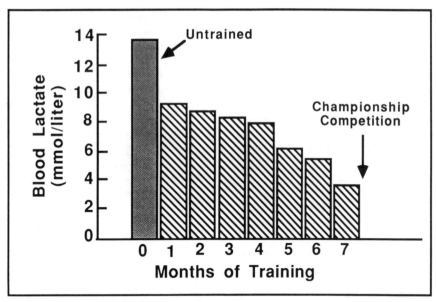

Figure 8–14 The relationship between blood lactate accumulation and swimming velocity before and after five months of training.

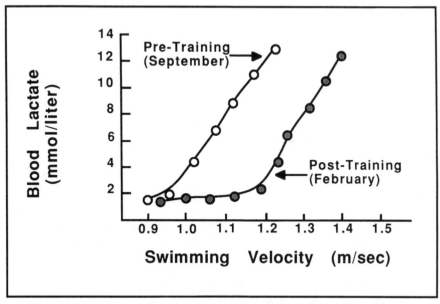

Figure 8–15 Effects of training on blood lactate concentration after a 200-meter swim at a predetermined speed. The lowest lactate values were recorded during the period when the swimmers performed their best.

single measurement of blood lactate requires expensive equipment and trained personnel. In addition, there is controversy regarding the use and interpretation of the findings from such testing. Should the results be used to vary the intensity of training? Precisely what physiological changes are responsible for changes in lactate threshold? These and other questions remain unanswered, but such information seems basic to the use and interpretation of tests to monitor the athlete's muscular adaptations to training.

SUMMARY

Both aerobic and anaerobic training produce remarkable adaptations in the skeletal muscle. Improvements in capillary blood flow and the muscle's energy systems appear to be a direct result of the intensity and duration of the specific exercise performed during training. Anaerobic training, for example, will enhance muscular strength, buffering capacity, and glycolytic energy production, but may have little effect on the aerobic capacity of the muscle. Aerobic activities, on the other hand, increase the muscle's respiratory capacity and capillarization, without altering its glycolytic potential or buffering capacity. Individuals who train solely for aerobic events may even show a decline in explosive muscular power. Little is known about the interaction between these two forms of training. Whether both systems can be trained simultaneously is not clear, although evidence suggests that it is possible to develop the aerobic and anaerobic benefits using various forms of intermittent and continuous exercise.

STUDY QUESTIONS

1. What effect does aerobic and anaerobic training have on muscle fiber composition?
2. How does endurance training improve oxygen delivery to the muscle fibers?
3. Describe the factors that are responsible for the improvements in muscle respiratory capacity (Q_{O_2}) with aerobic training.
4. What effect does endurance training have on the type of fuels used during exercise?
5. Describe the changes in muscle buffer capacity during aerobic and anaerobic training? How might this improve performance?
6. What changes occur in muscle during sprint training that might reduce its fatiguability in highly glycolytic exercise?
7. What changes might be expected in the anaerobic threshold as a result of aerobic training? Illustrate the relationship between running speed and blood lactate accumulation.
8. Outline a testing program to monitor the muscular adaptations during training for an 800-meter runner, marathoner, or swimmer.

REFERENCES

Åstrand, P. O., & Rodahl, K. (1986). *Textbook of work physiology* (3rd ed.) New York: McGraw-Hill.

Brooks, G. A. (1985). Response to Davis' manuscript. *Medicine and Science in Sports and Exercise, 17*, 19–21.

Costill, D. L. (1977). Adaptations in skeletal muscle during training for sprint and endurance swimming. In B. Eriksson & B Furberg (Eds.), *Swimming Medicine IV.* Baltimore: University Park Press, 233–248.

Costill, D. L. (1986). *Inside running: Basics of sports physiology.* Indianapolis: Benchmark Press.

Costill, D. L., Fink, W. J., Hargreaves, M., King, D. S., Thomas, R., & Fielding, R. (1985). Metabolic characteristics of skeletal muscle during detraining from competitive swimming. *Medicine and Science in Sports and Exercise, 17*, 339–343.

Costill, D. L., Fink, W. J., Ivy, J. L., Getchell, L. H., & Witzmann, F. A. (1979). Lipid metabolism in skeletal muscle of endurance-trained males and females. *Journal of Applied Physiology, 28*, 251–255.

Costill, D. L., Coyle, E. F., Fink, W. F., Lesmes, G. R., & Witzmann, F. A. (1979). Adaptations in skeletal muscle following strength training. *Journal of Applied Physiology, 46*, 96–99.

Costill, D. L. (1978). Adaptations in skeletal muscle during training for sprint and endurance swimming. B Eriksson & B. Furberg (Eds.). *Swimming Medicine IV.* Baltimore: University Park Press.

Davis, J. A. (1985). Anaerobic threshold: Review of the concept and directions for future research. *Medicine and Science in Sports and Exercise, 17*, 6–18.

Davis, J. A., Frank, M. H., Whipp, B. J., & Wasserman, K. (1979). Anaerobic threshold alterations caused by endurance training in middle-aged men. *Journal of Applied Physiology, 46*, 1039–1046.

Henriksson, J., & Reitman, J. S. (1977). Time course of changes in human skeletal muscle succinate dehydrogenase and cytochrome oxidase activities and maximal oxygen uptake with physical activity and inactivity. *Acta Physiologica Scandinavica, 99*, 91–97.

Hermansen, L. (1971). Lactate production during exercise. In B. Pernow & B. Saltin (Eds.), *Muscle metabolism during exercise.* New York: Plenum Press.

Holloszy, J. O., Oscai, L. B., Mole, P. A., & Don, I. J. (1971). Biochemical adaptations to endurance exercise in skeletal muscle. In B. Pernow & B. Saltin (Eds.), *Muscle metabolism during exercise.* New York: Plenum Press.

Lesmes, G. R., Costill, D. L., Coyle, E. F., & Fink, W. J. (1978). Muscle strength and power changes during maximal isokinetic training. *Medicine and Science in Sports, 10,* 266-269.

Saltin, B., & Rowell, L. B. (1980). Functional adaptations to physical activity and inactivity. *Federation Proceedings, 39,* 1506-1513.

Saltin, B., & Karlsson, J. (1971). Muscle ATP, CP, and lactate during exercise after physical conditioning. In B. Pernow & B. Saltin (Eds.), *Muscle metabolism during exercise.* New York: Plenum Press.

Saltin, B., Nazar, K., Costill, D. L., Stein, E., Jansson, E., Essen, B., & Gollnick, P. (1976). The nature of the training response: Peripheral and central adaptations to one-legged exercise. *Acta Physiologica Scandinavica, 96,* 289-305.

Sharp, R. L., Costill, D. L., Fink, W. J., & King, D. S. (1986). Effects of eight weeks of bicycle ergometer sprint training on human muscle buffer capacity. *International Journal of Sports Medicine, 7,* 13-17.

Wasserman, K. (1984). The anaerobic threshold measurement to evaluate exercise performance. *American Review of Respiratory Diseases, 129* (Suppl.), S35-S40.

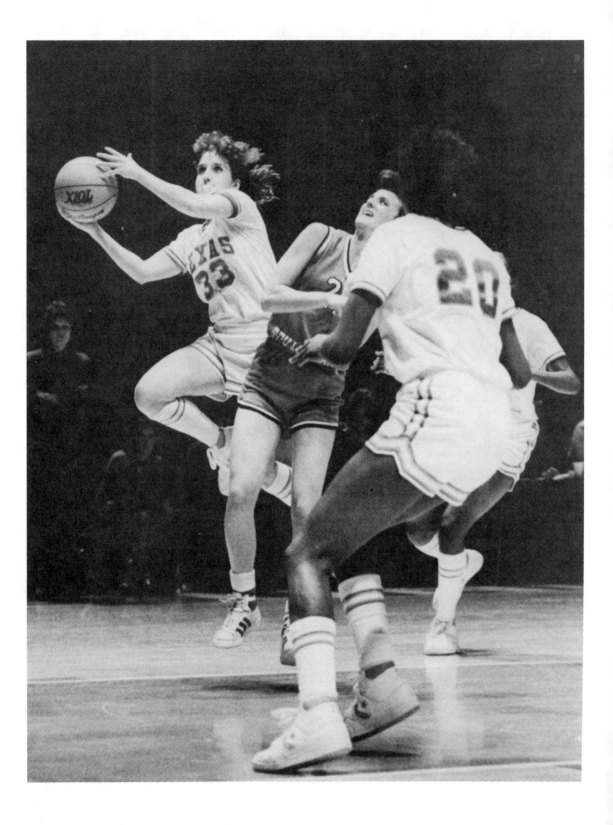

9

Cardiorespiratory Endurance and Aerobic Power

INTRODUCTION

Of the various components that comprise the total physical training program, endurance is probably the most underrated. It is given relatively little attention in the training programs of most non-endurance athletes. The football player fails to understand why the endurance component is an important part of his total training program. Football is perceived as an anaerobic activity, consisting of repeated bouts of high-intensity work of short duration. Seldom does a run exceed 40 to 60 yards, and even this is followed by a substantial rest interval. From all outward appearances, football is an anaerobic or burst-type of activity, and the need for endurance is not immediately obvious. Sport scientists, however, are beginning to recognize the importance of endurance training for all activities, whether burst-type, slow and skilled, or of an endurance nature. What the football player fails to realize is that this burst-type of activity must be repeated a number of times throughout the game. With a high level of muscular and cardiorespiratory endurance, the quality of the burst activity is maintained, and the athlete is still fresh at the start of the fourth quarter. It is now believed that those teams that fall apart in the final quarter are teams that have ignored the endurance component in their training programs. A similar case can be made for athletes

in most sports and will be presented in detail later in this chapter.

Endurance can be defined as the ability to perform prolonged bouts of work without experiencing fatigue or exhaustion. As was mentioned in both Chapters 2 and 8, endurance is comprised of two separate components, which are related but different in importance to athletic performance and in their manner of development through physical training. Muscular, or local, endurance refers to the ability of a single muscle or muscle group to sustain prolonged exercise, and is exemplified by the weight lifter, boxer, or wrestler. The exercise can be either of a rhythmical and repetitive nature, such as bench press and jabs, or of a static nature, such as sustained, isometric contraction, when trying to pin an opponent to the mat. The resulting fatigue is confined to the local group of muscles that was exercised. Cardiorespiratory endurance refers to the ability of the total body to sustain prolonged, rhythmical exercise. This type of endurance is typified by the runner who is able to run long distances at a fairly fast pace. Absolute muscular endurance is highly related to the muscular strength of the individual, while cardiorespiratory endurance is highly related to the development of the cardiovascular and respiratory systems. Muscular endurance was discussed in Chapter 8. This chapter will focus on cardiorespiratory endurance.

Although cardiorespiratory endurance is often one of the most neglected components in the athlete's training program, exercise physiologists recognize it as probably the most important component in the physiological profile of most athletes. Cardiorespiratory endurance has become synonymous with the term **physical fitness**. A minimal level of cardiorespiratory endurance is essential for any sport or activity, and current opinion is that even higher levels can improve the quality of the athlete's performance and reduce chances for serious injury.

Cardiorespiratory endurance can be assessed in the field or in the laboratory. The maximal oxygen uptake ($\dot{V}O_2$ max) is regarded by most sport scientists as the best objective laboratory measure of cardiorespiratory endurance capacity. As discussed in Chapter 2, $\dot{V}O_2$ max is defined as the highest attainable oxygen uptake value during maximal or exhaustive exercise. Just as the athlete reaches exhaustion, the volume of oxygen consumed ceases to increase and will plateau or decrease slightly. It is felt that the attainment of this plateau signals the end of the exercise, since the athlete has taxed his or her ability to deliver oxygen to the working muscles to its finite limit. This finite limit will dictate the level of work or the pace that the athlete can tolerate. One can continue for a brief period beyond the time at which $\dot{V}O_2$ max is attained by calling on one's anaerobic reserves, but these also have a finite capacity. With endurance training, this limit is increased following a six-month training program showing improvements in $\dot{V}O_2$ max of 20 percent or more (Pollock, Wilmore, & Fox, 1984). This results in the athlete being able to perform at higher rates of work or at a faster pace, thus improving his or her athletic performance potential.

ADAPTATIONS IN CARDIORESPIRATORY ENDURANCE AND AEROBIC POWER WITH PHYSICAL TRAINING

Training results in a number of changes that improve the transportation function of the cardiovascular and respiratory systems during exercise. These changes that occur consequent to endurance training, will be discussed as they relate to improved performance.

Heart Rate

The heart rate at rest will decrease markedly as a result of endurance conditioning. For a sedentary adult with an initial resting heart rate of 80 beats per min, the resting heart rate will decrease by approximately one beat per min for each week of training during the first few weeks. Following ten weeks of modest endurance training, the resting rate should drop to 70 beats per min. Highly conditioned endurance athletes typically have resting heart rates of 40 beats per min or lower, and several have had values below 30 beats per min. **Bradycardia** is a clinical term indicating a heart rate below 60 beats per min and in untrained individuals is commonly the result of an abnormal, or diseased, heart. Therefore, it is important to differentiate between a training-induced bradycardia, which is a natural response to endurance training, and a pathologically-induced bradycardia, which is cause for concern.

During exercise, the heart rate for the same rate of work will be less as one becomes more highly conditioned. This is illustrated in Figure 9–1. It is

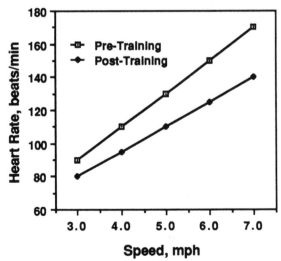

Figure 9–1 Changes in submaximal heart rate with endurance training.

not unusual to observe a 20 to 40 beat per min decrease in submaximal heart rate at a standardized rate of work following a six-month training program of moderate intensity. Since the work performed by the heart is a direct function of its rate of contraction, both at rest and during exercise, the reduced submaximal heart rate following training indicates that the heart is working more efficiently—doing less work.

At maximal levels of exercise, the maximal heart rate will remain approximately the same following endurance training. Several studies have suggested that there is a slight reduction in HR max in those individuals who have HR max values in excess of 180 beats per min. There is also a tendency for highly-conditioned, endurance athletes to have HR max values lower than untrained individuals of the same age. The major function of heart rate during exercise is to combine with stroke volume to provide the appropriate cardiac output for the rate of work being performed. Thus, it is entirely possible that at maximal or near-maximal rates of work, the body will adjust the heart rate to provide the optimal combination of heart rate and stroke volume to maximize cardiac output. If the heart rate is too fast, the diastolic filling period is reduced to a point where stroke volume is compromised. At a heart rate of 180 beats per min, the heart is beating three times per second; each cardiac cycle lasts for only 0.33 seconds (333 milliseconds). The period of diastole will be as short as 0.2 seconds (200 milliseconds) or less. It is possible that the heart rate at maximal rates of exercise is reduced to compensate for the increased stroke volume that results from training to provide the optimal combination of rate and stroke volume to maximize cardiac output.

The heart rate recovers from exercise at a much faster rate following a period of endurance training—there is a faster return of the heart rate to the pre-exercise level (see Figure 9-2). This is true following standardized, submaximal levels of exercise as well as maximal levels of exercise. The faster heart-rate recovery following endurance training has led to the use of the pulse-rate recovery as an index of cardiorespiratory fitness—the more fit individual will recover faster from a standardized rate of work. While the heart rate recovery curve is an excellent way to quantify

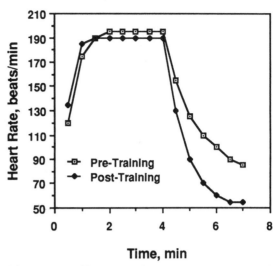

Figure 9-2 Changes in heart rate recovery with endurance training.

changes in your level of cardiovascular conditioning at different points in time as you endurance train, it is not a very accurate means of comparing one individual with another. Too many factors other than cardiorespiratory fitness are involved when absolute heart rate recovery values are compared among different people.

Stroke Volume, Cardiac Output, and Heart Volume

Changes in stroke volume are closely related to the changes in heart rate that result from training. At rest, the stroke volume is substantially higher following an endurance-training program. Similarly, stroke volume is higher at submaximal, standardized rates of work, as well as at maximal levels of exercise. This increase appears to be the result of a more complete filling of the heart during the period of diastole, resulting in a greater end-diastolic blood volume. In addition, the walls of the left ventricle tend to hypertrophy with training. This increased ventricular muscle mass allows an increased power of contraction (left ventricular contractility is increased). With increased contractility there is a decreased end-systolic volume, and

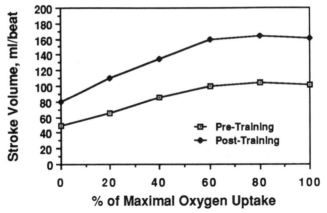

Figure 9-3 Changes in stroke volume with endurance training.

an increased ejection fraction (fraction or percentage of the end-diastolic volume expelled from the left ventricle). Thus, a stronger heart and the availability of greater blood volume (to be discussed later in this chapter), appear to account for these increases in resting, submaximal, and maximal stroke volumes. In turn, it appears that the increased stroke volume allows the heart to beat at a slower rate, both at rest and during submaximal levels of exercise. It is also possible that the increased stroke volume is the result of the decreased heart rate, rather than the reduced heart rate being the result of an increased stroke volume. Resting stroke volumes range from ≤70 ml for the untrained, ≤90 ml for the trained, or ≥130 ml for highly-trained, endurance athlete. Likewise, maximal stroke volumes vary from ≤125 ml for the untrained, ≤150 ml for the trained, and ≥220 ml for the highly-trained, endurance athlete. Changes in stroke volume with endurance training are illustrated in Figure 9-3.

Cardiac output is not greatly changed after training, either at rest or at standardized rates of submaximal work. For the same metabolic rate of work, such as 1.5 liters of oxygen per min, there may be a slight decrease in the cardiac output due to an increase in the a-v̄ O_2 difference, an increase in the mechanical or metabolic efficiency, or both. At maximal levels of work, however, the cardiac output is increased considerably. This is the result of the increase in maximal stroke volume since HR

max changes little, if at all. Maximal cardiac output ranges from 14 to 16 liters per min in untrained individuals, 20 to 25 liters per min for trained individuals, and up to 40 liters per min in large, highly-conditioned, endurance athletes. These relationships with training are illustrated in Figure 9-4.

The weight of the heart, the heart volume, and the size of the heart chambers, appear to increase as a result of endurance training. Cardiac muscle, like skeletal muscle, appears to undergo hypertrophy as a result of chronic endurance training. At one time there was great concern over the possible pathological consequences of cardiac hypertrophy induced by exercise, or the "athlete's heart," as it was called. It is now recognized that this is a normal adaptation to chronic endurance training. The left ventricle, which does most of the work, is the chamber most affected. It is not clear whether the endurance-trained heart experiences just an increased chamber size, or whether there is an increased wall thickness as well as chamber size.

Blood Flow, Blood Pressure, and Peripheral Vasculature

Blood flow through the muscle appears to be enhanced by endurance training. This is due to an increase in the number of capillaries in the trained muscle. Further, the muscle fibers tend to increase in size during training. Since the muscle fibers and

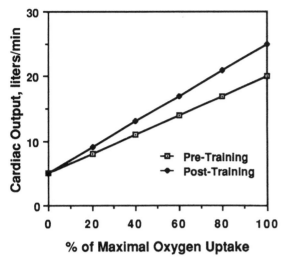

Figure 9-4 Changes in cardiac output with endurance training.

capillaries are in close proximity, a more favorable capillary-to-fiber ratio results. It is also possible that the increased blood flow is the result of the existing capillaries in the trained muscle opening up to a greater extent, providing better perfusion of the muscle. Since endurance training also increases the blood volume, this latter adaptation can occur without severely compromising the venous return.

Arterial blood pressure during standardized, submaximal rates of work, or at maximal rates of work, is altered very little following training. Resting blood pressure, however, is generally reduced with training for those individuals who are borderline or moderately hypertensive prior to training.

Blood Volume and Composition

As mentioned in the preceding section, blood volume increases with endurance training, with greater increases resulting from more intense levels of training. This is accomplished through an increase in both plasma and red blood cell volumes. The change in plasma volume, however, is usually much greater than that of the red blood cell volume, thus the hematocrit (ratio of cell volume to

total blood volume) actually decreases. It can decrease to the point where the trained athlete appears to be anemic on the basis of the relatively low concentration of red cells and hemoglobin. In fact, the total amount of hemoglobin and the total number of red blood cells (their absolute values), are typically above normal in the highly-trained athlete, even though their relative values are below normal. This condition leads to a reduction in the viscosity of the blood, which facilitates its movement through the blood vessels, particularly through the microcirculation. Recent research has pointed to the importance of a low blood viscosity in enhancing the delivery of oxygen to the active muscle mass.

The increase in plasma volume is possibly one of the most significant changes to occur with endurance training. An important study by Coyle and his associates (1986) indicates that one of the major adaptations that occurs with detraining is a reduction in plasma volume. Further, they found that the decreases in cardiovascular function associated with detraining could be largely reversed by simply expanding the plasma volume with a six percent dextran solution in saline, back to levels that had been achieved in the trained state. Stroke volume and $\dot{V}O_2$ max in the detrained state were returned to within two to four percent of the trained values by plasma volume expansion.

The oxygen content of the arterial blood changes very little with training. Even though total hemoglobin is increased in absolute terms, the amount of hemoglobin per unit of blood is the same, or even slightly reduced. The a-$\bar{v}$ O_2 difference is increased with training, particularly at maximal levels of exercise. This increase is the result of a lower, mixed venous oxygen content, which reflects both a greater extraction of available oxygen at the tissue level and a more effective distribution of total blood volume to the active tissue; for example, a lower percentage of the total blood volume is distributed to the inactive tissues.

Lactate threshold is increased with endurance training, thus blood lactate concentrations are lower at each level of a standardized, graded, exercise test following training. However, maximal blood lactate concentration at the point of exhaustion is increased following training. The increase in lactate threshold appears to be a result of several factors: a greater ability to clear lactate produced in the muscle and a shift in metabolic substrate as a result of training, which leads to reduced production of lactate for the same rate of work. Chapter 8 provides more details on this subject.

Pulmonary Function and Respiratory Changes

The static lung volumes change very little with training. There is a tendency for vital capacity to increase slightly and for residual volume to decrease by approximately the same amount. Thus, total lung capacity remains essentially unchanged.

Pulmonary ventilation is unchanged at rest, but is slightly reduced at standardized rates of work following training. Training substantially increases maximal pulmonary ventilation from values of 120 liters per min in the untrained, to 150 liters per min following training, to ≥ 180 liters per min in the highly-trained athlete. Endurance athletes with large builds can have maximal values in excess of 240 liters per min. Tidal volume is unchanged at rest and at standardized submaximal levels of exercise, but appears to increase at maximal levels of exercise. Respiratory rate is usually lowered at rest and during standardized submaximal exercise following training, although the reduction is small. During maximal levels of exercise, this rate is substantially increased following training. Ventilation is typically not considered to be a limiting factor for endurance exercise performance. However, recent work suggests that in the highly-trained individual, there will come a point in that individual's adaptation, where the capacity of the pulmonary system for oxygen transport will not be able to meet the demands imposed by the limbs and the cardiovascular system (Dempsey, 1986).

Pulmonary blood flow appears to be increased following training, particularly the flow to the upper regions of the lung when the individual is sitting or standing. This results in increased perfusion of the lung. Lung diffusion is unaltered at rest and during standardized submaximal exercise following training, but is increased during maximal exercise. This increase is probably due to both the enhanced perfusion and ventilation of the lung, which provides a larger and more efficient surface for gas exchange.

Metabolic Adaptations

The respiratory exchange ratio is decreased at both absolute and relative submaximal rates of work, but is increased at maximal levels following a period of endurance training. The changes in the submaximal responses are due to changes in substrate utilization, and are discussed in Chapter 8. The increase in the maximal respiratory exchange ratio reflects the ability of the individual to achieve a better, all-out maximal performance, which could reflect an increased psychological drive.

Oxygen consumption at rest is either slightly decreased or unaltered following endurance training. At submaximal levels of exercise, $\dot{V}O_2$ is either unchanged or slightly reduced. A decrease in $\dot{V}O_2$ at rest, during submaximal exercise, or both, would suggest an increase in metabolic and/or mechanical efficiency. While this might be a postulated change, conclusions from studies are divided as to whether this change does, in fact, occur. It is possible that researchers in those studies that demonstrated a reduced $\dot{V}O_2$ for the same rate of work following training, may have observed a practice effect on their testing devices. If not allowed prior practice on the cycle ergometer, treadmill, or other appropriate ergometer, the subject may perform at a lower energy cost the second or third time he or she exercises on that device, simply because of being more relaxed and accustomed to performing on the device, and knowing what is expected. Thus, the observed change may not be the result of training.

$\dot{V}O_2$ max is increased substantially with endurance training. Increases from four to 93 percent have been reported (Pollock, 1973). An increase of 15 to 20 percent is more typical for the average individual who was sedentary prior to training, and who had trained at 75 percent of his or her capacity, three times per week, 30 min per day for six months (Pollock, 1973). The $\dot{V}O_2$ max of a sedentary individual may increase from an initial value of 35 ml·kg^{-1}·min^{-1} to 42 ml·kg^{-1}·min^{-1} as a result of such a program. This is far below the values for world-class, endurance athletes, whose values generally range from 70 to 94 ml·kg^{-1}·min^{-1}. The better the initial state of conditioning, the smaller will be the relative improvement for the same program of training. In fact, it appears that in fully mature athletes, the highest attainable $\dot{V}O_2$ max is reached within 12 to 18 months of heavy, endurance training, indicating that each athlete has a finite level that can be attained. It has been suggested that this finite level is potentially influenced by training in early childhood, but this is purely conjecture at this point in time and needs substantiation by experimental research.

The factors responsible for this change in $\dot{V}O_2$ max have been identified, but there has been extensive controversy as to their relative importance. Two theories were at one time proposed to explain these increases with training. The first theory stated that endurance performance is not limited by the supply of oxygen coming into the tissue by way of arterialized blood, but, rather, by the lack of oxidative enzymes in the mitochondria. Proponents of this theory have provided impressive evidence that endurance-training programs increase these oxidative enzymes, allowing the active tissue to utilize more of the available oxygen, which would also result in a higher $\dot{V}O_2$ max. In addition, endurance training results in increases in muscle mitochondria. Thus, this theory argues that it is not solely a lack of oxygen coming into the active muscles that limits endurance performance, but it must also involve an inability of the existing mitochondria to utilize the available oxygen.

The second theory proposed that central and peripheral circulatory factors limited endurance capacity—an inability to deliver a sufficient amount of oxygen to the active tissue. In this theory, improvement in $\dot{V}O_2$ max following endurance training was believed to result from increases in blood volume, cardiac output (via stroke volume), and a better perfusion of blood in the active tissue. Again, impressive research evidence provided strong support for this theory. In one study, subjects breathed a mixture of carbon monoxide and air during exercise to exhaustion (Pirnay et al., 1971). The decrease in $\dot{V}O_2$ max was in direct proportion to the percentage of carbon monoxide breathed. The carbon monoxide molecules were bonded to approximately 15 percent of the total hemoglobin, which was exactly the same percentage as the reduction in $\dot{V}O_2$ max. In another study, approximately 15 to 20 percent of subjects' total

blood volume was removed, and the $\dot{V}O_2$ max decreased by approximately the same relative amount (Ekblom et al., 1972). Reinfusion of the packed red cells approximately four weeks later resulted in an increase in $\dot{V}O_2$ max above baseline, or control, conditions. In both of these studies, the reduction in the oxygen-carrying capacity of the blood, by either blocking hemoglobin or removing whole blood, resulted in less oxygen being delivered to the active tissues and a corresponding reduction in $\dot{V}O_2$ max. Similarly, studies have shown that breathing oxygen-enriched mixtures, in which the partial pressure of oxygen in the inspired air is substantially increased, results in large increases in endurance capacity.

These studies tend to indicate that it is the available oxygen supply that limits endurance performance. In an excellent review article, Saltin and Rowell (1980) conclude that the oxygen transport to the working muscles limits $\dot{V}O_2$ max, not the available mitochondria and oxidative enzymes. They argue that increases in $\dot{V}O_2$ max with training are largely attributable to increased maximal muscle blood flow and increased muscle capillary density. The major adaptations in skeletal muscle, including increased mitochondrial content and respiratory capacity of the muscle fibers, appears to be more closely related to the ability to perform prolonged high-intensity exercise (Holloszy & Coyle, 1984).

Although it was stated that the highest attainable endurance capacity, as represented by $\dot{V}O_2$ max, is usually reached within 18 months of intense endurance conditioning, endurance performance will continue to improve for many additional years with continued training. It is theorized that this improvement in endurance performance in the absence of improvements in $\dot{V}O_2$ max, might possibly be related to the ability to perform at increasingly higher percentages of $\dot{V}O_2$ max for extended periods of time. The mechanisms for this improvement are probably related to greater mechanical and metabolic efficiency, an increased lactate threshold, and greater utilization of fat as an energy source during exercise.

As an example, a young male runner, who starts training with an initial $\dot{V}O_2$ max of 52.0 ml·kg^{-1}·min^{-1}, reaches his genetically determined peak $\dot{V}O_2$ max of 71 ml·kg^{-1}·min^{-1} two years later and

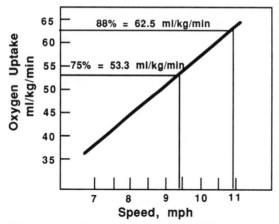

Figure 9-5 Change in race pace with continued training when maximal oxygen uptake fails to continue its increase.

is unable to increase it further, even with more intensive workouts. At this point, the young runner is able to run at 75 percent of his $\dot{V}O_2$ max $(0.75 \cdot 71.0 = 53.3 \text{ ml} \cdot \text{kg}^{-1} \cdot \text{min}^{-1})$ in a six-mile race. Following an additional two years of intensive training, the $\dot{V}O_2$ max is unchanged, but he is now able to compete at 88 percent of his $\dot{V}O_2$ max $(0.88 \cdot 71.0 = 62.5 \text{ ml} \cdot \text{kg}^{-1} \cdot \text{min}^{-1})$. Obviously, by being able to sustain an oxygen uptake of 62.5 ml $\cdot \text{kg}^{-1} \cdot \text{min}^{-1}$, he will be able to run at a much faster pace. Figure 9-5 illustrates this example.

The genetic aspects of $\dot{V}O_2$ max were originally demonstrated by Klissouras in a series of studies conducted in the late 1960s and early 1970s, and more recently by Bouchard and his colleagues (1986). Figure 9-6 illustrates the fact that identical, or monozygous, twins have nearly identical endurance capacity values, while the variability for

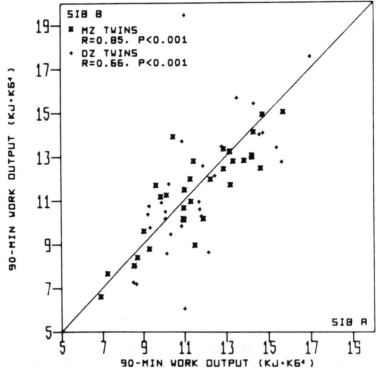

Figure 9-6 Comparison of endurance capacity, as defined by 90-minute endurance values, between monozygous and dizygous twins (data from Bouchard, et al., 1986).

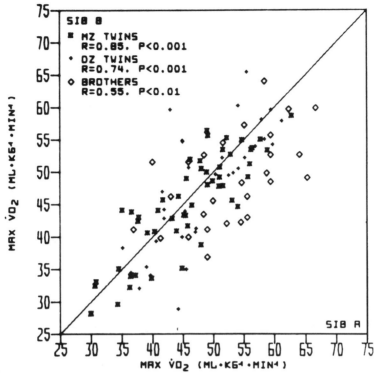

Figure 9-7 Comparison of $\dot{V}O_2$ max between monozygous and dizygous twins (data from Bouchard, et al., 1986).

dizygous, or fraternal, twins is much greater. Similar results have been found for $\dot{V}O_2$ max, as illustrated in Figure 9-7. Bouchard and Malina (1983) have concluded that heredity accounts for approximately 50 percent of the variance in $\dot{V}O_2$ max values. Åstrand (1973) has stated that the best way to become a champion Olympic athlete is to be selective when choosing your parents. World-class athletes who have been away from endurance training for many years continue to have high $\dot{V}O_2$ max values in their sedentary, deconditioned state. It appears that both genetic and environmental factors can influence $\dot{V}O_2$ max values. Genetic factors probably establish boundaries for the athlete, but endurance training can push the $\dot{V}O_2$ max value to the upper limit of these boundaries.

Age and sex can also influence $\dot{V}O_2$ max values. However, these values may lead to an improper interpretation of true age and sex differences. Figure 9-8 illustrates the $\dot{V}O_2$ max values of a group of older sprinters and distance runners between 40 and 74 years of age. Their $\dot{V}O_2$ max values do decrease with age, but they are considerably higher than the mean values for their particular age. Similar trends have been found in highly-conditioned, female endurance athletes when compared to the normal, sedentary population of females. In both cases, the average $\dot{V}O_2$ max values for the older individual and for the female are lower than they should be, due to the sedentary nature of the two populations. $\dot{V}O_2$ max values for athletes are listed in the Appendix by age, sex, and sport.

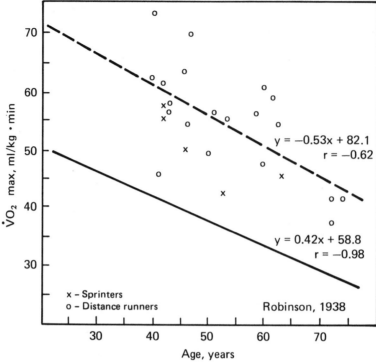

Figure 9-8 $\dot{V}O_2$ max values for a group of older sprinters and distance runners in comparison to normal values for the same age range.

TRAINING PROCEDURES FOR THE DEVELOPMENT OF CARDIORESPIRATORY ENDURANCE AND AEROBIC POWER

There are a number of specific endurance training programs, ranging from interval training to long, slow-distance (LSD) training, all of which provide similar results and take similar factors into consideration in their design. The factors to be considered in the development of any cardiorespiratory endurance program would be progressive overload, duration of each training session, frequency of the training sessions, intensity of the training sessions, the ratio of intense work to rest intervals, and the purpose of the training program. Progressive overload, as it applied to the development of strength, power, and muscular endurance, was discussed in Chapters 7 and 8. Progressive overload is also important to endurance conditioning and

simply implies that rate of work should be greater than (overload) that rate which can be comfortably performed continuously; this rate of work should be gradually increased as one becomes better conditioned (progressive overload).

The duration of the cardiorespiratory or aerobic portion of the training session will depend on several factors, including the sport or activity that is being pursued and the intensity of the individual training sessions. The competitive swimmer may need to spend five hours per day, five to seven days per week, in the water—a large percentage of this time will be spent on aerobic conditioning. The football player, however, may use jogging as a form of aerobic training for only 20 to 30 minutes per day, two to three days per week—a small percentage of his total training program. The frequency of the training sessions will depend on the nature of the training program. For general aerobic fitness, three to four days per week are sufficient, but for endurance competition, five to seven days per week will be necessary. The intensity of the training session will also depend on the purpose of the endurance training program—short-duration, high-intensity training for the middle-distance runner, long-duration, low-intensity training for the recreational jogger. The ratio of work to rest intervals depends on the philosophy of the training program. High-intensity training will necessitate frequent rest intervals, while no rest intervals are needed for low-intensity, continuous training.

With these factors in mind, the basic foundations of several endurance training systems will be explored in the following sections.

Interval Training

The concept of interval training has existed for a number of years in one form or another. Humphreys and Holman (1985) credit the famous German coach, Woldemar Gerschler, with the formalization of a structured system of interval training in the 1930s.

With interval training, short to moderate periods of work are alternated with short to moderate periods of rest, or reduced activity. The concept has a firm foundation in physiological principles. Researchers have demonstrated that athletes can perform a considerably greater volume of work by breaking the total work into short, intense bouts with rest, or reduced activity, intervals interspersed between consecutive work bouts. The intervals of work and rest are usually equal and can vary from several seconds to five minutes or more. The vocabulary of interval training includes the terms **set, repetition, training time, training distance,** and **frequency,** in addition to the **work interval** and the **rest, recovery,** or **relief interval.** These terms are comparable to the same terms used in previous sections of this book and will, therefore, not require further definition here. Interval training is frequently prescribed using the above terms and is illustrated in this example for a middle-distance runner:

Set 1: 6 × 400-m at 75 sec (90 sec jog)
Set 2: 6 × 800-m at 180 sec (200 sec jog-walk)

For the first set, an individual would run six repetitions of 400 meters each, completing the work interval in 75 seconds, and recovering for 90 seconds between work intervals with slow jogging. The second set consists of running six repetitions of 800 meters each, completing the work interval in 180 seconds, and recovering for 200 seconds between work intervals with slow jogging or walking.

The interval-training approach can be used in almost any sport or activity, but has received its greatest application in track, cross-country, and swimming. Interval procedures can be adapted to any sport or activity by selecting the form or mode of training and then manipulating the primary variables to fit the sport and athlete. Fox and Mathews (1974) have identified the following five variables that must be individually adjusted for each athlete:

- Rate and distance of the work interval
- Number of repetitions and sets during each training session
- Duration of the rest, recovery, or relief interval
- Type of activity during the rest interval
- Frequency of training per week.

Several methods can be used to determine a sufficient work rate or intensity. One that can be used with any form of physical activity is the monitoring of pulse rate. The athlete can be assigned a training pulse rate on the basis of his or her maximal heart rate. Since few people have access to a treadmill and electrocardiograph, this can be determined relatively accurately by having the athlete run an all-out, 400-meter run, monitoring the pulse rate during the first 15 seconds of recovery. It is assumed that the athlete attained maximal heart rate during the 400-meter run, and it is known that the first 10 to 15 seconds of recovery provide an accurate reflection of the heart rate during the last few seconds of exercise.

This procedure can be accomplished quite easily by locating the carotid pulse in the juncture of the head and neck, the radial pulse on the thumb-side of the wrist, or by simply placing the hand directly over the heart. With the second hand of a watch, start by counting the first pulse beat as zero and then proceed to count the number of beats in the following 15-second interval. This value multiplied by four will provide a reasonably accurate estimate of the maximal heart rate (HR max) in beats per minute. A set percentage of HR max can then be used to guide the rate or intensity of work during the work interval. A high-intensity work interval would be run at 95 percent of HR max, and a moderate-intensity work interval would be run at a rate between 85 and 95 percent of HR max. Frequently, the duration of the rest interval is dictated by the return of the HR to a pre-set level, such as 120 beats per min. When the heart rate reaches this level, the athlete starts the next work interval.

Another method for establishing the rate or intensity of the work interval is to assign a specific duration for a set distance, such as 30 seconds for 200 meters. Wilt (1968) has derived a simple way of establishing these durations, although his original procedures have been altered slightly to convert English to metric units. The times for distances between 50 and 200 meters are established by adding between 1.5 and 5.0 seconds, respectively, to the fastest time the athlete can run those distances from a running start. For the distance of 400 meters, one to four seconds should be subtracted from one-quarter of the athlete's fastest 1500-meter or mile time; for instance, for a five-minute, 1500-meter, 300 sec/4 = 75 sec − 4 = 71 sec. For distances over 400 meters, each 400 meters of the distance should be run at a speed equal to the average 800-meter time in the athlete's best 5000-meter run, minus four seconds; for instance, for an 800-meter interval and a 15-minute, 5000-meter best time, the athlete would run 144 sec/800 meters [(15-min/5000-meters) × 60 sec/min = 900 sec/5000 meters = 0.18 sec/meter or 144 sec for 800 meters].

The distance covered during the work interval can be varied from between 20 and 30 meters to distances in excess of several miles. The length of the interval will depend on the athlete. Athletes who run short distances, such as sprinters, basketball players, and football players, will utilize short intervals of 30 meters to 200 meters, although the 200-meter sprinter will frequently run over-distances of 300 to 400 meters. The 1500-meter runner may run intervals as short as 200 meters, but most of his or her training would be at dis-

tances of 400 meters, 800 meters, 1500 meters, and some over-distance work. In running over-distance intervals, the athlete extends the length of the interval beyond that distance normally run in competition. Theoretically, this type of training will allow the athlete to complete his or her racing distance at top speed, without experiencing fatigue or exhaustion towards the end of the run. While this is a widespread practice among coaches, and the theory appears sound, little research is available to substantiate the value of its use.

The number of repetitions and sets will also be largely determined by the sport, activity, or event of the athlete. Generally, the shorter and more intense the interval, the greater the number of repetitions and sets. As the training interval is lengthened in both distance and duration, the number of repetitions and sets is correspondingly reduced. Fox and Mathews (1974) have established a series of guidelines that can be followed in the selection of the number of repetitions and sets.

The duration of the rest interval will depend on how rapidly the athlete recovers from the work interval. This period of rest can be determined individually, using the athlete's pulse rate to dictate at what time he or she is recovered and physiologically ready to start the next work interval. For athletes 30 years of age and younger, it is a common practice to allow the pulse rate to drop to between 130 and 150 beats per min before starting the next repetition and to below 120 beats per min before starting the next set. For those over 30 years of age, since the maximum pulse rate declines with age, reduce the above pulse rate guidelines by one beat per min for every year over the age of 30. As an example, the 45-year-old, Masters-competition runner would use between 115 and 135 beats per min for a recovery pulse rate between intervals, and 105 beats per min for a recovery pulse rate between sets. Since absolute accuracy is not essential in determining these recovery rates, the pulse can be counted for a six-second period and multiplied by ten. This can result in a counting error as large as ten beats per min, but this is acceptable for these purposes. These pulse rate guidelines should be scaled down for swimmers since the heart rate in water is generally eight to ten beats per min lower for similar intensities.

The type of activity performed during the rest interval can vary from slow walking to rapid walking and jogging, or the equivalent of these activities in other sports. Generally, the more intense the work interval, the lighter or less intense the work performed in the rest interval. As the athlete becomes better conditioned, he or she will be able to increase the intensity or decrease the duration of the rest interval, or both.

The frequency of training will depend largely on the purpose of the interval training. The world-class sprinter or middle-distance runner will need to work out five to seven days per week, although not every workout will include interval training. The swimmer will use interval training almost exclusively. The athlete who plays team sports can benefit from two to four days of interval training per week when interval training is used only as a supplement to a general conditioning program. For general conditioning or for off-season conditioning programs, two to four days per week appear to be adequate, although the improvement gained from two days per week programs will be minimal.

Costill (1986) has made the important distinction between three types of interval training: aerobic, aerobic-anaerobic, and anaerobic. **Aerobic interval training** involves repeated short runs or swims at just below race pace, with very brief rest intervals of five to 15 seconds. As an example, for a runner preparing for a 10-kilometer race, he or she would perform 20 repetitions of 400 meters at a pace that is five to six seconds per minute slower than his or her best race pace. This type of interval training requires oxygen uptakes of approximately 65 to 75 percent of $\dot{V}O_2$ max and heart rates of 70 to 85 percent of HR max. Figure 9–9 illustrates the oxygen uptake and heart rate response to this type of an aerobic interval training workout. **Aerobic-anaerobic interval training** involves an intensity of training at speeds approximating race pace, which will require energy expenditures between 80 and 95 percent of $\dot{V}O_2$ max and heart rates between 85 and 100 percent of HR max (see Figure 9–10 on page 170); but the work intervals are shorter and the rest intervals are extended to between 60 and 90 seconds. **Anaerobic interval training** requires training at an

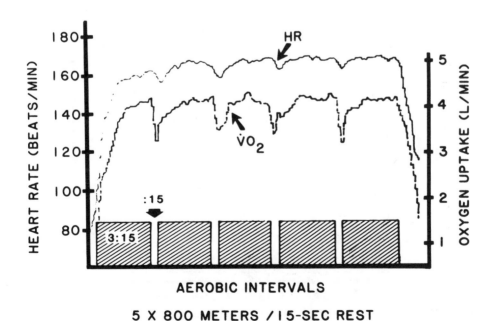

AEROBIC INTERVALS

5 X 800 METERS / 15-SEC REST

Figure 9–9 Heart rate and oxygen uptake during a series of aerobic intervals (from Costill, 1986).

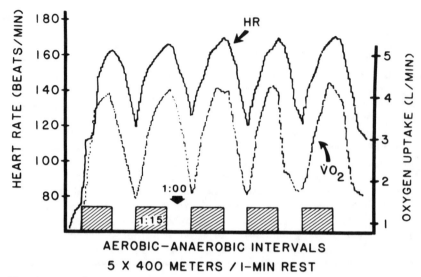

Figure 9-10 Heart rate and oxygen uptake during a series of aerobic-anaerobic intervals (from Costill, 1986).

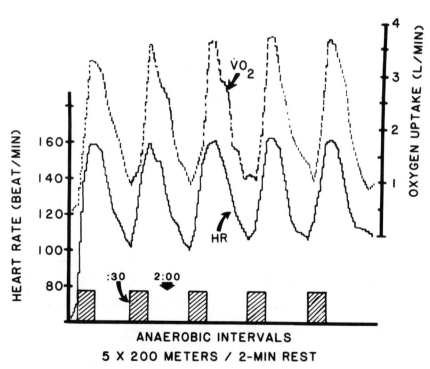

Figure 9-11 Heart rate and oxygen uptake during a series of anaerobic intervals (from Costill, 1986).

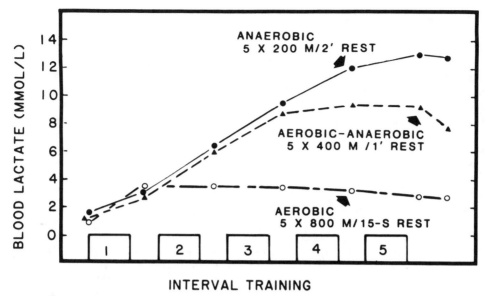

Figure 9-12 Blood lactate accumulation during aerobic, aerobic-anaerobic, and anaerobic interval training (from Costill, 1986).

intensity which exceeds race pace, but with even shorter work intervals and rest intervals of two minutes. Heart rate and oxygen uptake during these anaerobic intervals are similar to those observed in the aerobic-anaerobic intervals (see Figure 9-11), but the blood lactate responses are much higher (see Figure 9-12). Aerobic interval training builds a strong aerobic base, aerobic-anaerobic interval training develops speed and a sense of race pace, and anaerobic interval training develops leg strength, increases muscle buffering capacity, and increases the ability to clear lactate from the muscles. As mentioned earlier in this section, as the athlete becomes better conditioned, he or she increases the rate of the work interval and decreases the time of the rest, or recovery, interval.

The coach or athlete who is interested in the specific details of how to organize and administer an interval training program should refer to the excellent text by Fox and Mathews (1974) cited in the reference section of this chapter. These authors have provided many excellent examples of how interval training can be utilized for various types of conditioning programs. The text by Humphreys and Holman (1985) also provides an excellent, practical approach to interval training.

Continuous Training

Continuous training, as the name implies, involves continuous activity, without rest intervals. This has varied from high-intensity, continuous activity of moderate duration to low-intensity activity of an extended duration (long, slow distance, or "LSD" training). High-intensity, continuous activity is performed at work intensities that represent 85 to 95 percent of the individual's HR max. As an example, the middle-distance runner may run a total distance of five miles, averaging approximately a five min per mile pace, with an average pulse rate of 180 beats per min (HR max = 200 beats per min). The long-distance runner maintains a pace that is just below his or her racing pace, although this will depend on the competition distance and the distance of the training runs. This has been a very effective way of training endurance athletes without requiring high levels of work that are stressful and uncomfortable for the athlete. One advantage of this type of training for the competitive runner is the constant pace at near-competition levels. Running at an even pace during a race appears to be the most efficient way, physiologically, to attain the runner's best time. Therefore, this type of training would greatly aid the runner in preparing for actual competition. A word of caution should be introduced at this point, however, since the demands of this type of training program are extraordinary, particularly when extended over weeks and months. It is suggested that slower-paced variations, such as LSD or Fartlek (to be explained later in this section), be introduced periodically (for example, twice per week), to give the athlete some relief from the continuous level of exhaustive, high-intensity training.

LSD training became extremely popular during the latter part of the 1960s. Dr. Ernst VanAaken, a German physician and coach, is credited with introducing and popularizing this system of training. Dr. VanAaken's work in this area started in the 1920s, but has received widespread support only in the last 20 years. With LSD training, the athlete performs at a relatively low intensity, 60 to 80 percent of HR max. Pulse rates seldom get above 160 beats per min for the young athlete and 140 beats per min for the older athlete. Distance, rather than speed, is the main objective. Endurance runners may train 15 to 30 miles per day using LSD techniques, with weekly distances of 100 to 200 miles. The pace of the run is considerably slower than the maximum pace the individual can sustain. The individual capable of running a five min per mile pace will train at a seven to eight min per mile pace. While the cardiovascular and respiratory stress is considerably less and much more tolerable compared to high-intensity, continuous training, the extreme distances can result in significant muscle and joint discomfort, and actual injury. Further, the serious runner needs to either train or race at or near race pace on a regular basis to develop leg speed, leg strength, and the ability to clear lactate from the muscles.

LSD training is probably the most widely-used form of endurance conditioning for the jogger who wants to stay in condition for health-related purposes, the athlete who participates in team sports and endurance trains only for general conditioning, and the athlete who wants to maintain endurance conditioning during the off-season. For these purposes, the pace is kept at 60 to 80 percent of HR max, but the distance is reduced to three to five miles. This appears to be an excellent approach to general endurance conditioning, since it has been shown to be effective and can be performed at a comfortable level of work. For the middle-aged, or older, individual who is attempting to attain or maintain an acceptable level of physical fitness, from a medical viewpoint this is also the most judicious way to train. Vigorous exercise in the older individual is potentially dangerous and burst-types of activity should not be encouraged.

Fartlek training, or speed play, is another form of continuous exercise that has a flavor of interval training. This form of training was developed in Sweden in the 1930s and is used primarily by distance runners. The athlete varies the pace from high speed to jogging speed at his or her own discretion. This is a free form of training in which fun is the main goal and distance and time are not considered. Fartlek training is normally performed in the countryside where there are a variety of hills. Each athlete is free to run whatever course and speed he or she prefers, although periodically, the speed should reach high-intensity levels. Many coaches have used Fartlek training to supplement either high-intensity, continuous training, or interval training, since it provides variety to the normal training routine. Fartlek runs are normally performed for durations of 45 minutes or longer.

While the use of interval training methods is based on sound physiological principles, as was stated earlier in this chapter, it should be pointed out that the few studies that have compared interval training with continuous training have not found any differences in results between the two systems, but have found that both systems produce substantial gains in endurance capacity (Saltin, 1975). Additional research in this area is certainly necessary before any final conclusions can be drawn.

Interval-Circuit Training

A relatively new concept in training has been introduced in several of the Scandinavian countries. This concept combines interval and circuit training. The circuit may be one to five miles in length, with stations every 400 to 1,600 meters. The athlete jogs or sprints the distance between stations, stops at each station to perform a strength, flexibility, or muscular-endurance exercise in a manner similar to actual circuit training, and continues on, jogging or running, to the next station. These courses are typically located in parks or in the country where there are many trees and hills.

Combination Programs

Most training programs do not rely specifically on any one method or system of training. Each of the training methods presented in this chapter is unique and has inherent advantages or strengths not present in the other methods. Combining methods or systems gives both the coach and athlete variety in their total training program. Boredom is a real hazard in any intense training program, and variety tends to reduce the chances of the athlete becoming bored with a particular training routine.

Wilt (1968) has developed two tables to assist the coach and athlete in designing training programs for competitive runners. Tables 9–1 and 9–2 provide estimates of the training emphasis for various racing distances and the contributions of

Table 9–1 Training requirements for various running distances* (expressed relative to the percentage of emphasis).

Event	Speed	Aerobic endurance	Anaerobic endurance
Marathon	5	90	5
6 mi	5	80	15
3 mi	10	70	20
2 mi	20	40	40
1 mi	20	25	55
880 yd	30	5	65
440 yd	80	5	15
220 yd	95	3	2
100 yd	95	2	3

*From F. Wilt "Training for Competitive Running," in *Exercise Physiology*, edited by H. B. Falls. (New York: Academic Press, 1968.) Reproduced by permission of the publisher.

Table 9–2 Components of various systems of endurance and sprint training* (expressed relative to percentage involvement).

Type of training	Speed	Aerobic endurance	Anaerobic endurance
Repetitions of sprints	90	4	6
Continuous slow running	2	93	5
Continuous fast running	2	90	8
Slow interval	10	60	30
Fast interval	30	20	50
Repetition running	10	40	50
Speed play	20	40	40
Interval sprinting	20	70	10
Acceleration sprinting	90	5	5

*Adapted from F. Wilt "Training for Competitive Running," in *Exercise Physiology*, edited by H. B. Falls. (New York: Academic Press, 1968.) Reproduced by permission of the publisher.

these different training systems to major components of run-training—speed, aerobic endurance, and anaerobic endurance. On the basis of a survey of 20 to 30 top runners in each event conducted by *Runner's World* magazine, the most popular training patterns for each event were determined. A summary of this survey is presented in Table 9–3 on page 174. These data were published in 1974 and are likely to be outdated by present training standards.

It appears that a total program of training should include several different systems of training. This is true not only from the standpoint of variety, but also from a physiological point of view. It has been recently theorized that a combination program is essential for the success of the runner, irrespective of the distance of competitive runs. The sprinter may benefit greatly from endurance training, since it may allow maintenance of the quality of repeat sprints with interval training.

Table 9-3   *Runner's World* survey* of the training patterns of top-level runners.

Race	Avg. Time	Days/ Week	Miles/ Day	Types of Running† (% each)					Training Site (% each)		
				S.D.	F.D.	Int.	Flk.	Race	Track	Road	C-country
100 yards	9.8	5.8	4.8	17	16	49	12	6	50	30	20
220 yards	21.9	5.9	5.0	35	12	39	10	4	37	37	26
440 yards	48.8	5.9	7.5	40	12	35	9	4	44	33	23
880 yards	1:52	6.4	9.0	55	17	17	7	4	28	50	22
1 mile	4:10	6.8	10.5	55	19	15	6	6	22	52	26
2 miles	9:00	6.8	11.0	58	18	11	7	6	17	60	23
3 miles	13:50	6.8	12.8	53	26	9	8	4	18	50	32
6 miles	29:00	6.9	13.0	59	21	10	4	6	18	63	19
9-15 miles	—	6.9	13.0	51	21	5	15	8	17	54	29
Marathon	2:26	6.9	13.1	51	25	5	13	6	13	63	24

†S.D. = slow distance; F.D. = fast distance; Int. = intervals; Flk. = Fartlek.

*From *The Complete Runner*, Mountain View, Calif.: World Publications, 1974. Reproduced by permission of the publisher.

Likewise, the distance runner can benefit from speed work, since a finishing kick, or faster pace, is frequently required to complete the run. Undoubtedly, further research in this area will bring forward even better systems of training and a better understanding of the training needs for various sports, activities, or events.

RELATIONSHIP OF CARDIORESPIRATORY ENDURANCE TO ATHLETIC PERFORMANCE

Cardiorespiratory endurance is regarded by many as the most important component of physical fitness. Since all athletes should have above-average levels of physical fitness, endurance conditioning becomes an important part of their training program. Even the golfer, whose sport is considered relatively sedentary, will benefit from cardiovascular endurance conditioning. The gains in endurance from such conditioning will allow the golfer to complete a round of golf with less fatigue, and his or her legs will be better able to withstand the long periods of walking and standing. For the sedentary, middle-aged adult, this should be the primary emphasis of the training program. This will be discussed at length in Chapter 19.

For any athlete, fatigue represents a major deterrent to his or her best performance. Even minor, or low, levels of fatigue have negative influences on the athlete's total performance. Muscular strength is decreased, the reaction and movement times are prolonged, agility and neuromuscular coordination are reduced, the speed of total body movement is slowed, and the level of concentration and alertness is reduced. This latter factor is particularly important, for the athlete may become careless and more prone to serious injury, especially in contact sports. Even though this decrease in the athlete's performance may be small, it may be just enough to cause the individual to miss the critical free-throw in the basketball game, the three-point field goal in football, or the 20-foot putt in golf.

The extent of endurance training necessary will vary considerably from one athlete to the next, depending on his or her existing endurance capacity and the endurance demands of the sport. It is obvious that the marathon runner will use endurance training almost exclusively, with limited attention to strength, flexibility, and speed. The baseball player, however, has very limited demands placed on endurance capacity, so the training program will not emphasize endurance conditioning as much. Nevertheless, it is felt that the baseball player could gain substantially from endurance running, even if the periods are limited to three miles per day, three days per week at a moderate intensity. He would have little or no trouble with his legs (a frequent complaint of baseball players), and he would be able to complete a doubleheader with little or no fatigue. Many athletes in nonendurance sports, activities, or events have never incorporated even moderate endurance training into their training programs. Those who have incorporated endurance training, are generally well aware of their improved physical condition and its impact on their athletic performance.

SUMMARY

Cardiorespiratory endurance, in contrast to muscular endurance, is possibly the most important component of general physical fitness. As a result, it is an important area that should be developed in the training programs of most athletes. Cardiorespiratory endurance is defined as the ability of the total body to sustain prolonged, rhythmical exercise. The best measure of cardiorespiratory endurance capacity in the laboratory is the athlete's maximal oxygen uptake ($\dot{V}O_2$ max).

It is known that endurance capacity is influenced by genetic factors, sex, and age. In addition, it can be greatly influenced by physical training. The mechanisms by which the $\dot{V}O_2$ max is increased with endurance training include a combination of increased size and number of mitochondria and oxidative enzymes in the active tissue, as well as an increased blood volume, increased cardiac output, and better perfusion of the active tissue (increased capillarization and muscle blood flow). These latter factors are now considered to be the most important.

A number of specific training methods or systems exist for developing cardiovascular endurance. The two major classifications of training systems are interval training and continuous training. Interval training involves periods of high-intensity work with rest periods interspersed between the work bouts. In designing an interval training program, attention must be given to the rate and distance of the work interval, the number of repetitions and sets during each training session, the duration of the rest interval, the type of activity during the rest interval, and the frequency of training per week.

The use of interval training methods is based on sound physiological principles. Research has demonstrated that the total amount, or volume, of work accomplished in a given period of time is much greater if the work is broken into short, intense bouts of work with rest periods interspersed between them, as compared to continuous bouts of work without rest intervals. It should be pointed out, however, that the few studies that have compared interval training with continuous training have not found any differences in results between the two systems, but have found that both systems produce substantial gains in endurance capacity (Saltin, 1975). Additional research in this area is certainly necessary before any final conclusions can be drawn.

Continuous training involves continuous activity without rest intervals. This type of training can be of high intensity, or of moderate intensity, and an extended duration (LSD). A third type of continuous activity is the Swedish Fartlek system, which consists of jogging and bursts of sprinting as dictated by the will of the athlete. Interval circuit training involves an extended circuit one to five miles long, with several stations along the circuit for exercises for strength, flexibility, or muscular endurance.

Most coaches and athletes develop comprehensive training programs that combine two or more of the above systems. In this manner, the athlete can have more variety in his or her training, as well as gain from the strengths of the additional systems.

Cardiovascular endurance conditioning is a critical aspect of any athlete's training program. Low-endurance capacity leads to fatigue, even in the more sedentary sports or activities. Such a condition can only work to lower the performance potential of the athlete, since fatigue will reduce strength, speed, reaction and movement time, and will have a negative influence on agility and neuromuscular coordination. In addition, the athlete becomes more prone to serious injury, largely due to an inability to fully concentrate on his or her performance, because of the conditions just stated. Adequate cardiovascular conditioning must be the foundation of any athlete's general conditioning program.

STUDY QUESTIONS

1. Differentiate between muscular endurance and cardiovascular endurance.
2. What is maximal oxygen uptake or consumption ($\dot{V}O_2$ max)?
3. Of what importance is $\dot{V}O_2$ max to endurance performance?
4. Would a two-mile run at full speed be considered an anaerobic or an aerobic activity? Why?
5. How does the concept of progressive overload apply to cardiorespiratory endurance training?
6. What are the major factors that must be considered when developing a cardiorespiratory, endurance conditioning program?
7. Design an interval training program for a middle-distance runner.
8. How can work intervals be monitored when using interval training procedures?
9. How does high-intensity, continuous training differ from interval training?
10. Discuss the relative merits of both interval and continuous training.
11. Explain the two theories that were proposed to account for improvements in $\dot{V}O_2$ max. Which of these has the greatest validity today? Why?
12. Which is possibly the most important adaptation the body makes in response to endurance training, allowing for an increase in both $\dot{V}O_2$ max and performance?
13. How important is genetic potential in developing a young athlete?
14. Why would cardiovascular endurance conditioning be important for athletes in non-endurance sports?

REFERENCES

Åstrand, P. O. (1972, March-April). *Journal of Physical Education*, 129-136.

Åstrand, P. O., & Rodahl, K. (1986). *Textbook of work physiology*, (3rd ed.). New York: McGraw-Hill Book Co.

Bouchard, C., Lesage, R., Lortie, G., Simoneau, J. A., Hamel, P., Boulay, M. R., Pérusse, L., Thériault, G., and Leblanc, C. (1986). Aerobic performance in brothers, dizygotic, and monozygotic twins. *Medicine and Science in Sports and Exercise, 18,* 639-646.

Bouchard, C., & Malina, R. M. (1983). Genetics of physiological fitness and motor performance. *Exercise and Sport Sciences Reviews, 11,* 306-339.

Clausen, J. P. (1977). Effect of physical training on cardiovascular adjustments to exercise in man. *Physiological Review, 57,* 779-816.

Cooper, K. H. (1968). *Aerobics.* New York: M. Evans.

Costes, N. (1972). *Interval training.* Mountain View, CA: World Publications.

Costill, D. L. (1986). *Inside running: Basics of sports physiology.* Indianapolis, IN: Benchmark Press, Inc.

Coyle, E. F., Hemmert, M. K., & Coggan, A. R. (1986). Effects of detraining on cardiovascular responses to exercise: Role of blood volume. *Journal of Applied Physiology, 60,* 95-99.

Dempsey, J. A. (1986). Is the lung built for exercise? *Medicine and Science in Sports and Exercise, 18,* 143-155.

deVries, H. A. (1980). *Physiology of exercise for physical education and athletics* (3rd ed.). Dubuque, IA: William C. Brown Co.

Dowell, R. T. (1983). Cardiac adaptations to exercise. *Exercise and Sport Sciences Reviews, 11,* 99-117.

Edington, D. W., & Edgerton, V. R. (1976). *The biology of physical activity.* Boston: Houghton Mifflin Co.

Ekblom, B., Goldbarg, A. M., & Gullbring, B. (1972). Response to exercise after blood loss and reinfusion. *Journal of Applied Physiology, 33,* 175-180.

Fox, E. L. (1984). *Sports physiology* (2nd ed.). Philadelphia: W. B. Saunders Co.

Fox, E. L., & Mathews, D. K. (1974). *Interval training conditioning for sports and general fitness.* Philadelphia: W. B. Saunders Co.

Fox, E. L., & Mathews, D. K. (1981). *The physiological basis of physical education and athletics* (3rd ed.). Philadelphia: W. B. Saunders Co.

Holloszy, J. O., & Coyle, E. F. (1984). Adaptations of skeletal muscle to endurance exercise and their metabolic consequences. *Journal of Applied Physiology, 56,* 831-838.

Hudlicka, O. (1977). Effect of training on macro- and microcirculatory changes in exercise. *Exercise and Sport Sciences Reviews, 5,* 181-230.

Humphreys, J., & Holman, R. (1985). *Focus on middle-distance running.* London: Adam & Charles Black.

Jensen, C. R., & Fisher, A. G. (1979). *Scientific basis of athletic conditioning* (2nd ed.). Philadelphia: Lea & Febiger.

Jones, N. L., & Ehrsam, R. E. (1982). The anaerobic threshold. *Exercise and Sport Sciences Reviews, 10,* 49-83.

Klissouras, V. (1971). Adaptability of genetic variation. *Journal of Applied Physiology, 31,* 338-344.

Lamb, D. R. (1984). *Physiology of exercise: Responses*

and adaptations (2nd ed.). New York: Macmillan Publishing Co.

Laughlin, M. H., & Armstrong, R. B. (1985). Muscle blood flow during locomotory exercise. *Exercise and Sport Sciences Reviews, 13,* 95-136.

Pirnay, F., Dujardin, J., Deroanne, R., & Petit, J. M. (1971). Muscular exercise during intoxication by carbon monoxide. *Journal of Applied Physiology, 31,* 573-575.

Pollock, M. L. (1973). Quantification of endurance training programs. *Exercise and Sport Sciences Reviews, 1,* 155-188.

Pollock, M. L., Wilmore, J. H., & Fox, S. M. (1984). *Exercise in health and disease: Evaluation and prescription for health and rehabilitation.* Philadelphia: W. B. Saunders.

Robinson, S. (1938). Experimental studies of physical fitness in relation to age. *Arbeitsphysiology, 10,* 251-323.

Runner's World. (1974). *The complete runner.* Mountain View, CA: World Publications.

Saltin, B. (1975). *Intermittent exercise: Its physiology and practical applications.* Muncie, IN: Ball State University.

Saltin, B., & Rowell, L. B. (1980). Functional adaptations to physical activity and inactivity. *Federation Proceedings, 39,* 1506-1513.

Sharkey, B. J. (1979). *Physiology of fitness.* Champaign, IL: Human Kinetics Publishers.

Shepard, R. J. (1971). *Endurance fitness.* Toronto: University of Toronto Press.

Wilt, F. (1968). Training for competitive running. In H. B. Falls (Ed.), *Exercise physiology.* New York: Academic Press.

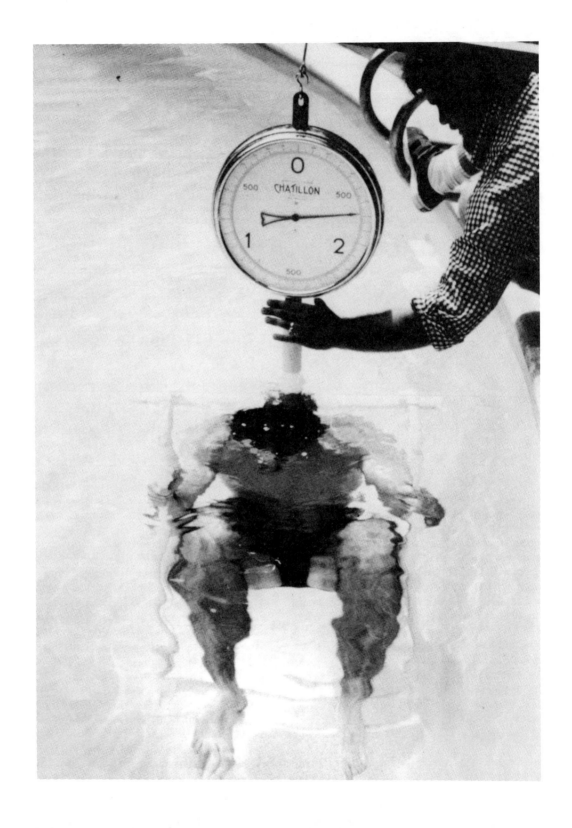

10

Body Build and Composition

INTRODUCTION

This chapter will focus on body build and composition as it relates to athletic performance. Body composition is also an important aspect of general fitness and good health, and will be discussed in detail in Chapter 18. Having the appropriate size, build, and body composition is of major importance to success in almost all athletic endeavors. It is obvious that the 7-foot 1-inch center in basketball could never have become a proficient jockey. Similarly, the 130-pound marathon runner would not be the ideal candidate for a starting assignment on the defensive line of the Dallas Cowboys professional football team. Each athlete has a genetic profile that predominantly dictates limits for both body build and composition. It is true that in most athletes, muscle training will develop substantial increases in muscle mass. Further, a combination of diet and vigorous exercise will lead to considerable losses in body fat. However, when compared to the broad range of body sizes and builds in the total arena of athletics, from the smallest gymnast to the largest Sumo wrestler, the range of potential variability for any one individual to develop is relatively small and quite restricted.

Athletes are then limited by what they have inherited from their parents. This does not imply

that they should dismiss this aspect of their physical profile with the feeling that nothing can be done to change or improve themselves. While body type or build can be altered only slightly, substantial changes can occur in body composition with diet and exercise, changes that can be of major importance to achieving optimal athletic performance.

What is the difference between body build, body size, and body composition? **Body build** refers to the morphology, or the form and structure, of the body. Somatotyping is a scientific procedure used to describe the morphology of the body in a quantitative manner. Most somatotyping systems utilize the concept that the body has three major components or dimensions: muscularity, linearity, and fatness. The three components have been termed **mesomorphy** for muscularity, **ectomorphy** for linearity, and **endomorphy** for fatness. A rating procedure was developed in which each person is rated in each of these three areas. The original system developed by Sheldon used a rating scale of one to seven to designate the degree that component was present, the higher the rating the more predominant the component. As an example, a rating of 2-7-2 (endomorphy-mesomorphy-ectomorphy) would indicate an individual who would be described as having a predominance of muscle, very little fat, and a stocky frame (lack of linearity).

179

Body size refers to the height and mass, or weight, of the individual. The distinctions of being classified as short or tall, large or small, heavy or light, depend entirely on the sport, position within a sport, or a particular event. A height of six feet three inches would be relatively short for a professional basketball player, but tall for a long distance runner. Similarly, a weight of 230 pounds would be heavy for a quarterback, just right for a linebacker, but light for a defensive end in professional football. Body size, therefore, must be considered relative to the sport, position, or event.

Body composition provides additional information to both the coach and the athlete. To know only the weight of an athlete has little meaning to either the athlete or the coach. To know that of a total weight of 200 pounds, ten pounds is fat and the remaining 190 pounds is lean, provides considerably more insight into this athlete. In this example, only five percent of his body weight [(10 lb/200 lb)·100 = 5] is fat, which is about as low as any athlete should go. This athlete would then realize that his body composition is ideal, and he should not try to lose weight, even though he may be overweight by the standard height-weight charts. A male athlete of the same weight, 200 pounds, who has 50 pounds of fat and 150 pounds of lean weight, would be 25 percent fat [(50 lb/200 lb)·100 = 25]. This would constitute a serious weight problem in that he would be overfat. If the amount of fat in proportion to an individual's total weight is high, it will have a negative influence on athletic performance; the higher the percentage of body fat, the poorer the performance. Thus, an accurate assessment of the athlete's body composition provides valuable insight into the best playing weight for that athlete for his or her sport, or event.

Total weight is composed of the fat weight and the lean weight. The lean weight is merely a convenient term to account for all of the body tissue that is not fat, including muscle, bone, skin, and internal organs. Fortunately, when working with athletes, weight gains and losses involve primarily the fat and muscle mass, and any changes in lean weight are generally reflective of changes in muscle mass.

ADAPTATIONS IN BODY BUILD AND COMPOSITION WITH PHYSICAL TRAINING

Body build can be altered slightly with physical training. However, previous research has suggested that somatotypes change very little during an individual's life span. In fact, studies have found that adult somatotypes can be predicted with a high degree of accuracy during preadolescence. As was stated earlier in this chapter, muscle mass can be lost with physical inactivity and gained with strength training, and body fat can be either gained or lost with manipulations in both diet and exercise. These changes are usually relatively small, and result in little or no change in the somatotype. This inability to substantially alter somatotype is largely the result of the inherited, or genetic, nature of body type.

Body composition can undergo substantial alterations with physical training. It has generally been stated by the masses, that physical activity has only a limited influence on changing body composition, and that even exercise of a vigorous nature requires the expenditure of too few calories to result in substantial reductions in body fat. Yet, research has conclusively demonstrated the effectiveness of exercise training in promoting major alterations in body composition. How do we account for this apparent conflict?

When estimating the energy cost of an activity, it is typical to multiply the steady-state rate of energy expenditure for a specific activity, times the minutes engaged in that activity. If the steady-state value for shoveling snow is 7.5 kcals/min, it would require a total of only 450 kcals for one hour of work (7.5 kcal/min · 60 min/hr). This would approximate a loss of 0.13 pounds of fat [approximately 3,500 kcal/lb of fat: 450 kcal/(3,500 kcal/lb) = 0.13 lbs]. However, the metabolism remains elevated during the post-exercise recovery period. The recovery back to pre-exercise levels can require several minutes for light exercise, several hours for heavy exercise, and between 12 and 24 hours, or sometimes longer, for prolonged, exhaustive exercise. The elevation of the metabolism above normal levels during the recovery period from intense or prolonged exhaustive exercise, can add up to a substantial energy expenditure when totaled over the entire period of recovery. If the oxygen consumption following exercise remains elevated by only 100 ml/min or 0.1 liter/min, this will amount to approximately 0.5 kcal/min or 30 kcal/hr. If the metabolism remains elevated for ten hours, this would amount to an additional expenditure of 300 kcal that would not normally be included in the calculated total energy expenditure for that particular activity. This major source of energy expenditure, which occurs during recovery but is directly the result of the exercise bout, is frequently ignored in most calculations of the energy cost of various activities. If the individual in this example exercised five days per week, he or she would have expended 1,500 kcal, or lost the equivalent of approximately 0.4 pounds of fat in one week, just from the recovery period alone.

The athlete who jogs three days a week for 30 minutes a day at a 7-mph pace, or slightly over 8½ minutes a mile, will expend approximately 14.5 kcal/min, or 435 kcal for the 30 minute run each day. This would result in a total expenditure per week of approximately 1,305 kcal, the equivalent of slightly over ⅓ pound of fat loss each week. One might conclude that exercise is a painfully slow way to significantly reduce body fat levels, and that there are better and easier ways to lose fat. However, in 52 weeks, providing energy intake remained constant, you would lose a total of 17 pounds!

Athletes often fall into the trap of discovering that they are considerably above their assigned playing weight with only a few weeks remaining before they have to report to training camp. Consider the 25-year-old professional football player who finds that his weight is 20 pounds above his weight the previous season. He must lose this excess poundage by the start of the pre-season training camp, four weeks away. Failure to lose this weight will result in a fine of $100 per day for each pound over his assigned weight. Obviously, exercise is of little value to him, for he would need between nine and 12 months to lose this much weight through exercise alone. He needs to lose five pounds per week, so he relies on a "crash" diet,

selecting whichever diet is in vogue at that time. It is well-known that it is possible to lose between six and eight pounds per week with these diets. What kind of success might this athlete have?

This example is not unique. Many athletes find themselves out of shape and overweight as a result of overeating and less activity during the off-season. Also, they typically wait until the last few weeks prior to reporting for their sport before attempting to attack the problem. In this example, the football player may be able to shed 20 pounds in four weeks as a result of a crash diet. However, much of this weight loss will be from his body's water compartment and very little from stored fat. Several studies have reported that substantial weight losses occur with very low calorie (500 kcal/day or less) diets, but of the total weight lost, over 60 percent comes from the body's lean tissue and less than 40 percent from the fat depots.

While much of the lean weight lost is from the body's water stores, a substantial amount of protein is lost as well. Most of these crash diets require a very low carbohydrate intake. As a result, the carbohydrate stores of the body become depleted. With every one gram of carbohydrate used, approximately three grams of water are lost. With a total body glycogen content of 800 grams, a depletion of the stored glycogen would result in a loss of approximately 2,400 grams of water, or slightly more than five pounds of total weight lost. Additional water is lost as a result of ketosis—ketone bodies accumulate in the blood from the breakdown of free fatty acids, a direct result of the body's reduced carbohydrate stores and the reduced availability of carbohydrates for energy. Much of this loss will occur during the first week of the diet. Figure 10–1 on page 182 illustrates these changes in body water, fat, protein, and carbohydrate over a period of 30 days of fasting.

It is literally impossible to lose more than four pounds of fat per week, even under conditions of total fasting. This can be demonstrated quite easily. Assuming that it requires a 3,500 kcal deficit to lose one pound of fat, this professional athlete could lose no more than 0.7 pounds per day on a total fast. His resting metabolic rate would be approximately 2,500 kcal/day, so he would have a

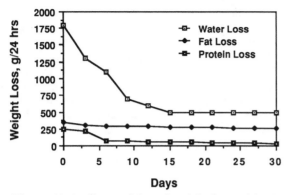

Figure 10-1 Composition of weight loss with 30 days of fasting.

2,500 kcal deficit per day if he fasted. However, during fasting, research indicates that the total body metabolism is reduced by 20 to 25 percent. A 20 percent reduction in this athlete's resting metabolic rate would lower his total deficit to only 2,000 kcal per day, or approximately 0.57 pounds of fat loss per day. In one week this would result in a loss of only four pounds of fat while totally fasting! Few people would be able to tolerate the discomfort associated with prolonged periods of fasting. By increasing his activity level he could add to this predicted rate of fat weight loss, but it would be impossible to train very hard with no intake of food and an almost total depletion of his glycogen stores.

The sensible approach to reduce body fat stores is to combine moderate dietary restriction with increased levels of exercise. The appetite is delicately balanced to meet the actual caloric needs of the body. Reducing dietary intake by just 100 kcal each day will result in a weight loss of ten pounds per year (100 kcal/day • 365 days), providing activity levels remain constant. Combined with a modest ¼- to ½-pound weight loss per week from a three-day per week jogging program, the total weight lost would amount to between 23 and 36 pounds in a single year, and most of the weight loss would be fat weight loss.

Figure 10-2 illustrates the results of one study in which 72 mildly obese male subjects were assigned to one of several treatment programs, which included either exercise or non-exercise in combination with different dietary treatments. While the exercise and non-exercise groups lost similar amounts of weight, the exercise group lost significantly more fat weight and did not lose lean weight. The non-exercising group lost a significant amount of lean weight (Pavlou, et al., 1985).

Thus, combining exercise with diet reduces the proportion of weight lost from the lean tissue to an insignificant level. In fact, the additional physical

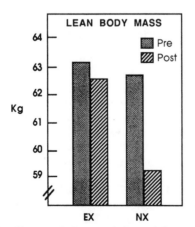

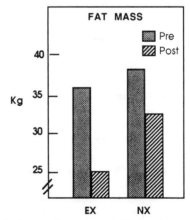

Figure 10-2 Changes in lean weight and fat weight with diet and exercise (EX) vs. diet and no exercise (NX) (adapted from Pavlou, et al., 1985).

activity might possibly even increase the lean weight over an extended period of time. The rapid weight losses experienced with crash diets are quickly regained, probably due to the fact that when a balanced diet is substituted for the low-carbohydrate diet, the water that was lost is quickly regained as the carbohydrate stores are repleted. Since the purpose of the weight-loss program is to lose body fat, and not lean tissue, the combination diet and exercise program is the preferred approach.

With respect to dietary modifications, a reduction of between 200 and 500 kcal/day from the athlete's normal diet will add up to a substantial weight loss over time. Weight losses of approximately one pound per week, which represents a realistic goal, can be achieved with such a modest reduction in calories, particularly in combination with a sound exercise program. It should be added that a balanced diet is essential to assure the necessary vitamins and minerals needed by that athlete. Vitamin supplementation may or may not be essential. Results of research at this time are in conflict. If there is any question about the nutri-

tional adequacy of the diet, a simple multivitamin that meets the recommended daily allowance (RDA) for that individual would be suggested.

When dieting, the total allotted calories should be consumed over at least three meals per day. Many athletes make the mistake of eating only one or two meals per day, skipping either breakfast or lunch, or both, and then consuming a very large dinner. Research in animals has demonstrated that, given the same number of total calories, the animals that eat their daily food ration in one or two meals gain more weight than those that nibble their ration throughout the day.

Another misconception that has been used frequently to discount the benefits of exercise in weight control is the contention that the exercise itself will stimulate the appetite to such an extent that voluntary food intake will be increased, accounting for the additional expenditure of energy through exercise. Jean Mayer, world-famous nutritionist, reported many years ago that in animals exercising for up to one hour per day, there is actually a decrease in appetite when compared to the appetites of sedentary animals (see Figure 10-3).

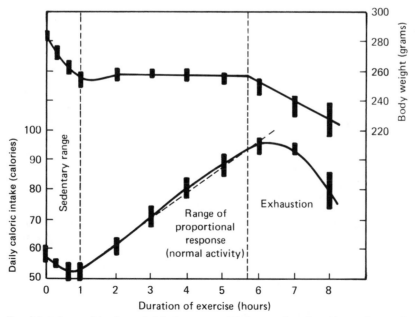

Figure 10-3 Food intake and body weight changes with increasing durations of exercise (from Mayer, et al., 1954).

Table 10-1　Caloric expenditure of running and jogging at different paces, on the basis of body weight.

	Calories per hour Pace per mile							
Weight	5:20	6:00	6:40	7:20	8:00	8:40	9:20	10:00
120	936	828	726	654	594	540	498	456
130	1,014	888	792	708	642	582	534	492
140	1,086	954	846	756	690	630	576	528
150	1,164	1,020	906	810	738	672	612	564
160	1,236	1,086	966	870	780	708	654	600
170	1,314	1,152	1,020	918	828	762	690	636
180	1,386	1,212	1,080	972	876	798	732	672
190	1,464	1,278	1,140	1,020	924	840	774	708
200	1,536	1,344	1,194	1,074	972	888	810	744
210	1,614	1,416	1,230	1,122	1,020	930	846	780
220	1,686	1,482	1,314	1,176	1,068	972	888	816

*Adapted from J. Henderson, "Planning High-Calorie Workouts." *Runner's World,* 9 (1974):24–25. Reproduced by permission of the publisher.

Mayer has concluded that when activity is reduced to below a minimum level, a corresponding decrease in food intake does not occur and the animal or human begins to accumulate body fat. This has led to the theory that a certain minimum level of physical activity is necessary before the body can precisely regulate, or fine-tune food intake to balance energy expenditure. A sedentary lifestyle may reduce the ability of the fine-tuning device to control food intake precisely, which would result in a positive energy balance.

Exercise does, in fact, appear to be a mild appetite suppressant, at least for the first few hours following intense training. Further, studies have shown that the total number of calories you consume per day does not change when you begin a training program. While some have interpreted this as evidence that exercise does not affect appetite, it may be more appropriate to conclude that appetite was affected, in that caloric intake did not increase in proportion to caloric expenditure.

From this discussion, it can be concluded that exercise plays an important role in weight-loss and weight-control programs. Further, exercise does not have to be of an extended and exhaustive nature to be effective. The athlete should select an endurance-type activity that is enjoyable, and participate in this activity for between 30 and 40 min

per day, four to five days per week, at an intensity of between 60 and 75 percent of his or her endurance capacity. Over time, this exercise program will produce the desired results. Table 10-1 provides an example of the caloric expenditure of running on the basis of the pace of running and body weight.

The role of exercise in spot weight-reduction is also a controversial area. Many individuals, including athletes, believe that by exercising a specific area, the fat in that localized area will be utilized, thus reducing the locally stored fat. Several early research studies reported results that tended to support the concept of spot reduction. However, later work suggested that spot reduction is a myth and that exercise, even when localized, draws from all of the fat stores of the body, not just from the local depots. Gwinup, et al. (1971) utilized outstanding tennis players to investigate the phenomenon of spot reduction, theorizing that tennis players would be ideal subjects for studying spot reduction since they could act as their own controls—the dominant arm exercises vigorously every day for several hours, while the nondominant arm is relatively sedentary. They postulated that if spot reduction was a reality, the nondominant (inactive) arm should have substantially more fat than the dominant (active) arm. In fact, while

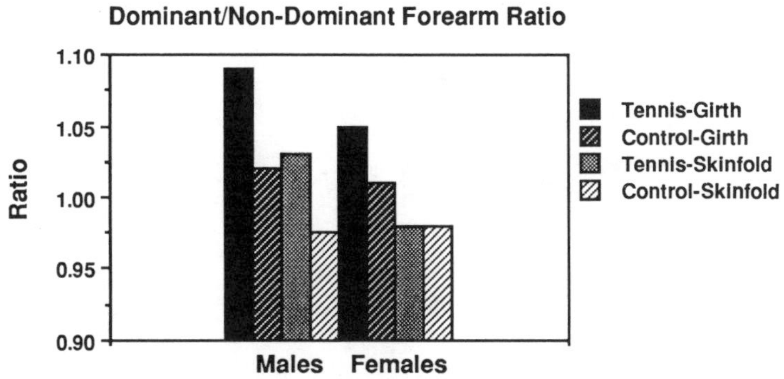

Dominant/Non-Dominant Forearm Ratio

Figure 10–4 The differences in muscle girth and skinfold fat between dominant and nondominant arms of professional tennis players (adapted from Gwinup, et al., 1971).

the arm girths were substantially greater in the dominant arm, due to exercise-induced muscle hypertrophy, there were absolutely no differences in the fat contents of the two arms, as assessed by subcutaneous skinfold fat thicknesses (see Figure 10–4). Katch, et al., (1984) reported no difference in the rate of change in adipose cell diameters at the abdomen, subscapular, and gluteal fat biopsy sites following a 27-day, intense sit-up training program. This indicates a lack of specific adaptation at the site of exercise training. Researchers now theorize that fat is mobilized from either those areas of highest concentration, or equally from all areas, thus negating the spot reduction theory.

Exercise can also lead to substantial weight gains. These gains appear to be predominantly, if not totally, increases in lean body weight. Strength and power training programs lead to the largest gains in lean weight, as a result of their relationship to muscle hypertrophy. Even limited muscle hypertrophy will result from endurance training programs. It is somewhat ironic that training programs will frequently lead to little or no change in total body weight, but body composition undergoes a marked change. Typically, the loss in body fat is masked, or hidden, by an increase of similar magnitude in lean tissue. This phenomenon can be deceptive since there is no change in scale weight even after months of hard work.

MECHANISMS OF CHANGE

It would appear that weight losses and weight gains are simply a matter of changing either energy input, energy expenditure, or both. To lose weight, one can reduce the caloric intake, increase the caloric expenditure, or combine the two. Likewise, with weight gains, one can increase the caloric intake, reduce the energy expenditure, or combine the two. Unfortunately, common observation and recent research suggest that energy balance is not that simple. Nearly everyone has known of individuals who can literally gorge themselves daily, yet remain lean. Or conversely, there are individuals who continue gaining body fat even though they eat only limited amounts of food, well below what would be expected to be their maintenance levels. Individuals do metabolize food differently, some more efficiently than others. Also, some individuals are more efficient in their expenditure of energy for fixed work tasks (see Chapter 2). These phenomena are not clearly understood at the present time, and considerably more research will be necessary to determine those factors that are involved and their relative importance. Researchers are now studying the thermogenic response, or increase in metabolic rate, to both food intake (dietary-induced thermogenesis) and exercise, and are beginning to demonstrate significant differences between selected populations—obese versus non-obese, trained versus untrained.

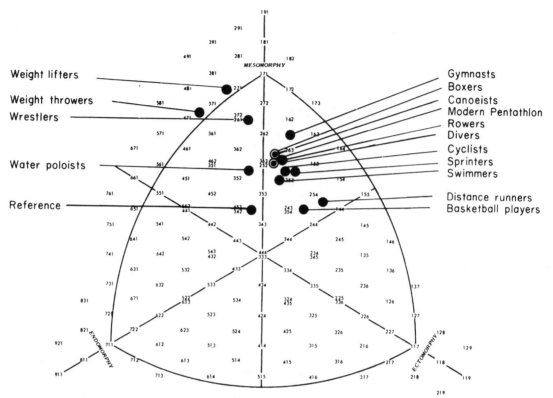

Figure 10–5 Somatogram of mean somatotypes for various male sports groups (from deGaray, et al., Reproduced by permission of the publisher).

With specific reference to exercise, it would appear that the reduction in fat by exercise is solely the result of an added expenditure of calories. Yet, the body might be expected to adapt to this additional expenditure by increasing the appetite to compensate for the deficit. This is a difficult problem that defies a simple solution. A number of research studies have pointed to the possible role of human growth hormone having responsibility for the increased fatty acid mobilization during exercise. Growth hormone levels do increase sharply with exercise and remain elevated for up to several hours in the recovery period. Other research has suggested that with exercise, the adipose tissue is more sensitive to the sympathetic nervous system or to the levels of circulating catecholamines, which would result in increased lipid mobilization. More recent research suggests that a specific fat-mobilizing substance found in the blood, which is highly responsive to elevated levels of activity, is responsible. At the present time, it is impossible to

state with certainty which factors are of greatest importance in mediating this response.

It was demonstrated in the previous section that exercise tends to attenuate appetite. While this has been demonstrated in male laboratory animals, it has been shown that exercise actually increases the appetites of female laboratory animals. The reason for this sex difference is not presently known. In humans, most of the research has been conducted on males, and the results indicate either no change in appetite with increased levels of exercise, or slight decreases. It is possible that the decrease in appetite occurs only with intense levels of work in which the increased catecholamine levels suppress the appetite. It is also possible that the increased body temperature that accompanies high-intensity activity, or almost any activity performed under hot and humid conditions, leads to a decreased appetite. When the weather is hot, or when there is an elevated body temperature as a result of illness, a loss of appetite results. This

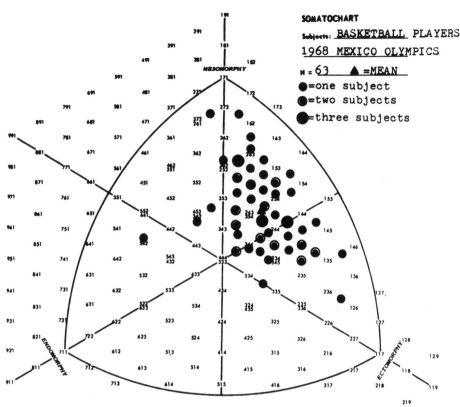

Figure 10-6 Somatogram illustrating the variation in somatotype for basketball players from various countries participating in the 1968 Olympic Games (from deGaray, et al., 1974. Reproduced by permission of the publisher).

might also explain why one can have little or no desire to eat after a hard running workout, but a relatively strong craving for food following a hard swimming workout. In the pool, providing the water temperature is well below core temperature, heat is lost very effectively, thus core temperature can be maintained within the desired range.

The gains in lean weight with exercise are undoubtedly due to increases in protein anabolism, or synthesis, which leads to muscle hypertrophy. In Chapter 7, the potential cause of muscle hypertrophy was explored, and found to be the result of increases in muscle fiber size, possibly due to an increased number of myofibrils. The potential for fiber splitting was also discussed. Without knowing the specific changes that occur within the muscle, it is difficult to postulate the possible mechanisms that trigger these changes. Again, since human growth hormone has anabolic properties,

its rise with exercise and its continued elevation during recovery have led several investigators to suggest that this might explain the gains in lean tissue. Obviously, further research is needed before the actual mechanisms for these changes can be adequately defined.

RELATIONSHIP OF BODY BUILD AND COMPOSITION TO ATHLETIC PERFORMANCE

Most sports require a certain body type for success. This is illustrated in Figure 10-5, which presents somatotype data for a number of sports from participants in the 1968 Olympic Games in Mexico City. Within any one sport, there is considerable variation in somatotype, as illustrated in Figure 10-6. From this information, it is obvious that to be successful, the athlete should select a sport in which his or her somatotype will be an asset. With few exceptions, almost all sports require a moderate-to-high rating in mesomorphy. Extreme endomorphs and extreme ectomorphs do very poorly in most sports.

Body composition must be considered equally as important to body build when attempting to maximize the athlete's performance potential. Several studies have found a high, negative relationship between performance in various activities and the relative amount of body fat. The higher the percentage of body fat, the poorer the performance of the individual. This is true of all activities in which the body weight has to be moved either vertically or horizontally through space, such as sprinting and long jumping. Many athletes are under the impression that they must be large in order to be good in their sport. Size has been associated with the quality of the athlete's performance—the larger the athlete, the better the performance. It is now recognized that this is true only if the size increase is due to an increase in the lean tissue. To add additional fat to the body just to increase the weight and overall size is detrimental to performance, with the possible exception of the heavyweight weight lifter. These individuals add large amounts of fat weight just prior to competition under the pretense that the additional weight will help lower their center of gravity and give them a greater mechanical advantage in lifting. The value of this additional fat weight has yet to be confirmed through research. Another notable exception to the theory that overall size is not the major determinant of athletic success, is the Sumo wrestler. The larger individual does have a decided advantage, but the wrestler with the higher lean weight should have the greatest overall success.

Rather than being concerned with overall weight, most athletes should be specifically concerned with their lean body weight. Eventually, techniques will be available that will allow a young athlete to undergo an extensive evaluation to provide an estimate of fat weight, lean weight, and a projected estimate of his or her potential for increasing lean body weight. In this way, the athlete could design a training program that would develop lean tissue to the projected maximum, while

maintaining fat content at relatively low levels. While this would be a desirable approach for the athlete dependent on strength, power, and muscular endurance, it would be counterproductive for the endurance athlete who is forced to move his or her total body mass horizontally for extended periods of time. Increased lean weight may prove to be a major detriment to successful performance by this athlete, since it is an additional load that must be carried. The same may also be true for the high jumper, long jumper, and triple jumper who depend on maximizing their vertical and horizontal distances. Additional weight, even though it is active lean tissue, may decrease rather than facilitate performance potential for these athletes.

An accurate assessment, or estimate, of the athlete's body composition is essential. Standard height-weight tables do not provide an accurate estimate of what the athlete should weigh. This fact was established in the original classic study relating body composition to athletics. Welham and Behnke studied the body compositions of 25 professional football players in 1942. Of these 25 professional athletes, 17 were physically unqualified for military duty or first-class insurance on the basis of their weight. Of the 17 "overweight" players, 11 were found to have very low levels of body fat, indicating that the overweight condition was the result of an excess of lean tissue and not excess fat. Wilmore and Haskell (1972) investigated the body composition of 44 professional football players according to the positions that they played. The defensive backs were the leanest, lightest, and shortest of the five groups analyzed, while the defensive linemen were the fattest, heaviest, and generally the tallest. The offensive backs and receivers were similar to the defensive backs, and the offensive linemen were comparable to the defensive linemen. The linebackers were unique and fell approximately between the linemen and backs relative to the observed variables. In comparison with the Welham and Behnke data for the 1942-era ball players, the linemen studied in 1969 through 1971 were taller and considerably heavier, but there were no substantial differences between the backs. The increased weight of the players studied in the 1960s and 1970s was due to an increase in both the lean and fat weights of the line-

Table 10-2 Body composition characteristics of professional football players grouped by position.

Position	Number	Height (in)	Weight (lb)	Fat (%)	Fat (lb)	Lean Weight (lb)
Defensive backs	26	71.9	187.0	9.6	18.1	168.9
Offensive backs and wide receivers	40	72.4	200.0	9.4	19.2	180.8
Linebackers	28	74.3	225.3	14.0	32.0	193.3
Offensive linemen and tight ends	38	76.0	248.3	15.6	38.7	209.0
Defensive linemen	32	75.8	258.2	18.2	47.0	211.2
Quarterbacks and kickers	16	72.8	198.7	14.4	28.7	170.0

men. These results, combined with additional results from 1972 through 1976, are summarized in Tables 10-2 and 10-3.

Body composition values tend to vary with the sport. Those sports or activities that have a high endurance component will typically have athletes who have low, relative body fats. Long-distance runners generally have less than ten percent body fat; by contrast, college-aged males and females will average 15 and 22 percent fat, respectively. However, even the better women endurance runners have body fat levels below ten percent. Is this the result of the natural selection of lean individuals for distance running, or is this the result of running 60 to 100 miles or more per week as a part

of their training program? Information is not available to answer this question at the present time, although it undoubtedly is a combination of both. Body composition values for athletes in selected sports are presented in the Appendix.

Of great concern to the medical and scientific community, as well as the involved coach and athlete, is the area of "making weight." While the major concern has been with the sport of wrestling, many schools, districts, or state-level organizations have organized their athletic programs on the basis of size, including weight as the predominant factor. The athlete attempts to get down to the lowest weight possible in order to gain an advantage over his or her opponent. In so doing,

Table 10-3 Comparison of the body composition of professional football players of the early 1940s with those of the late 1960s and early 1970s.

Position	Number	Height (in)	Weight (lb)	Fat (%)	Fat (lb)	Lean Weight (lb)
Backs						
1940—41	13	71.3	189.0	7.1	13.5	175.6
1960s—70s	66	72.2	194.9	9.5	18.8	176.1
Linemen						
1940—41	12	73.1	214.1	14.0	30.0	184.1
1960s—70s	70	75.9	252.8	16.8	42.5	210.0

many athletes have jeopardized their health. In a manner similar to using crash diets, as mentioned earlier in this chapter, these athletes will lose large amounts of weight predominantly through dehydration. They will exercise in rubberized sweat suits, sit in steam and sauna baths, chew on towels to lose saliva, and keep their food and fluid intake minimal. Such severe water losses compromise kidney and general cardiovascular function and are potentially dangerous. Losses of two to four percent of the athlete's total weight due to dehydration can impair performance. Standards should be established on the basis of the athlete's lean body weight. Total body weight for males should consist of not less than five percent fat. This would imply that 95 percent of the athlete's weight should be lean. Knowing lean weight, competition weight should not drop below the following weight:

Minimal competitive weight = Lean weight/0.95

Of course, as the lean weight is increased, the minimal competitive weight will increase. For females, a similar minimal competitive weight has not been defined. From the research literature, it would appear that females should not drop below eight to ten percent fat. In fact, because of the unique pattern of body fat in females, an allowance for even more body fat should be made for certain athletes. While this will be discussed in detail in Chapter 17, it is important to mention here that the female athlete can become too preoccupied with weight and develop serious weight and eating disorders. An overemphasis on low body weight by the coach, trainer, physician, parent, or teammate, can lead the intense competitor to serious performance and health problems brought on by the athlete's fixation on food and weight. While accurate statistics are not available, there is an increasing concern for problems such as anorexia nervosa and bulimia nervosa in the female athletic population. One study of 182 female collegiate athletes from two midwestern universities reported that 32 percent practiced at least one of the weight-control behaviors defined as pathogenic, which included self-induced vomiting, eating binges more than twice weekly, and the use of laxatives, diet pills, and/or diuretics (Rosen, et al., 1986).

Male athletes are not immune to problems associated with excessive weight loss and eating disorders. Steen and Brownell, from the University of Pennsylvania School of Medicine, conducted a survey in 1986 on 69 collegiate wrestlers representing 15 teams at the Eastern Intercollegiate Wrestling Association Championships. These wrestlers started wrestling at an average age of 10.9 years, started cutting weight at 13.5 years, and during a normal season, these wrestlers cut weight an average of 15 times per season. The average for the largest weight loss at any one time was 15.8

Table 10–4 The effects of the single and combined influences of food restriction, fluid deprivation, and thermal dehydration on selected parameters.

Parameters	Effects on Performance
Performance Factors	
• Aerobic power	Decreased
• Muscular strength	No change
• Muscular endurance	Decreased
• Muscular power	Unknown
• Speed of movement	Unknown
• Run time to exhaustion	Decreased
• Work performed	Decreased
Physiological Factors	
• Cardiac output	Decreased
• Blood volume	Decreased
• Plasma volume	Decreased
• Heart rate	Increased
• Stroke volume	Decreased
• Core temperature	Increased
• Sweat rate	Decreased
• Muscle water	Decreased
• Muscle electrolytes	Decreased

Adapted from C. M. Tipton and R. A. Oppliger, "The Iowa Wrestling Study: Lessons for Physicians." *Iowa Medicine* (Sept. 1984): 381–385.

pounds. For this championship meet, these wrestlers lost an average of 9.7 pounds in less than an average of three days. Wrestlers typically make weight by a combination of food restriction, fluid deprivation, thermal dehydration, and increased activity. The influence these practices have on performance and physiological function is outlined in Table 10–4. The potential health hazards of such practices led the American College of Sports Medicine to publish a position stand on *Weight Loss in Wrestlers* in 1976.

SUMMARY

It has become increasingly more evident that the athlete's body build and composition play a major role in determining athletic success. Body build refers to the form and structure of the body and is quantified by determining the athlete's somatotype. In somatotyping, the body is rated for each of three different components: endomorphy (adiposity), mesomorphy (muscularity), and ectomorphy (linearity). Body size simply refers to the height and body mass, or weight, of the individual. Body composition refers to the individual components that constitute the total body mass. Of primary concern to the athlete is the distinction between fat weight and lean weight; the latter refers to the fat-free weight of the body, which includes the weight of muscle, bone, skin, and organs, among others. Body composition can be measured in the laboratory, or estimated in the field.

Physical training has only a modest influence on the athlete's body build. The somatotype is established early in life and is primarily determined by the genetic constitution of the individual athlete. Body composition is changed markedly with physical training. With chronic exercise, the lean body weight is increased and the fat weight is decreased. The magnitude of these changes is largely dependent on the type of exercise used in the training program, with strength training facilitating gains in lean weight and endurance training facilitating losses in fat weight. For purposes of losing body fat, the athlete should combine a moderate endurance training program with a modest reduction in total caloric intake of between 200 to 500 kcal per day. A goal of one pound of weight loss per week is attainable and much more desirable than more rigid goals of three to four pounds of weight loss per week.

Exercise of up to one hour in duration does not markedly increase the appetite of the individual, and, in fact, may tend to suppress it. This could be the result of the increased levels of circulating catecholamines, which accompany moderate to heavy levels of exercise. These catecholamines may also have a fat-mobilizing effect on the adipose tissue, which may explain the fat loss normally experienced with chronic exercise. Human growth hormone may also play a significant role in the mobilization of fat and it may possibly be responsible for the increase of lean tissue with chronic exercise, due to its known anabolic action.

Spot reduction has been investigated in a number of studies and is now generally regarded as a myth. The body apparently mobilizes fat from the general body stores, calling first on those areas of highest concentration. Selective utilization of fat from isolated areas undergoing vigorous exercise has not been confirmed in recent research and is probably not possible.

Body build and composition are extremely important to the potential athlete. A certain body type is necessary for almost all sports, and each sport appears to require a different type. While mesomorphy is a predominant component for all athletes, few athletes are extreme endomorphs or ectomorphs. Body composition is of primary importance where the athlete must move his or her body vertically or horizontally through space. Many studies have found substantial negative correlations between athletic performance and relative fat—the higher the percentage of body fat, the poorer the athletic performance. While there is considerable variation between athletes in different sports with regard to relative fat values, it is generally felt that the lower the relative body fat, the greater the performance potential of the athlete, with only a few possible exceptions.

STUDY QUESTIONS

1. Differentiate between body build, body size, and body composition.

2. What is somatotyping? What are the three basic components of the somatotype and what do they represent?

3. How much will somatotype change with endurance training? Strength training?

4. What body tissues constitute the lean body weight?

5. Describe the appearance of a football player who is 22 percent fat and has a somatotype rating of 5-5-1.

6. How important is regular exercise in a weight reduction program? In a weight control program?

8. How much weight should an overweight athlete lose per week in order to maximize fat loss and minimize lean weight loss?

9. Why is there substantial water loss with most "crash" diets?

10. What effect does exercise have on the appetite?

11. Defend the use of spot-reducing techniques.

12. Of what importance is somatotype and body composition to athletic performance?

13. What is the lowest weight an athlete should be allowed to attain?

14. What potential problems are associated with a fixation on body weights that are too low?

REFERENCES

American College of Sports Medicine. (1976). Weight loss in wrestlers. *Medicine and Science in Sports, 8,* xi-xiii.

Behnke, A. R., & Wilmore, J. H. (1974). *Evaluation and regulation of body build and composition.* Englewood Cliffs, NJ: Prentice-Hall.

Bray, G. A., & Bethune, J. E. (1974). *Treatment and management of obesity.* New York: Harper and Row, Publishers.

Brownell, K. D., & Foreyt, J. P. (1986). *Handbook of eating disorders: Physiology, psychology, and treatment of obesity, anorexia, and bulimia.* New York: Basic Books, Inc.

Carter, J. E. L. (Ed.) (1982). *Physical structure of olympic athletes.* New York: S. Karger.

Cureton, T. K., Jr. (1951). *Physical fitness of champion athletes.* Urbana, IL: University of Illinois Press.

deGaray, A. L., Levine, L., & Carter, J. E. L. (Eds.). (1974). *Genetic and anthropological studies of olympic athletes.* New York: Academic Press.

Despres, J. P., Bouchard, C., Tremblay, A., Savard, R., & Marcotte, M. (1985). Effects of aerobic training on fat distribution in male subjects. *Medicine and Science in Sports and Exercise, 17,* 113–118.

deVries, H. A. (1980). *Physiology of exercise for physical education and athletics* (3rd ed.). Dubuque, IA: William C. Brown Co.

Fox, E. L. (1984). *Sports physiology* (2nd ed.). Philadelphia: W. B. Saunders Co.

Gwinup, G., Chelvam, R., & Steinberg, T. (1971). Thickness of subcutaneous fat and activity of underlying muscles. *Annals of Internal Medicine, 74,* 408–411.

Heath, B. H., & Carter, J. E. L. (1967). A modified somatotype method. *American Journal of Physical Anthropology, 27,* 57–74.

Hecker, A. L. (1984). *Nutritional aspects of exercise.* Clinics in Sports Medicine Series, Vol 3, #3. Philadelphia: W. B. Saunders Company.

Jackson, A. S., & Pollock, M. L. (1978). Generalized equations for predicting body density of men. *British Journal of Nutrition, 40,* 497–504.

Jackson, A. S., Pollock, M. L., & Ward, A. (1980). Generalized equations for predicting body density of women. *Medicine and Science in Sports and Exercise, 12,* 175–182.

Katch, F. I., Clarkson, P. M., Kroll, W., McBride, T., & Wilcox, A. (1984). Effects of sit-up exercise training on adipose cell size and adiposity. *Research Quarterly for Exercise and Sport, 55,* 242–247.

Katch, F. I., & McArdle, W. D. (1983). *Nutrition, weight control, and exercise* (2nd ed.). Philadelphia: Lea & Febiger.

Kuntzleman, C. T. (1975). *Activetics.* New York: Peter H. Wyden Publisher.

Mayer, J. (1968). *Overweight causes, cost, and control.* Englewood Cliffs, NJ: Prentice-Hall.

Mayer, J., Marshall, N. B., Vitale, J. J., Christensen, J. H., Mashayekhi, M. B., & Stare, F. J. (1954). Exercise, food intake, and body weight in normal rats and genetically obese adult mice. *American Journal of Physiology, 177,* 544–548.

Oscai, L. B. (1973). The role of exercise in weight control. *Exercise and Sport Sciences Reviews, 1,* 103–123.

Parizkova, J. (1977). *Body fat and physical fitness.* The Hague: Martinus Nijhoff B. V.

Parizkova, J., & Rogozkin, V. A. (1978). *Nutrition, physical fitness, and health.* Baltimore: University Park Press.

Pavlou, K. N., Steffee, W. P., Lerman, R. H., & Burrows, B. A. (1985). Effects of dieting and exercise on lean body mass, oxygen uptake, and strength. *Medicine and Science in Sports and Exercise, 17,* 466–471.

Roche, A. F. (Ed.). (1985). *Body composition assessments in youth and adults.* Columbus, OH: Ross Laboratories.

Rosen, L. W., McKeag, D. B., Hough, D. O., & Curley, V. (1986). Pathogenic weight-control behavior in female athletes. *Physician and Sportsmedicine, 14* (#1), 79–86.

Steen, S. N., & Brownell, K. D. (1986). Weight loss patterns and nutrition practices of collegiate wrestlers. *Abstracts, American Dietetics Association.*

Storlie, J., & Jordan, H. A. (Eds.). (1984). *Nutrition and exercise in obesity management.* Jamaica, NY: Spectrum Publications.

Stuart, R. B., & Davis, B. (1972). *Slim chance in a fat world: Behavioral control of obesity.* Champaign, IL: Research Press.

Stunkard, A. J., (Ed.). (1980). *Obesity.* Philadelphia: W. B. Saunders.

Tanner, J. M. (1964). *The physique of the olympic athlete.* London: George Allen and Unwin.

Welham, W. C., & Behnke, A. R. (1942). The specific gravity of healthy men. *Journal of the American Medical Association, 118,* 498–501.

Williams, M. H. (1983). *Nutrition for fitness and sport.* Dubuque, IA: William C. Brown Co.

Wilmore, J. H. (1983). Body composition in sport and exercise: Directions for future research. *Medicine and Science in Sports and Exercise, 15,* 21–31.

Wilmore, J. H., & Haskell, W. L. (1972). Body composition and endurance capacity of professional football players. *Journal of Applied Physiology, 33,* 564–567.

Wilmore, J. H., Parr, R. B., Haskell, W. L., Costill, D. L., Milburn, L. J., & Kerlan, R. D. (1976). Athletic profile of professional football players. *Physician and Sportsmedicine, 4* (10), 45–54.

Wilson, N. L. (Ed.). (1969). *Obesity.* Philadelphia: F. A. Davis.

Winick, M. (1975). *Childhood obesity.* New York: John Wiley & Sons.

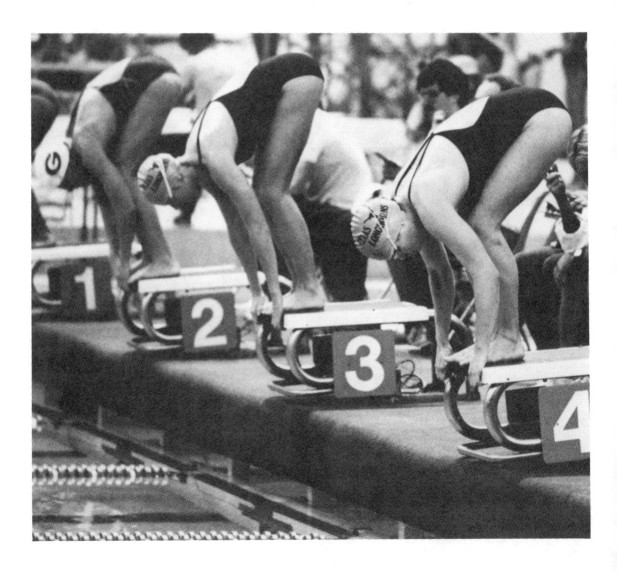

11

The Finer Points of Training

INTRODUCTION

Most coaches and athletes believe that the single most important requirement for success is hard, stressful training. While physical and psychological preparation for competition depends on the adaptations associated with physical training, many athletes fail to achieve their full potential as a result of poor management. Excessive overload may negate the benefits of months of hard training, leaving athletes unable to produce a performance representative of their potential. Likewise, individuals who interrupt their training for days and months may rapidly lose conditioning, and the ability to perform at a peak level. In this chapter we will discuss factors that must be monitored and properly managed for athletes to do their best.

OVERTRAINING

The ability to design a training regimen that provides the level of stress needed for optimal physiological improvement without exceeding the athlete's tolerance is a difficult task. Although most coaches employ a set of intuitive standards to judge the volume and intensity of each training session, few are able to assess the relative impact of the workout on the athlete. There are no preliminary symptoms to warn the athletes that they are on the edge of becoming overtrained. By the time coaches realize that they have pushed their athletes too hard, it is too late. The damage done by repeated days of excessive training and/or overstress can only be repaired by days and, in some cases, weeks of reduced training or complete rest.

It seems that the athletes most susceptible to overtraining or staleness, are those who are highly motivated, attempting to perform their best during every training session or competition. Sudden increases in training volume and intensity may emotionally and/or physically overload the athlete.

Though the symptoms of overtraining may vary from one individual to another, the most common are feelings of heaviness and the inability to perform well during training and competition. Physical symptoms may include one or more of the following:

- body weight loss with decreased appetite
- muscle tenderness
- head colds, allergic reactions, or both
- occasional nausea
- sleep disturbances, or
- elevated resting heart rate, blood pressure, or both.

The underlying causes of overtraining or **staleness** are often a combination of emotional and physical factors. Hans Selye (1956) has noted that a breakdown in one's tolerance of stress can occur as often from a sudden increase in anxiety as from an increase in physical distress. The emotional demands of competition, the desire to win, fear of failure, unrealistically high goals, and the expectations of coaches, parents, and others can be sources of intolerable emotional stress. In addition to the stress of exercise and training, factors such as environmental conditions (heat stress and altitude) and improper nutrition may lead to overtraining.

Day-to-day variations in the sensations of fatigue should not be confused with overtraining. It is not uncommon for the athlete to feel heavy after several days of hard training or after a stressful competition. Unlike the feelings of being overtrained, the short-lived sensations of heaviness are usually relieved with a day or two of easy training and a carbohydrate-rich diet. Overtraining, on the other hand, is accompanied by a loss in competitive desire and a loss in enthusiasm for training.

As noted, most of the symptoms associated with overtraining are subjective and identifiable only after the individuals have over-extended themselves. It has been observed that athletes who suddenly begin to perform very well during training may be on the verge of becoming overtrained. They feel so good during training sessions that they tend to extend themselves beyond their usual day-to-day tolerance, producing a performance breakdown.

Numerous investigators have used assorted physiological measurements in an effort to objectively diagnose overtraining in its early stages to prevent its occurrence. Unfortunately, none has proven totally effective. It is often difficult to differentiate whether the measurements are abnormal and related to overtraining, or simply the normal physiological responses to heavy training.

Measurements of blood enzyme levels have been used to diagnose overtraining with only limited success. Such enzymes as CPK (creatine phosphokinase), LDH (lactate dehydrogenase), and SGOT (serum glutamic oxalic transaminase) are important in muscle energy production but are generally confined to the inside of the cells. The presence of these enzymes in blood suggests some damage to or structural change in the muscle membranes. Following periods of heavy training, such enzymes have been reported to increase two to ten times above normal levels. Recent studies tend to support the idea that these changes in blood enzymes may reflect varied degrees of muscle tissue breakdown. As noted in Chapter 7, examination of tissue from the leg muscles of marathon runners has revealed that there is remarkable damage to the muscle fibers after training and marathon competition. The onset and time course of these muscle changes seems to parallel the degree of muscle soreness experienced by the runners.

Although the effects of muscle damage on performance are not fully understood, experts generally agree that they may be, in part, responsible for the localized muscle pain, tenderness, and swelling associated with muscle soreness. There is, however, no evidence that this condition is linked to the symptoms of overtraining. It is suspected that blood enzyme levels rise and muscle fibers are damaged frequently during eccentric exercise, independent of the state of overtraining. In addition to being expensive and difficult to measure, blood enzyme levels do not appear to be a valid indicator of overtraining.

White blood cells, or eosinophils, serve as a defense against foreign materials that enter the body or conditions that threaten the normal function of its tissues. Since the white blood cell count tends to rise during exhaustive exercise, some investigators have suggested that it may provide a warning signal for impending staleness. However, again it is not clear whether this change is a sign of overstress or simply a normal reaction to intense training. Acute and chronic changes in plasma water during training produce alterations in blood cell concentration (hemodilution or hemoconcentration), thereby altering the hematocrit and hemoglobin values without a change in the absolute number of red and white cells.

Early studies have reported abnormal resting electrocardiographic (ECG) tracings among swimmers who showed signs of overtraining. Typically, those swimmers who showed sudden decrements in performance often exhibited T-wave inversions. Since such ECG changes are associated with abnormal repolarization of the heart ventricles, it was suggested that these changes among training athletes may reveal signs of overuse. On the other hand, a number of the swimmers who clearly exhibited symptoms of overtraining had normal ECG tracings.

It has also been suggested that unusually high resting, blood lactate concentrations may be a sign of overstress. Many swimmers have been found to have high resting blood lactate concentrations when they are swimming poorly, and have normal concentrations when they are swimming well. Recent studies by Maglischo (1987), however, have failed to support this idea.

Despite various attempts to objectively diagnose overtraining, no single physiological measurement has proven 100 percent effective. Since performance is the most dramatic indicator of overtraining, it is not surprising to find that overtraining has a dramatic effect on the energy demands for a standard, submaximal exercise bout. When runners show symptoms of overtraining,

their heart rates and oxygen consumption during the runs are significantly higher.

Figure 11-1 compares a college cross-country runner when he was performing well and when he exhibited symptoms of being overtrained. When he was in good running form, he ran the treadmill at 16.1 km/hr (6 min/mile), he had an oxygen uptake of 49 ml/kg × min, and heart rate of 142 beats per minute, posting a best performance of 30 minutes and 53 seconds for 10 kilometers. Later in the season his 10-kilometer performance deteriorated to 32 minutes 10 seconds. At that time it cost him significantly more to run the 16.1 km/hr treadmill test—56 ml/kg × min (14 percent higher) with a heart rate of 168 beats per min (18 percent higher). Interestingly, his maximal oxygen uptake of 70 ml/kg × min^{-1} did not change, despite the diminished performance. While the first 16.1 km/hr run required him to work at 70 percent of his $\dot{V}O_2$ max, the same run when he exhibited signs of overtraining, required 80 percent of his $\dot{V}O_2$ max. In terms

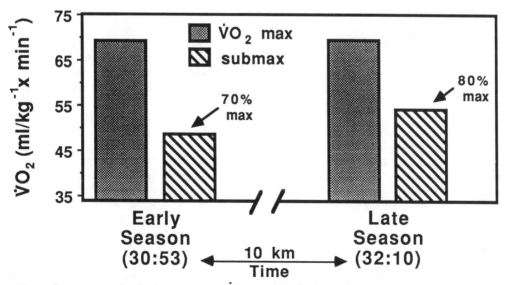

Figure 11-1 Oxygen uptake during maximal ($\dot{V}O_2$ max) and submaximal (16.1 km per hr) running during two periods of the season for a college cross-country runner. Note that there was no change in the runner's $\dot{V}O_2$ max, despite a marked decrement in his time for the 10-kilometer run. At the same time, the amount of energy needed to run at the submaximal speed was notably greater when he was overtrained (from Costill, 1986).

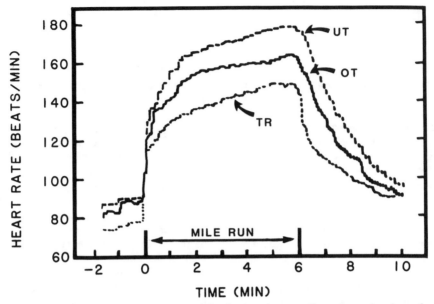

Figure 11-2 Heart rate responses during a standard, six-minute mile, submaximal run before training (UT), after eight weeks of training (TR), and during the period when the runner exhibited symptoms of being overtrained (OT) (from Costill, 1986).

of aerobic fitness, overtrained runners do not lose their conditioning, but they may demonstrate a deterioration in running form. Though the causes for this loss in skill are not fully understood, we might speculate that overtraining may cause some local muscular fatigue through selective glycogen depletion, forcing runners to alter their mechanics to achieve the same pace.

Although tests of oxygen consumption may be of little value to the coach or athlete, there are other ways to monitor the physical effort of exercise that may be a bit more practical. Current technology enables the coach to monitor the athlete's heart rate responses during a set exercise task. The data presented in Figure 11-2, for example, illustrate a runner's heart rate responses during a one mile run at a fixed pace of six min per mile at the onset of training (UT), after training (TR), and during a period when he demonstrated symptoms of being overtrained (OT). A similar test might be developed for swimmers and cyclists, in which the intensity (speed) of the exercise can be controlled. The advantage of this test is that it provides an

objective measurement of the athlete's physiological response to a given rate of work. Blood lactate measurements taken after this test correlate very closely with the individual's heart rate. Since heart rates are relatively simple to record and provide immediate information for the athlete and coach, such a test provides an objective way to monitor training and may provide a warning signal for overtraining.

Although the causes for deterioration in performance are not clear, it appears that the intensity, or speed, of training is a more potent stressor than volume of training. Relief from overtraining only comes with a marked reduction in training intensity or complete rest. Although most coaches suggest a few days of easy training, we are inclined to feel that athletes recover faster when they rest completely for three to five days, or engage in some other form of low-intensity exercise. In some cases, counseling may be needed to help the athletes cope with the stresses of their job, school, or social pressures. At other times the problem may simply be a matter of poor nutrition, insufficient sleep, or both. If the athlete shows continued signs of fatigue and substandard performances despite rest and counseling, medical help should be sought.

Prevention is always preferable to the task of attempting to cure an overtrained athlete. The best way to minimize the risk of overstressing is to follow cyclic training procedures by alternating easy, moderate, and hard periods of training. Although the tolerance limits vary from one individual to another, even the strongest athletes have periods when they are susceptible to overtraining. As a rule, one or two days of intense training should be followed by an equal number of easy, aerobic training days. Likewise, a week or two of hard training should be followed by a week of reduced effort with little or no emphasis on anaerobic exercise.

Endurance athletes (swimmers, cyclists, and runners) must give special attention to the dietary intake of carbohydrate in an effort to minimize the risk of chronic muscle glycogen depletion. As noted in Chapter 12, repeated days of hard training will result in a gradual reduction in muscle glycogen. Unless the athlete consumes extra quantities of carbohydrate-rich foods during these periods, muscle and liver glycogen reserves may be depleted, leaving the most heavily recruited muscle fibers incapable of generating the energy needed for exercise.

Reduced Training for Peak Performance

During periods of frequent competition, most athletes take several days of light training to boost their performances. In light of our previous discussions about training and overtraining, one might question whether these brief periods of tapering are adequate to promote optimal performance. Experience in sports, such as swimming, suggests that the **taper** period may need to cover two or more weeks for best results.

As noted earlier, in Chapter 7, periods of intense training reduce muscular strength, lessening the performance capacity of athletes. To compete at their peak, many athletes reduce their training for 5 to 21 days before a major competition. Although this regimen is widely practiced in a variety of sports, many coaches fear the loss of conditioning

and performance if they reduce training for such a long period before a major competition. A number of studies make it clear, however, that this fear is totally unwarranted (Costill, 1985).

Maximal oxygen uptake ($\dot{V}O_2$ max) can be maintained at the training level with a two-thirds reduction in training frequency. It appears that a greater amount of work is needed to increase $\dot{V}O_2$ max than to maintain it at the training level. Whereas $\dot{V}O_2$ max and the ability to perform exercise are measurably improved within one week of training, the rate of decline in physical performance with reduced training is much slower.

Swimmers who reduce their training from an average of 10,000 to 3,200 yards per day over a 15-day period show no loss in $\dot{V}O_2$ max or endurance performance. Measurements of blood lactate after a standard 200-yard swim were actually lower after the taper period than before. More importantly, the swimmers showed an average improvement in performance of 3.5 to 3.7 percent as a result of the reduced training.

But, what does this mean to athletes in other events? Unfortunately, there is little information to demonstrate the influence of tapering on performance in team sports and in long, endurance events like cycling and marathon running. Before guidelines can be offered for these athletes, research is needed to demonstrate that similar benefits can be generated by such periods of reduced training.

The most notable change during the taper period is a marked increase in muscular strength. As a consequence of reduced training, the previously mentioned swimmers demonstrated an increase in arm strength and power from 17.7 to 24.6 percent. This is a reasonable explanation for at least part of the improvement in performance seen with tapering. Similar benefits could be of significant value in events that rely on strength for optimal performance. Based on the discussion in Chapter 7, it is difficult to determine whether these improvements in muscle strength that result from tapering are the consequence of changes within the muscles' contractile mechanism or an improvement in muscle fiber recruitment. The underlying factors responsible for improved performance with tapering may be the focus of future studies, since it appears to play an important role in the fine-tuning of the athlete's skills.

DETRAINING

What happens to highly-conditioned athletes who have fine-tuned their performance skills to a peak level, only to have the competitive season and daily training come to a sudden end? Most athletes in team sports go into physical hibernation following the completion of their competitive season. Many have been working two to five hours per day in perfecting their skills and improving their levels of physical condition, and welcome the opportunity to completely relax, purposely avoiding any strenuous physical activity. How does total physical inactivity affect the highly-trained athlete? Does the body need this period of rest, or will it undergo rapid, physical deterioration? Are physical training programs necessary during the off-season to maintain the athlete's general physical condition? These and other related questions will be discussed in this section. The last section is devoted to a discussion of off-season, physical training programs.

Much of our knowledge about physical detraining comes from clinical research with patients who have been forced to be inactive as a result of injury or surgery. Additional information has been gained from aerospace research, on men in space, where the lack of gravity removes a number of physiological stresses which stimulate normal body functions. Humans have successfully adapted to the earth's environment and have extreme difficulty in adapting to the weightless state.

Most athletes agree that it is bad enough to suffer the pain of an injury, but it is even worse when the condition forces them to stop training. Most athletes fear that all they have gained through hard training will be lost after a few days or weeks of inactivity. Recent studies have made it clear that a few days of rest or a reduction in training will not impair, but may even enhance performance. It is logical, however, that at some point a reduction in training or complete inactivity will produce a deterioration in performance.

Physical detraining has been investigated through two major approaches: by observing changes following total bed rest for extended periods of time, and by observing changes in trained individuals as they cease formal physical training and become physically inactive. The results of these various studies will be discussed individually, according to the specific components of physical training.

Loss of Muscle Strength and Power

When an individual breaks an arm or a leg and the broken limb is placed in a rigid cast to render it completely immobile, changes immediately start taking place in both the bone and surrounding muscles. Within a period of only a few days, the cast, which was applied very tightly around the injured segment, becomes quite loose. By the end of several weeks, there is a large space between the cast and the limb. Is this the result of the cast expanding with use or does the limb decrease in size with disuse? It is now clearly understood that skeletal muscles will undergo a substantial decrease in size with inactivity. Accompanying this decrease in size is a considerable loss in strength and power. While total inactivity will lead to very rapid losses in both strength and power, even periods of reduced activity may lead to gradual losses that can become sizeable as the changes accumulate over long periods of time.

Research confirms that levels of strength, power, and muscular endurance are reduced once the athlete stops training. However, these changes are relatively small during the first few months following the cessation of training. No loss in strength is noted six weeks after cessation of a three-week training program. It has also been noted that 45 percent of the original strength gained from a 12-week training program was lost by the time the subjects were reevaluated one year later. Similar results have been found for muscular endurance.

Studies with collegiate swimmers revealed that the termination of training had no effect on arm and shoulder strength after up to four weeks of inactivity. Measurements of strength, using the

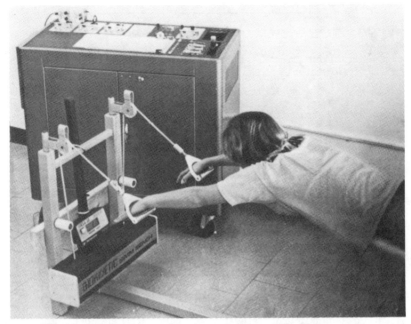

Figure 11-3 Swim bench apparatus for measuring arm strength and power.

semi-accommodating resistance device shown in Figure 11-3, have demonstrated no change with complete rest, or with one or three training sessions per week. However, when these same swim- mers were tested for power, using the swimming-specific apparatus shown in Figure 11-4, swimming power was reduced by 8 to 13.5 percent during the four weeks of reduced activity (see Figure

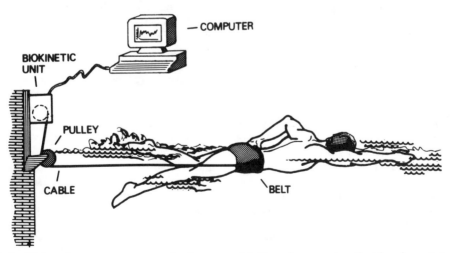

Figure 11-4 Swimming power measured using a semi-tethered apparatus that has been interfaced with a micro-computer.

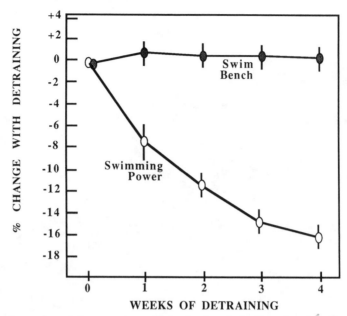

Figure 11-5 Percentage change in arm strength (swim bench test) and swimming power (swim power test) during four weeks of detraining. These measurements were made after five months of swim training in collegiate male swimmers.

11-5). This information suggests that the less-specific measurements of muscle strength on land, may not reflect the loss in performance experienced by the swimmers. That is, muscle strength may not diminish during four weeks of reduced training, but the swimmers may lose their ability to apply force during swimming. In terms used by swimming coaches, the swimmers appeared to lose their feel for the water.

In any event, it appears that the strength and muscular endurance gained during the training period for swimmers may be fully retained for periods up to six weeks, and approximately 50 percent of the strength gained with training will be retained for up to a year following the end of the training program. Also, studies have shown that it takes far less effort to regain the lost strength than it does to acquire it in the first place. In addition, it appears that by working out once every ten to fourteen days, athletes can maintain the strength, power, and muscular endurance that was gained through more vigorous and frequent training.

These findings tend to conflict with the observations noted earlier, that rather sizeable losses result in strength, power, muscular endurance, and muscle mass (**atrophy**). Atrophy results from periods of inactivity where a limb is totally immobilized. This conflict can be explained by the fact that most individuals get sufficient exercise through walking, climbing stairs, pushing, pulling, and lifting to allow a substantial retention of the strength previously gained through strength training. With immobilization, there is almost no activity at all within the muscle.

The physiological mechanisms responsible for the decline in muscle strength with immobilization and/or inactivity is not clearly understood. There is, however, a noticeable decrease in muscle mass and water content which accompanies muscle atrophy, and could, in part, account for a loss in maximal tension development. The disuse of muscle also reduces the frequency of neurological stimulation and normal pathways for the recruitment of fibers. Thus, part of the strength loss that is associated with detraining may be the result of an inability to activate some muscle fibers. This latter theory is supported by the fact that a sizeable strength gain is achieved with only a few training sessions, a period too brief to accommodate any significant structural development.

Evidently, the muscle requires only a minimal stimulus to retain the strength, power, endurance, and size of a muscle or muscle group. This has extremely important implications for the injured athlete. There will be a great savings in time and effort during the period of rehabilitation if the athlete can perform even a very low level of exercise in the injured segment, starting in the first few days of the recovery period. Simple, isometric contractions have been found to be very effective in this respect, since they can be graded in intensity and do not require movement at the joint. Any program of rehabilitation, however, must be worked out in cooperation with the supervising physician.

Loss of Muscular Endurance

The local adaptations in muscle during periods of inactivity are well documented. After a week or two of cast-immobilization, oxidative enzymes, such as succinate dehydrogenase (SDH), show a 40 to 60 percent decline in activity. As shown in Figure 11–6, the decline in the oxidative potential of muscle is much more rapid than the change in the subject's maximal oxygen uptake. After only two weeks of inactivity, endurance performance has been shown to decline. At this time there is insufficient evidence to determine whether the decline in performance is due to changes in the muscle or the result of a reduced cardiovascular capacity.

When swimmers stop training there is no change in their muscle glycolytic enzymes (phosphoralase and PFK) for at least four weeks, whereas the oxidative energy system seems to decline somewhat more quickly. With up to 84 days of detraining, Coyle, et al. (1985) observed no change in the muscle enzymes of glycolysis, but nearly a 60 percent decline for different oxidative enzymes. This may, in part, explain why performance times in sprint events are unaffected with a month or more of inactivity, whereas the ability to perform longer, endurance events may decline significantly with as little as two weeks of detraining.

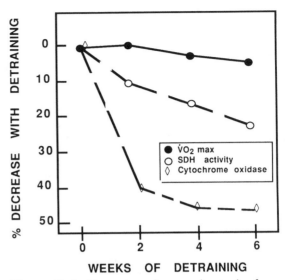

Figure 11–6 Percentage decrease in maximal oxygen uptake ($\dot{V}O_2$ max), muscle succinate dehydrogenase (SDH), and cytochrome oxidase activities during a six-week period of detraining.

Although it has been suggested that the capillary supply within the muscle may decrease with detraining, the findings are inconclusive. Muscle fiber composition does not appear to change during short periods of inactivity, however there have been some clinical cases that have reported dramatic changes in the percentage of slow-twitch and fast-twitch fibers in athletes who have undergone immobilization following surgery.

The only other notable change in the muscle with detraining is an alteration in glycogen content. As noted in Chapter 2, endurance-trained muscles tend to store substantially more glycogen than do untrained muscles. With periods of detraining, muscle glycogen levels have been shown to drop from 153 mmol/kg w.w. at the end of training to a value of 93 mmol/kg w.w. after four weeks of detraining. Figure 11–7 on page 203 illustrates the decline in muscle glycogen that accompanies four weeks of detraining in competitive collegiate swimmers.

Measurements of blood lactate and pH after a standard work bout have been used to assess the physiological changes that accompany training

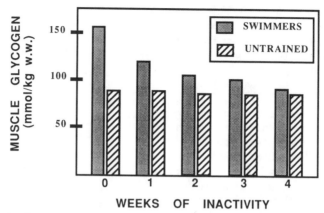

Figure 11–7 Changes in glycogen content of the deltoid muscle from competitive male swimmers during a four-week period of detraining. Note that muscle glycogen had returned to the untrained level at the end of this period of inactivity.

and detraining. For example, swimmers described in Table 11–1 were required to perform a standard-paced 200-yard swim, at 90 percent of their seasonal best. During the first few weeks of inactivity, there was little change in blood lactate, but they experienced a significant disturbance in acid-base balance by the fourth week of detraining. These findings support the theory that the muscle's oxidative and anaerobic energy systems change rather slowly, and are probably unaffected by only a few days of rest. Only during periods of complete inactivity (immobilization) do the changes impair performance within the first week or two.

Loss of Speed, Agility, and Flexibility

Physical training can influence speed and agility, but the degree of improvement will be far less than in the areas of strength, power, muscular endurance, flexibility, and cardiovascular endurance. Consequently, the loss of speed and agility with physical inactivity is relatively small, and peak levels can be maintained with only a limited amount of training. This does not imply that the sprinter in track can get by with training only a few days a week. Success in actual competition relies on factors other than basic speed, such as correct form, timing, and the finishing kick. It takes

Table 11–1 Blood lactate, pH, and bicarbonate (HCO_3^-) after a standard paced, 200-yard front crawl swim in eight collegiate swimmers undergoing detraining. The values reported at "Wk-0" represent the measurements taken at the end of five months of training. The other values are the results obtained after one (Wk-1), two (Wk-2), and four (Wk-4) weeks of detraining.

Measurement	Wk-0	Wk-1	Wk-2	Wk-4
Lactate	4.2 ±0.8	6.3 ±0.7	6.8 ±0.7	9.7 ±0.8*
pH	7.259	7.237	7.236	7.183*
HCO_3^-	21.1	19.5*	16.1*	16.3*
Swim Time (sec)	130.6	130.1	130.5	130.0

*Denotes a significant difference from the value at the end of training (Wk-0).

many hours of practice during the week to tune performance to its optimal level, but most of this time is spent in developing aspects of one's performance other than speed.

Flexibility, on the other hand, is lost rather quickly and must be worked on throughout the year. Stretching exercises, such as those outlined in Appendix B, should be incorporated into both the in-season and off-season training programs. While flexibility can be attained in a relatively short period of time, it is in the best interest of the athlete to maintain the desired levels of flexibility on a year-round basis. Many athletes, however, tend to ignore flexibility training during the off-season, since it can be regained so rapidly. It has been suggested that reduced flexibility may leave athletes more susceptible to serious injury, which could be a major factor in determining their longevity for participation in sports.

Cardiovascular Endurance

The heart, like all muscles in the body, strengthens itself in proportion to the force it must contract against. Likewise, periods of inactivity lead to substantial cardiovascular deconditioning. A simple reduction in the gravitational stress on the body, such as space flight and bed rest, is known to cause cardiovascular deterioration. Even limited activity provides considerable stress for the heart, since it must contract forcefully enough to circulate the blood throughout the body against the demands of gravity. In the weightless state, this is no longer necessary, and the work of the heart is reduced considerably. For this reason, astronauts in the series of Skylab flights during the early 1970s were required to perform daily bouts of exercise on a stationary bicycle ergometer or on an ingeniously designed "space treadmill." Such exercise was found to be essential in preventing serious cardiovascular deterioration.

Similar results have been observed in studies conducted on subjects undergoing long periods of total bed rest. In these studies, the subject was not allowed to leave the bed and physical activity was kept to an absolute minimum. Heart rates measured at a constant work load before and following a twenty-day period of bed rest, showed a considerable increase with detraining. This rise in heart rate was accompanied by a 25-percent decrease in stroke volume observed at this level of activity. In addition, the period of bed rest resulted in a 25-percent reduction in maximal cardiac output and a 27-percent decrease in maximal oxygen uptake ($\dot{V}O_2$ max) (see Figure 11-8 on page 206). This reduction in cardiac output and $\dot{V}O_2$ max appears to be the result of a smaller stroke volume, which was probably due to a combined decrease in heart volume, total blood and plasma volumes, and ventricular contractility.

Recent studies (Coyle, et al., 1986) have shown that the decline in cardiovascular function following a few weeks of detraining is largely due to a reduction in blood volume, which appears to diminish the stroke volume of the heart. Two to four weeks of inactivity following months of training for cycling and running resulted in a nine percent decline in blood volume and a 12 percent decrease in both stroke volume and plasma volume. As a result of these diminished blood, plasma, and stroke volumes, detraining produced a 5.9 percent drop in $\dot{V}O_2$ max. By infusing a dextran solution into the subjects after they were detrained, it was possible to expand their plasma and blood volumes to above their trained levels (see Table 11-2 on page 206). This produced an improvement in cardiovascular function and $\dot{V}O_2$ max, though it proved of little benefit to endurance performance.

It is interesting to note that two of the most highly-conditioned subjects shown in Figure 11-8 experienced larger decrements in $\dot{V}O_2$ max than the three sedentary men. Furthermore, the three sedentary subjects regained their initial, or pre-bed rest, level of conditioning within the first ten days of reconditioning, while the two physically active subjects needed about 40 days to regain their initial levels. This would tend to suggest that the more highly-trained individuals will not be able to afford long periods of inactivity with little or no endurance training. The athlete who totally abstains from physical training at the completion of the season will experience a great deal of difficulty in getting back into physical condition when the new season begins.

Studies have also observed changes in endurance performance of trained subjects during

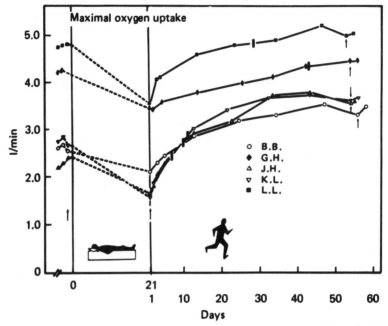

Figure 11–8 Reduction in maximal oxygen uptake with a twenty-day period of physical inactivity (bed rest) (from B. Saltin, et al., 1968. By permission of the American Heart Association, Inc.).

Table 11–2 Effects of detraining and blood volume expansion on maximal oxygen uptake ($\dot{V}O_2$ max), blood volume (BV), stroke volume (SV), maximal heart rate (HR_{max}), and exercise time (ET) to exhaustion (from Coyle, 1986).

	Normal BV		*Expanded BV detrained*
	trained	*detrained*	
BV (ml)	5,177	4,692	5,412
SV† (ml/stroke)	166	146*	164
$\dot{V}O_2$ max (liters/min)	4.42	4.16*	4.28
ET (min)	9.13	8.44	8.06**

*Denotes a significant difference from Trained (normal BV) and Detrained (expanded BV) values.

**Denotes a significant difference from the Trained (normal BV) value.

†Stroke volume measured during submaximal exercise.

periods of inactivity. This reduction is of considerably greater magnitude than the reduction observed in the areas of strength, power, and muscular endurance for the same period of inactivity. Drinkwater and Horvath (1972) studied seven female track athletes at the end of the competitive season and again three months after the cessation of formal training. During the three-month period following formal training, the girls participated in physical activities normal for their age group, including required physical education. They observed a 15.5 percent decrease in $\dot{V}O_2$ max over the three-month period, and noted that the new $\dot{V}O_2$ max levels were similar to those found in nonathletic girls of the same age. Similarly, Michael, et al. (1972) observed that three weeks of detraining after four months of training, resulted in an increase in heart rates recorded during a standardized submaximal exercise bout. These results are nearly identical to those illustrated in the bed rest study performed by Saltin, et al., (see Figure 11–8) for five men undergoing complete bed rest.

Brynteson and Sinning (1973) attempted to determine the amount of exercise necessary for the maintenance of these gains attained from a formal training program. The subjects exercised five days per week for five weeks to develop their initial training levels. They were then divided into four groups, exercising either one, two, three, or four times per week, to determine the minimal frequency that would maintain the initial training level. They found that cardiovascular fitness was maintained by exercising three times per week, and that there were significant losses in conditioning in the two groups that exercised only once or twice per week. Siegel, et al. (1970) found a 29 percent increase in $\dot{V}O_2$ max for nine men following 15 weeks of training (12 minutes per day, three days per week). At the end of training, five subjects continued to train once a week for an additional 14 weeks, at which time their $\dot{V}O_2$ max had decreased to only six percent above their initial control level. The remaining four subjects stopped training altogether, and their $\dot{V}O_2$ max values, following 14 weeks of detraining, dropped below their original control values. These studies make it clear that physical conditioning can be maintained by training as few as three times per week, but lesser training results in a significant loss in the benefits of physical conditioning.

Pate, et al. (1978) examined the ability of arm training or exercise to prevent a decline in conditioning that was achieved with leg training. Initially, the subjects trained on cycle ergometers for eight weeks. The subjects were then divided into one of three groups: arm training, continued leg training, and no training. After four weeks in one of the three subgroups, the subjects were retested. $\dot{V}O_2$ max continued to increase in the group that continued leg training (+3.7 percent), while the arm training group and the group that discontinued training decreased −2.6 percent and −6.8 percent, respectively. The authors concluded that arm training does not significantly affect the deterioration in metabolic response to leg work that occurs with the cessation of leg training.

Studies by Hickson, et al. (1985) have shown that training intensity plays a principal role in maintaining one's aerobic power during periods of reduced training. Their data suggest that the intensity of training must be at least 70 percent or more of $\dot{V}O_2$ max (probably 90 to 100 percent) to maintain the training-induced improvements in $\dot{V}O_2$ max. As little as a one-third reduction in training intensity for 15 weeks produced a significant decline in $\dot{V}O_2$ max, long-term endurance (80 percent $\dot{V}O_2$ max to exhaustion), and cardiac size in subjects who were previously trained for ten weeks. Short-term (four to eight minutes) endurance and body composition, on the other hand, did not decrease with a one-third reduction in training intensity. Although a decrease in training frequency and duration causes a decline in aerobic capacity, the losses are only significant when reduced by two-thirds of the prior training load. Nevertheless, the authors concluded that "some combination of the three training parameters are probably involved in maintaining certain adaptations to exercise."

From these and other studies, it is apparent that cardiovascular endurance capacity is lost very rapidly following the cessation of formal endurance training. While complete bed rest provides the most dramatic decreases, even periods of light activity or formal endurance training once or twice a week are not sufficient to prevent the loss of cardiovascular conditioning. Thus, the athlete must consciously work on maintaining his or her endurance capacity during the off-season, for once it is lost, it takes a considerable period of time to regain peak levels. The sooner the injured athlete can get back into some modified form of endurance exercise, the smaller will be the loss in cardiovascular endurance capacity. While it may be impossible to return to a running or swimming type of activity, stationary or regular bicycling are excellent cardiovascular conditioning exercises that will place less stress on the joints and muscles.

Changes in Body Composition. Changes in body composition with decreased physical activity are similar to those found for increased physical activity, except that the changes are in the reverse order. With inactivity, the lean body weight tends to decrease and total body fat tends to increase. Figure 11–9 illustrates the changes in subcutaneous fat, as measured by skinfold thicknesses, in a group of female gymnasts over a period of several

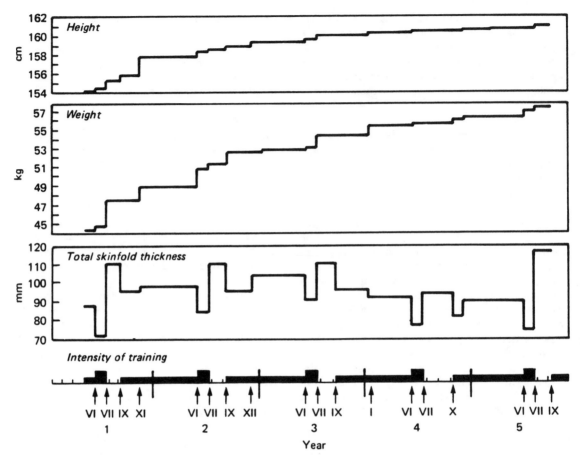

Figure 11-9 Changes in height, weight, and total skinfold thickness in young gymnasts as they progress from periods of limited, moderate, and heavy training (from Parizkova, 1963).

years, with indicated periods of total inactivity, moderate training, and intense training. A substantial variation in skinfold thickness occurred over this period of time, reflecting the influence of marked changes in activity patterns.

The degree of change in lean body weight and fat content will depend to a large extent on the initial size and composition of the individual and on the eating and activity habits of the athlete during the period of detraining. The athlete who has developed considerable muscle bulk from strength training activities during the season will lose a

considerable amount of lean weight once training has stopped. Losses of 10 to 20 pounds are not uncommon after a year or more of inactivity. The extremely lean athlete, such as the long-distance runner who trains 100 miles or more per week, will gain a considerable amount of fat if he becomes totally inactive.

Optimal body composition levels can be maintained during the off-season with a modest level of physical training and a conscious effort to control the diet. Although most athletes who work hard during the season can eat almost anything, and as much as they want to, they must watch their weight carefully during the off-season and regulate their diet accordingly.

RETRAINING

The recovery of the trained condition after a period of lay-off or forced immobilization, such as limb casting, is affected by the status of the individual's physical condition and the duration of inactivity. As noted in Figure 11-8, the most highly-trained individuals appear to experience the greatest loss of conditioning with a 20-day period of bed rest, and take considerably longer to regain their fitness than subjects who are less well-trained.

As noted earlier, 15 days of detraining produces significant decrements in oxidative enzymes (-13 to -24 percent), performance time (-25 percent), and $\dot{V}O_2$ max (-4 percent), whereas 15 days of retraining returned only the $\dot{V}O_2$ max to its original, trained level. That is, the oxidative enzymes did not improve with 15 days of retraining, and performance time was still 9 percent below the trained level after reconditioning. These findings suggest that, for very highly-trained athletes, even short periods of detraining result in significant changes in indices of physiological capacity and a longer period of retraining is necessary for them to regain their conditioning.

As noted earlier, muscles that have been immobilized by casting for a few days or several weeks lose much of their flexibility, strength, and endurance. After removal of the cast, most individuals cannot begin immediate activity because they lack sufficient joint mobility. Regaining the range of joint motion is a relatively slow process, often taking several months for full recovery.

Several procedures have been proposed to speed the recovery of muscle function following surgical immobilization. Use of a cast that allows some movement (20 to 60 degree range) in patients who had undergone anterior cruciate ligament reconstruction, produced full recovery of the range of joint motion within four weeks of retraining. This is in contrast to the 16 weeks to regain normal motion with an immovable cast. The movable cast-

brace resulted in minimal reduction of the muscle fibers' cross-sectional area, and no reduction in the oxidative enzyme activities (as with succinate dehydrogenase).

Other studies have revealed effective ways to limit the reduction in the aerobic capacity of the muscle following cast immobilization. Following cast removal, 20 to 60 minutes of daily cycling provides greater gains in muscle (vastus lateralis) aerobic capacity and improved knee-joint flexibility, as compared to only a strength-training program. Percutaneous electrical stimulation, while the muscles are immobilized in a cast, will prevent the loss in the muscle's oxidative capacity. It has also been suggested that electrical stimulation may be a method for preventing muscle fiber atrophy during casting.

In general, it is thought that the earlier a patient can resume active motion of the joint following an injury or surgery, the quicker will be the recovery of muscle function and, therefore, shorten the period of retraining. As shown in Figure 11-10, individuals who initiate an activity program, while

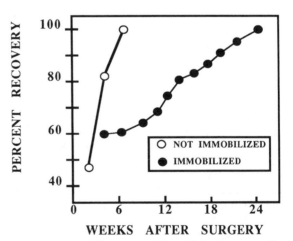

Figure 11-10 Recovery of quadriceps strength following surgical meniscectomy. The group that was immobilized for two weeks with an immovable cast showed a slow return to normal (24 weeks), compared to the rapid recovery (7 weeks) in the subjects that were not immobilized after surgery (from Sherman, et al., 1982).

they are still in the cast (two weeks), recover much more quickly than those who remain inactive during the same period. Sherman, et al. (1982) have proposed a two-phase, isokinetic training program for individuals who undergo knee surgery and limb immobilization. This training regimen concentrates on early post-surgery activity, with progressive stages of exercise intensity and range of joint motion.

OFF-SEASON TRAINING PROGRAMS

From the data in the previous section, it is obvious that the athlete undergoes considerable change as a result of periods of inactivity or detraining. Is this necessarily bad? The athlete can always start the reconditioning process several weeks before beginning a new season. Maybe the athlete needs several months of total inactivity to help pull things back together! While a definite answer to this question is not presently available, it appears that the athlete can receive great benefits from a comprehensive off-season conditioning program that is individually designed to meet personal needs and interests. The highly-conditioned athlete who becomes totally inactive, loses a considerable amount of that conditioning. Regaining this conditioning takes a considerable amount of time and effort, which could mean that the athlete might not regain peak form or performance potential until well into the competitive season. The inability to perform at optimal levels early in the season may prove costly, both in success and in potentially serious injuries. Observations of a number of professional athletes suggest that those who maintain themselves in reasonable condition throughout the year are able to continue their sport longer and more successfully than those who go into hibernation during the off-season.

In the previous discussion, it was demonstrated that peak levels of conditioning can be maintained by training at frequencies considerably less than those required during the season. Strength can be maintained by one full workout every ten to 14 days. Cardiovascular endurance, however, is maintained by training a minimum of three times per week. Therefore, an off-season program can be designed that would require no more than three days

of activity per week. In addition, the workout periods need not exceed one to two hours in length. This totals only three to six hours of training per week, which is a minimum investment of time for the resulting benefits.

The athlete and coach must give considerable thought to the design of the off-season conditioning program. All too frequently this is left strictly to chance. One of the most important factors to consider in off-season training is that it must be fun and enjoyable for the athlete. The activities that are selected should differ somewhat from those used during the season in order to prevent boredom. Occasional, or frequent, competition is suggested, since this provides additional motivation to participate. Many professional football teams have organized formal competition in basketball for their athletes as part of the off-season training program. This activity is physically demanding, has components of training that are similar to those for football, and the stimulus of competition maintains interest and enthusiasm.

The period of training during the off-season also allows the athlete to concentrate on the development of areas in which he or she is weak. The swimmer who lacks upper body strength can use this off-season time to concentrate on the development of strength in a way that will be applicable to performance in the pool. The wrestler who lacks cardiovascular endurance can use this time to develop endurance through running or bicycling. The off-season presents the athlete with a relatively free, unstructured period of time in which all aspects of performance can be worked on. As the athlete grows older, this off-season time becomes even more critical. He or she will notice that aging will gradually decrease peak levels of performance, and that it becomes increasingly more difficult to regain peak levels if his or her condition is allowed to deteriorate with periods of inactivity.

With this in mind, it is important that off-season conditioning programs be designed for the individual, whenever possible. Every off-season program must attend to the areas of strength, power, muscular endurance, flexibility, cardiovascular endurance, and body composition. An activity such as circuit training (Chapter 7) meets almost every need in each of these areas. An hour of circuit training, three days per week, combined with two to three hours of vigorous, game-type activities each week (basketball, handball, squash, or badminton), should provide a balanced off-season program for most athletes in team sports. If the athlete has a particular weakness, an additional hour or two can be devoted to developing this specific area. Another approach would be to combine running three to five miles per day, three days per week, with strength, power, and muscular endurance training exercises and selected flexibility exercises. Specific exercises should be selected on the basis of the needs of the individual and the demands of the sport.

Lastly, the athlete should receive sound nutritional counseling to assure a properly balanced diet which will provide essential vitamins and minerals, and assist in controlling weight. This is an area of considerable ignorance and a multitude of myths. Nutrition will be discussed in greater detail in Chapter 12.

In conclusion, it should be realized that the off-season training program is an extremely important aspect of the athlete's total training program, although it is frequently given little thought or attention, and is left strictly to chance. The coach and athlete should work closely together to design a program that will meet the needs of the athlete and provide him or her some variation from the traditional approach to training. The off-season provides an excellent opportunity to develop a basic foundation for each of the various components of physical training. For example, each program should devote at least some time to the areas of strength, power, endurance, flexibility, speed, agility, and nutrition. Ideally, athletes would be provided with an individualized program to follow, which would provide them with the opportunity to report at the beginning of the new season in peak physical condition.

IN-SEASON TRAINING PROGRAMS

Coaches and athletes have recently become concerned about the physical condition of the athlete during the season. Many athletes feel that they become deconditioned as the season progresses. In analyzing training programs in many sports, it is evident that once the competition begins, too little attention is given to physical conditioning. It is assumed that the competition alone will maintain the high level of conditioning that was developed in the pre-season conditioning program. While there has been no research to determine if, in fact, one does become deconditioned as the season progresses, it would seem reasonable to initiate in-season training programs to insure the maintenance of the athlete's fitness. Since so much time is needed during the season for skill and technique development, in-season conditioning programs must not require a great deal of time. These programs should, however, be designed to give attention to each of the areas previously mentioned.

Professional baseball and basketball are examples of sports which exhibit such a concern. For the athlete who is playing every day, there is reason to believe that the competition itself allows some maintenance of his or her physical condition. This may not be the case for a sport such as baseball or for reserve players in other team sports. For the eighth player on the basketball team, or the reserve catcher on the baseball team, games mean little more than riding the bench for several hours. Those individuals who are not playing regularly are most certainly undergoing deconditioning during the course of the season. It would seem wise to institute an in-season conditioning or maintenance program for all athletes, whether they are playing regularly or not. There will be a maximum return for a minimum investment.

SUMMARY

The preceding discussion has made it clear that in order to achieve maximal benefits from training, the athlete must be conscious of the negative effects of overtraining, yet realize that prolonged periods of reduced training will risk a loss in physical conditioning. On the other hand, the best possible performances can only be achieved following a period of reduced training (tapering). Thus, optimal training and maintenance for peak performance can only be achieved with a fine balance between intense training and proper rest. Since most athletes are highly motivated and tend to over-stress themselves, the most frequent error is on the side of over-training rather than under-training. Both the coach and athlete must be aware of this fault, since over-training will prevent the athlete from achieving his or her full potential.

Most athletes regard the conclusion of a long season of intense physical training and competition as the beginning of a welcomed and necessary period of rest and relaxation. While this rest and relaxation are certainly necessary and well-deserved, unfortunately many interpret this as a time to go into physical hibernation. Physical conditioning, however, cannot simply be put into storage and recalled at will when needed. If you don't use it, you lose it. Research evidence conclusively demonstrates that periods of physical inactivity will lead to losses in strength, power, muscular endurance, flexibility, and cardiovascular endurance. While the losses in strength and power are somewhat gradual, the loss in cardiovascular endurance capacity occurs very rapidly. Body composition will also change with inactivity, particularly without concomitant changes in diet. These changes would include a loss in lean body weight and an increase in fat weight, which would result in a substantial increase in relative fat.

To prevent or minimize the physiological changes that result from periods of physical inactivity, the athlete is strongly advised to participate in an off-season program of physical training. The off-season program should be varied so it includes activities that are enjoyable, but it should be sufficiently structured so each of the major components of physical training are stressed. The off-season program is also an opportune time to work on areas of weakness where supplemental training would be of considerable value. Circuit training provides one of the more versatile approaches to off-season conditioning, since it stresses each of the major components of training in a relatively brief workout. This type of activity, performed three times per week and coupled with a vigorous game-type of activity several days each week, would provide the athlete with an interesting, challenging, and physiologically rewarding program that would fully prepare him for the start of a new season.

STUDY QUESTIONS

1. What alterations occur in strength, power, and muscular endurance with physical detraining?
2. What alterations occur in speed, agility, and flexibility with physical detraining?
3. What changes occur in the cardiovascular system as one becomes deconditioned?
4. What are the causes of overtraining? How can it be identified? What is the proper treatment for overtraining?
5. During periods of reduced training, what factors (frequency, intensity, or duration) must be stressed in order to prevent a decline in long-term endurance and aerobic capacity?
6. How important is an off-season conditioning program for a football player? A swimmer? A gymnast?
7. Design an off-season conditioning program for a professional baseball player.
8. What changes occur in body composition during periods of detraining?
9. What changes take place in the muscle during periods of inactivity? During total muscle-limb immobilization (casting)?
10. How can the negative effects of muscle immobilization be reduced?
11. Design a retraining program for a distance runner who has been injured and unable to train for two months.

REFERENCES

Åstrand, P. O., & Rodahl, K. (1986). *Textbook of work physiology* (3rd ed.). New York: McGraw-Hill Book Co.

Brynteson, P., & Sinning, W. E. (1973). The effects of training frequencies on the retention of cardiovascular fitness. *Medicine and Science in Sports, 5,* 29-33.

Clarke, D. H. (1973). Adaptations in strength and muscular endurance resulting from exercise. *Exercise and Sport Sciences Reviews, 1,* 74–98.

Costill, D. L. (1985). Practical problems in exercise physiology. *Research Quarterly, 56,* 215–225.

Costill, D. L., King, D. S., Thomas, R., & Hargreaves, M. (1985). Effects of reduced training on muscular power in swimmers. *Physician and Sportsmedicine, 13,* 94–101.

Costill, D. L., Fink, W. J., Hargreaves, M., King, D. S., Thomas, R., & Fielding, R. (1985). Metabolic characteristics of skeletal muscle during detraining from competitive swimming. *Medicine and Science in Sports and Exercise, 17*, 339–343.

Coyle, E. F., Martin, W. H., III, Sinacore, D. R., Joyner, M. J., Hagberg, J. M., & Holloszy, J. O. (1984). Time course of loss of adaptations after stopping prolonged intense endurance training. *Journal of Applied Physiology, 57*, 1857–1864.

Coyle, E. F., Hemmert, M. K., & Coggan, A. R. (1986). Effects of detraining on cardiovascular responses to exercise: Role of blood volume. *Journal of Applied Physiology 60*, 95–99.

Drinkwater, B. L., & Horvath, S. M. (1972). Detraining effects in young women. *Medicine and Science in Sports, 4*, 91–95.

Fox, E. L. (1979). *Sports physiology*. Philadelphia: W. B. Saunders Co.

Hansen, K. N., Bjerre-Knudsen, J., Brodthagen, U., Jordal, R., & Paulev, P. E. (1982). Muscle cell leakage due to long distance training. *European Journal of Applied Physiology, 48*, 178–188.

Haggmark, T., Eriksson, E., & Jansson, E. (1986). Muscle fiber type changes in human skeletal muscle after injuries and immobilization. *Orthopedics, 9*, 181–185.

Henriksson, J., & Reitman, J. S. (1977). Time course of changes in human skeletal muscle succinate dehydrogenase and cytochrome oxidase activities and maximal oxygen uptake with physical activity and inactivity. *Acta Physiologica Scandinavica, 99*, 91–97.

Hickson, R. C., Foster, C., Pollock, M. L., Galassi, T. M., & Rich, S. (1985). Reduced training intensities and loss of aerobic power, endurance, and cardiac growth. *Journal of Applied Physiology, 58*, 492–499.

Jensen, C. R., & Fisher, A. G. (1979). *Scientific basis of athletic conditioning* (2nd ed.). Philadelphia: Lea & Febiger.

Maglischo, E. W. (1982). *Swimming faster*. Palo Alto, CA: Mayfield Publishing Co.

Mathews, D. K., & Fox, E. L. (1980). *The physiological basis of physical education and athletics* (3rd ed.). Philadelphia: W. B. Saunders Co.

Michael, E., Evert, J., & Jeffers, K. (1972). Physiological changes of teenage girls during five months of detraining. *Medicine and Science in Sports, 4*, 214–218.

Pate, R. R., Hughes, R. D., Chandler, J. V., & Ratliffe, J. L. (1978). Effects of arm training on retention of training effects derived from leg training. *Medicine and Science in Sports, 10*, 71–74.

Pollock, M. L. (1973). Quantification of endurance training programs. *Exercise and Sport Sciences Reviews, 1*, 155–182.

Saltin, B., Blomqvist, G., Mitchell, J. H., Johnson, R. L., Jr., Wildenthal, K., & Chapman, C. B. (1968). Response to submaximal and maximal exercise after bed rest and training. *Circulation, 38* (Suppl. 7).

Saltin, B., & Rowell, L. B. (1980). Functional adaptations to physical activity and inactivity. *Federation Proceedings, 39*, 1506–1513.

Selye, H. (1956). *The stress of life*. New York: McGraw-Hill.

Sherman, W. M., Plyley, M. J., Vogelgesang, D., Costill, D. L., & Habansky, A. J. (1981). Isokinetic strength during rehabilitation following arthrotomy: Specificity of speed. *Athletic Training, 16*, 138–141.

Sherman, W. M., Plyley, M. J., Pearson, D. R., Habansky, A. J., Vogelgesang, D. A., & Costill, D. L. (1983). Isokinetic rehabilitation after meniscectomy: A comparison of two methods of training. *Physician and Sportsmedicine, 11*, 121–133.

Siegel, W., Blomqvist, G., & Mitchell, J. H. (1970). Effects of a quantified physical training program on middle-aged sedentary men. *Circulation, 41*, 19–29.

Thorstensson, A. (1977). Observations on strength training and detraining. *Acta Physiologica Scandinavica, 100*, 491–493

SECTION C

Optimizing Sports Performance

Considerable variation exists both within and among athletes relative to their performance potential. This results from a number of factors, some of which are outside the control of either the coach or the athlete, for example, genetic constitution. However, many can either be controlled (taking water to prevent dehydration), or adaptations can be made to reduce or enhance the potential influencing factor (acclimatization to altitude or thermal stress). This section focuses on optimizing sports performance through attention to those factors that can make the difference between a successful and an unsuccessful performance.

First, Chapter 12 will discuss the importance of nutrition to athletic performance. Do we need to supplement our diets with vitamins and minerals? Protein? What is the carbohydrate loading? What should you drink to prevent dehydration and enhance performance? Chapter 13 discusses how performance can be improved by the use of various ergogenic or work-enhancing agents, and how other agents that are thought to be ergogenic in nature have a relatively small influence on the athlete's performance. This will include a discussion of drugs, oxygen, and blood doping. Finally, the various environmental factors that can influence athletic performance will be discussed in Chapter 14. How does the athlete contend with extreme variations in temperature, both hot and cold? How does humidity interact with temperature to influence the performance of the athlete? Can the athlete perform at moderate or even high altitudes without experiencing decrements in performance? What performance limitations does the athlete experience when exercising under increased atmospheric pressures, as in underwater diving? How can the athlete adapt to these environmental factors to improve performance under these conditions?

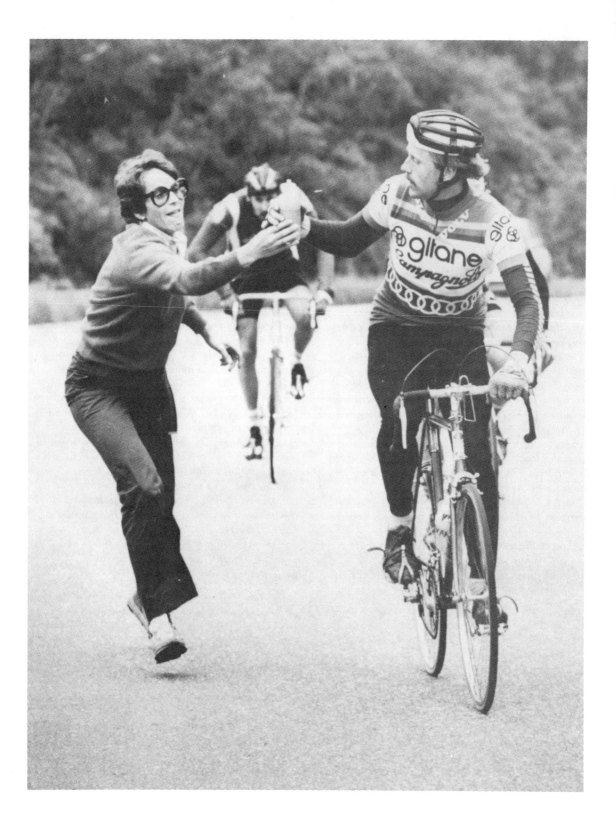

12

Nutrition and Optimal Performance

INTRODUCTION

Aside from the limits imposed by heredity and the physical improvements associated with training, no single factor seems to play a bigger role in sports performance than does diet. Despite the wealth of published information dealing with proper nutrition, few efforts have been made to describe the nutritional needs and the optimal dietary regimen for the training, competitive athlete. That is not to say that the area of nutrition has not been considered important by trainers, coaches, and athletes. In their quest for success, most athletes have at one time searched for the "magic food" that will produce a winning performance. Unfortunately, most efforts to manipulate diet have been prompted by suggestions from more successful performers, poorly designed research studies, invalid commercial advertising claims, and the misinterpretation of nutritional research. The net results are confusion and many claims that are not only unsound, but potentially dangerous. As an example, many elite athletes have attributed their athletic success to various nutritional practices. One of baseball's leading home run hitters in the early 1970s was relatively small in stature and did not appear overly muscular. When asked how he was able to generate the power necessary to hit the ball over the fence, he

responded by attributing his power to eating honey just prior to game time. Other athletes have advocated buffalo meat, dessicated liver, vitamins A, C, E, and B_{15}, bee's pollen, fructose, amino acid supplements, and various minerals, to name but a few. The American public, as a whole, is hungry for information on nutrition, spending billions of dollars each year on nutrition-related services or items. Billions of dollars are spent on the diet industry, including over a billion dollars per year spent on special diet food. It is important that more effort be placed on consumer education, making the public aware of the tremendous potential for fraud, misrepresentation, and misguided zeal.

The intent of the following discussion, therefore, will be to take an objective look at the nutrient needs of the athlete, and to present the current state of knowledge relative to the dietary demands of the athlete before, during, and after competition and training.

BASIC NUTRITIONAL NEEDS

Simply defined, food includes all the solid and liquid materials taken into the digestive tract that are utilized to maintain and build body tissues, regulate body processes, and supply body heat.

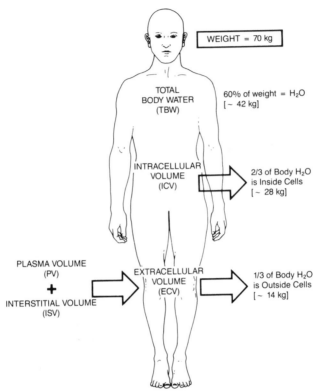

WEIGHT = 70 kg

TOTAL
BODY WATER
(TBW)

60% of weight = H_2O
[~ 42 kg]

INTRACELLULAR
VOLUME
(ICV)

2/3 of Body H_2O
is Inside Cells
[~ 28 kg]

PLASMA VOLUME
(PV)
+
INTERSTITIAL VOLUME
(ISV)

EXTRACELLULAR
VOLUME
(ECV)

1/3 of Body H_2O
is Outside Cells
[~ 14 kg]

Figure 12–1 Body water content. The three water compartments within the body are plasma (plasma volume), between and around the cells (interstitial volume), and within the cells (intracellular volume).

Food can be categorized into six classes of nutrients, each with a unique chemical structure and a specific function within the body. The six categories include **water, minerals, vitamins, proteins, fats,** and **carbohydrates.** Each of these will be briefly discussed relative to their importance in general body function.

Water

Seldom is water thought of as a food. While it has no caloric value, and does not provide any of the other nutrients, water is second in importance only to oxygen in maintaining life. As noted in Figure 12–1, water constitutes about 60 percent of the total body weight, with two-thirds of the water con-

tained within the body tissues (**intracellular**) and one-third outside the cells (**extracellular**). While we can survive for weeks, or even months, without food, we cannot tolerate water deprivation for more than a few days. It has been estimated that we can lose up to 40 percent of our body weight in fats, carbohydrates, and proteins and still survive, while a 15- to 20-percent loss in body water can be fatal.

Water is necessary for digestion, absorption, circulation, and excretion. With respect to exercise, water plays two critical roles. First, it is important in maintaining the electrolyte balance in the body. Second, it is a transporter of nutrients and by-products to and from the cells, via the circulatory system. Its role in circulation was discussed earlier in Chapters 4 and 9.

Water intake is controlled largely by thirst sensations which are received by a regulatory center in the hypothalamus. These sensations are activated by an increase in the concentration of particles (proteins, minerals, etc.) in body fluids. This is called osmotic pressure. It should be mentioned, however, that the body's thirst mechanisms do not always keep up with the body's need for water. This has been referred to as **voluntary dehydration** and occurs when working or exercising in hot climates. This phenomenon is not completely understood, but it is known that although there are no serious consequences after a single day of exercise, repeated exposures to exercise in the heat may be cumulative and can have serious, if not fatal, consequences. Large volumes of water are lost via sweating in order to maintain a normal body temperature. Men who live and work in the desert are able to adequately replace their daily water losses when allowed to drink water *ad libitum*. Because of our sluggish drive to replace body water, however, it is generally recommended that we drink more fluid than our thirst mechanisms dictate in an attempt to avoid voluntary dehydration. If too much water is ingested, the body can adapt readily by passing off the excess in urine.

Water is normally ingested directly, in other fluids, or as a part of ingested food. The normal water intake of the average adult in a moderate climate will be approximately two liters per day. This will obviously increase in direct proportion to the fluid loss experienced by the individual through exercise and increased environmental temperature. With respect to foods, water constitutes 96 percent of the total content of lettuce, 88 percent of an orange, 87 percent of milk, 74 percent of eggs, 60 percent of lean beef, and only 4 percent of dry cereals and soda crackers. In addition to the water contained in the ingested food, water is also a by-product of the metabolism of stored food. The oxidation of 100 grams of fat, carbohydrate, and protein yields 107, 55, and 26 grams of water, respectively, which is referred to as metabolic water.

Ingested water is rapidly absorbed by the intestines, but it must first be emptied from the stomach. Considerable research has shown that when materials are dissolved in the solutions we drink, they tend to be delayed as they pass through the stomach, slowing the replacement of body water.

Thus, to increase water absorption in the intestines, it is important to ingest either water, or solutions that have few dissolved particles, such as sugar or minerals. Details about the fluids for rehydration will be discussed later in this chapter.

Minerals

Minerals refer to the elements in their simple inorganic form. While there are more than 20 mineral elements in the body, approximately 17 have been proven to be essential in the diet. Approximately four percent of one's body weight is in the form of minerals, and most of this is in bone. Minerals such as calcium, phosphorus, and magnesium, are needed in relatively large amounts, and are referred to as macrominerals. Potassium, sulfur, sodium, and chlorine also fall into this category. **Macrominerals,** by definition, are minerals that are needed by the body in amounts of more than 100 milligrams per day. **Microminerals,** or trace elements, are those minerals needed in amounts of less than one hundred milligrams per day, and include iron, zinc, selenium, manganese, copper, iodine, molybdenum, cobalt, fluorine, and chromium. Several of the more important macrominerals will be discussed briefly. In addition, Table 12-1 on pages 220-221 provides a list of the seventeen essential minerals, their location in the body, their major function, the best food source, and the 1980 recommended daily dietary allowance for each.

Calcium is the most abundant mineral in the body, constituting 1.5 to 2.0 percent of the total body weight and approximately 40 percent of the total minerals present in the body. Of the total calcium in the body, 99 percent is found in the bones and teeth. The major function of calcium is to build and maintain bones and teeth. It is essential for muscle contraction, blood clotting, control of cell membrane permeability, and nervous control of the heart. Milk and other dairy products are the best sources of calcium.

Phosphorus is closely linked to calcium, and constitutes approximately 22 percent of the total mineral content of the body. About 80 percent of phosphorus is found in combination with calcium in the form of calcium phosphate, which provides

Table 12-1 Mineral elements in the body.

Mineral	Primary Location in Body	Primary Function	Food Sources	1980 Recommended Dietary Allowance (units/day)
Calcium	Bone and teeth	Blood clotting, bone formation, transportation of fluids, muscle contraction	Milk and milk products, broccoli, sardines, clams, and oysters	1200 milligrams for ages 11–18 years, and 800 milligrams for adults
Phosphorus	Bone and teeth	Bone formation, body's energy system, pH regulation	Cheese, egg yolk, milk, meat, fish, poultry, whole-grain cereals, legumes, and nuts	1200 milligrams for ages 11–18 years, and 800 milligrams for adults
Magnesium	Bone and inside cells	Activates enzymes	Whole-grain cereals, nuts, meat, milk, green vegetables, and legumes	300–400 milligrams for teens and adults
Sodium	Bone and extracellular fluid	Regulation of body fluid osmolarity, pH, and body fluid volume	Table salt, seafood, milk and eggs; abundant in most food, except fruits	900–3,300 milligrams for teens and adults
Chloride	Extracellular fluid	Buffer and enzyme activation	Table salt, seafood, milk, meat, and eggs	1,400–5,100 milligrams for teens and adults
Potassium	Intracellular fluid	Regulation of body fluid osmolarity, pH, and cell membrane transfer	Fruits, meat, milk, cereals, vegetables, and legumes	1,525–5,625 milligrams for teens and adults
Sulfur	Amino acids	Oxidation-reduction reactions	Protein foods, including meat, fish, poultry, eggs, milk, cheese, legumes, and nuts	None
Iron	Hemoglobin, liver, spleen, and bone	Oxygen transportation	Liver, meat, egg yolk, legumes, whole or enriched grains, dark green vegetables, shrimp, and oysters	10–18 milligrams for teens and adults

Table 12–1   (continued)

Mineral	Primary Location in Body	Primary Function	Food Sources	1980 Recommended Dietary Allowance (units/day)
Zinc	Most tissues, with higher amounts in liver, muscle, and bone	Constituent of essential enzymes and insulin	Milk, liver, shellfish, herring, and wheat bran	15 milligrams for teens and adults
Copper	All tissues, with larger amounts in the liver, brain, heart, and kidney	Constituent of enzymes	Liver, shellfish, whole grains, cherries, legumes, kidney, poultry, oysters, chocolate, and nuts	2.0–3.0 milligrams for teens and adults
Iodine	Thyroid gland	Essential constituent of thyroxin	Iodized table salt, seafood, water, and vegetables	150 micrograms for teens and adults
Manganese	Bone, pituitary, liver, pancreas, and gastrointestinal tissue	Constituent of essential enzymes	Grains, nuts, legumes, fruit, and tea	2.5–5.0 milligrams for teens and adults
Fluoride	Bone	Reduces dental caries and may reduce bone loss	Drinking water, tea, coffee, soybeans, spinach, gelatin, onions, and lettuce	1.5–2.5 milligrams for teens, and 1.5–4.0 milligrams for adults
Molybdenum	Enzymes	Constituent of essential enzymes	Legumes, cereal grains, dark green leafy vegetables, and organs	0.15–0.5 milligram for teens and adults
Cobalt	In cells	Essential to normal function of all cells	Liver, kidney, oysters, clams, poultry, and milk	None
Selenium	In the cell	Fat metabolism	Grains, onions, meats, milk, and vegetables	0.05–0.2 milligram for teens and adults
Chromium	In the cell	Glucose metabolism	Corn oil, clams, whole-grain cereals, meats, and drinking water	0.05–0.2 milligram for teens and adults

strength and rigidity to the bones and teeth. It is also an essential part of metabolism, cell membrane structure, and the buffering system to maintain the blood at a constant pH. Meat, poultry, fish, eggs, and milk are the major sources of phosphorus.

Iron is present in the body in relatively small amounts, 35 to 50 milligrams per kilogram of body weight. Iron plays an extremely critical role in the transportation of oxygen throughout the body. As was mentioned in Chapters 3 and 4, oxygen is carried in the blood primarily by its attachment to hemoglobin, an iron-containing protein. The iron combines with oxygen in the lungs and releases the oxygen at the level of the tissues. The myoglobin found in muscle, similar to hemoglobin, is also an iron-containing protein.

Iron deficiency is considered to be very prevalent throughout the world, with some estimates as high as 25 percent of the world's population. The major problem associated with iron deficiency is iron-deficiency anemia, where there is a reduction in the oxygen-carrying capacity of the blood and a resulting feeling of general tiredness and lack of energy. The major dietary source of iron is liver. However, oysters, shellfish, lean meat, and other organ meats provide good sources, as do leafy green vegetables and egg yolks.

Sodium, potassium, and chloride are classified as electrolytes and are found distributed throughout all body fluids and tissues, with sodium and chloride found predominantly extracellularly and potassium intracellularly. These electrolytes function to maintain normal water balance and distribution, normal osmotic equilibrium, normal acid–base balance, and normal muscular irritability. The major sources of sodium and chloride are table salt, seafood, milk, and meat. Potassium is found most readily in fruits, milk, meat, cereals, and vegetables.

Vitamins

Vitamins are defined as a group of unrelated organic compounds that perform specific functions to promote growth and to maintain health. They are needed in relatively small quantities, but they are essential for specific metabolic reactions within the cell, and for normal growth and mainte-

nance of health. Vitamins function primarily as catalysts in chemical reactions within the body. They are essential for the release of energy, for tissue building, and for controlling the body's use of food. Vitamins can be classified into one of two major categories: fat soluble or water soluble. Fat-soluble vitamins A, D, E, and K, are stored by the body in lipids. Because they are stored by the body, there is the possibility that excess dosages could lead to vitamin toxicity. Vitamin C and the B-complex vitamins are water soluble, and when taken in excess will be excreted, mainly in the urine. A brief discussion of the major vitamins related to sports, and their functions, will follow. Refer to Table 12–2 for a more complete list of each vitamin, its sources and functions, and the 1980 recommended daily dietary allowance.

The first fat-soluble vitamin to be discovered was vitamin A, or Retinaol in 1913. Natural vitamin A is usually found esterified with a fatty acid. It is essential for night vision, as an integral part of the visual purple of the retina. It is also essential for maintaining normal epithelial structure, and is thus important in the prevention of infection. It is also important for healthy skin, normal bone development, and tooth formation. The major dietary sources of vitamin A are liver, kidney, butter, egg yolk, whole milk, fruits, and leafy dark green and yellow vegetables. Approximately 90 percent of the stored vitamin A is found in the liver. Toxicity results in bone fragility and stunted growth, loss of appetite, coarsening and loss of hair, scaly skin eruptions, enlargements of the liver and spleen, irritability, double vision, fatigue, and skin rashes.

Vitamin D was discovered in 1930. In its ingested state, it is absorbed with fats from the intestine, but it can also be absorbed from the skin directly into the blood. It is stored in the liver, skin, brain, and bones. It is essential for normal growth and development, and for normal bone and tooth formation. Rickets results from vitamin D deficiency, and toxicity leads to excessive calcification of bone, kidney stones, headache, nausea, and diarrhea. Major dietary sources for Vitamin D are fish, eggs, fortified dairy products, liver, and a natural source, sunlight.

Vitamin E, discovered in 1922, consists of four different tocopherols (viscous oils): alpha, beta,

Table 12–2   Vitamins and their primary functions, sources, and recommended daily allowance.

Vitamin	Primary Function	Sources	1980 Recommended Dietary Allowance units/day
Fat-Soluble Vitamins			
A	Adaptation to dim light, resistance to infection, prevention of eye and skin disorders, promotion of bone and tooth development	Liver, kidney, milk, butter, egg yolk, yellow vegetables, apricots, cantaloupe, and peaches	800 and 1,000 micrograms for females and males, respectively—teens and adults
D	Facilitates absorption of calcium; bone and tooth development	Sunlight, fish, eggs, fortified dairy products, and liver	10 micrograms for ages 11-18; 5-7.5 micrograms for adults
E	Prevents oxidation of essential vitamins and fatty acids, and protects red blood cells from hemolysis	Wheatgerm, vegetable oils, green vegetables, milk fat, egg yolk, and nuts	8-10 milligrams for teens and adults
K	Blood clotting	Liver, soybean oil, vegetable oil, green vegetables, tomatoes, cauliflower, and wheat bran	70-140 micrograms for teens and adults
Water-Soluble Vitamins			
B₁ (thiamine)	Energy metabolism, growth, appetite, and digestion	Pork, liver, organ meats, legumes, whole-grain and enriched cereals and breads, wheatgerm, and potatoes	1.0-1.5 milligrams for teens and adults
B₂ (riboflavin)	Growth, health of eyes, and energy metabolism	Milk and dairy foods, organ meats, green vegetables, eggs, fish, and enriched cereals and breads	1.2-1.7 milligrams for teens and adults
Niacin	Energy metabolism and fatty-acid synthesis	Fish, liver, meat, poultry, grains, eggs, peanuts, milk, and legumes	13-19 milligrams for teens and adults
B₆ (pyridoxine)	Protein metabolism and growth	Pork, glandular meats, bran and germ cereals, milk, egg yolk, oatmeal, and legumes	1.8-2.2 milligrams for teens and adults

continued on next page

Table 12–2 Vitamins and their primary functions, sources, and recommended daily allowance. (continued)

Vitamin	Primary Function	Sources	1980 Recommended Dietary Allowance units/day
Water-Soluble Vitamins			
Pantothenic acid	Hemoglobin formation, and carbohydrate, protein, and fat metabolism	Whole-grain cereals, organ meats, and eggs	4–7 milligrams for teens and adults
Biotin	Carbohydrate, fat, and protein metabolism	Liver, peanuts, yeast, milk, meat, egg yolk, cereal, nuts, legumes, bananas, grapefruit, tomatoes, watermelon, and strawberries	100–200 micrograms for teens and adults
Folic acid (folacin)	Growth, fat metabolism, maturation of red blood cells	Green vegetables, organ meats, lean beef, wheat, eggs, fish, dry beans, lentils, asparagus, broccoli, and yeast	400 micrograms for teens and adults
B_{12} (cobalamin)	Red blood cell production, nervous system metabolism, and fat metabolism	Liver, kidney, milk and dairy foods, and meat	3.0 micrograms for teens and adults
C (ascorbic acid)	Growth, tissue repair, tooth and bone formation	Citrus fruits, tomatoes, strawberries, potatoes, melons, peppers, and pineapple	50–60 milligrams for teens and adults

gamma, and delta. Alpha tocopherol is biologically more active than the other three, and delta tocopherol is the most potent antioxidant. Vitamin E functions in metabolism and helps to enhance the activity of vitamins A and C. Major dietary sources are wheatgerm, vegetable oils, green vegetables, milk fat, egg yolk, and nuts. Vitamin E deficiency in humans is rare, and few serious toxic effects have been identified. Many claims have been made for vitamin E with respect to the prevention and treatment of rheumatic fever, muscular dystrophy, coronary artery disease, sterility, menstrual disorders, and spontaneous abortion,

among others, but the claims for cures or benefits for any of these areas lacks the support of scientific evidence. Its most important function is probably that of an anti-oxidant, particularly in the lungs when exposed to air pollutants.

The B-complex vitamins were at one time considered to be the single most important vitamin in the prevention of the disease beriberi. At the present time, however, more than a dozen B-complex vitamins have been identified, which have very specific functions within the body (see Table 12–2 for a complete listing). B-complex vitamins play an essential role in the metabolism of all living cells, serving as co-factors in the various enzyme systems involved in the oxidation of food and the production of energy. The B-complex vitamins have such a close interrelationship, that a deficiency in one may impair the utilization of the others. Dry yeast is the single best source of the B-complex vitamins. Table 12-2 lists other major food sources for each of the B-complex vitamins.

Vitamin C, or ascorbic acid, was isolated in 1928, and is both the prevention and cure for scurvy. Vitamin C functions as either a co-enzyme or co-factor in metabolism. It is required for the production and maintenance of collagen, and has been postulated to assist in wound healing, combat fever and infection, and prevent or cure the common cold. Vitamin C deficiency is characterized by general weakness, poor appetite, anemia, swollen and inflamed gums and loosened teeth, shortness of breath, swollen joints, and neurotic disturbances.

Proteins

Proteins are nitrogen-containing compounds formed by amino acids, and they constitute the major structural component of the cell, antibodies, enzymes, and many hormones. Protein is necessary for growth, but it is also necessary for the repair and maintenance of body tissues; the production of hemoglobin (iron and protein); the production of enzymes, hormones, mucus, milk, and sperm; the maintenance of normal osmotic balance; and protection from disease through antibodies. Proteins are also potential sources of energy, but they are generally spared when fats and carbohydrates are available in ample supply. Over 20 amino acids have been identified, and of these, eight or nine are considered to be essential as a part of the daily food intake. While many of the amino acids can be manufactured or synthesized by the body, the essential, or indispensable, amino acids either cannot be synthesized by the body or cannot be synthesized at a rate sufficient to meet the body needs, and thus need to be obtained through dietary intake. If any one of these essential amino acids is absent from the diet, protein cannot be synthesized or body tissue maintained. Protein sources in the diet which contain all of the essential amino acids in the proper ratio and in sufficient quantity, are referred to as **complete pro-**

teins. Meat, fish, and poultry are the three primary complete proteins. The proteins in vegetables and grains are referred to as **incomplete proteins,** as they do not supply all of the essential amino acids in appropriate amounts. This concept becomes important for individuals on vegetarian diets. This will be discussed in much greater detail in the next section of this chapter.

Approximately five to 15 percent of the total calories consumed per day in the United States are in the form of protein. This is considered by many to be two to three times the actual amount of protein necessary for proper body function. The daily recommended allowance published in 1980 by the National Research Council, is 45 and 56 grams per day for the teenage and adult male, respectively, and 44 to 46 grams per day for the teenage and adult female. Since the allowance is dependent on the individual's body weight, an allowance of 0.8 gram per kilogram of body weight is considered appropriate for the adult. These recommendations are substantially lower than the 1968 recommendations.

Fats

Fats, or **lipids,** are composed of about 98 percent triglycerides, with the remainder including traces of mono- and diglycerides, free fatty acids, phospholipids, and sterols. Triglycerides are composed of three molecules of fatty acids and one molecule of glycerol. While fat has generally been thought of in negative terms—a person is considered too fat or the blood fats are elevated placing the person at risk for coronary artery disease—fat provides many useful functions in the body. It is an essential component of cell walls and nerve fibers; a primary energy source, providing up to 70 percent of the total energy when the body is in the resting state; a support and cushion for vital organs; involved in the absorption and transport of the fat-soluble vitamins; and an insulative layer subcutaneously for the preservation of body heat.

There are two types of fatty acids: saturated and unsaturated. The difference between the two is in the bonding between carbon and hydrogen atoms. Unsaturated fats contain one (monounsaturated) or more (polyunsaturated) double bonds between carbon atoms in a chain of carbon atoms. Each double bond in the chain takes the place of two hydrogen atoms. When the carbon chain is saturated with hydrogen atoms, two hydrogen atoms or more for each carbon atom, this is called a saturated fatty acid. In practical terms, a saturated fat is in the form of a solid (animal fat), and an unsaturated fat is in the form of a liquid (fish and vegetable oil). Saturated fats are derived primarily from animal sources and unsaturated fats from plant sources. Saturated fats have been associated with an increased risk of coronary artery disease.

Fat supplies approximately 40 to 45 percent of the total caloric intake of the American population, and this represents a substantial increase over the percentage of fat consumed in the early 1900s. In addition, fat from animal sources has increased markedly, and that from vegetable sources has decreased. Most nutritionists recommend approximately 25 percent of the caloric intake in the form of fat, but this should not exceed 30 to 35 percent. While many agree that the reduction of fat intake should come from saturated fats, there is presently a great deal of controversy on specific recommendations for the intake of saturated fats, particularly in reference to egg and dairy products.

Carbohydrates

Carbohydrates are composed of sugars and starches, and are classified as either **monosaccharides, disaccharides, oligosaccharides,** or **polysaccharides.** Monosaccharides are the simple sugars (glucose and fructose are the primary simple sugars) that cannot be hydrolyzed to a simpler form. Disaccharides can be hydrolyzed into two molecules of the same or different monosaccharide, such as sucrose that we commonly use as table sugar. Oligosaccharides can be hydrolyzed to yield three to ten monosaccharide units, and polysaccharides can provide more than ten monosaccharide units. The major polysaccharides are starch, dextrin, cellulose, and glycogen, which are composed completely of glucose units. Glucose serves many functions in the body. First, it is a major source of energy, particularly during high-intensity exercise. Glucose also exerts an influence on both protein and fat metabolism, sparing the use of protein as an energy source, and controlling the

utilization of fat. Glucose is the sole source of energy for the nervous system.

In the early 1900s, carbohydrates constituted over 55 percent of the total caloric intake. In the 1970s, this figure dropped to approximately 45 percent. In the early 1900s, starches constituted 68 percent of the total carbohydrate intake, but this has dropped to below 50 percent today. Sugar intake, conversely, increased from 32 percent to over 50 percent of the diet over the same time period. The major sources of carbohydrates are grains, fruits, vegetables, milk, and concentrated sweets. Refined sugar, syrup, and cornstarch are examples of pure carbohydrates. Many of the concentrated sweets such as candy, honey, jellies, molasses, and soft drinks contain few, if any, other nutrients.

THE ATHLETE'S DIET

Since athletes place considerable demands on their bodies every day they train and compete, it is important that the body be as finely tuned as possible. This, by necessity, must include optimal nutrition. Too often, athletes spend considerable time and effort in perfecting skills and attaining top physical condition, only to ignore proper nutrition and sleep. It is not uncommon to trace the deterioration of an athlete's performance back to poor nutrition.

Unfortunately, we know very little about the actual eating habits of athletes. To gain a little insight, the diets for a group of highly-trained distance runners were recorded during a period of training and during the three days before a marathon. The 22 runners (11 men and 11 women) who were studied, included a wide spectrum of running abilities, from international-level runners to recreational competitors.

The findings revealed that there was little difference between what elite and average runners ate. Diet did not appear to be a determinant of success or failure among these performers. Although specific items in the diets varied—from pork chops to pasta, from collard greens to candy bars—differences were small when each runner's food intake for several days was analyzed for its percentages

Table 12–3 A comparison of the twenty-two runners' diets with the RDA (Recommended Dietary Allowance). Figures shown in parentheses represent estimates of the average values in the American diet, which may or may not be healthy. Even where the figure is low (as with folic acid and vitamin E), that does not necessarily suggest a deficiency since the RDA is somewhat arbitrary, with a large safety factor.

Diet Composition	Runner's Average	RDA
Calories (kcal/day)	3,012	(2,000)
Carbohydrate (gm)	375	(250)
Protein (gm)	112	(70)
Saturated fats (gm)	42	(26)
Unsaturated fats (gm)	64	(54)
Total fat (gm)	122	(66–100)
Cholesterol (mg)	377	(300)
Fiber (gm)	7	(3–6)
Vitamin A (IU)	10,814	5,000
Vitamin B$_1$ (mg)	1.9	1.3
Vitamin B$_2$ (mg)	2.5	1.6
Vitamin B$_6$ (mg)	2.2	2
Vitamin B$_{12}$ (ug)	3.8	3
Folic acid (mg)	0.23	0.4
Niacin (mg)	27.3	16
Pantothenic acid (mg)	5.3	7.5
Vitamin C (mg)	205	55
Vitamin E (mg)	5.2	14
Iron (mg)	25	14
Potassium (gm)	4.3	2.5
Calcium (gm)	1.3	1.0
Magnesium (gm)	0.4	0.3
Phosphorus (gm)	2.0	1.0
Sodium (gm)	2.6	(6.0)

of fats, proteins, and carbohydrates, or amounts of vitamins and minerals. One interesting finding was how closely runners came to meeting the RDA, the standard considered necessary for good health.

The diet for this cross-section of runners contained 50 percent carbohydrates, 36 percent fats, and 14 percent proteins. In light of the need for a high carbohydrate diet when training for distance running, the carbohydrate intake of these runners might be considered to be low. These runners actually ate more than enough carbohydrate to meet the energy needed for training. Since their total caloric intake was nearly 50 percent higher than would be expected for individuals of similar size (145 pounds), their total carbohydrate intake was well above average (see Table 12–3).

It was also observed that these runners consumed adequate vitamins and minerals to at least equal the RDA, which contains a built-in cushion. Unless a runner's vitamin intake falls well below the RDA for an extended period of time, no effects on performance would be expected. Although diets rich in simple carbohydrates tend to be deficient in some of the B-complex vitamins, only two runners appeared to consume too little vitamin B$_{12}$.

Although some experts have suggested that we need 1,000 milligrams of vitamin C per day, the RDA is only 60, well below that consumed by the runners in our survey. Most of the runners studied did not use vitamin supplements, contrary to some recent surveys about the habits of runners. These participants also obtained more-than-adequate amounts of minerals, including iron, as well as ample fiber, another item associated with good health.

In the last three days before a marathon, our subjects changed both their training and eating habits. Where previously they had averaged 8.5 miles per day, they reduced their daily mileage to an average of 2.3 miles. In an apparent attempt to load their muscles with glycogen, the runners increased their daily caloric intake from 3,012 kilocalories (kcal) during training to a pre-marathon average of 3,730. Several ate more than 5,000 kcal, nearly twice their rate of caloric expenditure during that period.

Such overeating might hurt their performances. Since the marathoners had reduced their mileages, they were burning only about 2,526 kilocalories per day (kcal/day), while eating 3,730 kcal per day. The result was a daily surplus of 1,204 kcal that might have resulted in the storage of one extra pound of unnecessary and unproductive fat (3,600 kcal equals one pound of fat). From the standpoint of performance, however, it is probably better to eat a bit too much food, principally carbohydrates, than to risk not being fully loaded with muscle and liver glycogen at the time of competition.

Thus, these findings and other available evidence suggests that the dietary requirements of the athlete are no different than the requirements of the non-athlete, with the exception of the total number of calories consumed. Thus, the optimum diet for athletes, as for non-athletes, must contain adequate quantities of water, calories, proteins, fats, carbohydrates, minerals, and vitamins in the proper proportions, independent of the sport or the event within a sport. In other words, a well-balanced diet appears to be all that is necessary!

What is a well-balanced diet? In the early 1940s, the Food and Nutrition Board of the National Research Council of the National Academy of Sciences was formed to define the nutrient requirements of the American population. At the conclusion of their deliberations, they published a report that became known as the "Recommended Dietary Allowances," or the RDA. The allowances were designed to provide a guideline for planning and evaluating food intake. In 1980, the National Research Council published its most recent of a number of revisions. The allowances for minerals and vitamins are listed in Tables 12-1 and 12-2; the protein allowance was discussed in the previous section. With respect to energy intake, males 11 to 50 years of age should consume between 2,700 and 2,900 kcal, and females between 2,000 and 2,200 kcal. These figures are calculated on the basis of the average height and weight of the population, for individuals doing light work. Obviously, athletes in intensive training would have considerably higher energy-intake demands, as was discussed in Chapter 2.

One of the problems associated with the RDA was the inability of the average individual to understand the specific allowance value, its units of measure, and to translate this information into meaningful terms. This led to a grouping of foods,

and the simplified "Basic Seven Food Plan." In 1956, this was simplified even further into the "Four Food Group Plan," which was published in the U. S. Department of Agriculture's publication, *The Essentials of an Adequate Diet*. The "Four Food Group Plan" consists of the following four groups: milk and milk products, meat and high-protein foods, fruits and vegetables, and cereal and grain foods. Table 12-4 outlines the basics of the "Four Food Group Plan," including the number of servings per day and the major contributions of each food group. These suggestions are based on the minimal requirements, and will have to be increased either by larger servings, or more servings, for individuals who are active and expend a considerable amount of additional energy each day. This basic dietary plan is recommended as a base or foundation, as it will assure the athlete of a well-balanced diet, with no deficiencies, providing the energy intake matches the energy expenditure. With respect to the balance between the basic food groups, protein should constitute 10 to 20 percent of the total caloric intake, fats 25 to 35 percent, and carbohydrates 50 to 55 percent. For athletes who are training to exhaustion on successive days, the carbohydrate fraction could be as high as 70 percent.

Vegetarian Diets

More people appear to be reducing their intake of meat and increasing their intake of vegetables. In some cases, people have made the complete transition to vegetarianism. Vegetarian diets are chosen for a number of reasons, including health, ecological, and economical reasons. Most vegetarians eat any food from plant sources. However, there are several types of vegetarians. **Vegans** are strict vegetarians and eat only food from plant sources. **Lacto-vegetarians** eat plant foods plus dairy products. **Ovo-vegetarians** eat plant foods plus eggs, and **lacto-ovovegetarians** eat plant foods, dairy products, and eggs. **Fruitarians** eat fruits, nuts, olive oil, and honey.

Can athletes survive on a vegetarian diet? The answer is a qualified yes. If the athlete is a strict vegan, he or she must be very careful in the selection of the plant foods eaten in order to provide a good balance of the essential amino acids, and

Table 12–4 The basic four food group plan.

Food Group	Daily Amounts for Adults	Nutritional Contribution
Milk and milk products	Two or more servings per day, either as a milk beverage or a milk product, such as cheese and ice cream. A serving would be one cup or its equivalent.	Protein Calcium Riboflavin Vitamin D
Meat and high-protein products	Two or more servings of meat, fish, poultry, eggs, or vegetables, such as dried beans, lentils, peas, and nuts. A serving of meat, fish, or poultry would be 3.5 ounces of lean and boneless meat.	Protein Thiamin Iron Niacin Riboflavin
Fruit and vegetables	Four or more servings per day of ½ cup or more.	Vitamin A Vitamin C Folic acid
Cereal and grain	Four or more servings per day with one serving equal to one slice of bread, ½ to ¾ cup of cooked cereal, macaroni, spaghetti, etc.	Protein Thiamin Riboflavin Niacin Iron

adequate sources of vitamin A, riboflavin, vitamin B_{12}, vitamin D, calcium, iron, and sufficient calories. More than one professional athlete has noted significant deterioration in athletic performance after switching over to a strict vegetarian diet. The problem was later traced to an unwise selection of plant foods. Inclusion of milk and eggs is highly recommended, since their inclusion will lessen the likelihood of nutritional deficiencies. Anyone contemplating a switch from a normal to a vegetarian diet would be well-advised to read authoritative reference material on the subject, written by qualified nutritionists, or to consult a registered dietition.

Special Diets and Supplements

Athletes are always looking for an edge, something that will give them an advantage. Since the difference between winning and losing can often be measured in fractions of a second, no athlete wants to feel that he or she did not try everything possible to achieve his or her best performance. Manipulating the diet and taking extra quantities of various vitamins and minerals seem to be relatively harmless methods to make the body work at its best. But do these efforts really help?

As noted earlier, vitamins are essential for normal body function. Unfortunately, athletes have no way to judge their vitamin levels until they become deficient. Only then do the rather unpleasant symptoms appear. The characteristic sores and loss of vision associated with a deficiency in vitamin B_2 (riboflavin), for example, are a rare event in our society and unheard of among athletes. Earlier evidence has shown that, on the average, most athletes consume equal or greater amounts of vitamins than the RDA. Some individuals, however, have been observed to consume diets containing less than the RDA for vitamins B_6, B_{12}, pantothenic acid, and folic acid. Some distance runners were found to be taking less than 50 percent of the recommended amount for these vitamins, based on the number of calories they were eating. One explanation for the low levels may be that some of the athletes studied were vegetarians, or ate diets low

Table 12–5 Electrolyte concentrations and osmolarity in sweat, muscle, and plasma.

	Electrolytes (mEq/liter)				Osmolality (mOsm/liter)
	Na^+	Cl^-	K^+	Mg^{++}	
Sweat	40–60	30–50	4–5	1.5–5	80–185
Plasma	140	101	4	1.5	302
Muscle	9	6	162	31	302

Notes: Na^+ = sodium; Cl^- = chloride; K^+ = potassium; Mg^{++} = magnesium

in such animal products as meats, cheese, milk, and eggs, which are the principal sources of B_6, B_{12}, and panothenic acid.

There have been a number of studies that found increased endurance with megadoses of vitamins C, E, and B-complex, but there are far more studies demonstrating that vitamins in excess of the RDA will not improve performance in either strength or endurance activities. Experts generally agree that popping vitamins will not make up for a lack of talent or training, or give one an edge over the competition.

As a matter of fact, too much of a good thing can be harmful. Extremely large doses of vitamins A and D may produce some undesirable effects. Overdoses of vitamin A, for example, may cause a loss of appetite, loss of hair, enlargement of the liver and spleen, swelling over the long bones, and general irritability—scarcely ideal conditions for any athlete. These symptoms, however, have never been reported in athletes, even those taking two to three times the RDA for these vitamins.

All in all, it appears that the RDA values for the various vitamins are about optimal for normal body operations, though possibly on the conservative side. Certainly, there is no convincing evidence to prove that vitamin pills taken to supplement a balanced diet will improve athletic performance. Megadoses of vitamins may be of some value, if for some reason one wants to increase the vitamin content of his or her urine, since that is where most of the excess ends up. Perhaps that is why it is said that athletes produce the most expensive urine in the world.

Minerals are the second most widely used diet supplement by athletes. Since perspiration tastes salty, many athletes fear a large loss of body salts during periods of heavy sweating. Actually, sweat is quite dilute when compared to other body fluids (see Table 12–5). There is, however, a wide individual variation in the quantity of electrolytes lost in sweat. Although fewer electrolytes are lost in the sweat of highly-trained and heat-acclimatized runners than in untrained individuals, the mineral content of the diet can have an effect on the electrolyte concentration of sweat. A low-salt diet results in a low-salt sweat. The body adjusts the electrolyte content of sweat to keep pace with dietary intake. It seems that even without mineral supplements, the body can get all it needs from the natural minerals in food.

Iron is an essential component of hemoglobin, the oxygen-carrying component of blood, and of myoglobin, the oxygen-transporting pigment of muscle. Since iron-deficiency anemia is known to impair endurance performance, it is important to distinguish between true anemia and the plasma volume dilution associated with repeated days of training in warm weather. Training tends to increase the volume of plasma more than the number of red blood cells, producing a drop in hemoglobin concentration with no apparent effect on oxygen transport or endurance. As noted in Figure 12–2, plasma water changes dramatically with both acute and chronic exercise, whereas the number of red cells remains relatively constant. Thus, changes in plasma volume can alter the concentration of red blood cells and hemoglobin, giving the false impression of anemia or an excess of blood cells.

Several studies have reported that between 36 and 82 percent of female runners are anemic or iron deficient. In light of this high frequency of iron deficiency in females, it seems logical to suggest that

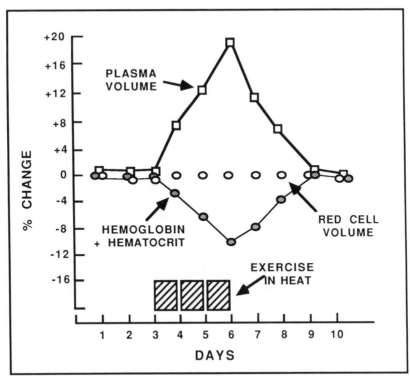

Figure 12-2 Changes in plasma water content during acute and chronic exercise. Note that the volume of red blood cells remains constant, while the concentration of red cells (hematocrit) and hemoglobin change significantly.

they include iron-rich foods in their diets. In addition, athletes suspected to be anemic or iron-deficient should be tested for serum ferritin, a measure of the body's iron stores and a method to determine the athlete's need for extra dietary iron. Iron supplementation should, however, be directed by a physician, since prolonged administration of iron can cause an iron overload, a potentially serious condition.

Many athletes wish to lose body fat while continuing to train hard. Unfortunately, to lose excess fat the body must be forced to rely more heavily on its fat reserves for energy, while taking in little fuel. This results in a caloric deficit and a gradual reduction in the body's fat weight. Although such a diet-exercise regimen accelerates the rate of fat-loss, it fails to allow for adequate replacement of muscle and liver glycogen stores. As a result, the

athlete may feel heavy and is easily fatigued, able to train only at a relatively slow pace and with a reduced total work output.

During periods of voluntary weight loss, the individual must take care to obtain the essential vitamins and minerals while consuming fewer than required calories. Malnutrition among these individuals may occur when they consume foods low in these necessary ingredients. Under these conditions it may be helpful to use vitamin and mineral supplements.

Attempts to lose weight should be scheduled for periods when the athletes are not preparing for competition. During those periods they can afford to perform lower intensity exercise for longer periods, thereby stimulating the burning of calories, mostly fat. Although exercise will aid in losing weight, the only known way to insure the removal of body fat is partial starvation. Too bad it isn't as easy or as enjoyable to get rid of body fat as it is to put it on!

Pre-contest Meal

For years, the athlete has been given the traditional steak dinner several hours prior to competition. Possibly, this practice originated from the early belief that the muscle consumed itself as fuel for muscular activity and that steak provided the necessary protein to counteract this loss. It is now recognized that this is probably the worst possible meal that the athlete could eat prior to competition. Steak contains a high percentage of fat, which takes many hours to be fully digested. The digestive process competes with the muscles used in the contest for the available blood. Because of this, the pre-contest meal, no matter what its content, should be given no later than three hours prior to the contest. Another factor to consider is the emotional climate at the time of this meal. Extreme nervousness is frequently present, and even the choicest steak is not enjoyed. The steak would be psychologically more satisfying to the athlete either the night before, or the night following the contest.

Nathan J. Smith, in his book, *Food for Sport*, lists five goals that should be considered in planning the pre-contest diet. These are as follows:

1. Energy intake should be adequate to ward off any feeling of hunger or weakness during the entire period of the competition. Although pre-contest food intakes make only a minor contribution to the immediate energy expenditure, they are essential for the support of an adequate level of blood sugar, and for avoiding the sensations of hunger and weakness.
2. The diet plan should ensure that the stomach and upper bowel are empty at the time of competition.
3. Food and fluid intakes prior to and during prolonged competition should guarantee an optimal state of hydration.
4. The pre-competition diet should offer foods that will minimize upset in the gastrointestinal tract.

5. The diet should include food that athletes are familiar with, and are convinced will "make them win."

It is also important that the athlete not eat anything with a high sugar content two hours or less before competition. Some athletes will ingest two or three candy bars 30 to 60 minutes prior to competition. With such a heavy sugar load, the body reacts by substantially increasing the insulin levels in the blood. In some individuals, the body overreacts and produces more insulin than is needed. This results in a very sharp decrease in the blood sugar level, causing the athlete to become hypoglycemic. This condition may reduce the performance potential of the athlete. Research has found that glucose feedings 30 to 45 minutes before endurance exercise increased the rate of carbohydrate oxidation and impeded the mobilization of free fatty acids, thereby reducing the exercise time to exhaustion by 19 percent (see Figure 12-3).

Many athletes are starting to use a liquid pre-game meal, since it is palatable, digests relatively easily, and is less likely to result in nervous indigestion, nausea, vomiting, and abdominal cramps. Those who have experimented with liquid meals before a contest have found them to be highly satisfactory. At the present time, this would appear to be the best available choice as a pre-game meal.

DIETARY AIDS TO PERFORMANCE

Ergogenic aids are substances, or phenomena, that elevate or improve the performance of the individual above that expected. The subject of ergogenic aids will be discussed in detail in Chapter 13. In this chapter, however, we will look at the ergogenic properties of various nutrients. Although some attention has already been given to the role of food supplements in athletic performance, this section will focus on those substances taken by athletes to enhance performance.

Is it possible to manipulate the diet to achieve improvement in performance? The answer is a qualified yes, although improvement is limited to manipulation in only one or two nutritional areas,

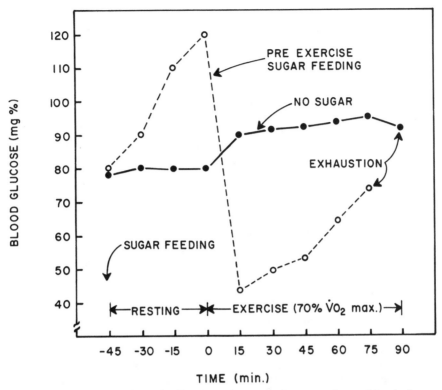

Figure 12-3 Effects of a carbohydrate feeding 45 minutes before exercise on blood glucose concentration. Note the rapid drop in blood glucose during the first 10 minutes of exercise when the subjects begin the activity with an elevated glucose concentration (from Costill, et al., 1977).

and the degree of improvement is still debatable. Unfortunately, much of the research that has been conducted in this area has lacked adequate controls. Despite this rather major limitation, however, a great deal of information has accumulated that provides valuable insights for the coach and athlete.

Protein

Is it necessary for athletes, who are training for strength and muscle bulk, to increase their normal dietary intake of protein? Protein is essential for the growth and development of the various tissues of the body, since amino acids are the body's "building blocks." For many years, it was thought that protein had to be supplemented in rather

large quantities. In fact, at one time it was thought that the muscle consumed itself as fuel for its own contractions, and that protein supplementation was essential to prevent the muscles from wasting away. It is now recognized that little protein is consumed as fuel for muscular work. If fats or carbohydrates are available, they are selected in preference to proteins as sources of energy.

Does protein supplementation enhance athletic or work performance? Horstman (1972) has concluded that the average diet in the Western culture provides adequately for the protein needs of the athlete. When the energy expenditure of heavy exercise exceeds 20.9 MJ (5,000 kcal/day), the diet should provide adequate protein. Although this would appear to be theoretically sound, studies are equivocal relative to the protein intake levels of athletes. Several of these studies will be reviewed. The reader is referred to a recent paper by Haymes (1983) for a more comprehensive review of this area of protein supplementation and athletic performance.

Early studies found little or no difference in performance between diets low, normal, and high in protein. Darling, et al. (1944) studied the effects of a low protein diet (53 g/day) on endurance performance, compared with diets containing normal (95 to 113 g/day) and high (151 to 192 g/day) levels of protein. No differences between diets were found for endurance, serum protein, erythrocyte count, or hemoglobin content. Pitts, et al. (1944) reported no reduction in endurance following a diet low in protein as compared to diets of normal and high protein content.

Rasch and Pierson (1962) investigated the effects of a 25 g protein supplement on increases in strength and muscle hypertrophy following six weeks of strength training. Strength was significantly increased in both the protein supplement and placebo groups, but there were no changes in arm girth or volume in either group. Rasch, et al. (1969) studied the influence of protein supplementation on physical performance in two groups of marines who were undergoing a four week physical training program, consisting primarily of weight training, calisthenics, field maneuvers, sports, and running for about four hours per day. One group was given 0.69 g of protein/kg of body weight per day whereas the other group received a placebo. No significant differences were noted between the groups for any of the performance variables, which were basically strength and muscular endurance items, or for serum total protein, blood urea nitrogen, or albumin.

Several studies have reported an increased protein requirement with exercise training. Yoshimura, et al. (1980), in a summary of their previous work, demonstrated a close association between the anemia identified during hard physical training, which they have referred to as sports anemia, and protein-intake levels. They reported a decrease in hemoglobin and plasma protein over the course of strenuous training while consuming a diet containing 1.3 g of protein/kg per day. They found that by taking more than 2.0 g protein/kg per day

they could prevent this sports anemia. It could also be prevented by changing the protein source from approximately 30 percent fish protein and 70 percent vegetable protein, to 57 percent animal protein, maintaining the protein intake at 1.2 to 1.3 g/kg per day. They concluded that sports anemia is the result of an osmotic fragility caused by chemical hemolysis.

Studies examining nitrogen balance in exercising subjects have also found evidence that a protein intake of 1.0 g/kg per day may not be adequate. Gontzea, et al. (1974, 1975) have found negative nitrogen balances in subjects during exercise training with a protein intake of 1.0 g/kg per day, with the major increase in nitrogen excretion occurring through the sweat. Celejowa and Homa (1970) reported that five of ten weight lifters had a negative nitrogen balance with a protein intake of 2 g/kg per day. Laritcheva, et al. (1978) also found that protein intakes of 2 g/kg per day were inadequate to maintain protein balance when weight lifters were preparing intensely for an important competition.

Marable, et al. (1979) investigated four groups of college men who consumed two levels of protein (0.8 or 2.4 g/kg per day) for 28 days while serving either as controls or subjects in a weight training program. Urinary nitrogen, expressed relative to protein intake, decreased significantly in the exercising subjects and was more pronounced in the group taking 0.8 g/kg per day. They concluded that the decreases in urinary nitrogen for the exercising subjects at both protein levels could account for sufficient extra nitrogen retention to allow for synthesis of approximately 2 kg of lean weight in 28 days. However, the magnitude of decrease required for the low protein intake group suggested that the protein intake of this group was marginal during muscle-building exercise. Consolazio, et al. (1975) studied two groups of men consuming two levels of protein (1.4 and 2.8 g/kg per day) during a 40-day experimental period of intense physical training. Although urinary nitrogens were fairly constant across the two groups, and both groups remained in nitrogen balance, only the group on the high-protein diet increased lean body mass significantly, by 3.3 kg. Although not reported directly in this study, the authors

Table 12-6 Effects of dietary carbohydrate on muscle glycogen stores and endurance performance.

CHO Intake (gm/24 hr)	Glycogen Content (mmol/kg muscle)	Exercise Time to Exhaustion (min)
100	53	57
280	100	114
500	205	167

concluded that the additional body protein did not enhance work performance.

In her comprehensive review, Haymes (1983) has concluded that a protein intake of 1.0 g/kg per day may be inadequate for the diets of athletes in training. Increased protein intake may be important during the early stages of training to support increases in muscle mass, myoglobin, enzyme content, and erythrocyte formation, and the optimal intake during this period may be as low as 1.2 g/kg per day. For weight lifters, or athletes undergoing intense strength training, optimal intake may be as high as 2.0 g/kg per day.

Carbohydrates

Early studies demonstrated that when men ate a diet containing a normal amount of carbohydrates, about 55 percent of total caloric intake, their muscles stored approximately 100 millimoles of glycogen per kilogram of muscle (mmol/kg). As shown in Table 12-6, diets low in carbohydrate (less than 15 percent of the total calories) resulted in storage of only 53 mmol/kg, whereas a rich carbohydrate diet produced a muscle glycogen content of 205 mmol/kg. When these men were asked to exercise to exhaustion at 75 percent of their maximal oxygen uptake, their exercise times were proportional to the amount of glycogen present in the muscles before the test (see Table 12-6). Carbohydrate in the diet clearly has a direct influence on muscle glycogen stores and the ability to train and compete in endurance events.

Studies from Scandinavia in the mid-1960s indicated that muscle glycogen was restored to muscle within 24 hours if athletes ate a carbohydrate-rich diet after the exhaustive exercise. Continuing this diet for two additional days was found to elevate the muscle glycogen to twice the pre-exercise level. More recent studies have shown that glycogen replacement and storage is not so simple. Sherman, et al. (1983) observed that seven days after a marathon race in which muscle glycogen dropped from 196 to 26 mmol/kg, muscle glycogen had only recovered to 125 mmol/kg (see Figure 12-4 on page 236).

This delayed recovery of muscle glycogen seems to be characteristic of distance running, since it does not occur after exhaustive cycling or swimming. Although the cause has not been fully explained, the muscle trauma which occurs in distance running may inhibit the mechanisms normally responsible for the uptake and storage of glucose by the muscle.

Although the amount of carbohydrate in the diet determines, to a large extent, the rate of muscle glycogen storage, there are also special enzymes, **glycogen synthase,** that facilitate the conversion of glucose molecules into glycogen. The activity of glycogen synthase is very high when the muscle glycogen is low, promoting glycogen storage (see Figure 12-4). As the glycogen reserves begin to refill, the synthase activity declines, lessening the drive for further glycogen formation. Even in the presence of a high glycogen synthase activity, muscle glycogen replacement is slow and incomplete unless the dietary intake is rich in carbohydrate.

As noted in Figure 12-5 on page 236, athletes who train intensely and eat low-carbohydrate diets (40 percent of total calories), often experience a day-to-day decline in muscle glycogen. When the same subjects consume high-carbohydrate diets (70 percent of calories) of equal total caloric content, muscle glycogen replacement is nearly complete within the 22 hours between training bouts.

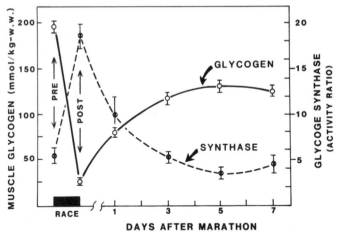

Figure 12-4   Leg muscle glycogen levels before and during seven days of recovery from a marathon competition (Sherman, et al., 1983).

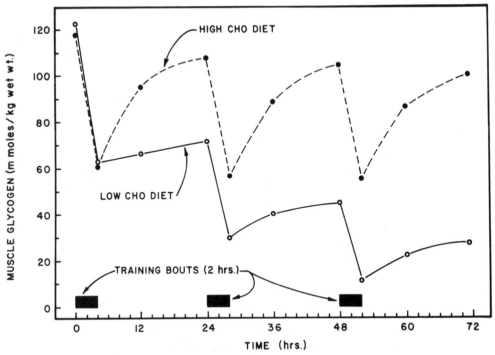

Figure 12-5   Muscle glycogen content of the vastus lateralis (thigh) during three successive days of heavy training with diets whose caloric compositions were 40 percent carbohydrate (Low CHO) and 70 percent carbohydrate (High CHO) (from Costill & Miller, 1980).

In addition, the athletes perceive the training as much less difficult when muscle glycogen was maintained, than when it was lowered with training.

When athletes eat only as much food as they desire, *ad libitum,* they often underestimate their caloric needs and fail to consume enough carbohydrate to compensate for levels used during training or competition. This discrepancy between glycogen use and carbohydrate intake may explain, in part, why some athletes become chronically fatigued and need 48 hours or longer to completely restore muscle glycogen. Individuals who train exhaustively on successive days must consume a diet rich in carbohydrates to reduce the heavy, tired feeling associated with a deficit in muscle glycogen.

Although athletes need supplemental carbohydrates during intense training periods, untrained individuals who consume excessive carbohydrates under normal conditions may elevate their plasma triglyceride levels, a factor often associated with a high risk of heart disease. In the endurance athlete, supplemental carbohydrates usually restore muscle and liver glycogen, rather than form blood fats.

The type of carbohydrate, simple or complex, also has a bearing on the formation of blood cholesterol and other fat-related molecules (glycerides). When subjects eat simple sugars such as glucose or sucrose, serum cholesterol and glyceride concentrations increase more than they do when subjects eat the same number of calories in the form of starch. Since the simple sugars are absorbed rather quickly, their ingestion results in hyperglycemia, a sudden rise in blood glucose, which overloads the cells' energy-producing system, favoring the formation of blood fats and cholesterol. Complex carbohydrates, such as starch, produce a smaller rise in blood glucose and cholesterol.

Since these observations were confined to relatively inactive subjects, it is speculative to suggest that the same patterns will occur among trained distance runners. In fact, endurance-trained athletes generally demonstrate a smaller rise in blood glucose and a lower insulin response, even to a feeding of sucrose. Endurance athletes divert the majority of carbohydrate foods to glycogen storage with little disturbance in their blood lipid (fat and cholesterol) profiles.

In light of the differences in simple and complex carbohydrates, we might anticipate differences in the rate and quantity of glycogen formation following the intake of diets rich in either glucose or starch. Tests of this theory, however, are inconclusive. Men, who were fed diets principally composed of either simple sugars or starches (70 percent of calories) for two days following exhaustive exercise, revealed no significant difference in muscle glycogen formation for the two diets, although there was a trend toward greater glycogen storage when the men consumed starch. Recent studies, on the other hand, have shown that simple carbohydrates facilitate glycogen storage to a greater extent than do complex carbohydrates. In light of these conflicting reports, the preferential use of either simple or complex carbohydrates for muscle glycogen replacement is unclear.

In the preceding discussion we have established that different diets can markedly influence muscle glycogen stores and that endurance performance depends in part on the glycogen content at the onset of exercise. Based on muscle biopsy studies in the mid-1960s, a plan was proposed to help runners store the maximum amount of glycogen possible, a process known as **glycogen loading.**

It has been proposed that endurance athletes prepare for competition by completing an exhaustive training bout seven days before the event. For the three days following, they should eat fat and protein almost exclusively in order to deprive the muscles of carbohydrate and drive up glycogen synthase. The athlete is then recommended to eat a carbohydrate-rich diet for the remaining days. The intensity and volume of training during this six-day period should be markedly reduced to prevent additional consumption of muscle glycogen and to maximize liver and muscle glycogen reserves.

While this regimen has been shown to elevate muscle glycogen to twice the normal level, it is somewhat impractical for most highly-trained competitors. During the three days of low carbohydrate intake, athletes generally find it difficult to train, are often unable to perform mental tasks, are irritable, and show the usual signs of low blood sugar. In addition, exhaustive, depletion bouts of exercise, performed seven days before the competition is of little training value and may impair glycogen storage rather than enhance it. This depletion exercise also exposes the individual to possible injury or overtraining when they are already susceptible to breakdown.

Considering these limitations, it is proposed that the "depletion run" and low carbohydrate aspects of this regimen be eliminated, and that the athlete simply reduce the training intensity and eat a normal, mixed diet containing 55 percent of the calories from carbohydrate, until the final three days before the competition. In the 48 to 72 hours before the competitive event, training should be reduced to a daily warm-up of 10 to 15 minutes, accompanied by the ingestion of a rich, carbohydrate diet. Following this plan, glycogen will be elevated to 200 mmol/kg muscle, a level equal to that attained with the regimen described by Åstrand (1979) (see Figure 12-6).

Diet also plays an important role in preparing the liver for the demands of distance running. Studies have shown that liver glycogen stores will decrease rapidly when an individual is deprived of carbohydrates for only 24 hours, even when at rest. As a result of strenuous exercise lasting 60 minutes, liver glycogen was found to decrease from 244 mmol/kg to 111 mmol/kg, a 55 percent reduction. Thus, in combination with a low carbohydrate diet, hard training may empty the liver glycogen stores. A single carbohydrate meal, however, will quickly restore liver glycogen to normal. Clearly, a rich-carbohydrate diet in the days preceding competition will insure a large, liver-glycogen reserve and minimize the risk of hypoglycemia during the endurance event.

Water is stored in the body at a rate of roughly 2.6 grams of water for each gram of glycogen. Consequently, the increase or decrease in tissue glycogen generally produces a change in body weight of from one to three pounds. It has been proposed that muscle and liver glycogen stores can be moni-

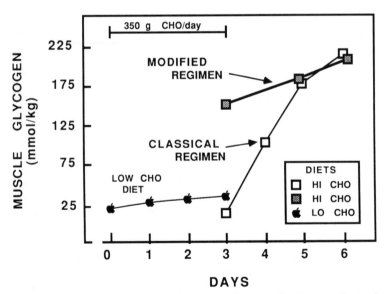

Figure 12-6   A comparison of the results of the modified glycogen loading regimen described by Sherman, et al. (1981) and the results of the classical method of glycogen loading developed by Scandinavian researchers.

tored by recording the athlete's early morning weight immediately after rising, after emptying the bladder, and before eating breakfast. Any sudden drop in weight may reflect a failure to replace glycogen, a deficit in body water, or both.

Fat

Since the muscle and liver glycogen stores are limited, encouraging the muscles to use fat in the form of **free fatty acids (FFA)** as an alternative fuel, can spare muscle glycogen and prevent premature exhaustion. Unfortunately, eating fat does not stimulate the muscles to burn fat. Fatty foods only tend to elevate plasma triglycerides, a complex fat molecule that must be broken down to FFA before it can be used to produce energy.

Aside from endurance training, the only known stimulus to increase FFA use is to elevate its concentration in the blood. Laboratory studies have demonstrated that when the blood levels of FFA are elevated following the injection of heparin, an anticoagulant that prohibits the clotting of blood, exercising muscles tend to use more fat and spare their glycogen reserves. The amount of glycogen used during 30 minutes of treadmill running was reduced by 40 percent when the blood FFA was first elevated using the anticoagulant drug.

Dietary attempts to elevate plasma FFA have been relatively unsuccessful. Some foods that contain caffeine, a stimulant to the nervous system, promote fat use and improve performance in prolonged, exhaustive exercise when consumed one hour before exercise. Caffeine ingestion of four to five milligrams per kilogram of body weight lessens the subjective feelings of effort during the exercise, which is similar to the effect of amphetamines. Twenty percent of the individuals tested experienced a negative reaction to caffeine, with no improvements in performance.

Despite the potential performance advantages offered by drinking tea or coffee, the ethical use of these items is questionable since they offer an unnatural advantage. Although international governing bodies, such as the International Olympic Committee, have attempted to ban the use of such stimulants, policing their use is difficult and impractical.

NUTRITION DURING EXERCISE

Studies conducted early in this century noted the occurrence of low blood glucose during exhaustive long-distance running and cycling. Although it seems reasonable to assume that such a decrease in blood glucose might contribute to the sensations of fatigue, recent studies have suggested that hypoglycemia may not be directly to blame. Although 142 minutes of exhaustive exercise dropped blood glucose from normal levels of 5.0 millimoles per liter to 2.5 millimoles per liter in 30 to 40 percent of the subjects, the intake of glucose during exercise did not consistently delay exhaustion or alter the subjective sensations of exertion.

In contrast, several studies have noted improvements in performance when the subjects were given carbohydrate feedings during exercise lasting one to four hours. Although none of these studies noticed any differences in performance during the early phase of the exercise when carbohydrates were given, the subjects were able to perform better over the final stage of the experiments. Recent investigations have observed that repeated carbohydrate feedings during four hours of cycling reduced muscle glycogen depletion and improved the ability to sprint at the end of the activity. Elevating blood glucose via carbohydrate feedings enables the muscles to obtain more of their energy from the available glucose, thereby lessening the demand on muscle glycogen. Endurance athletes can, therefore, go longer before the muscle glycogen stores become exhausted.

One may wonder why carbohydrate feedings during exercise don't produce the same hypoglycemic effects observed with the pre-exercise feedings? Sugar feedings during exercise result in smaller rises in both blood glucose and insulin, lessening the threat of an overreaction and sudden drop in blood glucose. The cause for this finer control on blood glucose during exercise may be related to the fact that the muscle fibers become more permeable, allowing glucose to enter the muscle with the aid of less insulin. As a result, less insulin is released from the pancreas and the rise in blood glucose is smaller.

The only complication associated with sugar feedings during endurance exercise is a delay in absorption. Before sugar solutions can be absorbed into the blood, they must pass through the stomach and into the small intestine. Since most carbohydrate solutions are held in the stomach for a short period, the first traces of any sugar solution do not appear in the blood for five to seven minutes after consumption. This delay is caused by the stomach's attempts to dilute the solution, delivering fluids that can be rapidly absorbed by the intestine.

DEHYDRATION

The ability to lose body heat during exercise depends, for the most part, on the formation and evaporation of sweat. The amount of sweat lost during exercise, in turn, depends on one's running pace, body size, and the environmental heat stress. Exercising in warm weather may evoke sweat losses in excess of two quarts per hour. Despite efforts to drink fluids during an event such as the marathon, sweating and the loss of water in the air we exhale may reduce body water content by 13 to 14 percent (see Chapter 14).

Studies have shown that dehydrated individuals are quite intolerant of exercise and heat stress. Distance runners, for example, are forced to slow their pace by two percent for each percent of weight lost as a consequence of dehydration. Both heart rate and body temperature are elevated during exercise when the individual is dehydrated more than two percent of body weight.

As noted in Chapter 4, the impact of dehydration on the cardiovascular system is quite predictable. Plasma volume is lost and the ability to provide adequate blood flow to the skin and muscles is reduced. Under such circumstances, it is common for subjects to collapse, showing the usual symptoms of heat exhaustion. It is difficult to understand how some athletes tolerate several hours of hard running in warm weather. In addition to the body water lost during endurance events, many nutrients are known to escape with sweat. The following discussion will examine the effects of heavy sweating on body water and the mineral composition of body tissues.

Human sweat has been described as a filtrate of plasma, since it contains many of the items present in the water portion of blood, including sodium, chloride, potassium, magnesium, and calcium. However, even though sweat tastes salty, it actually contains far fewer minerals than do body fluids. Sweat is considered hypotonic, meaning it is a very dilute version of body fluids.

Sodium and chloride are the ions primarily responsible for maintaining the water content of the blood. Table 12-5 shows that the concentrations of sodium and chloride in sweat are roughly one-third those found in plasma and five times those found in muscle. The ionic concentration of sweat may vary markedly between individuals and is strongly influenced by the rate of sweating and the athlete's state of training and heat acclimatization.

At the high rates of sweating reported during endurance events, sweat contains relatively high levels of sodium and chloride, but little potassium, calcium, and magnesium. A sweat loss of nearly nine pounds, representing a 5.8 percent reduction in body weight, resulted in sodium, potassium, chloride, and magnesium losses of 155, 16, 137, and 13 milliequivalents (mEq), respectively. Based on estimates of the athlete's body mineral contents, such losses would only lower the body's sodium and chloride content by roughly five to seven percent. At the same time, total body levels of potassium and magnesium, two ions principally confined to the inside of the cells, would decrease by about one percent.

The other major source of mineral loss is routine urine production. In addition to cleaning the blood of cellular waste products, the kidneys also control the body's water and electrolyte content. Under normal conditions, the kidneys excrete about 1.7 ounces of water per hour. During exercise, however, blood flow to the kidneys decreases and urine production drops to near zero. Consequently, electrolyte losses by this avenue are quite diminished during exercise.

There is another facet of the kidneys' management of electrolytes. If an individual eats 250 mEq of sodium and chloride per day, normally the kidneys will excrete an equal amount of those electrolytes to keep their levels constant. Heavy sweating and dehydration, however, cause the release of aldosterone, a hormone from the adrenal gland that stimulates the kidneys to reabsorb sodium and chloride.

Since the body loses more water than electrolytes during heavy sweating, the concentration of these minerals in the body fluids rises. That means that instead of showing a drop in plasma electrolyte concentrations, there is actually an increase. Although this may seem confusing, the point is that during periods of heavy sweating, the need to replace body water is far greater than the need to replace electrolytes.

REHYDRATION

There are obvious benefits to drinking fluids during prolonged exercise, especially during hot weather. Drinking will minimize dehydration, lessen the rise in internal body temperature, and reduce the stress placed on the circulatory system (see Figure 12-7). Even warm fluids, near body

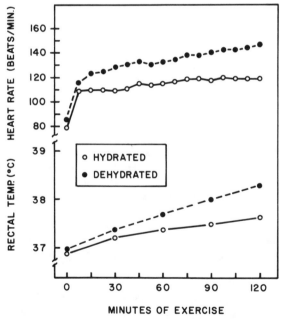

Figure 12-7 Rectal temperature and heart rates during two hours of treadmill running when normally hydrated and when dehydrated by about 3.5% of body weight (from Costill, 1986).

temperature, provide some protection against overheating, but cold fluids seem to enhance body cooling. It takes some of the deep body heat to warm a cold drink to the temperature of the stomach and blood.

As noted earlier, the fluid composition of the drink has an effect on the rate that it empties from the stomach. Since little exchange of water occurs directly from the stomach, the fluids must pass into the intestine before entering the blood. In the intestine, absorption is rapid and unaffected by exercise, provided that the activity does not exceed 75 percent of the runner's $\dot{V}O_2$ max. Many factors affect the rate at which the stomach will empty, including its volume, temperature, acidity, and the number of particles it contains (osmolality).

Although large volumes of up to 600 milliliters (ml) empty faster from the stomach than small portions, most athletes find it uncomfortable to exercise with a nearly full stomach, since this may interfere with breathing. Drinking 100 to 175 ml at 10- to 15-minute intervals tends to minimize this effect. Since there are wide individual variations in the rate of stomach emptying, the suggestions offered here are based on averages, and may not be appropriate for every individual.

Cold drinks have been found to empty more rapidly from the stomach than warm fluids. Although fluids at refrigerator temperatures of from 38 to 40° Fahrenheit may reduce the temperature of the stomach from 99 to 50° Fahrenheit, they do not appear to cause stomach cramps. Such stomach distress occurs more often when the volume of the drink is unusually large. It has been suggested that cold fluids may upset the normal electrical activity of the heart, thus threatening the health of the athlete. It is true that some electrocardiographic changes have been reported in a few individuals following the ingestion of ice-cold drinks at 33 to 35° Fahrenheit, but the medical significance of these changes has not been established. It seems that drinking cold fluids during distance running seems to pose no threat to a normal heart.

Another factor known to regulate the rate at which the stomach empties is the drink's osmolality, the number of dissolved substances in the solution. Drink osmolalities above 200 mOsm/liter tend to move out of the stomach more slowly than those below that level. The addition of electrolytes and other ingredients that raise the osmolality, slow the rate of water replacement. Since dehydration is the primary concern during hot weather running, water seems to be the preferred fluid. Under less stressful conditions where overheating and large sweat losses are not as threatening, runners might use liquid feedings to supplement their carbohydrate supplies.

A number of "sports drinks," containing electrolytes and carbohydrates are currently on the market, grossing more than $100 million each year. Unfortunately, many of the claims used to sell these drinks are based on misinterpreted and often inaccurate information. Electrolytes, for example, have long been touted as important ingredients in sports drinks. But, as noted earlier, these claims may be exaggerated, since a single meal can usually replace the electrolytes lost during exercise. The body needs water to bring its concentration of the electrolytes back into balance. While the importance of minerals such as sodium, potassium, and magnesium should not be underestimated, blood and muscle biopsy studies have shown that heavy sweating has little or no effect on water and electrolyte concentrations in body fluids during events that last for several hours.

One might wonder if the intake of too much water could overdilute the blood electrolytes, leading to a body deficit? Apparently not. Even marathoners who lose six to nine pounds of sweat and drink nearly half a gallon of water, retain normal plasma sodium, chloride, and potassium concentrations. Marathoners and ultra-marathoners who run 15 to 25 miles per day in warm weather and do not season their food, do not develop electrolyte deficiencies.

Some experts have suggested that during an ultra-marathon (50 miles or more) run, some individuals may experience unusually low blood sodium levels. A case study of two runners, who collapsed after an ultra-marathon race in 1983, revealed that they had blood sodium values of 123 and 118 mEq/liter, remarkably lower than the normal values of 135 to 148 mEq/liter. One of the runners experienced a grand mal seizure; the other man became disoriented and confused.

Although the cause of these after-effects is unclear, the initial diagnosis tends to implicate the lack of body sodium. An examination of the runners' fluid intake (21 to 24 liters) and estimates of their sodium intake (224 to 145 mEq) during the run suggested that they diluted their body sodium levels by consuming fluids that contained little sodium. Nevertheless, studies during the marathon and exercise bouts lasting up to six hours, suggest that electrolytes are not an essential ingredient for sports drinks.

There is evidence to support putting some carbohydrates in sports drinks, including several types of sugar. While even small amounts of glucose tend to slow the emptying of the stomach, small amounts of fructose can be used without inhibiting the stomach's action. Aside from this point, there is little difference as to whether the carbohydrate in the drink is glucose or fructose, since both take five to seven minutes before they first appear in the blood.

In early studies, it was suggested that the sports drinks should have less than 2.5 grams of sugar per 100 milliliters of water to speed its removal from the stomach. Unfortunately, this small amount of carbohydrate contributes little to the energy reserves. Even if you drank 200 milliliters of such a drink every 15 minutes during a long run, you would only take in 20 grams of carbohydrate per hour. Recent studies suggest that to improve performance with the aid of a carbohydrate drink, the athlete should consume at least 50 grams of sugar per hour.

Most of the sports drinks on the market contain only about 0.6 grams of carbohydrate per ounce. An endurance athlete would need to drink half a gallon of these drinks every hour to get enough carbohydrates to be of benefit. Most people can drink only nine to 15 ounces per hour during exercise. Thus, it would take a drink containing 3.8 grams of carbohydrate per ounce to be of any value. Such a rich mixture, however, may be delayed in the stomach, draw water from the stomach's lining, and cause an uncomfortable feeling of fullness.

Recent technological advances in the manufacture of carbohydrates have made it possible to combine many glucose molecules into one large molecule called a **glucose polymer.** A drink containing glucose polymer does not cause such a negative effect on the stomach and can replace both water and carbohydrates.

Finally, athletes will not drink solutions that taste poor. Unfortunately, we all have different taste preferences. To confuse the issue even further, what tastes good before and after a long, hot bout of exercise will not necessarily taste good during the event. Recent studies have tested the taste preferences of runners and cyclists during 60 minutes of exercise. Those studies demonstrated that most of the 50 subjects chose a drink with a relatively light flavor without a strong aftertaste. Nearly all of the commercial sports drinks failed this criterion.

So what should the athlete drink during training and competition? Under the extreme stress of hot weather, water is the primary need and the preferred drink. It empties from the stomach with minimal delay, is easy to obtain, and reduces the dehydration associated with heavy sweating. Under cooler conditions, a carbohydrate drink will provide the energy lift needed for peak performance in events lasting an hour or longer. In events lasting less than an hour, there is less need for water ingestion and little benefit from the intake of carbohydrates.

It is important to remember that human thirst is a poor indicator of the body's water and electrolyte balance. No matter how efficiently the kidneys do their job, body fluid balance depends on a strong thirst sensation to stimulate fluid intake. Unfortunately, man's drive to replace body fluids is far less effective than that seen in other animals. Burros, for example, will replace a 40-pound loss of body water in five to six minutes of continuous drinking whereas humans, who sweat away six to eight pounds, are satisfied after drinking only a pint of fluid. If the athlete's thirst is used as the only gauge of water need, it may take 12 to 24 hours to replace such a sweat loss. During exercise and heavy sweating, athletes should be encouraged to drink more than their thirst demands.

SUMMARY

For hundreds of years, it has been assumed that nutrition can influence the quality of one's athletic performance. The present chapter, in reviewing the six classes of nutrients—water, minerals, vitamins, proteins, fats, and carbohydrates—discussed the importance of each, relative to general nutrition. This provided the background for a discussion of the athlete's diet. It was concluded that the optimum diet for athletes, as for non-athletes, must contain adequate quantities of water, calories, proteins, fats, carbohydrates, minerals, and vitamins in the proper proportions. In addition, diet is generally independent of the sport, or the event within a sport. A well-balanced diet, as exemplified by the "Four Food Group Plan" appears to provide the base or foundation for the athlete, assuring him or her that there will be no deficiencies, providing the total caloric intake is sufficient. Athletes can do very well on vegetarian diets providing they make a careful selection of their plant food sources, in order that they receive a good balance of the essential amino acids and adequate sources of vitamin A, riboflavin, vitamin B_{12}, vitamin D, calcium, iron, and sufficient calories. Finally, the pre-contest meal should be light, taken at least three hours prior to the contest, and easily digestible. A liquid pre-contest meal appears to have many advantages over solid food.

Does food have special ergogenic qualities, or can you alter what you eat to improve performance? While it appears that the average athlete consumes a sufficient quantity of protein and supplementation has little additional effect, there is evidence to indicate that carbohydrate loading is an effective, nutritional, manipulative technique, which can increase general cardiovascular endurance by increasing the storage of muscle glycogen. The technique of carbohydrate loading is discussed in detail. Various vitamins and minerals have been proposed as ergogenic aids. From the available research, it appears that the B-complex vitamins, and vitamins C and E, may have ergogenic properties, but the evidence is not conclusive and additional research is needed. Finally, water is definitely an ergogenic aid for endurance activities, though there appears to be little need for mineral replacement during exercise bouts lasting only two to four hours.

STUDY QUESTIONS

1. What are the six categories of nutrients?
2. What role does water play in body function?

Why is it classified as a nutrient?

3. What are the major macrominerals of importance to sport and activity?

4. What are the major functions of the primary macrominerals?

5. What are the major roles of vitamins in the body?

6. Which vitamins are fat soluble? Why is this important?

7. What are the major food sources for the individual vitamins?

8. What are essential amino acids? Why are they important relative to food intake?

9. What is an appropriate protein allowance for the adult male? Female?

10. What is the difference between saturated and unsaturated fats?

11. What is the difference between glucose and glycogen?

12. Describe an ideal athlete's diet for football. For swimming.

13. Can an athlete survive on a vegetarian diet?

14. Describe the ideal pre-contest meal.

15. Discuss the ergogenic properties of the various nutrients. Which nutrients have definite ergogenic properties?

REFERENCES

Ahlborg, G., & Hagenfeldt, L. (1977). Effect of heparin on the substrate utilization during prolonged exercise. *Scandinavian Journal of Clinical Laboratory Investigation, 37,* 619-624.

Åstrand, P. O. (1967). Diet and athletic performance. *Federation Proceedings, 26,* 1772-1777.

Åstrand, P. O. (1979). Nutrition and physical performance. In M. Rechcigl (Ed.), *Nutrition and the world food problem.* Switzerland: S. Karger, Basel.

Bergstrom, J., Hermansen, L., Hultman, E., & Saltin, B. (1967). Diet, muscle glycogen, and physical performance. *Acta Physiologica Scandinavica, 71,* 140-150.

Celejowa, I., & Homa, M. (1970). Food intake, nitrogen and energy balance in Polish weight lifters during a training camp. *Nutrition and Metabolism, 12,* 259-274.

Christensen, E. H., & Hansen, O. (1939). Zur methodik der respiratorischen quotient-bestimmungen in ruhe und bei arbeit. *Skandinavian Archieves of Physiology, 81,* 137-143.

Consolazio, C. F., Johnson, H. L., Nelson, R. A., Dramise, J. G., & Skala, J. H. (1975). Protein metabolism during intensive physical training in the young adult. *American Journal of Clinical Nutrition, 28,* 29-35.

Costill, D. L. (1972). Water and electrolytes. In W. P. Morgan (Ed.), *Ergogenic aids and muscular performance.* New York: Academic Press.

Costill, D. L., Bennett, A., Branam, G., & Eddy, D. (1973). Glucose ingestion at rest and during prolonged exercise. *Journal of Applied Physiology, 34,* 764-769.

Costill, D. L., & Saltin, B. (1974). Factors limiting gastric emptying during rest and exercise. *Journal of Applied Physiology, 37,* 679-683.

Costill, D. L., Coyle, E., Dalsky, G., Evans, W., Fink, W., & Hoopes, D. (1977). Effects of elevated plasma FFA and insulin on muscle glycogen usage during exercise. *Journal of Applied Physiology, 43,* 695-699.

Costill, D. L., Dalsky, G. P., & Fink, W. J. (1978). Effects of caffeine ingestion on metabolism and exercise performance, *Medicine and Science in Sports, 10,* 155-158.

Costill, D. L., Fink, W. J., Getchell, L. H., Ivy, J. L., & Witzmann, F. A. (1979). Lipid metabolism in skeletal muscle of endurance-trained males and females. *Journal of Applied Physiology, 47,* 787-791.

Costill, D. L., & Miller, J. (1980). Nutrition for endurance sport: Carbohydrate and fluid balance. *International Journal of Sports Medicine, 1,* 2-14.

Costill, D. L. (1986). *Inside running: Basics of sports physiology.* Indianapolis: Benchmark Press.

Coyle, E. F., Hagberg, J. M., Hurley, B. F., Martin, W. H., Ehsani, A. A., & Holloszy, J. O. (1983). Carbohydrate feedings during prolonged strenuous exercise can delay fatigue. *Journal of Applied Physiology, 55,* 230-235.

Dairy Council Digest. (1975). *Nutrition and athletic performance, 46,* 7-10.

Dairy Council Digest. (1980). *Nutrition and human performance, 51,* 13-17.

Darling, R. C., Johnson, R. E., Pits, G. C., Consolazio, F. C., & Robinson, P. F. (1944). Effects of variations in dietary protein on the physical well-being of men doing manual work. *Journal of Nutrition, 28,* 273-281.

Farrell, P. M., & Bieri, J. G. (1975). Megavitamin E supplementation in man. *American Journal of Clinical Nutrition, 28,* 1381-1385.

Fordtran, J. S., & Saltin, B. (1967). Gastric emptying and intestinal absorption during prolonged severe exercise. *Journal of Applied Physiology, 34,* 331-335.

Foster, C., Costill, D. L., & Fink, W. J. (1979). Effects of pre-exercise feedings on endurance performance. *Medicine and Science in Sports, 11,* 1-5.

Golding, L. A. (1973). Drugs and hormones. In W. P. Morgan (Ed.), *Ergogenic aids and muscular performance.* New York: Academic Press.

Gontzea, I., Sutzescu, P., & Dumitrache, S. (1974). The influence of muscular activity on nitrogen balance and on the need of man for proteins. *Nutrition Reports International, 10,* 35-43.

Gontzea, I., Sutzescu, P., & Dumitrache, S. (1975). The influence of adaptation to physical effort on nitrogen balance in man. *Nutrition Reports International*, 11, 231–236.

Haymes, E. M. (1983). Proteins, vitamins, and iron. In M. H. Williams (Ed.), *Ergogenic aids in sport*. Champaign, IL: Human Kinetics Pub., Inc., 27–55.

Hickson, R. C., Rennie, M. J., Conlee, R. K., Winder, W. W., & Holloszy, J. O. (1977). Effects of increased plasma fatty acids on glycogen utilization and endurance. *Journal of Applied Physiology*, 43, 829–833.

Helgheim, I., Hetland, O., Nilsson, S., Ingjer, F., & Stromme, S. B. (1979). The effects of vitamin E on serum enzyme levels following heavy exercise. *European Journal of Applied Physiology*, 40, 283–289.

Horstman, D. H. (1972). Nutrition. In W. P. Morgan (Ed.), *Ergogenic aids and muscular performance*. New York: Academic Press.

Howald, H., & Segesser, B. (1975). Ascorbic acid and athletic performance. *Annals of the New York Academy of Science*, 258, 458–464.

Ivy, J. L., Costill, D. L., Fink, W. J., & Lower, R. W. (1979). Influence of caffeine and carbohydrate feedings on endurance performance. *Medicine and Science in Sports*, 11, 6–11.

Karlsson, J., & Saltin, B. (1971). Diet, muscle glycogen, and endurance performance. *Journal of Applied Physiology*, 31, 203–206.

Krause, M. V., & Hunscher, M. A. (1972). *Food, nutrition, and diet therapy* (5th ed.). Philadelphia: W. B. Saunders Co.

Lawrence, J. D., Bower, R. C., Riehl, W. P., & Smith, J. L. (1975). Effects of alpha-tocopherol acetate on the swimming endurance of trained swimmers. *American Journal of Clinical Nutrition*, 28, 205–208.

Londeree, B. (1974). Pre-event diet routine. *Runner's World*, 9, 26–29.

Marable, N. L., Hickson, J. F., Korslund, M. K., Herbert, W. G., Desjardins, R. F., & Thye, F. W. (1979). Urinary nitrogen excretion as influenced by a muscle-building exercise program and protein intake variation. *Nutrition Reports International*, 19, 795–805.

Piehl, K. (1974). Time course for refilling of glycogen stores in human muscle fibers following exercise-induced glycogen depletion. *Acta Physiologica Scandinavica*, 90, 297–302.

Perkins, R., & Williams, M. H. (1975). Effect of caffeine upon maximal muscular endurance of females. *Medicine and Science in Sports*, 7, 221–224.

Sherman, W. M., Costill, D. L., Fink, W. J., & Miller, J. M. (1981). Effects of exercise-diet manipulation on muscle glycogen and its subsequent utilization during performance. *International Journal of Sport Medicine*, 2, 1–15.

Sherman, W. M., Costill, D. L., Fink, W. J., Armstrong, L. E., & Hagerman, F. C. (1983). The marathon: Recovery from acute biochemical alterations. *Biochemistry of Exercise*, 13, 312–317.

Smith, N. J. (1976). *Food for sport*. Palo Alto, CA: Bull Publishing Company.

Vellar, O. D. (1968). Studies on sweat losses of nutrients. Iron content of whole body sweat and its association with other sweat constituents, serum iron levels, heatological indices, body surface area and sweat rate. *Scandinavian Journal of Clinical Laboratory Investigation*, 1, 157–167.

Williams, M. H. (1976). *Nutritional aspects of human physical and athletic performance*. Springfield, IL: Charles C. Thomas.

Young, D. R. (1977). *Physical performance fitness and diet*. Springfield, IL: Charles C. Thomas.

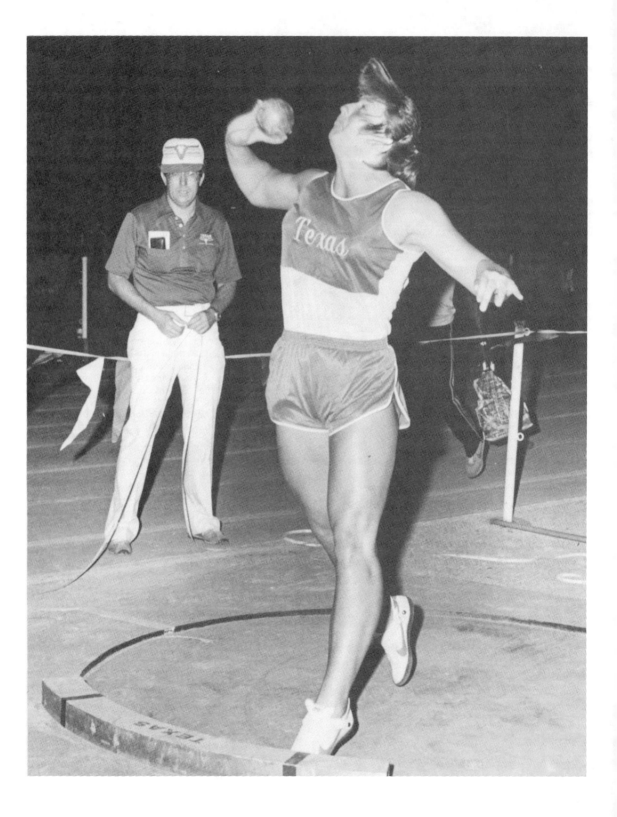

13

Ergogenic Aids in Sports

INTRODUCTION

As the skill level of athletes in various sports improves from year to year, and as athletic records reach new heights, the margin between success and failure in the world of sports becomes smaller. Consequently, both coach and athlete look for that slight edge that might assure victory and avoid defeat—a special diet, altering psychological states, or trying various hormones or pharmacological agents to alter physiological states. Substances or phenomena that elevate or improve the performance of the athlete, or even the non-athlete, above expected levels are referred to as **ergogenic aids** (Morgan, 1972). Weight lifters have taken anabolic steroids in an attempt to increase muscle mass and strength; distance runners have loaded up on carbohydrates two to three days prior to competition in an attempt to pack extra glycogen into the active muscles; a number of athletes have undergone hypnosis in an attempt to overcome specific hang-ups; and the home team, with the cheers of the crowd in support, may have a distinct advantage over the visiting team.

While a number of substances and phenomena have been labeled as ergogenic aids, it must be proven that they actually facilitate the athlete's performance before they can legitimately be classified as ergogenic. The purpose of this chapter is to investigate the various substances and phenomena that have been used by athletes in order to determine their ergogenic potential. Simply because a professional, superstar athlete consumes large quantities of a particular substance several hours prior to game-time and attributes a successful performance to this behavior, it does not prove that this substance has mystical, power-inducing qualities that will assure other athletes similar success. While science, with carefully controlled investigations, does not have all of the answers, this is an area in which scientific studies are essential in order to differentiate between a truly ergogenic response and a pseudo-ergogenic response in which the performance is improved simply because the athlete expects it to improve.

This psychological, or placebo, effect was clearly demonstrated in one of the earliest studies of anabolic steroids (Ariel and Saville, 1972). Fifteen male athletes volunteered to be part of a weight training experiment using anabolic steroids. They were told that those who made the greatest gains in strength over a preliminary sixteen-week period would be selected for the second phase of the study in which the subjects would be given anabolic steroids. Following this preliminary period, eight of the fifteen subjects were randomly selected to enter the treatment phase. Only six of these subjects passed all medical screening tests and were

247

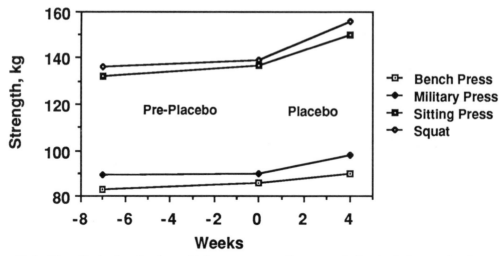

Figure 13-1 The effect of a placebo, which was supposedly an anabolic steriod, on gains in muscular strength (adapted from Ariel & Saville, 1972).

allowed to continue into the treatment phase. The treatment phase consisted of a four-week period in which the subjects were told that they would receive ten mg of Dianabol per day, when in fact they received a placebo. Strength data were collected over seven weeks of the pre-treatment period, and over all four weeks of the treatment (placebo) period. Even though the subjects were experienced weight lifters, they continued to gain impressive amounts of strength during the pre-treatment period. However, the gains in strength while on the placebo were substantially greater than the pre-treatment period! For four lifts—bench press, military press, sitting press, and squat—the group improved a total of 10.2 kg (2.3%) during the pre-treatment period, but improved 45.1 kg (10.0%) during the treatment, or placebo, period (see Figure 13-1).

DRUGS AND HORMONES

Numerous drugs and hormones have been suggested as having ergogenic properties. This section will be confined to a review of the facts that

have been determined related to the use of alcohol, amphetamines, and anabolic steroids—three major drugs or hormones that have received widespread use and national attention. Caffeine, considered a stimulant drug, was discussed in Chapter 12. Little is known about the influence of the so-called recreational drugs, cocaine and marijuana, on athletic performance. Two recent reviews by Lombardo (1986) and Cantwell and Rose (1986) address the tremendous health risks associated with the use of cocaine, including death, with no known benefits to performance. Nicotine has also been used as a stimulant, but it has generally been found to be detrimental to most athletic performances. Used recreationally, nicotine has been found to have very serious long-term effects on health, being associated with various cancers and heart disease. Fortunately, there has been a significant decline in the number of individuals who smoke cigarettes. However, the use of smokeless tobacco, in the form of loose leaf chewing tobacco, snuff (dipping), or compressed tobacco (plug) appears to have increased, and is all too common among athletes. There are significant health risks associated with the use of smokeless tobacco, particularly cancers of the mouth, larynx, and pharynx.

Alcohol

Cooper, in 1972, stated that alcohol is the number one drug problem in the United States. While others consider alcohol a food, Cooper feels that alcohol is correctly classified as a drug, due to its influence on the central nervous system. Unfortunately, little is known about the influence of varying amounts of alcohol on athletic performance. Obviously, alcohol intoxication results in erratic, unpredictable performance; however, the influence of small amounts of alcohol just prior to, or during a contest, is not clearly understood.

Studies have been conducted in the laboratory to observe the effects of small and moderate doses of alcohol on strength, muscular endurance, and cardiovascular endurance. The results from these studies conflict somewhat since several found improved performance and several found decreased performance, but the majority found no difference in performance. It would appear safe to conclude that alcohol has little, if any, ergogenic properties, but that it could be detrimental to optimal performance if taken in sufficient quantity. Recently, there has been increasing awareness and concern for the growing number of athletes who are becoming alcoholics as a result of indiscriminate consumption. Most professional teams in all sports have now established alcohol and drug rehabilitation programs, with professional groups to assist in the treatment of their athletes who admit to, or who are identified as, having a problem with substance abuse. The American College of Sports Medicine published a position statement in 1982 on *The Use of Alcohol in Sports*, which presents an excellent summary of the literature and general recommendations regarding alcohol use and abuse.

Amphetamines

Amphetamines are prescription drugs that stimulate the central nervous system. They have been used under close medical supervision as appetite suppressants for individuals on weight-loss programs. Used during World War II by army troops to combat fatigue and to improve endurance, they soon found their way into the athletic arena as a stimulant with possible ergogenic properties. Amphetamines have been referred to as "pep pills," "uppers," "bennies," "greenies," and "dexies," just to name a few. Athletes have found amphetamines readily available, even though they are a prescription drug. Supposedly, amphetamine usage by an athlete will help him or her run faster, throw farther, jump higher, and prolong the time it takes to reach total fatigue, or exhaustion. Do controlled scientific research studies support these claims?

Amphetamines are both sympathomimetic (mimics sympathetic nervous system stimulation) and central nervous system stimulants (Ivy, 1983). Physiologically, amphetamines are known to reduce one's sense of fatigue; increase vasoconstriction, both systolic and diastolic blood pressure, and heart rate; redistribute blood flow to the skeletal musculature; elevate blood sugar; and increase muscle tension. Because amphetamines stimulate the central nervous system, increasing the state of arousal, this leads to a sense of increased energy, self-confidence, and faster, more efficient, thought and decision making. Does this insure that the drug will aid physical performance?

In 1963 Golding and Barnard conducted one of the better designed and controlled studies in this area. They used a double-blind procedure in which either 15 mg of d-amphetamine sulfate, or a placebo, were administered three times each. Approximately two to three hours after either the drug or the placebo was administered, the subject was given two treadmill tests to exhaustion; the second test following the first by 12 minutes. Since amphetamines supposedly abolish or delay the onset of fatigue, the purpose of two treadmill tests to exhaustion was to determine whether amphetamines would "pick up" the subject after one exhaustive bout and make him more tolerant of the second bout. Two groups of subjects were used—one considered to be conditioned, a second considered to be unconditioned. The results concluded no differences between the placebo and amphetamine treatments for either the first or second treadmill runs, for either the conditioned or the unconditioned groups.

Chandler and Blair (1980) conducted a well-designed, highly controlled, and comprehensive,

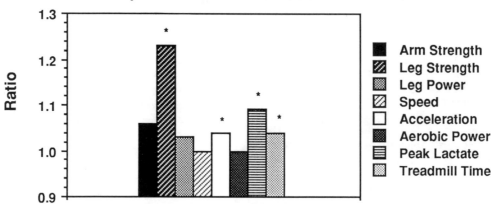

Figure 13-2   Physical and physiological performance changes with the use of amphetamines (adapted from Chandler & Blair, 1980).

double-blind, placebo-controlled study of the effects of amphetamines on arm and leg strength, leg power, running speed, acceleration, aerobic power, anaerobic capacity (peak lactates), and treadmill time. The subjects received either a placebo, or 15 mg of Dexedrine per 70 kg of body weight, two hours prior to testing. When testing followed amphetamine administration, improved performance was found in knee extension strength, acceleration, peak lactates, time to exhaustion, and pre-exercise and maximum heart rates (see Figure 13-2). Even though the time to exhaustion on the treadmill was increased, there were no differences in aerobic power. In studies dealing with fatigue or with the sensation, or feeling of fatigue, administration of amphetamines may have a small, but significant effect.

While many of the earlier studies suggested that amphetamines do little to facilitate performance, a number of the more recent studies have reported significant improvements in performance. Ivy (1983), in his excellent and extensive review of the literature in this area, concludes that amphetamines extend aerobic endurance and hasten recovery from fatigue, although reduced endurance results from the administration of high concentrations. Further, he concludes that amphetamines increase static muscular strength, although there is

little consistent information on dynamic strength or power.

It is quite possible that the laboratory tests used in most studies do not accurately duplicate the conditions encountered in the playing situation. Treadmill-running time, reaction time, and oxygen debt may be unrelated to the actual stress the athlete faces in the sport or event. Future studies must take this factor into account. Also, it is quite possible that athletes in actual play may be consuming far greater doses of amphetamines than allowed in controlled, research studies. If future studies show amphetamines to be potent ergogenic aids, the moral and ethical issue of whether they should be allowed in sports must be considered, as well as the critical problem of the potential medical risks associated with acute and extended usage of amphetamines.

Are amphetamines potentially harmful? Experience would tend to suggest that they are inherently dangerous. Deaths have been attributed to excessive amphetamine usage where athletes have pushed themselves beyond the normal state of exhaustion. One of the claims for amphetamines is that they delay the onset of fatigue. It is possible that, rather than delaying the onset, they delay the sensation of fatigue, enabling the individual to push dangerously beyond normal limits to the point of circulatory failure. Amphetamines can be highly toxic and they can also be physically addictive if taken regularly. Extreme nervousness, acute anxiety, aggressive behavior, and insomnia are frequently mentioned side effects of regular usage.

Anabolic Steroids

Androgenic-anabolic steroids are nearly identical to the male sex hormones. The androgenic properties of these hormones accentuate the development of secondary sex characteristics. The anabolic properties are responsible for acceleration of growth through an increased rate of bone maturation and increased development of muscle mass. Anabolic steroids have been given for years to youngsters with delayed growth patterns to normalize their growth curves. Synthetic steroids have been altered to reduce the androgenic properties and increase the anabolic effects. Theoretically, steroid administration will result in increased weight as well as increased strength. Consequently, the athlete who is dependent on size and strength would naturally be interested in steroids. Two questions need to be asked: First, are anabolic steroids ergogenic in nature (can they facilitate the actual performance of the athlete)? Second, and of greater importance, what are the inherent medical risks associated with taking steroids?

Research studies have been evenly balanced between those that have found no statistically significant change in body size and physical performance attributable to taking steroids, and those that have found steroids to have a considerable influence on weight and strength. How can this basic inconsistency be explained? It may be due to the following: lack of proper controls, a lack of an adequate number of subjects in the study, failure to use a protein supplement, differences in the athletic ability of the subjects used, the use of different drugs, dosages, or methods of drug administration, a combination of these causes, or any of a number of other possibilities.

In his comprehensive review of the research literature, Wright (1981) concluded that in inexperienced subjects (subjects not experienced in weight training), therapeutic doses have little or no effect on total or lean body weight, strength, or aerobic power. In this same group of subjects, combining therapeutic doses with strength training does appear to provide additional increases in strength above levels observed with placebo. By adding a protein supplement, one can enhance weight gain. For experienced subjects, Wright concluded that even therapeutic doses enhance increases in weight, lean weight, and strength, above that seen with placebo comparisons.

One basic problem with almost all of the present research is the inability to scientifically observe the effects of the drug dosages that are actually being used in the athletic world. It is estimated that some athletes are taking five to ten times the recommended maximum daily dosage. For obvious reasons, it would be unethical to design a study that used a dosage that exceeded the recommended dosage.

Hervey and colleagues (1981) observed the effects of high doses of anabolic steroids on seven male weight lifters. A dose of 100 mg of methandienone per day was given alternately with a placebo in a double-blind crossover experiment. Two treatment periods lasting six weeks each were separated by a six-week interval without treatment: half of the subjects received the placebo during the first six-week treatment period and the steroid during the second six-week treatment period; the other half received the medications in reverse order—steroid first, then placebo. When the data were analyzed, they found that body weight, potassium and nitrogen, muscle size, and leg performance and strength increased significantly during training while on the drug, but not during the placebo period. These results are summarized in Figure 13–3 on page 252.

Forbes (1985) observed body composition changes (^{40}K) in a professional body builder and a competitive weight lifter who were on self-prescribed high doses of steroids for 140 and 125 days respectively. The average increase in lean body mass was 19.2 kg, with a loss of almost ten kg in fat weight. Forbes concluded that only minimal increases in lean body mass ($\leq$ 1 to 2 kg) occur with up to approximately 2,535 mg total steroid use over the duration of the treatment period.

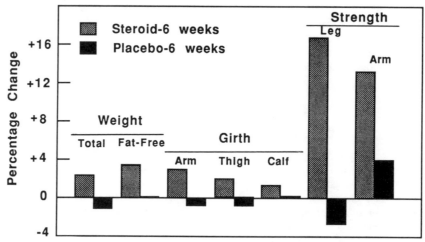

Figure 13–3 Alterations in body size, composition, and strength as a result of using anabolic steroids (adapted from Hervey, et al., 1981).

Beyond this total dosage there is a marked increase in lean body mass.

Even if anabolic steroids are shown to be beneficial for athletic performance, two questions must be resolved. First, is it morally and ethically right for the athlete to artificially induce changes in his or her performance potential? Most athletes feel it is wrong for their competition to do anything that might artificially improve performance, yet many of these same athletes feel they are forced to take steroids in an effort to "keep up" with the other athletes in their sport or event who are chronic steroid users. It has been estimated that 80 percent of all weight lifters, shot putters, discus throwers, and javelin throwers of national caliber are using anabolic steroids, and this is considered by many to be a conservative estimate. It is difficult to be the only athlete in an event at a particular meet who has not been using steroids. This places considerable pressure on that athlete to start taking steroids. It is now well-known that female athletes are taking anabolic steroids in an attempt to increase both performance and size of the lean body mass. Although the pressures on the athlete are great, are the potential gains worth the possible risks associated with steroid use?

This leads to the second question, what are the potential risks associated with taking anabolic

steroids in such massive doses? First, there is evidence to conclude that the use of steroids by individuals who are not fully mature will lead to an early closure of the epiphysis of the long bones. Since steroid use is also associated with an increase in the rate of growth of the long bones, it is difficult to determine whether the individual's final height will be less than, greater than, or the same as the height that would have been achieved without steroids. At least the potential for a reduced height exists.

Secondly, several side effects may result from the use of large doses of anabolic steroids: suppression of the natural secretion of gonadotropin, possibly causing atrophy of the tubules and interstitial tissue of the testes, and possibly atrophy of the testicles themselves; enlargement or hypertrophy of the prostate; liver damage from a form of chemical hepatitis; and markedly depressed HDL-cholesterol levels of up to 50 percent (see Figure 13–4). HDL-cholesterol is known to have anti-atherogenic properties, with high levels providing protection from coronary artery disease and heart attacks, and low levels being associated with a high risk for coronary artery disease and premature heart attacks. Neither scientists nor physicians know the potential long-term effects of chronic steroid use. The American College of

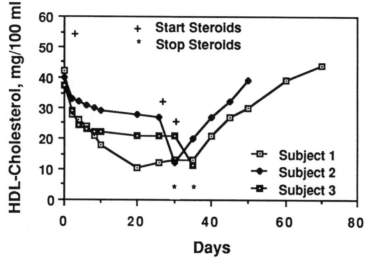

Figure 13-4 Alterations in HDL-cholesterol as a result of using anabolic steroids (adapted from Costill, et al., 1984).

Sports Medicine issued a position statement on the use of steroids in 1977, which contains a comprehensive review of the existing research literature up to that time. The extensive review by Wright in 1981 provides the most current summary of our knowledge in this area.

During the 1980s, athletes started investigating the potential of human growth hormone as a possible substitute for or compliment to their use of anabolic steroids. As with steroids, there is considerable concern for the potential risks associated with the use of human growth hormone. To date, there is little information available concerning potential benefits, or potential or known risks, although acromegalia has been reported (enlargement of the bones of the head, hands, and feet, and enlargement of the nose and lips).

NUTRITION

The possible influence of nutrition on athletic performance was discussed in great detail in Chapter 12, providing evidence to indicate that certain nutritional manipulations can substantially alter athletic performance.

OXYGEN

During the televised, professional football game of the week, it is not uncommon to see the star running back break-loose for a 35-yard touchdown, struggle back to the bench, grab a face mask, and start breathing 100 percent oxygen. How much does he gain over a normal recovery, breathing the surrounding air?

Initial attempts to scientifically investigate the ergogenic properties of oxygen began in the early 1900s, but it was not until the 1932 Olympic Games that oxygen was considered to be a potential ergogenic aid for athletic performance. At that time, Japanese swimmers won great victories, and many attributed their success to the fact that they breathed pure oxygen prior to competition. Was this success due partly or totally to their use of oxygen, or was it solely due to the fact that they were better athletes at the time of competition?

Oxygen can be supplemented in one of three ways: increasing the partial pressure of oxygen in the inspired gas mixture, using the normal concentration of oxygen in air under compression, or using an increased partial pressure of oxygen in the inspired gas mixture that is under compression.

Oxygen can be administered immediately prior to competition, during competition, during recovery from competition, or during any combination of these three.

Oxygen breathing prior to exercise has a limited effect on that exercise. If the bout is of a short duration, the total amount of work performed or the rate of work can be increased by breathing oxygen; submaximal work can be performed at a lower pulse rate, providing it occurs within seconds following supplemental oxygen breathing. For exercise bouts in excess of two minutes, or when the interval between the oxygen breathing and actual performance exceeds two minutes, the influence of breathing oxygen is greatly diminished. This simply reflects the limits of the body's oxygen storage potential.

When oxygen is administered during the exercise, definite improvements in performance are noted. The amount of work performed and the rate of work are substantially increased. Likewise, submaximal work is performed more economically, at a lower physiological cost to the individual. Interestingly, peak blood lactate levels are depressed following exhaustive exercise with oxygen breathing, even though considerably more work can be performed.

During the recovery period, studies have been unable to demonstrate any clear advantage to oxygen breathing, both with respect to facilitating recovery and to improving subsequent performance. In an unpublished study in our laboratory, subjects performed an exhaustive, all-out work bout for 60 seconds on a cycle ergometer and then were immediately switched to breathing a gas mixture of either oxygen or air for a two-minute recovery period. This was immediately followed by a second all-out 60-second bout. Neither the recovery during the two minutes between exhaustive bouts, nor the total work accomplished in the second bout, were facilitated by oxygen breathing. This is illustrated in Figure 13-5.

From a practical standpoint, oxygen administration prior to exercise would have little value because of the relatively short time interval during which the oxygen stores would remain elevated above normal levels. Most sports or events would not provide the opportunity to go immediately

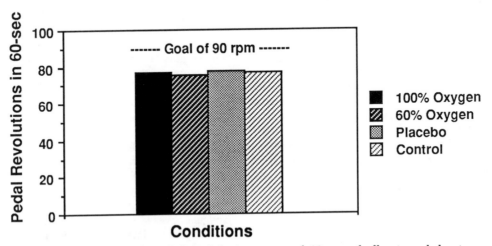

Figure 13-5 Pedal revolutions accomplished during a second 60-second all-out work bout on a cycle ergometer. This second bout was performed two minutes following the first all-out work bout of 60 seconds, with either oxygen (60 percent and 100 percent) or room air being administered during the period between bouts. The conditions were administered on a double-blind basis. Subjects attempted to achieve 90 revolutions in 60 seconds in both work bouts.

from oxygen breathing directly into competition. Likewise, administration during exercise would have limited value, for obvious reasons—during which sport or event could you carry an oxygen source, such as a cylinder, without the source greatly restricting movement? Oxygen breathing during the recovery period has not been demonstrated to have any benefit or value, other than a possible placebo, or psychological effect. The recovery period would appear to be the only practical time to administer oxygen, but only if it speeded up the recovery process, allowing the athlete to re-enter the contest or game in a more fully-recovered state, something which has not been substantiated by research.

BLOOD DOPING

Ekblom, Goldbarg, and Gullbring (1972) created quite a stir in the sports world in the early 1970s. Their research indicated that by withdrawing between 800 and 1,200 ml of blood from a subject and then reinfusing the red cells back into that subject some four weeks later, a considerable improvement in $\dot{V}O_2$ max and treadmill performance time could be demonstrated. The subjects in this study were divided into two groups: Group I had 800 ml of blood withdrawn in a single day, and Group II had 1,200 ml of blood withdrawn over an eight-day period. Immediately following the blood withdrawal, both hemoglobin concentration and $\dot{V}O_2$ max decreased by 13 percent in Group I and 18 percent in Group II, while both groups decreased 30 percent in treadmill performance. At the end of four weeks, the red cells were reinfused. Treadmill performance time increased 23 percent, and $\dot{V}O_2$ max increased nine percent over those values prior to the initial blood withdrawal.

Williams (1975), in a review of all research on blood doping through 1975, concluded that while there were several studies that supported the enhancement of athletic performance with blood doping, the bulk of evidence did not substantiate that contention. Shortly after Williams' review article, Ekblom, et al. (1976), in a second study of blood doping, reported results that were in agreement with their initial study in 1972—an increase of

eight percent in $\dot{V}O_2$ max following reinfusion of the red blood cells. In 1978, Williams, Lindhjem, and Schuster found no significant differences in ratings of perceived exertion or in treadmill time to exhaustion following reinfusion of red blood cells. In this study, two groups of subjects were used, both having 460 ml of blood withdrawn following the initial testing sessions. However, only one of the two groups had their red blood cells reinfused. The other group received 460 ml of normal saline (placebo).

A study by Buick, et al. (1980) used a well-conceived, double-blind design, in which 11 highly-trained distance runners were studied before the blood withdrawal, following the normal restoration of the red blood cells, following a sham reinfusion of 50 ml of saline, and following the actual reinfusion of 900 ml of blood which had been originally withdrawn and freeze-preserved. They also conducted one more observation on these subjects, once their elevated red blood cell levels had returned to normal. They found a substantial increase in $\dot{V}O_2$ max following the reinfusion of the red blood cells, and no change following the sham reinfusion. The results of this study are summarized in Figure 13-6.

Gledhill provided a comprehensive summary of the research literature on blood doping in his excellent 1982 and 1985 review articles. In his discussion of the early controversy in this area, where several studies reported blood doping improved treadmill time and $\dot{V}O_2$ max while others were unable to confirm these findings, he points to the importance of the total volume of red blood cells withdrawn and reinfused, the time interval between withdrawal and reinfusion, and the method for storing the blood after it has been withdrawn.

First, it appears that you must withdraw and reinfuse 900 ml or more of whole blood. Increases in $\dot{V}O_2$ max and performance are not nearly as great when smaller volumes are used. Second, it appears that you must wait for at least five to six weeks, and possibly as long as ten weeks, prior to reinfusion. This time interval is based on the time it takes to return hematocrit and hemoglobin concentrations back to pre-withdrawal levels. Once they have returned to normal levels you then initiate reinfusion to maximize the effect.

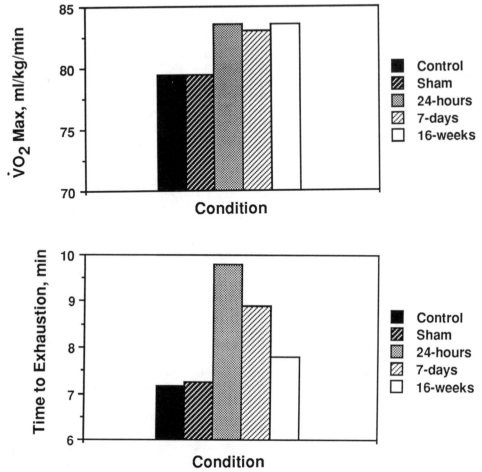

Figure 13–6 Alterations in maximal oxygen uptake and running time to exhaustion following reinfusion of red blood cells (adapted from Buick, et al., 1980).

Finally, the early studies refrigerated the blood which had been withdrawn. Maximum storage time under conditions of refrigeration is approximately three weeks. Further, with refrigeration, approximately 40 percent of the red blood cells are destroyed or lost, thus only 60 percent are available post-infusion. Later studies have used the freeze technique for storage. Freezing allows unlimited storage time, and there is only a loss of approximately 15 percent of the red blood cells.

Gledhill has concluded that under optimal conditions of 900 ml of blood reinfusion or more, a five to six week minimum interval between withdrawal and reinfusion, and with the freeze technique, blood doping does result in significant improvements in both $\dot{V}O_2$ max and endurance performance. Further, he has shown that these improvements are directly the result of the increase in hemoglobin as opposed to an increased cardiac output due to an expanded plasma volume. This is illustrated in Table 13–1.

Does an increase in $\dot{V}O_2$ max and treadmill time translate into an increase in the performance of the endurance athlete? Two studies have addressed this issue. Williams and his associates (1981) recorded the times for a five-mile treadmill run by a

Table 13–1 The interrelationships among total body Hb (TBHb), Hemoglobin Concentration (*[Hb]*), Blood Volume (BV), $\dot{V}O_2$ max, and Physical Performance (Perf).

Blood Volume	TBHb	[Hb]	BV	$\dot{V}O_2$ max	Perf
Hypervolemic anemia	0 or −	−	+	0 or −	−
Normovolemic anemia	−	−	0	−	−
Hypovolemic anemia	−	−	−	−	−
Hypervolemic normocythemia	+	0	+	0	0
Normovolemic normocythemia	0	0	0	0	0
Hypovolemic normocythemia	−	0	−	0 or −	0 or −
Hypervolemic erythrocythemia	+	+	+	+	+
Normovolemic erythrocythemia	+	+	0	+	+
Hypovolemic erythrocythemia	0	+	−	0 or −	0 or −

0 = no change; − = decreased; and + = increased.

(Adapted from N. Gledhill, "The Influence of Altered Blood Volume and Oxygen Transport Capacity on Aerobic Performance," *Exercise and Sports Science Review, 13,* 75–93, 1985).

group of 12 experienced distance runners, before and after saline (placebo) and blood infusions. The five-mile runs on the treadmill were significantly faster following blood infusion but this difference became significant only over the last 2.5 miles. The difference was 33 seconds (3.7 percent) or greater over the last 2.5 miles (average time of ~15 min, 7 sec), or 49 seconds (2.7 percent) over the full 5.0 miles (average time of ~30 min, 15 sec) when the blood infusion trials were compared to the other three conditions. In a second study, Goforth and his associates (1982) reported a decrease of 23.7 seconds in three-mile run time by a group of six trained distance runners following blood doping, a decrease which was significantly different from their blinded control conditions.

While this procedure is relatively safe in the hands of competent physicians, it has inherent dangers associated with it. The potential risks of such a procedure seem to outweigh any potential benefits, above and beyond the ethical issue involved.

WARM-UP AND TEMPERATURE VARIATIONS

Most athletes warm up prior to competition. For some this may consist of simple stretching, while for others it may be a time for an intensive bout of work. Does this precompetition activity facilitate the athlete's performance during the competition, or is this merely a traditional formality that has been carried down through the years? Before this question can be answered, it is important to recognize the different forms of warm-up. Warm-up activities can be identical to those used in competition, or they can be directly related (free-throw shooting drill without the stress of actual competition) or indirectly related (calisthenics for some muscle groups). Lastly, warm-up can be passive, such as hot showers or a massage.

Attempting to determine the specific effects of warm-up is extremely difficult, since the effect appears to differ with the activity, as well as with the form of the warm-up. Franks (1983) has provided an outstanding summary of the research through the early 1980s. There is evidence supporting both the beneficial and detrimental effects of warm-up, as well as a number of studies showing that warm-up has no effect on performance. Studies that have shown the beneficial effects of warm-up have found improved accuracy, movement time, range of motion, and strength in movements of selected parts of the body, while reaction time does not appear to be affected. Sprints and distance runs are generally improved with warm-up, but agility runs are not. Baseball throwing speed and softball distance throw are improved with warm-up, but not the accuracy of the throw.

Although many coaches and athletes feel the warm-up is essential to prevent injuries, there is little direct research evidence to support this contention. This lack of supporting evidence is true for burst-type activities, as well. However, until this critical aspect of warm-up can be explored more fully, it would seem wise to continue using the warm-up as a precautionary, preventive procedure.

It appears that the efficacy of the warm-up depends on the type of warm-up as well as on the sport. The coach or athlete who has questions about a particular sport should refer directly to the specific research studies dealing with that sport. Unfortunately, no general conclusions can be drawn at this time.

Passive hot and cold applications have also been proposed as potential ergogenic aids. Falls (1972) concludes that cold applications are more likely to provide an ergogenic effect than hot applications. The benefit of a cold application, such as a shower, lies in its effect on circulatory function. Cold causes a peripheral vasoconstriction and possibly a reflex vasodilation within the muscle, which makes more blood available for the active tissues. In addition, the cold application cools the body surface, which enhances its ability to dissipate body heat. Heat applications have the opposite effect and tend to reduce efficiency in performances of an endurance nature. Heat applications that are used for warming and loosening a joint, such as the shoulder of a pitcher in baseball, may have a substantial effect, but this depends largely on the individual.

OTHER SUBSTANCES OR PHENOMENA

Other substances, or phenomena, have been identified as having either suspected or proven ergogenic properties. The use of bicarbonates to increase blood and muscle bicarbonate levels has been proposed as an effective technique for improving short-term anaerobic power and capacity. This was discussed in detail in Chapter 3. The use of phosphate loading, salts of aspartic acid, and dichloroacetate (DCA) have also been proposed as

potential ergogenic aids, but sufficient research has not been conducted to substantiate any possible benefits. The use of mandibular orthopedic repositioning appliances (MORA) has also been proposed as an ergogenic aid, with claims of marked gains in strength with the realignment of the jaw. Research has failed to substantiate these claims.

Several social and psychological factors have either known or postulated ergogenic properties. Since the emphasis of this book is on the physiological aspects of performance, these factors will not be reviewed. For more information about this topic, refer to excellent reviews which have been written on hypnosis (Morgan, 1972; Morgan & Brown, 1983); mental practice (Corbin, 1972) or covert rehearsal strategies (Silva, 1983); and social facilitation (Singer, 1972).

SUMMARY

In the never-ending search for excellence and improved performance, the athlete has tried numerous drugs, hormones, and diets, as well as many other physical substances and phenomena, such as hypnosis and mental practice. Often, the athlete has used these aids indiscriminately with complete disregard for health and safety. Furthermore, if an athlete becomes successful after using one of these substances or phenomena, the word spreads quickly, and, soon, athletes in all parts of the world are using the substance or phenomena without waiting for evidence of its effectiveness or information about its side-effects. Just as important are the moral and ethical considerations.

This chapter has reviewed the more widely used physiological substances and phenomena thought to have ergogenic properties. With regard to drugs and hormones, it was concluded that alcohol has no apparent effect on athletic performance when consumed in small doses, but that it can have a substantial detrimental effect when consumed in large doses. Amphetamines have been shown to improve, as well as to have no influence on athletic performance, which suggests a need for further study of a more highly-controlled nature. Anabolic steroids have been shown to cause great increases in lean weight and strength in individual athletes who have taken extremely high doses. However, controlled research studies, using only the recommended daily dosage have shown both increases, as well as no change, in weight and strength, depending on the experience of the population tested. With both amphetamines and steroids, the potential medical risks must be given serious consideration.

One of the areas that receives the greatest attention and interest among athletes who are concerned with improving their performance, is nutrition. This was discussed in detail in Chapter 12.

Oxygen is an ergogenic aid when administered immediately before a short-duration contest (less than two minutes in length), or during the contest or work bout. These ergogenic properties are not present when oxygen is administered during the period of recovery. The issue of blood doping has now been resolved, recent evidence suggesting that it is an ergogenic aid.

Warm-up and hot and cold applications were also discussed as potential ergogenic aids. While warm-up appears to be beneficial for most activities or contests, for others, it either has no effect or it can actually be detrimental. Cold applications, such as cold showers, do appear to improve the cardiovascular function of the individual during controlled bouts of exercise.

STUDY QUESTIONS

1. What is the meaning of the term ergogenic aid?
2. What is presently known about the use of amphetamines in athletic competition? What are the potential risks?
3. Does the use of alcohol in moderate or large doses improve or negatively affect athletic performance?
4. What are anabolic steroids? What are the differences between the androgenic and anabolic properties of steroids?
5. Does the use of anabolic steroids result in improved athletic performance? How and why?
6. What are some of the medical risks of steroid use?

7. How beneficial is the breathing of oxygen prior to the start of competition, during competition, and during the recovery from competition?
8. What is blood doping? Does blood doping improve athletic performance?
9. What factors account for the inconsistent findings of earlier versus later studies of blood doping?
10. How important is warm-up in improving athletic performance? Is it essential for injury prevention?
11. How do heat or cold applications affect performance? What physiological mechanisms are involved?
12. Discuss the moral and ethical issues involved in the use of any ergogenic aid.

REFERENCES

American College of Sports Medicine Position Statement. (1977). The use and abuse of anabolic-androgenic steroids in sports. *Medicine and Science in Sports, 9,* xi–xiii.

American College of Sports Medicine Position Statement. (1982). The use of alcohol in sports. *Medicine and Science in Sports and Exercise, 14,* ix–xi.

Ariel, G., & Saville, W. (1972). Anabolic steroids: The physiological effects of placebos. *Medicine and Science in Sports, 4,* 124–126.

Buick, F. J., Gledhill, N., Froese, A. B., Spriet, L., & Meyers, E. C. (1980). Effect of induced erythrocythemia on aerobic work capacity. *Journal of Applied Physiology, 48,* 636–642.

Cantwell, J. D., & Rose, F. D. (1986). Cocaine and cardiovascular events. *Physician and Sportsmedicine, 14,* (#11), 77–88.

Chandler, J. V., & Blair, S. N. (1980). The effect of amphetamines on selected physiological components related to athletic success. *Medicine and Science in Sports and Exercise, 12,* 65–69.

Cooper, D. L. (1972). Drugs and the athlete. *Journal of the American Medical Association, 221,* 1007–1011.

Corbin, C. B. (1972). Mental practice. In W. P. Morgan (Ed.), *Ergogenic aids and muscular performance* (pp. 293–320). New York: Academic Press.

Costill, D. L. (1972). Water and electrolytes. In W. P. Morgan (Ed.), *Ergogenic aids and muscular performance.* New York: Academic Press (pp. 293–320).

Costill, D. L., Pearson, D. R., & Fink, W. J. (1984). Anabolic steroid use among athletes: Changes in HDL-C levels. *Physician and Sportsmedicine, 12* (#6), 113–117.

Ekblom, B., Goldbarg, A. N., & Gullbring, B. (1972). Response to exercise after blood loss and reinfusion. *Journal of Applied Physiology, 33,* 175–180.

Ekblom, B., Wilson, G., & Åstrand, P. O. (1976). Central circulation during exercise after venesection and reinfusion of red blood cells. *Journal of Applied Physiology, 40,* 379–383.

Falls, H. B. (1972). Heat and cold applications. In W. P. Morgan (Ed.), *Ergogenic aids and muscular performance* (pp. 119–158). New York: Academic Press.

Forbes, G. B. (1985). The effect of anabolic steroids on lean body mass: The dose response curve. *Metabolism, 34,* 571–573.

Franks, B. D. (1983). Physical warm-up. In M. H. Williams (Ed.), *Ergogenic aids in sports* (pp. 340–375). Champaign, IL: Human Kinetics Publishers.

Gledhill, N. (1982). Blood doping and related issues: A brief review. *Medicine and Science in Sports and Exercise, 14,* 183–189.

Gledhill, N. (1985). The influence of altered blood volume and oxygen transport capacity on aerobic performance. *Exercise and Sport Sciences Reviews, 13,* 75–93.

Glover, E. D., Edmundson, E. W., Edwards, S. W., & Schroeder, K. L. (1986). Implications of smokeless tobacco use among athletes. *Physician and Sportsmedicine, 14* (#12), 95–105.

Goforth, H. W., Jr., Campbell, N. L., Hodgdon, J. A., & Sucec, A. A. (1982). Hematologic parameters of trained distance runners following induced erythrocythemia. *Medicine and Science in Sports and Exercise, 14,* 174 (abstract).

Golding, L. A. (1972). Drugs and hormones. In W. P. Morgan (Ed.), *Ergogenic aids and muscular performance* (pp. 367–397). New York: Academic Press.

Golding, L. A., & Barnard, R. J. (1963). The effect of d-amphetamine sulfate on physical performance. *Journal of Sports Medicine and Physical Fitness, 3,* 221–224.

Hervey, G. R., Knibbs, A. V., Burkinshaw, L., Morgan, D. B., Jones, P. R. M., Chettle, D. R., & Vartsky, D. (1981). Effects of methandienone on the performance and body composition of men undergoing athletic training. *Clinical Science, 60,* 457–461.

Horstman, D. H. (1972). Nutrition. In W. P. Morgan (Ed.), *Ergogenic aids and muscular performance,* (pp. 343–365). New York: Academic Press.

Hurley, B. F., Seals, D. R., Hagberg, J. M., Goldberg, A. C., Ostrove, S. M., Holloszy, J. O., Wiest, W. G., & Goldberg, A. P. (1984). High-density-lipoprotein cholesterol in bodybuilders vs. powerlifters: Negative effects of androgen use. *Journal of the American Medical Association, 252,* 507–513.

Ivy, J. L. (1983). Amphetamines. In M. H. Williams (Ed.), *Ergogenic aids in sports* (pp. 101–127). Champaign, IL: Human Kinetics Publishers.

Johnson, L. C., & O'Shea, J. P. (1969). Anabolic steroid: Effects on strength development. *Science, 164,* 957–959.

Karpovich, P. V. (1959). Effect of amphetamine sulfate on athletic performance. *Journal of the American Medical Association, 170,* 558–561.

Lamb, D. R. (1983). Anabolic steroids. In M. H. Williams (Ed.). *Ergogenic aids in sports* (pp. 164–182). Champaign, IL: Human Kinetics Publishers.

Lombardo, J. A. (1986). Stimulants and athletic performance: Amphetamines and caffeine. *Physician and Sportsmedicine, 14* (#11), 128–142.

Lombardo, J. A. (1986). Stimulants and athletic performance: Cocaine and nicotine. *Physician and Sportsmedicine, 14* (#12), 85–91.

Moore, T. J., Santa Maria, D. L., Hatfield, B. D., Ryder, M. N., & Weiner, L. B. (1986). The mandibular orthopedic repositioning appliance and its effect on power production in conditioned athletes. *Physician and Sportsmedicine, 14* (#12), 137–145.

Morgan, W. P. (Ed.). (1972). *Ergogenic aids and muscular performance.* New York: Academic Press.

Morgan, W. P. (1972). Hypnosis and muscular performance. In W. P. Morgan (Ed.), *Ergogenic aids and muscular performance,* (pp. 193–233). New York: Academic Press.

Morgan, W. P., & Brown, D. R. (1983). Hypnosis. In M. H. Williams (Ed.), *Ergogenic aids in sports* (pp. 223–252). Champaign, IL: Human Kinetics Publishers.

Morris, A. F. (1983). Oxygen. In M. H. Williams (Ed.), *Ergogenic aids in sports* (pp. 185–201). Champaign, IL: Human Kinetics Publishers.

Silva, J. M., III. (1983). Covert rehearsal strategies. In M. H. Williams (Ed.), *Ergogenic aids in sports* (pp. 253–274). Champaign, IL: Human Kinetics Publishers.

Singer, R. N. (1972). Social facilitation. In W. P. Morgan (Ed.), *Ergogenic aids and muscular performance* (pp. 263–289). New York: Academic Press.

Smith, G. M., & Beecher, H. K. (1959). Amphetamine sulfate and athletic performance. *Journal of the American Medical Association, 170,* 542–557.

Strauss, R. H., Liggett, M. T., & Lanese, R. R. (1985). Anabolic steroid use and perceived effects in ten weight-trained women athletes. *Journal of the American Medical Association, 253,* 2871–2873.

Strauss, R. H., Wright, J. E., Finerman, G. A. M., & Catlin, D. H. (1983). Side effects of anabolic steroids in weight-trained men. *Physician and Sportsmedicine, 11* (#12), 87–98.

Webb, O. L., Laskarzewski, P. M., & Glueck, C. J. (1984). Severe depression of high-density lipoprotein cholesterol levels in weight lifters and body builders by self-administered exogenous testosterone and anabolic-androgenic steroids. *Metabolism, 33,* 971–975.

Williams, M. H. (1975). Blood doping—does it really help athletes? *Physician and Sportsmedicine, 3,* 52–56.

Williams, M. H. (1983). *Ergogenic aids in sports.* Champaign, IL: Human Kinetics Publishers.

Williams, M. H. (1983). Blood doping. In M. H. Williams (Ed.), *Ergogenic aids in sports* (pp. 202–219). Champaign, IL: Human Kinetics Publishers.

Williams, M. H., Lindhjem, M., & Schuster, R. (1978). The effect of blood infusion upon endurance capacity and ratings of perceived exertion. *Medicine and Science in Sports, 10,* 113–118.

Williams, M. H., Wesseldine, S., Somma, T., & Schuster, R. (1981). The effect of induced erythrocythemia upon five-mile treadmill run time. *Medicine and Science in Sports and Exercise, 13,* 169-175.

Wilmore, J. H. (1972). Oxygen. In W. P. Morgan (Ed.), *Ergogenic aids and muscular performance* (pp. 321-342). New York: Academic Press.

Wright, J. E. (1981). Anabolic steroids and athletics. *Exercise and Sport Sciences Reviews, 8,* 149-202.

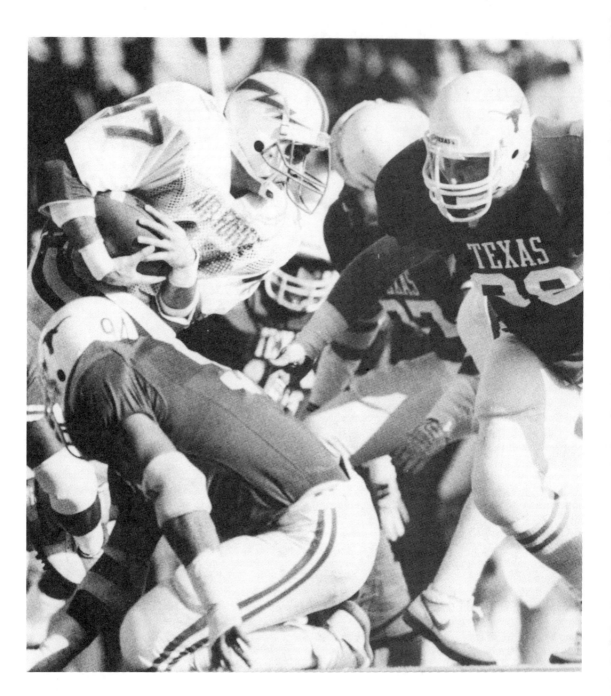

14

Environmental Factors

INTRODUCTION

Athletes are often expected to perform under less than optimal environmental conditions. The athletes who train at sea level, for example, are forced to make rather extensive physiological adjustments when they attempt to compete at high altitudes. Hot, humid climates, on the other hand, place unusual demands on the circulatory system and limit the athlete's ability to perform long term exercise. Training in cool climates does little to prepare athletes to compete under conditions of extreme heat and humidity. Similarly, sudden exposure to cold can have a dramatic influence on the athlete's performance if he or she has not had an opportunity to acclimatize to the colder environment.

Although the environment dictates to a large extent the quality of an athlete's performance, the body is capable of extensive adaptations that will accommodate the physiological stresses of heat, cold, and altitude. The purpose of this chapter is to provide information that will help the athlete prepare for these environmental variations. This chapter will be of limited value for those sports that are performed in a controlled indoor environment, such as basketball, wrestling, and swimming, with the exception of competition at high altitudes. However, for sports such as cross-country, football, and soccer, the importance of preparing for radical changes in environmental conditions must be recognized. Football provides an excellent example of a sport that requires the athlete to adapt to varied environmental conditions.

The football season usually starts in July or August, depending on the region and the level—high school, college, or professional. In most regions of the United States, this is the hottest season of the year. The combination of high humidity and heat poses a potentially lethal environment. The padding and clothing worn by football players add another stress, since they create a closed microenvironment in which it is difficult to lose body heat. Even under moderately cool conditions, this equipment and clothing create potential problems of heat stress. During one three-year period, seven high school and five college football players died as a result of heat stress. At the other extreme, but of considerably less consequence, football players are exposed to subfreezing temperatures in certain regions of the United States as the season draws to a close. This, too, can create many problems, such as frostbite and other weather-related injuries.

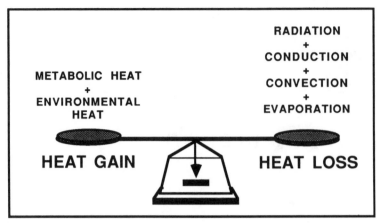

Figure 14-1   The balance of body heat production and dissipation. Note that under resting conditions in a thermoneutral environment, most of the heat removed from the body is accomplished by radiation.

VARIATIONS IN TEMPERATURE AND HUMIDITY

The topic of body temperature regulation was briefly mentioned in Chapter 2. As noted, the body is substantially less than 100 percent efficient, resulting in the production of a considerable amount of heat as it generates energy for muscular activity. In cold environments, this metabolic heat production is necessary to assist in maintaining the body temperature. In hot environments, however, it is a liability, since it adds to the body's heat load.

As noted in Figure 14-1, heat dissipation from the body is dependent on the transfer of heat from the metabolically active tissues to the environment. Heat produced during energy metabolism is transported by the blood to the skin where it is removed by the combination of **conduction, convection, radiation,** and **evaporation** (see Figure 14-2). At rest, the internal body temperature is kept at approximately 99.2° F, but during exercise the body is often unable to dissipate heat as rapidly as it is being produced. As a result, the athlete may develop a fever in excess of 105° F, with muscle temperature above 108° F. Although a small rise in muscle temperature aids the muscle's energy systems by making them more efficient, temperatures above 104° F can affect the nervous sys-

tem and the body's mechanisms of temperature regulation. The removal of heat from the body is regulated by the hypothalamus, a small mass of nervous tissue seated at the base of the brain. Functioning as a thermostat, the **hypothalamus** triggers a sweating response and directs blood flow to the skin in an effort to dissipate the excess body heat. Although surprisingly effective, this system of cooling is not without limitations; often it is no match for the high rate of heat produced during exercise.

When the temperature regulatory mechanisms fail or when the environmental conditions result in excessive heat storage, the athlete is placed in a potentially lethal situation. Therefore, a basic knowledge of how the body performs under various environmental temperatures and how to cope with environmental extremes is essential for both the coach and the athlete.

Exercise in the Heat

The ability of the athlete to successfully perform in the heat depends on the air temperature, humidity, air movement, the intensity and duration of effort, and the individual's tolerance to such environmental conditions. Also of major importance is the athlete's fluid and mineral intake schedule

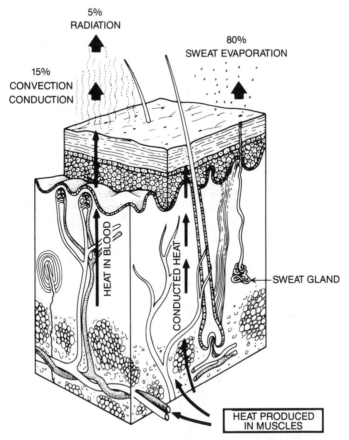

Figure 14-2 The removal of heat from the skin. Note that heat is delivered to the body shell via the arterial blood, which loses heat to the subcutaneous layers of skin.

both prior to and during competition. Each of these factors must be considered when preparing the athlete for competition in the heat.

One of the primary responsibilities of the circulatory system is to transport heat from the muscles to the surface of the body where the heat can be transferred to the environment. Since the volume of blood is limited, exercise poses a complex problem for the circulatory and temperature regulatory systems. During exercise in the heat, a large part of the cardiac output must be shared by the skin and working muscles. An increase in the demand for blood flow to one tissue will automatically decrease flow to the other.

Any factor that tends to overload the cardiovascular system or interfere with the transfer of heat from the body to the environment will drastically impair the athlete's performance and increase the risk of overheating. Running at a fast pace, for example, will require more oxygen and blood flow to the muscles, with a concomitant increase in muscle heat production. In spite of this increase in heat production, blood flow to the skin decreases, resulting in an inability to move the heat to the shell of the body.

The higher the ambient, or existing temperature, the greater the stress placed on the athlete. At rest, with a neutral temperature of 70 to 80° F, the average individual gives off an excess of 80 kcal of heat per hour as the by-product of energy production. Of this, approximately 25 percent or 20 kcal per hour are removed from the body by evaporation; the remainder is lost by radiation, convection, and conduction. As the athlete exercises at different levels of intensity up to exhaustion, the metabolic needs of the body increase in a linear manner and up to 900 kcal per hr or more can be produced as a by-product of metabolism. Consequently, nearly 80 percent of the heat production is removed by sweat evaporation. This presents the body with a greater challenge to dissipate this excess heat. As noted in Figure 14-3, the demands placed on sweat production increase in increments with exercise intensity (heat production) and environmental heat stress.

Studies by Fink, et al. (1975) demonstrated that in addition to raising body temperature and heart rate, exercise in the heat also increased the uptake of oxygen, causing the working muscles to use more glycogen and produce more lactate (see Figure 14-4). This results in an earlier onset of fatigue and a marked reduction in performance in events of long duration.

When exercising in a cold environment, heat production is actually beneficial, assisting in the maintenance of normal body temperature. However, even when the exercise is conducted in a thermally neutral environment, between 70 and 80° F, the metabolic heat load places a considerable burden on the cardiovascular system, as the body attempts to transport heat from the center of the body out to the skin.

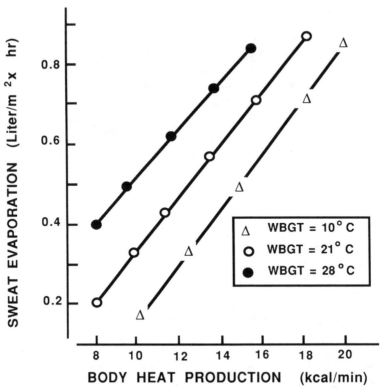

Figure 14-3 The interaction between body heat production, environmental heat stress, and the rate of sweating. The WBGT is a combined measurement of environmental heat stress—air temperature, humidity, and radiant heat from the sun.

The gradient between the athlete and the environment decreases as the temperature of the surrounding environment increases. Under some conditions the temperature of the environment approaches, and can exceed, the skin and deep body temperature. This results in an even greater reliance on evaporation as the major avenue of heat loss, since radiation, convection, and conduction lose effectiveness as the environmental temperature increases. Evaporation requires sweating, therefore, an increased dependence on evaporation means an increased demand for sweating. Since a high percentage of the fluid lost in sweat comes from the blood plasma, an even greater demand is imposed on the cardiovascular system. As the environmental temperature increases, more blood is needed to transport heat to the skin. The high rate of sweating reduces the existing blood volume, which is available to deliver nutrients to the muscles and to prevent a build-up

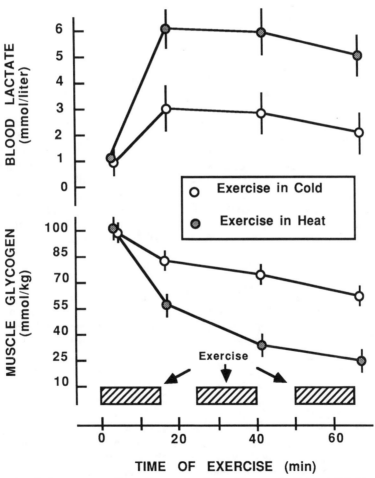

Figure 14-4 The rate of glycogen use from the vastus lateralis muscle (lateral thigh) and blood lactate accumulation during cycling exercise in the heat (41° C, 15% humidity) and cold 9° C, 55% humidity) (modified from Fink, et al., 1975).

of heat. This results in a reduction in the athlete's performance potential, particularly for activities of an endurance nature. In long-distance runners, sweat losses may approach six to ten percent of their body weight. Such severe dehydration may limit subsequent sweating and makes the athlete susceptible to heat cramps, heat stroke, or heat exhaustion.

Radiation, conduction, and convection, while working to cool the athlete on cool days when there is a breeze and partial or total cloud cover, can actually contribute to the heat load of the body if the climatic conditions are right. The athlete exercising at 75° F on a bright, sunny day with no measurable wind will notice considerably more heat stress than when exercising at the same temperature but with a cloud cover and a slight breeze. At temperatures above 88 to 92° F, radiation, convection, and conduction will substantially add to the heat load rather than act as an avenue of heat loss.

Clothing is an important consideration for the problem of heat stress. Obviously, the more clothing worn, the smaller the available area for evaporation to take place. The foolish practice of exercising in a rubberized suit to promote weight loss is an excellent illustration of how a microenvironment (environment inside the suit) can be created. Temperature and humidity can reach a sufficiently high level within this microenvironment to cause heat stroke or exhaustion if exercise is continued. A football uniform provides a similar microenvironment that is inherently dangerous in hot weather. It is strongly advocated by exercise scientists and sports physicians that the athlete wear as little clothing as possible when heat stress is a potential problem. Where clothing is necessary or required, it should be of loose weave to allow the skin beneath to breathe.

Humidity. The amount of water vapor in the air surrounding the athlete, **relative humidity,** is an additional factor that must be considered important in the regulation of body temperature during exercise in the heat. Sweating contributes to the loss of body heat only if the sweat evaporates from the skin. The conversion of sweat from a liquid to a gaseous state (evaporation) requires heat, which

is drawn from the body. The evaporation of one milliliter of water requires 0.58 kcal. Thus, the evaporation of a liter (approximately a quart) of sweat would remove 580 kcal of heat from the body. Humans are capable of sweating up to three liters or more per hour. If the surrounding air is totally saturated with water vapor, 100 percent humidity, it is impossible for sweat to evaporate, since there is no room in the surrounding air to hold the water molecules from the skin. An example of this is the contrast between the bodily sensations in the middle of the desert at a temperature of 100° F, and ten percent relative humidity compared to those in Houston, Texas at 80° F, and 95 percent relative humidity. In the former, the body sweats profusely, but evaporation occurs so rapidly that you are not conscious of the fact that you are sweating. In the latter situation, only a limited amount of sweat can evaporate, since 95 percent of the surrounding air is filled with water vapor. The result is a continuous bath of sweat that drips from the body, thereby removing very little heat.

This example points to the stress imposed by humidity on athletic performance. In the previous section, it was stated that evaporation is the major method of regulating body temperature in the heat. If the air is saturated with water vapor, no evaporation can occur even at lower environmental temperatures; at higher temperatures, the body has no way of losing heat, so the body temperature will rise to critical levels, risking the health of the athlete.

It is clear that air temperature alone is not an accurate index of the total physiological stress imposed on the athlete. Humidity, air velocity, the degree of cloud cover (radiation), as well as temperature, all directly influence the degree of stress felt by the athlete. The relative contribution of these factors to the total heat stress is not clearly understood, since they probably vary with changing environmental conditions. Efforts have been made to quantify these four factors into a single index. In the 1920s, the effective temperature index was developed, which was later altered to account for the effect of radiation. The latter index was called the corrected effective temperature. In the 1970s, a wet globe thermometer (WGBT) was devised to simultaneously account for conduction, convection, evaporation, and radiation, providing a single temperature reading to estimate the potential cooling capacity of the surrounding environment. Unfortunately this instrument has not been widely used to monitor the environmental conditions for most athletic events.

Dehydration. One of the greatest problems associated with exercise in the heat, particularly under conditions of high humidity, is dehydration. Since sweating is the major avenue of heat loss during exercise, the total amount of fluid lost becomes very important as the duration of the activity is extended over time. Humans are able to sweat at the rate of two liters per hour for short periods of time and are able to sustain sweating at the rate of one liter per hour, or more, for periods of three hours or longer. Marathon runners commonly lose five to seven pounds as a result of the 26.2-mile race, even though they may drink freely during the race. Along with water, salts and other critical electrolytes are lost at a substantial rate. The following section will discuss the effects of heavy sweating on body fluids, and the importance of body water balance on performance.

As noted earlier, dehydration presents a serious threat to the athlete's performance and health. It is estimated that the deep body temperature will rise from 0.3 to 0.5° F for every percent loss in body weight. This rise is the result of several factors, one of which is the loss in blood volume. Figure 14-5 illustrates the contribution of water from each of the body's fluid compartments during varied levels of dehydration. In general, about half of the water lost in sweat comes from inside the cells, intracellular water, whereas about ten percent is taken from the plasma. The balance of the water loss is taken from the fluids that surround the

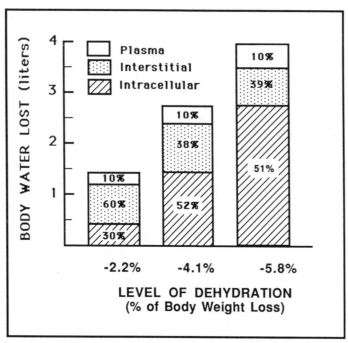

Figure 14-5 Contribution of water from intracellular, vascular, and interstitial compartments to the sweat lost during varied levels of dehydration (from Costill, et al., 1976).

Table 14-1 The influence of dehydration (hypohydration) and hyperhydration on selected physiological parameters and performance in strength and endurance events.

Measurement	Hypo-hydration	Hyper-hydration
Performance		
Strength	Unchanged	Unchanged
Sprint Running	Unchanged	Unchanged
Reaction Time	Small Increase	No Information
Endurance	Decrease	Unchanged
Submaximal Exercise		
Heart Rate	Increased	Unchanged
Oxygen Uptake	Unchanged	Unchanged
Body Temp.	Increased	Decreased
Blood Lactate	Increased	Unchanged
Maximal Exercise		
$\dot{V}O_2$ max	Decreased	Unchanged
Heart Rate	Unchanged	Unchanged
Blood Lactate	Higher	Unchanged

body cells, interstitial water. Although plasma volume would seem to be the compartment least affected by dehydration, it is also the compartment that is most sensitive to losses. A reduction in plasma volume impairs the transport of heat from the core to the skin, and impairs the supply of blood to the exercising muscles.

Since dehydration has a most profound influence on the oxygen transport system, it is not surprising that endurance activities are affected more than are strength and power events. Table 14-1 and Figure 14-6 describe the importance of body water on performance in a variety of events. Whereas excess amounts of body water (hyperhydration) has no influence on performance, dehydration has a negative effect on most measurements of endurance. Armstrong, et al. (1985) have shown that running performance is slowed four to 6.7 percent with a three percent loss in body weight. Since runners who sweat heavily for an hour can lose this amount of body water, it follows that

their time for a ten kilometer run might slow from 40 minutes to over 42 minutes, 30 seconds; a major performance deficit.

The problem of dehydration is not unique to those athletes competing under conditions of thermal stress. In 1967, a county medical society in Iowa recommended that high school wrestling be abolished as a sport. This group of physicians was concerned with the hazardous health practices used by high school wrestlers to "make weight" for a specific weight class. This recommendation created a major wave of hysteria that quickly spread to other states. In the athletic world, Iowa and wrestling are considered inseparable. To ban wrestling in Iowa would be comparable to banning skiing in Colorado, swimming in California, or football in Texas.

Why were these physicians concerned? A group of researchers from the University of Iowa set out to define the problem and recommend a solution. They found that the high school wrestlers were losing a considerable amount of body weight over a period of 17 days, some losing nearly 30 pounds, or almost two pounds per day! In addition, they found that most of the weight loss occurred in the last few days prior to certification and that the greatest weight loss occurred in the youngest boys and lightest weight classes. Simple calculations indicated that most of the weight that was lost came from dehydration, not from a loss of body fat. Analysis of the wrestlers' urine samples confirmed the fact that substantial dehydration had occurred. In addition to impairing performance, such chronic periods of dehydration have been suggested to expose the athlete to the risk of kidney damage.

Thus, it appears that voluntary dehydration, exemplified by the wrestler, is an undesirable practice and should be discouraged. This would apply to any athlete trying to make weight through a rapid loss of body fluids—football players, boxers, and even jockeys. The advantages gained are far out-weighed by the disadvantages; the primary danger is the potential for serious medical complications. The athlete should focus on weight loss as a long-term process, losing no more than one to two pounds of excess fat per week. A 10- to 15-pound weight loss over a 7- to 14-day period is essentially a loss of body fluids, not fat. A fat loss

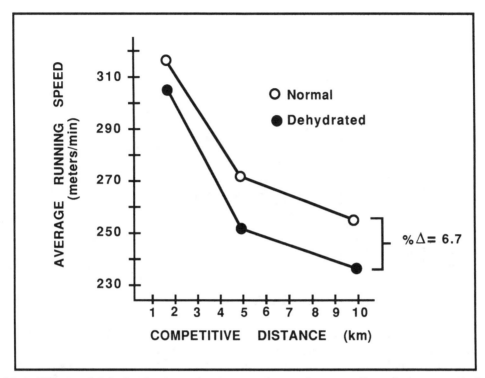

Figure 14-6 Effects of dehydration on endurance running performance (from Armstrong, et al., 1985).

should be the desired goal, since excess fat reduces the athlete's performance potential, while the body fluids are essential for optimal performance.

Fluid and Mineral Replacement. For many years, it was considered dangerous for athletes to stop and drink water or other fluids, either during practice or competition. It was feared that the intake of fluids would cause cramping of the stomach and intestine. Therefore, all fluids were generally withheld until after the practice or competition. In the late 1960s coaches began to realize that with copious sweating, large quantities of salt were being lost, and salt losses were associated with muscle cramps. This led to the practice of requiring athletes to take indiscriminant amounts of salt tablets, yet fluids were still withheld! From our present knowledge of dehydration and fluid ingestion during exercise, we are now aware of how dangerous and foolish such practices were.

Ingestion of fluids during exercise is essential whenever dehydration is a potential problem. Fluid intake, both before and during exercise in the heat, has been shown to reduce the increase in rectal temperature, as exercise is prolonged up to two hours (see Figure 14-7 on page 272). For the same level of work and thermal stress, exercise with fluid ingestion results in a deep body temperature that is approximately 1.5° F lower than the same conditions with no fluid ingestion.

Most teams with sound medical leadership are now periodically stopping during practice for a fluid break. Both water and drinks that contain small amounts of carbohydrate are absorbed and distributed freely throughout the body. The frequency of such breaks is dictated by the climatic conditions: the more severe the heat stress and subsequent dehydration, the more frequent the breaks. In the game situation, fluid should be made available at all times when the athlete is not

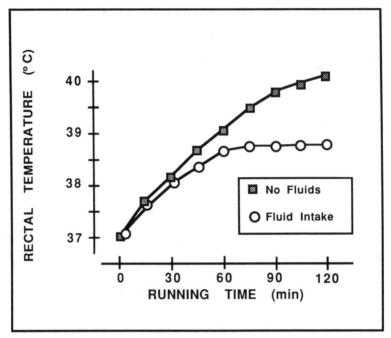

Figure 14-7   Effects of fluid intake on internal (rectal) body temperature. Note that the intake of fluids appeared to have no influence on rectal temperature during the first 45 minutes of exercise. After that time, however, the rate of body heat storage slowed when fluids were given (modified from Costill, et al., 1970).

in competition, and he or she should be encouraged to drink as much as possible. Since research shows that you do not drink as much as you should to replace the fluid that is lost, athletes should be told to drink even more than their thirst tells them they need. Fluid intake prior to competition or practice should be encouraged. Additional information about fluid replacement was described in Chapter 12.

It has been suggested that the athlete drink 200 to 300 ml (approximately one-half of a pint) of fluid every fifteen to twenty minutes. Since it is essential to replace as much fluid as possible, the glucose and mineral content of the solutions should be kept to a minimum (see Chapter 12). The drink should be cool, slightly hypotonic (few dissolved particles), and palatable to the individual. As emphasized in our earlier discussion, the loss of salt in sweat is usually insignificant compared to the water lost. The liberal use of salt at meal time is the most effective method of replacing the lost salt.

Acclimatization. How can we prepare the athlete for competition in the heat? Does training in the heat make the athlete more tolerant of this thermal stress? Many studies have investigated this problem and have concluded that repeated exposure to heat causes a gradual adjustment that enables the athlete to perform better in hot conditions.

Prolonged and repeated exercise bouts in the heat cause a gradual improvement in the athlete's ability to eliminate excess body heat, thereby reducing the risk of heat exhaustion and heat stroke. This process, termed **heat acclimation**, results in a number of adjustments in the distribution of blood flow and sweating. Although the amount of sweat produced during exercise in the heat does not always change with heat acclimation, the distribution of sweating over the skin often increases in those areas that have the greatest exposure and are most effective in dissipating body heat. In addition, the sweat that is produced is a more dilute sweat, thus conserving the body's mineral stores. There is a lowered skin and body temperature for the same level of work, and the heart rate response to a standardized, sub-maximal level of exercise is reduced. This latter response is the result of either or both an increased blood volume and a reduction in skin blood flow, both of which would increase the stroke volume. In addition, more work can be accomplished prior to reaching the point of fatigue or exhaustion.

As shown in Figure 14-8, heat acclimation is generally characterized by reductions in heart rate and rectal temperature during exercise in the heat. These physiological adjustments improve rapidly with successive days of training in the heat, being fully improved within eight to 12 days. It has been noted that heat acclimation is dependent on the rate of internal heat production (for instance, running speed), the duration of heat exposure, and the environmental conditions during each exercise session.

The adaptations to the heat, however, seem to require more than just exposure to a hot environment. While the research literature is not in total agreement on this point, it does appear that exercise in a hot environment is required in order to attain acclimatization that will carry over to exercise in the heat. For individuals or teams that are training in environments cooler than those in which they will be competing, it is important to achieve thermal acclimatization prior to the contest or event. This would improve the individual's performance, in addition to reducing the associated physiological stress. Normal workouts in the

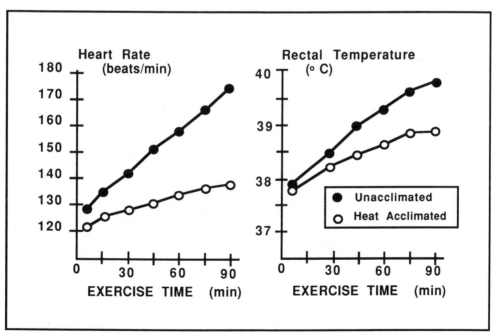

Figure 14-8 Effects of repeated days of exercise in the heat (90 minutes/day; 39°C; 60% $\dot{V}O_2$ max; eight days) on heart rate and rectal temperature during a standard heat-exercise test (from King, et al., 1985).

heat for five to seven days should provide nearly total acclimatization, although the intensity of the workout should be reduced to between 60 and 70 percent during the first few days to prevent excessive heat stress.

Improved heat tolerance is associated with an earlier onset of sweating at the beginning of the exercise. As a result, skin temperatures are lower, and the difference between the temperatures of body and skin are greater. Thus, less blood flow to the skin is required to transfer excess body heat. Although some investigators have found an increase in blood volume with heat acclimation, this change is somewhat temporary, and is probably related to the body's efforts to retain sodium, thereby expanding the plasma volume.

What does all this mean to the athlete, and how can he or she train to gain the greatest degree of heat acclimation? Although most individuals must be exposed to the heat to gain full adjustment, they can gain partial heat tolerance by training in a cooler environment. It is interesting to note that when athletes become acclimated to a given level of heat stress, they will also be able to perform better in cooler weather. If they must compete in hot weather, then at least part of their training should be conducted in the warmest part of the day. Of course, care must be taken to guard against heat injuries such as heat stroke and heat exhaustion. Early morning and evening training runs will not fully prepare an athlete to tolerate the heat of midday.

One possible side effect of exercise in the heat is the stress it places on muscle glycogen stores. As we noted earlier, exercise at a given load in the heat will require a greater use of muscle glycogen than the same effort in cooler air. As a result, repeated days of training in the heat may result in a rapid depletion of muscle glycogen and the symptoms of chronic fatigue. Heat acclimation, on the other hand, reduces this rate of glycogen use by as much as 50 to 60 percent, thereby reducing the risk of exhaustion due to a depletion of the muscle's energy reserves (see Figure 14-9).

Heat Disorders and their Prevention. When the body is unable to successfully adapt to heat stress, three forms of failure exist. **Heat cramps,** the least

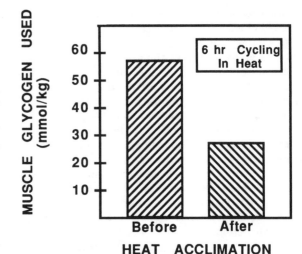

HEAT ACCLIMATION

Figure 14-9 Amount of muscle glycogen used during six hours of exercise in the heat of 102° F before and after eight days of heat acclimation. Note the smaller amount of glycogen used after heat acclimation.

serious of the three heat disorders, is thought to result from dehydration and the mineral loss that accompanies high rates of sweating. It is characterized by severe cramping of the skeletal muscles, primarily those muscles used in the exercise. **Heat exhaustion** is the second type of heat disorder, which is characterized by a body temperature of 101 to 104° F, extreme tiredness, breathlessness, dizziness, and tachycardia, or rapid pulse. These symptoms appear to be the result of reduced sweat production, thus limiting the body's major avenue of heat loss.

Heat stroke is the most serious of the three heat disorders and is characterized by a body temperature of 104 to 106° F or higher, cessation of sweating, and total confusion or unconsciousness. A number of studies have reported rectal temperatures higher than 104° F after marathon races conducted on only moderately warm days. Following a 10,000-meter race in the heat (85° F, 80 percent relative humidity, and bright sun), for example, the rectal temperature of 109.5° F was observed in a 40-year-old man who collapsed only

100 yards from the finish (Costill, 1986). Without proper medical attention, such fevers result in permanent damage to the central nervous system and in some cases death. Fortunately, this man was rapidly cooled with ice and recovered without complications. Since body heat production during exercise is dependent on exercise intensity and body weight, heavier individuals run a higher risk of overheating than lighter athletes when they are exercising at the same rate.

There is little we can do about environmental conditions, but it is obvious that athletes must decrease their rate of energy expenditure to reduce heat production and the risk of overheating. All athletes, coaches, and sports organizers should be able to recognize the symptoms of a high internal fever. There is a fair relationship between subjective sensations and body temperature (see Table 14-2). Although there is generally little concern when the rectal temperature rises to between 101 and 104° F during prolonged exercise, athletes who have a throbbing pressure in their head and chills should realize that they are rapidly approaching a dangerous stage that could prove fatal if they continue to exercise.

To prevent heat disorders, several simple precautions should be taken. Competition and practice outdoors should not be held when the wet bulb temperature is over 78° F. Wet bulb temperature

reflects the humidity as well as the absolute temperature, therefore, it is a more sensitive indication of physiological stress. Scheduling practices and contests either in the early morning or at night is one way of overcoming the severe heat stress of midday. Fluids should be made readily available and the athlete required to drink as much as he or she can, stopping every ten to twenty minutes in the higher temperatures for a fluid break. Clothing should be as brief as possible, loose-weaved, and of a light color, since dark colors absorb heat while light colors reflect. The athlete should always under-dress, because the metabolic heat load will soon make extra clothing an unnecessary burden.

The American College of Sports Medicine has provided some guidelines to help distance runners prevent these heat-related injuries in the publication *Prevention of Thermal Injuries During Distance Running*, (*Medicine and Science in Sports Exercise, 16*, ix-xiv, 1984). A modified list of these recommendations are as follows:

1. Distance races of greater than ten kilometers should not be conducted when the combination of air temperature, humidity, and sun raise the WBGT temperature above 82° F.

   $WBGT = 0.7(TWB) + 0.2(TG) = 0.1(TDB)$
   where TWB = temperature of wet bulb; TG = temperature of black globe; and TDB = temperature of dry bulb.

2. Summer events should be scheduled before 8 A.M. or after 6 P.M., to minimize the heat of the sun.

3. An adequate supply of water or other fluids should be available before the race and at two to three kilometer intervals during the race. Runners should drink 100 to 200 milliliters at each feeding station.

4. Runners should train adequately for fitness and become heat-acclimatized.

5. Runners should be aware of the early symptoms of heat injury, including dizziness, chilling, headache, and awkwardness.

6. Race sponsors should make prior arrangements with medical personnel to care for heat injuries. Responsible and informed personnel should supervise each feeding station. Organizational

Table 14-2 Subjective symptoms associated with overheating (from Costill, 1986).

Rectal Temperature	Symptoms
104–105°F	Throbbing pressure in head, cold sensation over stomach and back, with piloerection (goose bumps).
105–106°F	Muscular weakness, disorientation, and loss of postural equilibrium.
Above 106°F	Diminished sweating, loss of consciousness.

personnel should reserve the right to stop runners who exhibit clear signs of heat stroke or heat exhaustion.

Exercise in the Cold

Exercise in the cold presents far fewer problems of a severe medical nature. Additional clothing can always be worn during the athletic contest to maintain the athlete in a warm and comfortable environment. The extremities, particularly the hands and feet, are most susceptible to discomfort and injury from exposure to cold.

As with heat, the temperature alone is not a valid index of the degree of stress felt by the individual. The wind creates a chill factor, and the more moist the surrounding air, the greater the physiological stress. A dry, still day at 10° F in the direct sun can be quite comfortable, yet on a moist, windy day with complete cloud cover at 40° F, the cold can be quite penetrating. Table 14-3 lists equivalent temperatures for various absolute, dry bulb temperatures and wind velocities.

The ability to acclimatize to cold is open to question. If acclimatization does occur as a result of repeated exposures, it seems to be of relatively little value with regard to athletic performance. Of much greater significance are the protective measures taken by physicians, trainers, and coaches to assure the most favorable circumstances for the athlete. Proper protective clothing is important. Tightly woven garments will help maintain a small heat pocket between the skin and clothing. Gloves, hats or caps, and double pairs of stockings are also helpful. Thermal underwear is recommended for the arms, legs, and torso in extreme cold, but as the temperature rises and metabolic heat builds, a serious heat problem could develop. Once the ath-

Table 14-3 Wind-chill factor chart.

Estimated wind speed (mph)	Actual thermometer reading (°F)											
	50	40	30	20	10	0	−10	−20	−30	−40	−50	−60
	Equivalent temperature (°F)											
Calm	50	40	30	20	10	0	−10	−20	−30	−40	−50	−60
5	48	37	27	16	6	−5	−15	−26	−36	−47	−57	−68
10	40	28	16	4	−9	−24	−33	−46	−58	−70	−83	−95
15	36	22	9	−5	−18	−32	−45	−58	−72	−85	−99	−112
20	32	18	4	−10	−25	−39	−53	−67	−82	−96	−110	−124
25	30	16	0	−15	−29	−44	−59	−74	−88	−104	−118	−133
30	28	13	−2	−18	−33	−48	−63	−79	−94	−109	−125	−140
35	27	11	−4	−20	−35	−51	−67	−82	−98	−113	−129	−145
40	26	10	−6	−21	−37	−53	−69	−85	−100	−116	−132	−148
	Green			Yellow			Red					
(Wind speeds greater than 40 mph have little additional effect.)	LITTLE DANGER (for properly clothed person). Maximum danger of false sense of security.			INCREASING DANGER Danger from freezing of exposed flesh.			GREAT DANGER					
Trenchfoot and immersion foot may occur at any point on this chart.												

*Adapted from *Runner's World*, 8 (1973):28. Reproduced by permission of the publisher.

lete starts to warm up and starts to sweat, he or she should remove excess clothing. Sweat-soaked clothing can create problems in a dry environment where evaporation occurs naturally with its resultant cooling effect.

ALTITUDE

With the selection of Mexico City as the site of the 1968 Olympic Games came a number of questions and a great deal of confusion as to what influence competition at 7,340 feet would have on athletic performance. Physiologists had been interested in altitude as a physiological stressor for a number of years prior to this time, but with the reality of Olympic competition only a few years away, physiologists, athletes, and coaches alike began to realize that little was known about athletic competition at moderate and high altitudes. Would performance in all activities suffer, or would altitude influence only the endurance activities? Would performance in the long jump, high jump, pole vault, shot put, javelin, discus, and hammer be improved due to the lower density of the surrounding air? Would those who live at altitude have an advantage when competing at altitudes, and if so, could the sea level resident move to altitude for several weeks or a month and achieve acclimatization? These and many other questions stimulated a great deal of research between 1963 and 1968, research which has continued to the present time.

Oxygen Transport

The major problem associated with competition at altitude is the reduced availability of oxygen at the tissue level. The surrounding air has the same percentage of oxygen as that found at sea level (20.93 percent), but due to the lower total pressure, the partial pressure of oxygen is reduced in inverse proportion to the increase in altitude. At sea level, the partial pressure of oxygen is 159 mmHg (760×0.2093), while at 8,000 feet the total pressure drops from 760 to 564 mmHg, and the partial pressure of oxygen drops to 118 mmHg. This only reduces the saturation of hemoglobin from 97 percent at sea level to approximately 92 percent at

8,000 feet. It was once thought that it was this small drop in saturation that reduced $\dot{V}O_2$ max approximately 15 percent at this altitude. However, it is also important to remember that the partial pressure of oxygen in the arterial blood drops from about 94 mmHg at sea level to 60 mmHg at 8,000 feet. Assuming a tissue partial pressure of 20 mmHg, the pressure differential drops from 74 to 40 mmHg, or nearly a 50 percent reduction in the diffusion gradient. If the tissue partial pressure were to drop to 10 mmHg, which may be possible for small localized areas of tissue under conditions of exhaustive exercise, the respective gradients would be 84 and 50, or a 40 percent reduction in the diffusion gradient. Since the diffusion gradient is responsible for driving the oxygen from the blood into the tissue, this is an even greater consideration than the small five-percent reduction in hemoglobin saturation.

From the data, it appears that the oxygen delivery system is restricted in direct proportion to the decrease in total pressure, or in inverse proportion to the altitude. Are similar decrements noted in performance and in the various physiological parameters assessed during exercise?

Physical Performance at Altitude

Sprint-type or anaerobic activities are generally not influenced to a great extent by altitude. These are activities that require only a matter of seconds for completion. Consequently, the demands on the oxygen transport system are minimal, which explains why performance is generally unaffected. It has been postulated that at the higher altitudes, 8,000 feet and above, sprint-type or throwing performances may even be enhanced due to the decreased air density, which reduces the frictional resistance of air to running, or to the objects being thrown. Limited experience tends to support this theory.

Activities requiring a longer duration, those with a higher aerobic component, are affected most by increases in altitude. It appears that the greater the aerobic component, the more the activity will be influenced by altitude, and the higher the altitude, the greater the decrement in performance. The decrement in performance is approxi-

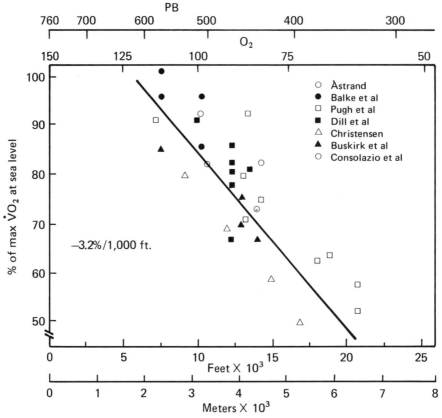

Figure 14-10   Reduction in maximal oxygen uptake in relation to increases in altitude, and a decrease in the barometric pressure (PB) and partial pressure of oxygen in the ambient air (pO₂). The symbols represent data of various authors (from Buskirk, et al., 1967).

mately proportional to the decrease in maximal oxygen uptake.

Physiological Function at Altitude

As previously mentioned, there is a reduction in maximal oxygen uptake in inverse proportion to the increase in altitude. This is illustrated in Figure 14-10. Consequently, at submaximal levels of work, the individual will be working at a higher percentage of his or her capacity. It also appears that the individual calls on his or her anaerobic metabolism, (reaches anaerobic threshold) at a much lower absolute level of work but probably at approximately the same relative level.

The pulmonary ventilation is increased at higher altitudes, both at rest and during exercise. Since the air at higher altitudes is less dense, the increase in ventilation is a compensatory mechanism to bring the same number of molecules of oxygen into the lung as the individual would take in at sea level. Since the number of molecules of oxygen for a given volume of air is less at higher altitudes, an additional volume of air is necessary to supply the same total number of molecules of oxygen. This increased ventilation acts much the same as hyperventilation at sea level, in that the carbon dioxide in the alveoli is reduced, causing more carbon dioxide to diffuse from the blood, which results in an increase in pH of the blood. This is referred to as a **respiratory alkalosis** and is compensated for by the kidneys where the excess bicarbonate is removed to normalize the blood pH.

The cardiovascular system also undergoes substantial changes to compensate for the increase in altitude and decrease in partial pressure of oxygen. The heart rate at standardized submaximal levels of work is elevated in direct proportion to the decrease in oxygen partial pressure. The stroke volume appears to be uninfluenced by altitude, since some studies have shown no change in stroke volume for the same absolute level of work when sea-level values are compared with values at different altitudes. However, this point is unresolved at the present time, since there are some studies which have also shown slight increases, as well as decreases, in stroke volume for the same level of work at higher altitudes as compared to sea level. This apparent conflict is probably the result of the methodological problems of obtaining accurate estimates of stroke volume from determinations of cardiac output. However, since the change in stroke volume, if real, is small at best, the elevated heart rate at submaximal levels of work results in an increase in cardiac output. Thus, since the amount of oxygen available to the tissues from a certain volume of blood is limited due to the reduced partial pressure of oxygen and the subsequent drop in diffusion gradient, a greater volume of blood is delivered to the exercising tissues.

This discussion of cardiovascular alterations refers only to submaximal levels of work. At maximal or exhaustive levels, the maximal stroke volume does not appear to be influenced, but the peak or maximal heart rate is reduced at higher altitudes. This results in a decrease in the maximal cardiac output. With a decrease in the diffusion gradient to push oxygen across the membrane from the blood into the tissues along with this reduction in maximal cardiac output, it is not difficult to understand why both maximal oxygen uptake ($\dot{V}O_2$ max) and performance in aerobic activities are affected by increases in altitude. The reason for the decrease in maximal heart rate is not known at the present time.

Acclimation. As one extends his or her exposure to altitude for days and weeks, the body gradually adjusts to the lower oxygen tension in the air. The athlete is never able to completely compensate for the increased elevation. While performance will improve with continued exposure, it will never reach the level that the athlete could attain at sea level, providing his or her general level of conditioning has not changed.

One of the first adaptations made at altitude is an increase in the number of circulating red blood cells. The actual amount of increase is not completely understood, however, as there is also a substantial loss in plasma volume due to a generalized dehydration. This causes a concentration of the existing red cells, referred to as hemoconcentration. Along with the increase in red cells there is an increase in hemoglobin. The net effect of both the red cell and hemoglobin increase is to increase the oxygen-carrying capacity of a fixed volume of blood.

The loss in plasma volume that occurs immediately upon arriving at a higher altitude is a transient response. After a week or more at this altitude, the plasma volume will start to increase back to sea-level values. Whether it fully returns to sea-level values is not clear on the basis of existing research. Several studies have shown a complete recovery, others have shown only a partial recovery, while still others have shown an increase above sea-level values.

Maximal oxygen uptake is decreased upon first reaching higher altitudes, but the adaptive changes in blood volume, red cell mass, and hemoglobin will gradually increase the maximal oxygen uptake, but not to the pre-altitude, sea-level values. Performance in activities of a predominantly aerobic nature will show a similar improvement as the athlete becomes acclimatized, but the ultimate performance will still be below that observed at sea level.

Altitude Training. Researchers in several early studies on the influence of altitude on athletic performance, trained athletes at higher altitudes and found, on returning to sea level, that their performances had improved over their pre-altitude, sea-level performances. Athletes themselves have noted similar improvements following altitude training. Frederick (1974) stated that altitude training has become a basic ingredient of success for many world-class distance runners. He further stated that every gold medal in the 1972 Munich Olympic Games, from the 1,500 meters through the marathon, was won by an altitude-trained athlete.

While these practical examples are impressive, they are not totally supported by controlled research studies. Several studies have shown no improvement in sea-level performance following altitude training. In several studies where altitude training was found to have an influence on post-altitude, sea-level performance, the subjects were not well-trained prior to going to altitude, so it is difficult to discern how much of their post-altitude improvement was due solely to training, independent of altitude.

The research literature is in apparent conflict on this matter. Even so, it is possible to construct a strong theoretical argument for altitude training. First, altitude training evokes a substantial tissue hypoxia (reduced oxygen supply), which is felt to be essential for initiating the conditioning response. Second, the major adaptations of increased red blood cell mass and hemoglobin levels will provide a major advantage with regard to oxygen delivery on return to sea level. While evidence suggests these latter changes are transient, lasting only several days, this would still provide an advantage for the athlete. Maximum ventilation volume appears to be enhanced, so does maximum cardiac output, although the latter is not well-documented. Putting all of these adaptations together would give the endurance athlete a distinct advantage upon returning to sea level.

Despite these theories, research studies do not support the idea that altitude training will improve sea-level performance. Studies by Adams, et al. (1975) have shown that there is no difference in the effects of hard endurance-training at 7,500 feet and equivalently severe sea-level training on $\dot{V}O_2$ max or two-mile performance time among runners who were already well-conditioned. This is not to say that training at altitude will not improve performance at altitude. To the contrary, after 20 weeks of training at altitude the runners showed marked improvements in their performance at altitude. Sea-level performance, on the other hand, was unchanged as a result of the altitude training.

There is no evidence to support the concept that breathing gases low in oxygen content for brief periods of exercise (one to two hours/day) will induce even a partial adaptation to altitude. It has, however, been demonstrated that this procedure may enhance the maximal exercise-breathing capacity. Since most athletes cannot afford the time or expense involved in long stays at altitude, it is pertinent to consider the value of intermittent visits to altitude on acclimation. Daniels and Oldridge (1970) observed that alternate periods of training at 7,500 feet (seven to 14 days per session) and at sea level (five to 11 days each) were adequate stimuli for altitude acclimation. Sea-level stays of up to 11 days did not interfere with the usual adjustments to altitude as long as training was maintained.

Athletes who wish to prepare for competition at moderate altitude must realize:

1. Full adaptation may require several months
2. Work capacity will be reduced during the initial days at altitude
3. The rate of acclimatization is unaffected by brief periods at sea level
4. Short exposure to gases containing reduced levels of oxygen will not stimulate adaptation to altitude
5. Sea-level performance is not improved by altitude training in runners who are already well-trained.

What about the athlete who normally trains at sea level and must compete at altitude? What can he or she do to prepare most effectively for competition? While the research is not clear on all aspects of this question, it appears that the athlete should either compete within 24 hours of arrival at higher altitudes, or train at higher altitudes for at least two weeks prior to competition. Even two weeks, however, is not sufficient for total acclimatization. That would require a minimum of four to six weeks. Competing within the initial 24 hours does not provide much in the way of acclimatization, but the exposure is brief enough that the classic symptoms of altitude sickness have not become totally manifest.

When training at higher altitudes, the coach or athlete should select an altitude between 5,000 and 10,000 feet, since the former is considered the lowest level at which an effect will be noticed, and the latter is the highest level for efficient conditioning. When first reaching higher altitudes, the magnitude of the workout should be reduced to between approximately 60 and 70 percent of the intensity of the sea-level workout schedule, gradually working up to a full workout within ten to fourteen days. Symptoms of altitude sickness, such as shortness of breath, headache, dizziness, nausea, and disturbed sleep, may persist for a few days, but they will gradually disappear.

AIR POLLUTION

During the past fifteen years, there has been increasing concern relative to the possible problems associated with exercising in polluted air. Ambient air in many cities is contaminated with small quantities of gases and particulates that are not among its normal constituents. When air becomes stagnant or when a temperature inversion occurs, some of these air pollutants reach levels of concentration that produce significant detrimental effects on athletic performance. Carbon monoxide, photochemical oxidants, and sulfur oxides are the major contaminants of concern.

Carbon monoxide is essentially an odorless gas that is rapidly absorbed from inspired air due to the high affinity of hemoglobin for carbon monoxide. The affinity of hemoglobin for carbon monoxide is approximately 240 times greater than its affinity for oxygen. Several studies have reported an inverse, linear decrease in $\dot{V}O_2$ max with increases in blood levels of carbon monoxide, and the blood levels of carbon monoxide are a direct function of the levels of carbon monoxide in the inspired air. Literature reviews in 1979 (Raven) and 1984 (Folinsbee and Raven) of this topic concluded that the reduction in $\dot{V}O_2$ max is not statistically significant until blood carbon monoxide levels exceed 4.3 percent, although performance time on the treadmill has been found reduced at levels as low as 2.7 percent. Submaximal performance does not appear to be greatly affected until the blood levels exceed 15 percent. This would correspond to oxygen uptake values between 35 and 60 percent of maximum.

Ozone is the primary photochemical oxidant that produces many subjective complaints when breathed at high ambient levels of concentration.

Eye irritation, chest tightness, a feeling of breathlessness, coughing, and a feeling of nausea are the primary complaints. Ozone has its primary influence on the lungs and respiratory tract. Decrements in lung function occur with increasing concentrations of ozone, as well as with increases in time of exposure and level of ventilation. $\dot{V}O_2$ max has been found to be significantly decreased following two hours of intermittent exercise exposure to 0.75 parts/million (ppm) of ozone. This decrease in $\dot{V}O_2$ max is thought to be associated with a reduced oxygen transfer at the lung resulting from a reduced alveolar air exchange.

Sulfur dioxide is the major sulfur oxide contaminant of concern during exercise. While the research on sulfur dioxide and exercise is limited, it is certain that ambient levels above 1.0 ppm will cause significant discomfort and will prove detrimental to performance (Raven, 1979). Sulfur dioxide is primarily an upper-airway and bronchial irritant.

Certain cities have initiated air pollution or smog alerts. These are usually color-coded with the colors indicating the degree of severity of pollution. Standards need to be established nationally, and the air monitored accordingly. Increasing evidence is pointing to the wisdom of canceling all games and practices when pollution levels reach a certain point. Hopefully, current and future research will provide a clearer understanding of the limitations imposed by air pollutants.

EXERCISE IN THE WATER

As one takes to water, an entirely different physical and physiological environment is encountered, which requires a full understanding on the part of swimmers and divers. As they descend below the surface of water, the swimmer is subjected to an increasing pressure; while at higher altitudes, the problem is one of a decreasing pressure. Fresh water weighs 62.4 pounds per cubic foot while salt water, due to the salt content, weighs 64.0 pounds per cubic foot. Descending to a level of 33 feet produces 14.7 pounds per square inch (psi) pressure on the diver from the water alone. Since the atmosphere provides an additional 14.7 psi, the total pressure on the diver would be 29.4 psi (water pressure plus air pressure). As the diver descends to 66 feet, the water pressure doubles from 14.7 to 29.4 psi which, when added to the air pressure of 14.7 psi, makes a total pressure of 44.1 psi. While this increased pressure has little direct effect on body fluids, air in the lungs, sinus, and intestinal tract are compressed. Air taken into the lungs at the surface of the water will be compressed to one-half its volume at a depth of 33 feet. Conversely, air taken into the lungs at a 33-foot depth will expand to twice its original volume by the time the swimmer reaches the surface. If breathing from a self-contained underwater breathing apparatus (SCUBA), it would be extremely dangerous for the diver to take in a deep breath at a depth of 33 feet and to hold this breath as he or she ascended to the surface. As illustrated in Figure 14–11, over-

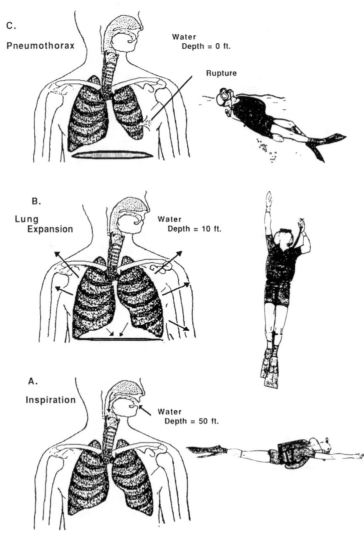

Figure 14–11 Changes in lung volume during ascent and descent in the water.

distension of the lung would result in rupturing the aveoli and pulmonary hemorrhage. If air bubbles end up in the circulatory system as a result of this extensive damage, emboli develop and can block major vessels, leading to extensive tissue damage, if not death. Thus, it is important for the diver to always blow out or exhale as he or she ascends to the surface.

An additional factor that must be considered relative to the increased pressure with dives is the increased partial pressure of the individual gases—oxygen, nitrogen, and carbon dioxide. Breathing air at a depth of 33 feet doubles the partial pressure of each of the gases. At depths approaching 100 feet, the partial pressures are four times greater than on the surface. It is at 100 feet, when breathing air, that problems of nitrogen narcosis develop. Nitrogen narcosis is known as the "rapture of the deep." The diver develops symptoms similar to those of alcohol intoxication, in which the effect is primarily on the central nervous system. Judgment is distorted, and foolish decisions frequently result in serious injury, or death.

Another problem caused by the high partial pressures at the lower depths is oxygen poisoning. Breathing high concentrations of oxygen for long periods of time during deep dives drives a great deal of oxygen into solution. The oxygen in solution is used preferentially over that carried in combination with hemoglobin in the red blood cell. Consequently, oxygen is not released from the red cell and a carrier is not available to remove the CO_2 produced. An excess of both O_2 and CO_2 develops in the tissues, causing visual distortion, confusion, rapid and shallow breathing, and convulsions. The use of oxygen in diving is to be avoided whenever possible.

The high partial pressures of nitrogen in diving will force nitrogen into the blood and tissues. If the diver attempts to ascend too rapidly, this additional nitrogen cannot be delivered to and released through the lungs quickly enough, and it becomes trapped as bubbles in the circulatory system and tissues, causing discomfort and pain. While the joints and ligaments are most often involved, occasionally emboli can form in the circulatory system causing more serious complications. This is referred to as decompression sickness, or the bends. Treatment involves placing the diver into a recom-

pression chamber, where the pressure of nitrogen is increased again and then gradually returned to the ambient pressure. This period of recompression forces the nitrogen back into solution and the gradual decrease in pressure then allows the nitrogen to escape through the respiratory system. To prevent this condition, charts have been created that provide the necessary information relative to the time sequence for ascending from various depths. Strict adherence to the respective timetable for the depth submerged will allow a safe ascent without the problem of decompression sickness.

One last word of caution: annually, a number of deaths result from underwater swimming. Typically, the diver forcefully hyperventilates and then attempts to swim as far as possible on a single breath of air. Unfortunately, the individual may lose consciousness and drown before realizing he or she is in trouble and needs to come to the surface for a breath of air. In hyperventilating, the carbon dioxide levels are greatly reduced. Since carbon dixoide is a potent stimulus for breathing, its reduction in the blood decreases the stimulus for breathing and the oxygen concentration drops below critical levels, resulting in a loss of consciousness. While hyperventilation will allow new records to be set in underwater swimming, it is a practice that must be strongly discouraged because of this inherent danger.

SUMMARY

Frequently, athletic competition is conducted under environmental conditions that are less than optimal. Heat, cold, humidity, altitude, air pollution, and underwater swimming each present unique problems for the athlete, which need not seriously handicap performance if he or she understands the situation and plans in advance the proper preventive and precautionary procedures.

This chapter attempts to briefly summarize the nature of these various environmental stresses and to provide the coach and athlete with suggestions for coping with them more successfully. In hot environments, performance is compromised in proportion to the severity of the heat stress. Evaporation becomes the most important avenue of heat loss, but this presents potential problems of dehydration if the fluid loss is not rapidly replaced. As the humidity increases, the problem becomes considerably more serious. Practicing in the heat for a week or two will almost fully acclimatize the athlete to the heat stress. In addition, ingestion of fluids before practice, and frequently during practice and competition, will reduce the degree of heat stress and aid performance. In cold environments, acclimatization does not significantly contribute to the athlete's performance, but proper clothing can play a major role. It is important to dress warmly but not to overdress, for this can cause heat stress.

Altitude directly influences the oxygen transport system. As the altitude increases, the total atmospheric pressure decreases, and this results in a proportional decrease in the partial pressure of the respiratory gases. The decrease in the partial pressure of oxygen reduces slightly the degree of saturation of the arterial blood with oxygen, but more importantly, it decreases the partial pressure of oxygen in the arterial blood, thus substantially lowering the diffusion gradient between the blood and active tissues. The result is a decreased maximal oxygen uptake and a decrement in performances of an aerobic nature. Acclimatization will reduce the magnitude of these performance decreases but will not totally overcome the influences of altitude—performance will not equal that at sea level. There appears to be little or no benefit associated with altitude training with respect to subsequent performance at sea level.

Air pollution is another area of concern relative to athletic performance. Carbon monoxide, ozone, and sulfur dioxide are the primary contaminants that can have a detrimental effect on athletic performance when their concentrations reach critical threshold levels. Activities of an endurance nature are those primarily affected.

Lastly, diving involves another unique environment for performance in which the major consideration is the increased pressure under the surface of the water. This increased pressure will have a substantial influence on the breathing pattern of the diver and will also affect the amounts of nitrogen and oxygen that are driven into solution in the tissues and blood. If these are too great, they can lead to problems of nitrogen narcosis, decompression sickness, and oxygen poisoning.

STUDY QUESTIONS

1. What are the four major pathways available for loss of body heat?
2. Which of the above four pathways is most important for controlling body temperature during exercise and under resting conditions?
3. What happens to the body temperature during exercise, and why?
4. Why is humidity an important factor when performing in the heat?
5. What is the purpose of a wet globe thermometer (WBGT)? What does it measure?
6. What is the relationship between dehydration and increasing body temperature during exercise?
7. How important is fluid ingestion before and during practice or competition in the heat?
8. What physiological adaptations occur allowing one to acclimate to exercise in the heat?
9. Differentiate between heat cramps, heat exhaustion, and heat stroke.
10. What factors should be considered to provide maximum protection when exercising in the cold?
11. How does altitude influence athletic performance? Does it influence all sports or events to the same degree?
12. Physiologically, how does altitude affect endurance performance?
13. Would an endurance athlete profit by training at altitude with respect to subsequent sea-level performance? Why or why not?
14. With underwater diving, what specific problems must one be aware of to avoid serious injury or death?
15. How is endurance-exercise performance affected by high concentrations of air pollutants?

REFERENCES

Adams, W. C., Bernauer, E. M., Dill, D. B., & Bomar, J. B. (1975). Effects of equivalent sea-level and altitude training on $\dot{V}O_2$ and running performance. *Journal of Applied Physiology, 39,* 262-266.

Armstrong, L., Costill, D. L., & Fink, W. J. (1985). Influence of diuretic-induced dehydration on competitive running performance. *Medicine and Science in Sports and Exercise, 17,* 456-460.

Åstrand, P. O., & Rodahl, K. (1986). *Textbook of work physiology* (3rd ed.). New York: McGraw-Hill Book Co.

Balke, B. (1968). Variation in altitude and its effect on exercise performance. In H. B. Falls (Ed.) *Exercise physiology.* New York: Academic Press.

Buskirk, E. R., Kollias, J., Piconreatique, E., Akers, R., Prokop, E., & Baker, P. (1967). In R. F. Goddard (Ed.), *The effects of altitude on physical performance,* pp. 65-71. Chicago: Athletic Institute.

Costill, D. L., Kammer, W. F., & Fisher, A. (1970). Fluid ingestion during distance running. *Archives of Environmental Health, 21,* 520-525.

Costill, D. L. (1974). Hazards of the heat. In *The complete runner.* Mountain View, CA: World Publications.

Costill, D. L. (1979). *A scientific approach to distance running.* Los Altos, CA: Track and Field News.

deVries, H. A. (1974). *Physiology of exercise for physical education and athletics* (2nd ed). Dubuque, IA: William C. Brown Co.

Daniels, J., & Oldridge, N. (1970). Effects of alternate exposure to altitude and sea level on world-class middle-distance runners. *Medicine and Science in Sports, 2,* 107-112.

Fink, W., Costill, D. L., Van Handel, P., & Getchell, L. (1975). Leg muscle metabolism during exercise in the heat and cold. *European Journal of Applied Physiology, 34,* 183-190.

Folinsbee, L. J., Wagner, J. A., Borgia, J. F., Drinkwater, B. L., Gliner, J. A., & Bedi, J. F. (Eds.). (1978). *Environmental stress: Individual human adaptations.* New York: Academic Press.

Folinsbee, L. J., & Raven, P. B. (1984). Exercise and air pollution. *Journal of Sports Sciences, 2,* 57-75.

Fox, E. L. (1979). *Sport physiology.* Philadelphia: W. B. Saunders Co.

Fox, E. L. (1980). *The physiological basis of physical education and athletics.* (3rd ed.). Philadelphia: W. B. Saunders Co.

Frederick, E. C. (1974). Training at altitude. In *The complete runner.* Mountain View, CA: World Publications.

Gisolfi, C. V. (1975). Exercise, heat, and dehydration don't mix. *Rx for Sports and Travel, 2,* 23-25.

Karpovich, P. V., & Sinning, W. E. (1971). *Physiology of muscular activity* (7th ed.). Philadelphia: W. B. Saunders Co.

King, D. S., Costill, D. L., Fink, W. J., Hargreaves, M., & Fielding, R. A. (1985). Muscle metabolism during exercise in the heat in unacclimatized and acclimatized humans. *Journal of Applied Physiology, 59,* 1350-1354.

Lenfant, C., & Sullivan, K. (1971). Adaptation to high altitude. *New England Journal of Medicine, 284,* 1298-1309.

Margaria, R. (Ed.). (1967). *Exercise at altitude.* Amsterdam: Excerpta Medica Foundation.

Nadel, E. R. (Ed.) (1977). *Problems with temperature regulation during exercise.* New York: Academic Press.

Raven, P. B. (1979). Heat and air pollution: The cardiac patient. In M. L. Pollock & D. H. Schmidt (Eds.), *Heart disease and rehabilitation.* Boston: Houghton Mifflin.

Robertshaw, D. (1977). *Environmental physiology II.* Baltimore: University Park Press.

Sharkey, B. J. (1979). *Physiology of fitness.* Champaign, IL: Human Kinetics Publishers.

Tipton, C. M., Zambraski, D. J., & Tcheng, T. K. (1974). Iowa wrestling study: Lessons for physicians. *Rx for Sports and Travel, 1,* 19-22.

Van Handel, P. (1974). Drinks for the road. *Runner's World, 9,* 29-31.

SECTION D

Special Considerations

This section deals with special considerations, focusing on those unique needs and concerns facing the child and young athlete; the older individual and the masters athlete; and the girl, woman, and female athlete. Much of what has been discussed throughout this book is directly applicable to each of these special populations. However, there are a number of issues that have not been discussed, and others that require further elaboration, that apply directly to one or more of these three distinct groups.

Chapter 15 discusses the child and the young athlete. How do you train a youngster? Is weight training appropriate for this age group? What growth and development concerns should we have when working with this population? Do the physiological systems grow and develop in concert, or do they have their own unique patterns? The older individual and the masters athlete are the topics of Chapter 16. Is it possible to continue to compete when you are in your 40s? 50s? 60s? 70s? or even in your 80s? What special concerns do we have when training the older individual? How do older people adapt to training; do they differ significantly from younger people? Chapter 17 will discuss the girl, woman, and female athlete. What physical limitations should be placed on the developing girl, the young woman athlete, the older woman athlete? Are women biologically inferior to men with respect to athletic ability? How can we explain performance differences between the sexes when they are equally matched by training status. Chapter 18 addresses the issue of physical activity for health and fitness. How important is it to be active throughout your life? Are there health risks associated with a sedentary lifestyle? This chapter looks specifically at the role of physical activity in the prevention and treatment of cardiovascular diseases, heart disease in particular, and obesity. This is followed by a discussion of how to get started on an exercise program, detailing those factors that constitute the exercise prescription. The final chapter deals with the assessment of human performance, providing detailed information on how the various components of fitness and performance are measured.

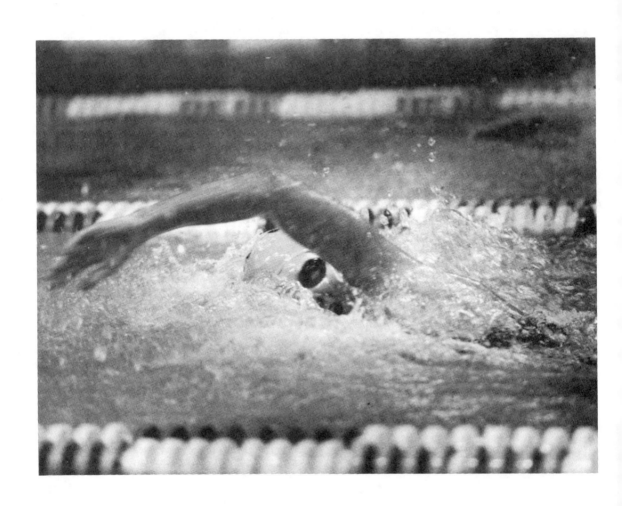

15

The Young Athlete

INTRODUCTION

Age-group competition has grown considerably over the last decade and is now a major force in the world of sport. Little League baseball and Pop Warner football are examples of this type of sport or activity for boys, as is Bobby Sox and Little League softball for girls, and mini-bike racing, swimming, track and field, and long-distance running for youngsters of both sexes.

With this tremendous interest in age–group competition, many questions have been raised. Is competition physically or psychologically harmful for the preadolescent? Should preadolescents be competing in long-distance running, or in strength training activities? Does pitching a baseball place traumatic stress on the elbow of the youngster's pitching arm? These and many other questions of a similar nature will be addressed in this chapter as we focus attention on the growth and development process.

GROWTH AND DEVELOPMENT OF THE TISSUES

This section will address those issues related to height and to the growth and development of selected tissues of the body. The focus will be on those areas of greatest concern to the child during sport and activity.

Height and Bone

During the first two years of life there is a rapid increase in height, with 50 percent of adult height reached by the age of two years. This is followed during childhood by a progressive decline in the rate of change in height. Just prior to puberty, there is a marked increase in the rate of change in height, followed by an exponential decrease until full height is attained at a mean age of 16½ years in girls and 18 years in boys. These trends are illustrated in Figure 15–1 on page 290.

The characteristics and development of bone were discussed in detail in Chapter 1. There is a wide variation in the average age at which the different bones reach full growth or maturity, ranging from the preteens to the early twenties. On the average, girls achieve full maturity of their bones several years before boys. Exercise is regarded as essential for proper bone growth. While exercise appears to have little or no influence on the growth in length of long bones, it does increase the width of bone, gives the bone greater tensile strength, and lays down more mineral in the bone matrix.

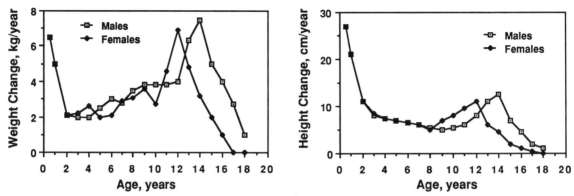

Figure 15–1 Changes in the rate of change in weight and height with age in both males and females between the ages of 6 months and 18 years.

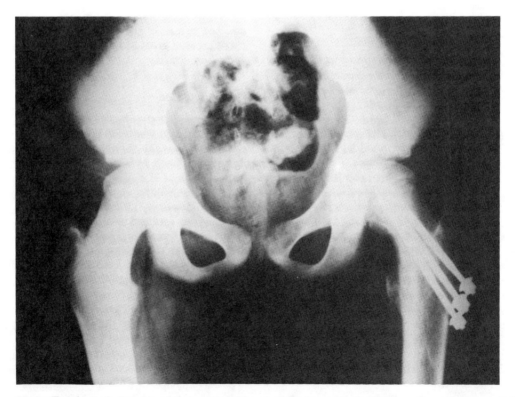

Figure 15–2 Epiphyseal slippage at the proximal head of the femur in the left leg of an eight-year-old girl injured while playing competitive soccer (from Murray Robertson, M.D., Tucson, AZ, with permission).

In this chapter, we are interested in the process of bone growth primarily for the purpose of understanding the potential for injury. An injury to an immature bone could result in the premature cessation of growth, resulting in a shorter bone. Disruption of the growth of the femur, as an example, would lead to a difference in the lengths of the two legs, with the involved leg being much shorter. The greatest concern is with the potential for injury at the epiphyses, since a fracture at the epiphysis and growth plate could disturb the blood supply and disrupt the growth process. Fortunately, such injuries are relatively rare and seldom occur in sports. In one study of 31 epiphyseal injuries, only 23 percent were sports-induced, the remainder resulting from falls and vehicular accidents (Larson, 1974). Figure 15-2 illustrates a slipped epiphysis of the distal head of the femur in an eight-year-old girl, whose presenting symptoms were initially diagnosed as a groin pull. The injury occurred during a championship soccer match.

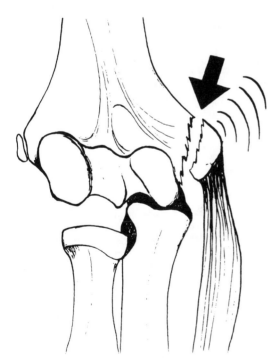

Figure 15-3 An example of a separation of the epiphysis (from Larson, 1974).

One type of serious epiphyseal injury that occurs in athletics is called **traumatic epiphysitis.** One form is "Little Leaguer's elbow," a condition resulting from repetitive strains to the medial epicondylar epiphysis of the humerus. According to Larson, studies have shown that 12-year-old boys can throw a baseball up to 70 mph. This can cause a sudden pull on the epiphysis, which anchors the tendons of the involved muscles, which may result in its separation (see Figure 15-3). The repetitive stress of throwing may produce an inflammatory response, referred to as traumatic epiphysitis. In a well-controlled study published in 1965, Adams found epiphysitis by X-ray examination in all 80 pitchers in a group of 162 young boys, while only a small percentage of the nonpitchers and the control group of nonplayers exhibited similar changes. Subsequent studies have not substantiated this initial study, in that a much lower percentage of those with epiphysitis has been reported.

Larson and McMahan (1966) reviewed 1,338 consecutive athletic injuries seen by a group of four orthopedists in one major sports medicine practice. They reported that 20 percent of these injuries were in the age range of 14 years and younger. Only six percent of all injuries in 15-year-olds and younger involved the epiphysis. They also stated that this type of injury does not always result in crippling, or permanent, trauma and that early recognition is important.

Of all the sports, competitive baseball appears to be the most dangerous because of its potential for serious injuries, which largely result from the pitching motion. Some leagues have replaced the pitcher with a pitching machine. This would seem to be the only sensible approach until the youngster reaches an age at which pitching is not a major source of injury. Pop Warner football and the other competitive sports and activities have a relatively good record with regard to bone injury. While the potential for injury in football is generally considered high, apparently the small size of the player, the matching of children by size, and good protective equipment provide a relatively safe environment for the young football player. Inappropriate equipment, and mismatching players by size and ability, creates an environment with a high potential for injury.

Muscle

The ultrastructure and growth characteristics of muscle tissue were discussed in detail in Chapter 1. From birth through adolescence there is a steady increase in the muscle mass of the body that parallels the youngster's gain in weight. The total muscle mass in males increases from 25 percent of body weight at birth to 40 percent or more in the adult. Much of this gain occurs at puberty, when there is a peak acceleration in the development of muscle, which corresponds to the sudden, approximately tenfold increase in testosterone production. Girls do not experience this period of rapid acceleration at puberty, but their muscle mass does continue to increase at a rate considerably below that of boys. Once a girl reaches puberty, her estrogen levels increase, which promotes the deposition of body fat. The increases in muscle mass with age appear to result primarily from hypertrophy of existing fibers, with little or no hyperplasia (increase in fiber number). The hypertrophy is the result of increases in the myofilaments and myofibrils. As bones grow in length, muscle length increases. Increases in the number of sarcomeres, which are added at the junction of muscle and tendon, and increases in the length of existing sarcomeres, result in this increase in muscle length.

When the female reaches 16 to 18 years of age and the male 18 to 22 years, the muscle mass is at its peak, unless it is increased further through exercise, diet, or both. The muscle mass will remain relatively stable from this age through the ages of 30 to 40 years, if physical activity levels remain constant and do not decrease. With older age, there is a decrease in the total muscle mass, which may result from both atrophy of selected muscle fibers, generally Type II, and a decrease in the number of muscle fibers. The decrease in fibers may be the result of nerve fiber degeneration.

Fat

Fat cells form and fat starts to deposit in these cells early in the development of the fetus and continues indefinitely. Each fat cell has the ability to increase in size at any age, from birth to death. Initial studies suggested that the number of fat cells became fixed early in life, thus it was considered important to keep the total fat content of the body low during this early period of development. In this way, the total number of fat cells would be minimized, and the chances of extreme obesity as an adult would be greatly reduced. More recent evidence, however, suggested that fat cells can continue to increase in number throughout life (Bjorntorp, 1986). The most recent evidence suggests that as fat is added to the body, existing fat cells continue to fill with fat to a certain critical level, at which point new cells are formed from pre-

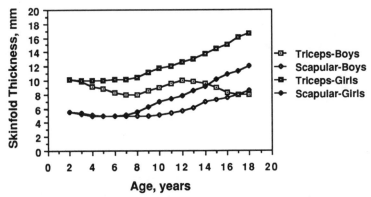

Figure 15-4 Changes in triceps and subscapular skinfold thickness (subcutaneous fat) with age, from 2 years to 18 years (data from the NHANES-I, National Center for Health Statistics).

adipocytes of undifferentiated cells. Thus, it is important to maintain good dietary and exercise habits throughout life!

The degree of fat accumulation with growth and aging will depend entirely on your dietary and exercise habits, in addition to heredity. While heredity is unchangeable, diet and exercise can be manipulated to either increase or decrease the fat stores. At birth, 10 to 12 percent of your body weight is fat, and by the time you reach physical maturity, the fat content reaches 15 to 25 percent of the total body weight for males and females, respectively. Figure 15-4 illustrates the relationship between subcutaneous fat at the triceps and subscapular sites, and age for males and females, with subcutaneous fat being representative of total body fat.

Nervous System

As the child grows, he or she develops better agility and coordination, which is a direct function of the development of both the central and peripheral nervous systems. During the early stages of development, myelination of the nerve fibers must be completed before fast reactions and skilled movement can occur. Conduction velocity along a nerve fiber is considerably slower if myelination is absent or incomplete. Late in life, as aging progresses, conduction velocity along a nerve fiber may tend to slow. Speed of reaction and movement both decrease with aging due to an increased conduction velocity in the peripheral nervous system, both sensory and motor.

GENERAL PERFORMANCE AND PHYSIOLOGICAL FUNCTION

In almost all of the physiological systems, function appears to improve until maturity, or shortly before, and then plateaus for a period of time, before starting to decline with old age. This section will focus on changes in motor ability, strength, cardiovascular function, aerobic capacity, and anaerobic capacity that accompany the growth and development process.

Motor Ability

The motor skill ability of boys and girls generally increases with age, from six years to 17 years, although girls tend to plateau at about the age of puberty for most items tested. This is illustrated in Figure 15-5 on page 294 and Figure 17-5 on page 327. These improvements are the result of the development of the neuromuscular and endocrine systems that occur with growth and development, and secondarily to the increased activity patterns of these children. The plateau observed in the girls at puberty is most likely explained by two factors. With puberty, the increase in estrogen levels, or in the estrogen/testosterone ratio, leads to a greater deposition of body fat. As fat levels increase, performance tends to decrease. Probably of greater importance, however, is the fact that many girls assume a much more sedentary lifestyle coincident with puberty. As these girls become less active and more sedentary, their motor abilities tend to plateau.

Strength

Changes in strength with age parallel the increases that occur in muscle mass. Peak strength is usually attained by the age of 20 years in females and between 20 and 30 years in males. Rather marked increases in strength occur at the time of puberty in the male resulting from sudden changes in the hormonal status, up to tenfold increases in the androgens, that lead to increased deposition of muscle. Brooks and Fahey (1984) have also made the important observation that the extent of the development and performance of muscle is dependent on the relative maturation of the nervous system. High levels of strength, power, and skill are impossible if the child has not reached neural maturity. Since myelination of nerves is incomplete until sexual maturity, the neural control of muscle function will be limited. Figure 15-6 on page 294 illustrates changes in leg strength in a group of boys from the Medford Growth Study followed longitudinally for a period of 12 years, from the age of eight years to 18 years. There is a noticeable increase in the rate of strength gain at about the age of 12 years, which is coincident with the onset of puberty. Similar longitudinal data for girls is

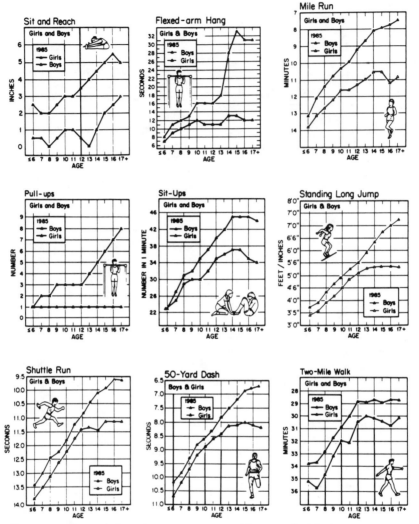

Figure 15-5 Changes in means of performance scores of boys and girls from ages 6 to 17 years (data from the President's Council on Physical Fitness and Sports, 1985).

not available. From cross-sectional data, however, girls experience a more gradual increase in strength, and do not exhibit a marked change in the rate of strength gain with puberty.

Basal Metabolic Rate (BMR)

The BMR, or lowest metabolic rate that the individual attains during a 24-hour day, decreases at a rate of approximately three percent per decade from the age of three through 80. Longitudinal studies that have followed the same individuals over 20-year periods, or longer, suggest a more conservative decrease of only one to two percent per decade. Up to the age of 20 to 30 years, this decrease is assumed to reflect a more efficient metabolism. Beyond 30 years of age, this decrease could be a result of the decrease in lean body

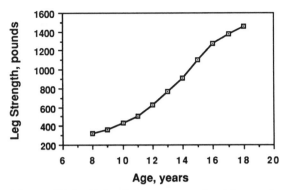

Figure 15-6 Gains in leg strength with age in young boys followed longitudinally over a 12-year period. Data from the Medford Growth Study (from Clarke, H. H., 1971).

The changes in these volumes and flow rates are matched by the changes in maximal ventilatory capacity during exhaustive exercise. Maximal expiratory ventilation ($\dot{V}E$ max) will increase with age to the point of physical maturity, and then it will decrease with the aging process. From cross-sectional data for males, the $\dot{V}E$ max, for four- to six-year-old boys, will average about 40 liters per min, increase to from 110 to 140 liters per min at full maturity, and decrease from 60 to 80 liters per min for 60- to 70-year-olds. Females follow the same general pattern, although their absolute values will be considerably lower for each age level, due, primarily, to their smaller stature.

Cardiovascular Function

A number of changes occur in cardiovascular function as the child ages. There is a linear decrease in maximal heart rate with age. Young children, under ten years of age, frequently exceed 210 beats per min, while the average 20-year-old has a maximal heart rate of approximately 195 beats per min. It has been estimated that the maximal heart rate decreases by slightly less than one beat per year as the individual ages. The submaximal heart rate response to the same absolute rate of work on a cycle ergometer is higher in the child compared to the adult. This higher submaximal heart rate is a partial compensation for a lower stroke volume which results from a smaller heart size and smaller total blood volume. As the child ages, heart size and blood volume will increase parallel with increases in body size, and stroke volume will thereby increase for the same absolute rate of work. The higher submaximal heart rate does not totally compensate for the lower stroke volume in the child, thus the cardiac output will be somewhat lower in the child compared to the adult for the same absolute rate of work. The child, to maintain adequate oxygen uptake for these submaximal levels of work, further compensates by increasing the arterio-mixed venous oxygen difference. These submaximal relationships are illustrated in Figure 15-7. Blood pressure at rest and during submaximal levels of exercise is lower in the child compared to the adult, but will progressively increase to reach adult values during late pubescence.

weight. It would be interesting to determine if physically active individuals, particularly those performing heavy-resistance exercise on a regular basis, have this same decrease in BMR. Likewise, it would be interesting to determine whether increasing muscle mass through heavy-resistance weight training would increase the BMR in older people. An increased BMR might reduce the degree of fat accumulation that seems to accompany the aging process.

Pulmonary Function

A number of cross-sectional studies have demonstrated that lung function is markedly altered by age. During the period of growth, the static lung volumes, as well as the volumes determined during functional pulmonary tests, increase to the time of physical maturity. Shortly after reaching this peak, however, there is a gradual reduction with age. Vital capacity, $FEV_{1.0}$ (the greatest volume of air that can be exhaled in the first second of a forced vital capacity test), residual volume, and forced expiratory flow rate, all exhibit a linear increase with age, up to the age of 20 to 30 years. These changes are associated with the growth in size of the pulmonary system, which parallels the growth patterns of the child.

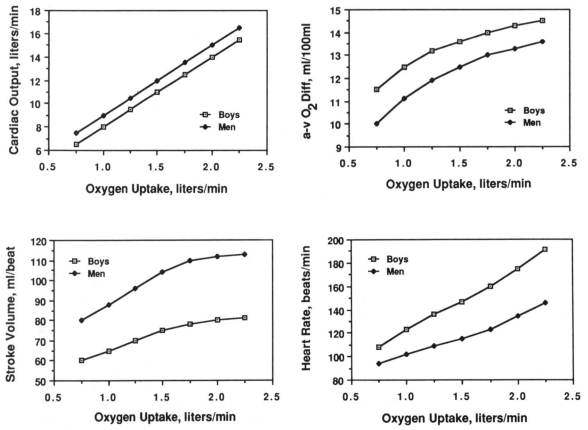

Figure 15-7 Submaximal heart rate, stroke volume, cardiac output, and arterio-venous oxygen difference in boys and men at fixed rates of oxygen uptake.

Blood flow to active muscle may be increased during exercise in the child as compared to the adult, due to a reduced peripheral resistance.

During maximal levels of exercise, the smaller heart of the child limits the maximal stroke volume that can be achieved. While the child has a higher maximal heart rate, this higher rate is unable to fully compensate for the lower maximal stroke volume, thus maximal cardiac output is lower in the child. This will be a limitation in the performance of high absolute rates of work, such as a fixed rate of work on a cycle ergometer, since the capacity for oxygen delivery will be less. However, for high relative rates of work, where the child is only responsible for moving his or her body mass, this will not be as serious a limitation.

Maximal Aerobic Capacity

The purpose of the basic pulmonary and cardiovascular adaptations that are made in response to varying levels of exercise, or rates of work, is to accommodate the need of the exercising muscles for oxygen. Thus, the increases in pulmonary and cardiovascular function with growth suggest that aerobic capacity, or $\dot{V}O_2$ max, experiences a similar increase with age. Robinson, in 1938, demonstrated this phenomenon in a cross-sectional sample of boys and men ranging in age from six to 91 years. He found that $\dot{V}O_2$ max attained its peak value at 17 to 20 years of age and then decreased as a linear function of age. Others have subsequently reported results that confirm these origi-

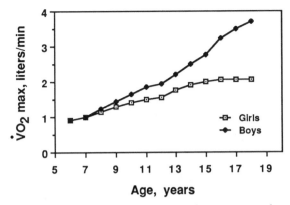

Figure 15-8 Changes in maximal oxygen uptake with age with values expressed in liters $\cdot$ min^{-1}.

nal observations. Studies of girls and women have shown essentially the same trend, although the female starts her decline at a much younger age (refer to Chapter 17), probably due to an earlier assumption of a sedentary lifestyle. The changes in $\dot{V}O_2$ max with age, expressed in liters$\cdot$min^{-1}, are illustrated in Figure 15-8.

When $\dot{V}O_2$ max values are expressed relative to body weight, a considerably different picture emerges (see Figure 15-9). Values appear to change very little in boys from the age of six years to young adulthood. For girls, however, there appears to be little or no change from six years to 13

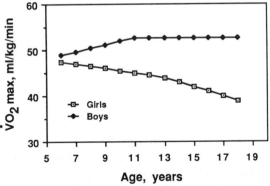

Figure 15-9 Changes in maximal oxygen uptake with age with values expressed relative to body weight (ml $\cdot$ kg^{-1} $\cdot$ min^{-1}).

years, but from 13 years to young adulthood there is a gradual decrease in aerobic capacity.

How do these changes in aerobic capacity with growth affect the child's performance? For any activity that requires a fixed rate of work, for example, cycling on an ergometer, the low $\dot{V}O_2$ max expressed in absolute liters$\cdot$min^{-1} will present limitations to endurance performance. However, for activities where the body weight is the major resistance to movement, as in distance running, the child should not be at a disadvantage, since his or her $\dot{V}O_2$ max, expressed relative to body weight, is already at or near adult values. Does this mean that a child should be able to run as fast as an adult? The answer to this question is "no," due to basic differences in mechanical efficiency between the child and the adult. For the same speed on a treadmill, the child will have a substantially higher submaximal oxygen consumption. If the child's lactate threshold occurred at the same relative oxygen consumption as an adult (the same percentage of their respective $\dot{V}O_2$ max), the child would be running at a much slower pace.

Anaerobic Capacity

The child has limited ability to perform anaerobic types of activities. This is demonstrated in several ways. First, the child is not able to achieve adult concentrations of lactate in either muscle or blood for submaximal, maximal, and supramaximal rates of exercise. It has been suggested that this reflects a low concentration of the key, rate-limiting enzyme of glycolysis, phosphofructokinase. This is also apparent in the inability of the child to achieve high respiratory exchange ratios during maximal or exhaustive exercise—the maximal values are seldom above 1.10, and are frequently below 1.00. Lactate threshold, however, when expressed as a percentage of $\dot{V}O_2$ max, does not appear to be a limiting factor in the child, as his or her values are similar, if not somewhat higher, than those of similarly trained adults.

Anaerobic mean and peak power output, as determined on the Wingate anaerobic test (see Chapter 19) is also lower in the child as compared to the adult. Figure 15-10 illustrates this fact on 306 males who performed the Wingate test with both

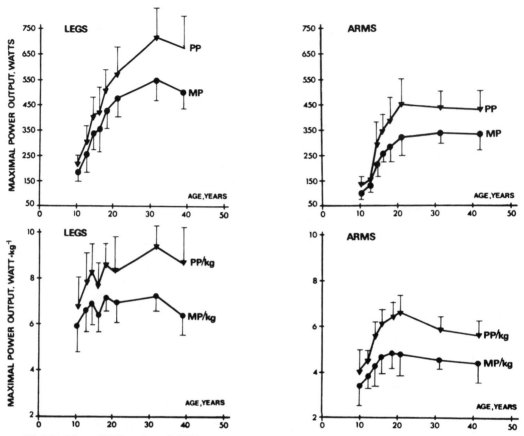

Figure 15-10   Mean (MP) and peak (PP) anaerobic power changes with age, expressed in absolute terms (watts) and relative to body weight (watts·kg^{-1}) (reprinted with permission from Inbar & BarOr, 1986).

arms and legs. Mean power output was the average power output for the entire 30-second test. Peak power output was the highest power output attained during any one five-second interval during the 30-second test. Anaerobic power does increase with growth and development, even when the values are expressed relative to body weight, as watts·kg^{-1}.

TRAINING THE YOUNG ATHLETE

Must special consideration be given to the young athlete when developing individualized programs of training? Generally, the youngster will adapt

well to the same type of training routine used to train the mature athlete. This section will look at the specific areas of strength, aerobic and anaerobic training, addressing those issues that are of concern to this age group.

Strength

One area of major controversy with regard to muscle development in youngsters is the use of weight training to increase muscular strength and endurance. For many years, young boys and girls were discouraged from using weights for fear that they might injure themselves and prematurely stop their growth processes. Studies on animals suggest that heavy-resistance exercise would lead to a stronger, broader, and more compact bone. However, since it is nearly impossible to load these animals to the same extent as youngsters, it has not been practical to design an experiment that accurately defines the risks associated with heavy-resistance exercise in youngsters. It would appear that the potential for injury and structural damage from heavy-resistance exercise is extremely low, but since the future of the youngster is at stake, it is appropriate to take a conservative approach until additional studies can be conducted. Thus, a program using low weights and high repetitions would be preferred to one using high weights and low repetitions. One of the safest techniques for strength training in youngsters would be to use the isokinetic concept, in which resistance is matched to the force applied, so that the youngster does not have to contend with actual weights, such as a barbells and dumbbells. Refer to Chapter 7 for a more detailed description of this technique.

It has been suggested that since young, prepubescent boys have relatively low circulating androgen levels, there is no reason to expect them to be able to benefit from strength training at this early age. Several recent studies have demonstrated that prepubescent boys can not only participate in this form of activity safely, but they can also gain substantial increases in strength. In a study conducted by Sewall and Micheli (1986), prepubescent boys and girls took part in a nine-week progressive, resistance-strength training program, 25 to 30 minutes per day, three days a week. They experienced a mean strength increase of 42.9 percent compared to a 9.5 percent increase in a non-training control group. Weltman and his colleagues (1986) followed 26 prepubertal males with a mean age of 8.2 years through a 14-week strength training program using isokinetic techniques with hydraulic resistance. Isokinetic strength increased between 18 and 37 percent in these young boys. Only one injury was reported which the authors felt was related to the strength training routine. As a result, the boy missed three training sessions. An additional six subjects reported injuries resulting from activities of daily living, independent of the strength training program. No boy demonstrated any evidence of damage to epiphyses, bone, or muscle as a result of strength training.

Aerobic and Anaerobic Training

Do prepubescent boys and girls benefit from aerobic training (training to improve the cardiorespiratory systems)? This has also been a highly controversial area as several early studies indicated that training prepubescent children did not affect changes in $\dot{V}O_2$ max. Interestingly, even without significant increases in $\dot{V}O_2$ max, these children had substantial improvements in performance, for example, reduced time for running a fixed distance. From the research studies that have been conducted to date, it seems appropriate to conclude that there will be only small increases in aerobic capacity with training in youngsters ten years of age and younger, even though their performances in aerobic activities are improved. More substantial changes in $\dot{V}O_2$ max appear to occur once the child has reached puberty. The reasons for these findings are not well-defined at this time. Since stroke volume appears to be the major limitation to aerobic performance in this age group, it is quite possible that further increases in aerobic capacity are dependent on growth of the heart.

Anaerobic training does appear to improve the anaerobic capacity of children. Following training, children have increased resting levels of creatine phosphate, ATP, and glycogen, and they have an increased activity of phosphofructokinase, and increased maximal lactate levels in the blood.

PSYCHOLOGICAL ASPECTS

Is formal, organized competition or participation in vigorous physical activity damaging to the emotional health and psychological development of the athlete? For the mature athlete, this presents no major problem, but many parents, educators, physicians, and psychologists have expressed concern over the potential for undesirable emotional experiences in the developing young athlete. The question has been raised whether children who compete in formal, highly-organized activities are likely to develop undesirable behavior patterns or psychological damage as a result of the pressures to win and be successful by adult standards. Does the 11-year-old boy competing on the all-star Little League team experience pressures and situations that could lead to immediate or future behavior or emotional problems?

Only limited research has been conducted in this area. Skubic (1954, 1955) studied both Little League and Middle League (13 to 15 years of age) baseball athletes in a small community in California. Using parents' opinions and the Galvanic skin-resistance measurement, she found essentially no difference between the athletes in formal competition compared to those who participated informally in physical education softball. There were few athletes who had any serious emotional problems that could be related to the stress of competition. Generally, her results suggested that formal competition at this age level was not detrimental to the child, but actually facilitated social and emotional growth.

On the other hand, Sherif, et al. (1961) conducted a fascinating study, which has been referred to as the "Lord of the Flies" or "Robber's Cave" experiment. In this study, a group of boys at summer camp were divided into two subgroups. During the initial part of the study, the groups were separated during much of the day, but they had periods of interaction. No problems between the groups developed during this part of the study. For the second phase of the study, the groups were put into situations where they were always in competition with each other in camp life, as well as in sports and games, both for recognition and for tangible rewards. During this phase, members of the individual groups developed strong allegiances to their own group and extreme hostility toward the other group. Night raids, cheating, and other forms of aggressive behavior began to develop. This phase of the study was discontinued when several members of both groups started developing serious psychological disturbances. During the third, and last, phase of the experiment, an attempt was made to bring the two groups back together in cooperative ventures, removing all forms of competition between the groups. It took considerable time to achieve the goal of working in a genuinely cooperative effort.

From these examples, it can only be concluded that competition can have both positive and negative influences on the emotional development of the youngsters. Of major importance is the climate in which the competition takes place. If the climate is such that winning is the only goal and parents are allowed to say and do whatever they please without giving the child sound guidance in coping with the stress of the situation, the child will be likely to have a negative experience. In short, the nature of the child's experience will depend almost entirely on the local situation. If competition is organized with this in mind, and the goal is to satisfy the needs of the child and not the adult, the experience should be positive and facilitate sound emotional growth and psychological development.

SUMMARY

This chapter has outlined those physiological and body composition alterations that accompany the growth and development process from birth to maturity. In addition, potential physiological and psychological problems associated with competition in the young athlete were discussed. It appears that strenuous physical exercise and intense competition can be of considerable value to athletes of all ages providing that the athletes have proper medical clearance and guidance and that the goals of competition are adjusted to serve the needs of the athlete.

STUDY QUESTIONS

1. What is the major concern when a bone that has not reached full growth breaks?
2. What is traumatic epiphysitis?
3. From the aspect of serious injury, which sport, baseball or football, places the youngster at higher risk?
4. At what age does lean body weight reach its peak in both males and females?
5. How dangerous is weight training in young boys and girls? What advice could be given to these youngsters if they wanted to improve their strength? Can they improve strength?

6. What typical changes occur in fat cells with growth and development?
7. As one ages, what happens to the basal metabolic rate?
8. How does pulmonary function change with growth?
9. What changes occur in stroke volume for a fixed rate of work as the child grows? What factors explain these changes?
10. What changes occur in cardiac output for a fixed rate of work as the child grows? What factors explain these changes?
11. What changes occur in submaximal and maximal heart rate as the child grows?
12. Why does absolute cardiovascular endurance capacity increase with age from the age of six to 20 years?
13. What happens to aerobic capacity as the prepubescent child trains aerobically?
14. What happens to anaerobic capacity as the prepubescent child trains anaerobically?
15. What does research tell us with respect to the psychological problems associated with competition at early ages?

REFERENCES

Adams, J. E. (1965). Injury to the throwing arm. *California Medicine, 102,* 127–132.

Albinson, J. G., & Andrew, G. M. (1976). *Child in sport and physical activity.* Baltimore: University Park Press.

Åstrand, I. (1967). Aerobic work capacity: Its relation to age, sex, and other factors. New York: *American Heart Association Monograph, No. 15.*

Bar-Or, O. (1983). *Pediatric sports medicine for the practitioner: From physiologic principles to clinical applications.* New York: Springer-Verlag.

Berg, K., & Eriksson, B. O. (Eds.). (1980). *Children and exercise IX.* Baltimore: University Park Press.

Binkhorst, R. A., Kemper, H. C. G., & Saris, W. H. M. (Eds.). (1985). *Children and exercise XI.* Champaign, IL: Human Kinetics Publishers, Inc.

Bjorntorp, P. (1986). Fat cells and obesity. In K. D. Brownell & J. P. Foreyt, *Handbook of eating disorders: Physiology, psychology, and treatment of obesity, anorexia, and bulimia.* New York: Basic Books, Inc., Publishers.

Boileau, R. A. (Ed.) (1984). *Advances in pediatric sport sciences, Volume 1.* Champaign, IL: Human Kinetics Publishers, Inc.

Brooks, G. A., & Fahey, T. D. (1984). *Exercise physiology: Human bioenergetics and its applications.* New York: John Wiley & Sons.

Clarke, H. H. (1971). *Physical and motor tests in the Medford boys' growth study.* Englewood Cliffs, NJ: Prentice-Hall, Inc.

Cronk, C. E., & Roche, A. F. (1982). Race- and sex-specific reference data for triceps and subscapular skinfolds and weight/stature^2. *American Journal of Clinical Nutrition, 35,* 347–354.

Espenshade, A. S., & Eckert, H. M. (1967). *Motor development.* Columbus, OH: Charles E. Merrill Publishing Co.

Faust, I. M., Johnson, P. R., Stern, J. S., & Hirsh, J. (1978). Diet-induced adipocyte number increase in adult rats: A new model of obesity. *American Journal of Physiology, 235,* E279–E286.

Forbes, G. B. (1964). Growth of the lean body mass during childhood and adolescence. *Journal of Pediatrics, 64,* 822–827.

Inbar, O., & Bar-Or, O. (1986). Anaerobic characteristics in male children and adolescents. *Medicine and Science in Sports and Exercise, 18,* 264–269.

Larson, R. L. (1974). Physical activity and the growth and development of bone and joint structures. In G. L. Rarick (Ed.), *Physical activity: Human growth and development,* pp. 32-59. New York: Academic Press.

Larson, R. L., & McMahan, R. O. (1966). The epiphyses and the childhood athlete. *Journal of American Medical Association, 196,* 607–612.

Malina, R. M. (1975). *Growth and development: The first twenty years.* Minneapolis: Burgess Publishing Company.

Rarick, G. L. (1973), *Physical activity: Human growth and development.* New York: Academic Press.

Robinson, S. (1938). Experimental studies of physical fitness in relation to age. *Arbeitsphysiologie 10,* 251–323.

Sewall, L., & Micheli, L. J. (1986). Strength training for children. *The Journal of Pediatric Orthopaedia Strabismus, 6,* 143–146.

Shephard, R. J. (1982). *Physical activity and growth.* Chicago: Year Book Medical Publishers, Inc.

Sherif, M., Harvey, O. J., White, B. J., Hood, W. R., & Sherif, C. W. (1961). *Intergroup conflict and cooperation: The robber's cave experiment.* Norman, OK: University of Oklahoma Book Exchange.

Skubic, E. (1954). Studies of Little League and Middle League Baseball. *Research Quarterly, 27,* 97–110.

Skubic, E. (1955). Emotional responses of boys to Little League and Middle League competitive baseball. *Research Quarterly, 26,* 342–352.

Smith, N., Ogilvie, B., Haskell, W., & Gaillard, B. (1978). *Handbook for the young athlete.* Palo Alto, CA: Bull Publishing Co.

Stull, G. A., & Eckert, H. M. (Eds.), (1986). *Effects of physical activity on children.* Champaign, IL: Human Kinetics Publishers, Inc.

Weltman, A., Janney, C., Rians, C. B., Strand, K., Berg, B., Tippitt, S., Wise, J., Cahill, B. R., & Katch, F. I. (1986). The effects of hydraulic resistance strength training in pre-pubertal males. *Medicine and Science in Sports and Exercise, 18,* 629–638.

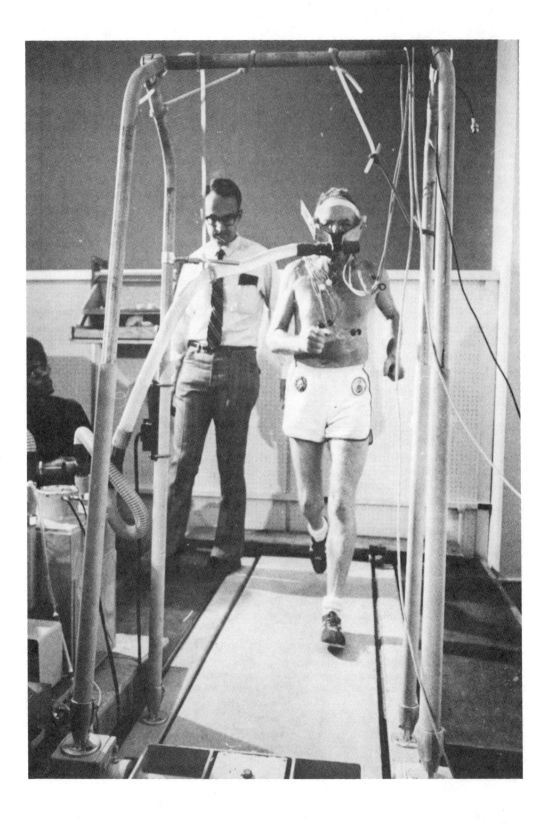

16

The Masters Athlete

INTRODUCTION

The number of adult men and women participating in competitive sports has increased dramatically over the past ten years. Although a great many of these "masters athletes" engage in competition for recreation and fitness, there are many who train with the same enthusiasm and intensity as young Olympians. Opportunities for competition are now available for adult athletes in a wide variety of activities, ranging from marathon running to weight lifting.

It should be recognized that such voluntary participation in strenuous physical activity is an unusual pattern of behavior, not observed in other aging animals. Studies have shown that, on the average, both man and lower animal forms tend to decrease their physical activity levels as they grow older. When rats, for example, were allowed to exercise freely, they ran 24 to 25 miles per week during the first five months of life, but covered only two to four miles per week during the final months of life. Consequently, it is difficult to distinguish between the effects of aging and reduced activity when studying the life-long changes in physiological function and performance. It is also difficult to understand why some older individuals choose to remain physically active when the natu-

ral tendency is to become sedentary. The psychological factors that motivate masters athletes to compete are not clearly defined, but their goals probably do not differ substantially from their younger counterparts.

Participation in sports competition and intense physical training beyond high school and college age raises a number of questions relative to the effects of aging on performance. What effect does aging have on sports performance? What physiological changes occur during aging that affect exercise tolerance? What health risks are posed by intense physical activity in aging men and women? Does exercise influence longevity? How trainable are middle-aged and older adults?

PERFORMANCE AND AGING

Records for running, swimming, and weight lifting suggest that the "best years of our lives" are between 20 and 30 years of age. National and world records for masters athletes in these events allow us to examine the effects of aging on the best performers. Unfortunately, this approach offers little information about the longitudinal effects of aging on physical performance. Few studies have been

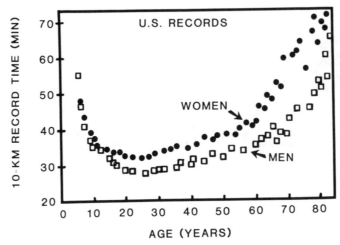

Figure 16-1 United States records for the 10-km for male and female runners ranging in age from 5 to 83 years. Note that males and females have similar records until approximately age 14 or 15 years, and that the best performances for both sexes are attained between 20 and 30 years of age (from Costill, 1986).

done which enable us to follow physical performance and aging in select individuals over the span of their athletic careers. Consequently, most of our knowledge of the effects of aging on physical performance have been drawn from cross-sectional studies.

Based on data from running records, it appears that the rate of decline in performance with aging

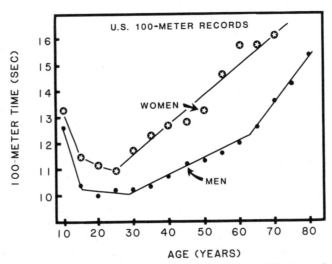

Figure 16-2 U. S. national records for the 100-meter dash for men and women between the ages of 10 and 80 years (Costill, 1986). Note that the best performances occur between the ages of 20 and 30 years, followed by a gradual decline in performance (+ 1.0 percent per year) until the age of 60.

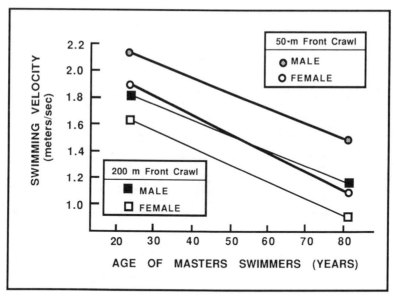

Figure 16–3 Changes in the velocity of swimming records with aging. The values shown here are those for men and women record-holders in the 50- and 200-meter front crawl swimming events. Note that the rate of decline in swimming speed is about the same for men and women, and the slope of these lines is approximately the same for both events.

is independent of the competitive distance. Performance records for 100 meters, 10-kilometer, and the marathon show a decrease of about 1 percent per year from the age of 25 to 60 years, at which time the rate of decline in performance accelerates to nearly 2 percent per year (see Figures 16–1 and 16–2). Thus, aging appears to affect both speed and endurance to the same degree. The following discussion describes the physiological changes that can be blamed for these age-related decreases in performance.

Swimming performance is affected by the aging process in much the same manner as endurance running. As noted in Figure 16–3, the average velocities for the record performances in the 50-yard and 200-yard freestyle events decline at about one percent per year for both men and women between the ages of 25 and 85 years. Because success in this sport depends on both muscular power and mechanical skill, some masters swimmers are able to achieve personal best performances well into middle-age. As an example, the data in Table 16–1 on page 306 illustrate the best performances for

a male swimmer at the ages of 20 and 50 years. Despite a 30-year lapse in swimming training, this swimmer was able to achieve his best performances at 50 years of age. Although the precise reasons for these improvements are unknown, it is logical to assume that they are the result of combined improvements in swimming technique, training methods, and swimming facilities, with little decline in physiological capacity.

Nevertheless, it is generally agreed that athletic performance declines at a steady rate during middle and advanced aging, the result of decrements in muscle strength and endurance. In the following discussion, attention will be directed toward the underlying physiological causes for these changes.

Factors of Endurance

The first studies of aging and physical fitness were performed by Sid Robinson in the late 1930s. He demonstrated that maximal oxygen uptake ($\dot{V}O_2$ max) in normally active men, declined steadily between 25 and 75 years of age. The average values

Table 16-1 Swimming performances at age 20 and 50 years for a male masters swimmer. Note that the best freestyle swimming (front crawl stroke) times were achieved at age 50, despite the fact that the swimmer was an accomplished collegiate swimmer between the ages of 18 and 21 years. It is also interesting to mention that this swimmer trained by swimming about 1,500 meters per day at the age of 20 years and 2,500 meters per day at age 50 years.

| | Best performance (seconds) | | Percent (%) |
Distance (meters)	*20 years*	*50 years*	*improvement*
50 m	27.2	26.5	2.6
100 m	62.7	60.3	3.8
200 m	147.8	137.7	6.8
400 m	318.8	288.9	9.4
1500 m	1403	1227	12.5

reported by Robinson (1938) for different age groups were as follows:

Age (years)	$\dot{V}O_2$ max (ml/kg × min)
25	47.7
35	43.1
45	39.5
52	38.4
63	34.5
75	25.5

Although investigators have since confirmed these findings in relatively inactive men and women, there have been few opportunities to study athletes over a long period of time to determine the impact of lifelong training on $\dot{V}O_2$ max levels. One notable exception is a recent study by Pollock, et al. (1987), who studied 24 master track athletes between the ages of 50 and 82 years of age, to evaluate the relationship between age and training over a ten year period. During that period, only 11 of the athletes (COMP) remained highly competitive, whereas the other 13 participants in the study became non-competitive (NON-COMP) and reduced their training intensity. The results showed that the COMP individuals maintained their $\dot{V}O_2$ max (54.2 to 53.3 ml/kg × min^{-1}), whereas the NON-COMP subjects showed a significant decline (52.5 to 45.9 ml/kg × min^{-1}) over the ten year period. Maximum heart rate, on the other hand, declined similarly (-7 beats/min) for both groups. During the ten years of this study, all of the subjects showed a slight decline in body weight (70.0 to 68.9 kg) and a significant increase in body fat content (13.1 to 15.1 percent). The authors have concluded that aging, per se, may not cause a decline in aerobic capacity. Rather, when the intensity and volume of training are kept at a high level, as was the case for the COMP group, $\dot{V}O_2$ max is unchanged.

Figure 16–4 illustrates the changes in $\dot{V}O_2$ max levels among groups of untrained men and women, joggers, and highly-trained runners. Although endurance training appears to offer substantial aerobic advantage, aging seems to induce a similar decline in $\dot{V}O_2$ max during middle age. Some caution must be used in drawing conclusions from these findings, since it is probable that the older runners and joggers did not train with the same intensity and duration as their younger counterparts. At least part of the decline in this aerobic endurance with age may be related to the nature of training.

Laboratory data covering 13 years have been reported for a national-level, distance runner (Costill, 1986). During that period, this runner occasionally trained at the same relative intensity as he did when he was 21- to 25-years old. Despite variations in his training regimen, his $\dot{V}O_2$ max has remained relatively constant (Table 16–2). It was also interesting to note that his running economy, or oxygen uptake while running at eight minutes per mile, remained between 32 and 33 ml/kg × min^{-1} over

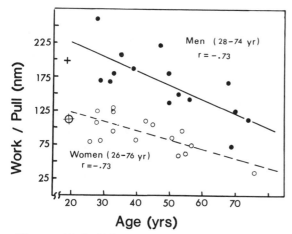

Figure 16-4 Relationship between aging and maximal oxygen uptake ($\dot{V}O_2$ max) for inactive men and women, joggers, and highly-trained runners. These cross-sectional data suggest that after the age of 20 to 25 years, $\dot{V}O_2$ max declines at a steady rate for all adults, regardless of their activity level.

that may be determined as much by heredity as by the training regimen.

One of the most notable long-term studies with distance runners and aging was conducted by D. B. Dill and his colleagues from the Harvard Fatigue Laboratory. Don Lash, world record-holder for the two-mile (8 min, 58 sec) in 1936, was among those studied by the Harvard group. Although few of the former runners continued to train after leaving college, Lash was still running approximately 45 minutes per day at the age of 49. Despite this activity, his $\dot{V}O_2$ max had declined from 81.4 ml/kg × min^{-1} at age 24 years, to 54.4 at age 49, a 33 percent decline. As expected, those runners who did not continue to train during middle-age showed much larger declines. On the average, their aerobic capacities declined by about 43 percent from the age of 23 to 50 years (70 to 40 ml/kg × min^{-1}). These data suggest that prior training offers little advantage to endurance capacity in later life, unless the individual continues to engage in some form of vigorous activity.

Bengt Saltin and Gunnar Grimby (1968) have shown that former athletes who have been out of training for more than ten years, still have a 20 percent advantage in $\dot{V}O_2$ max compared to untrained non-athletes. A group of untrained former athletes ranging in age from 50 to 59 years had a $\dot{V}O_2$ max of 38 ml/kg × min^{-1}, while a randomly-selected age-matched group of untrained, non-athletes averaged 30 ml/kg × min^{-1}. It is impossible, however, to determine whether the higher $\dot{V}O_2$ max values of the former athletes' are due to their earlier periods of training, to differences in life-

this 13-year period. It is not surprising, therefore, that his performances for the 10-kilometer and marathon distances have declined very little.

Are the individual examples given here for the masters swimmer and runner exceptions to the natural rules of aging? Can other athletes reduce the effects of aging on their endurance by continuing to train intensely? Much depends on the training adaptability of the masters athlete, a factor

Table 16-2 Laboratory tests results for an elite masters distance runner (from Costill, 1986).

Year	Age (yr)	Weight (kg)	$\dot{V}O_2$ max (ml/kg × min)	HR max (beats/min)
1968	36	67.5	67.6*	163
1971	39	65.4	62.7	158
1974	43	64.7	64.9	152
1979	48	63.5	65.8	156
1980	49	63.9	64.0	155
1981	50	62.7	63.7	155

*Denotes that the runner was training for the 1968 Olympic marathon trial at the time of this test.

style, inherited factors, or a combination of these factors.

Again the questions must be asked: How much of the observed decrease is a result of biological aging? How important is the habitual level of physical activity in determining the rate of decline? Andersen and Hermansen (1965) gained insight into these questions when they compared the $\dot{V}O_2$ max values for a group of 63 cross-country skiers, between 50 and 66 years of age, with a group of office workers and a group of industrial workers of similar ages, and with a group of 20- to 30-year-old students. They found the following:

Group	Age Range (years)	$\dot{V}O_2$ max (ml/kg × min)
Skiers	50–66	46
Office workers	50–60	36
Industrial workers	50–60	34
Students	20–30	44

These data support the contention that the decline in $\dot{V}O_2$ max with age, demonstrated in several studies, is not strictly a function of age, although the possibility that heredity might be an important factor in the high $\dot{V}O_2$ max values of the older skiers should not be discounted. Results of a similar study add support for this conclusion. A group of 25 of the best sprint and distance runners over 40 years of age in the United States was brought into the laboratory for a comprehensive series of tests. While their $\dot{V}O_2$ max values were considerably higher than those of average men of the same age, the relative rate of decline with age closely paralleled the rate of decline illustrated by Robinson's 1938 data for normal men. Were these older athletes genetically superior, or can their comparatively high values be attributed to their training programs? The answer to these questions will have to await studies of a longitudinal nature, though data by Pollock, et al. (1987) suggest that a decade of aging may have little effect on aerobic capacity if the training intensity and volume are maintained.

What are the underlying causes for the decline in endurance with aging? A number of cross-sectional studies have demonstrated that lung function is markedly altered by age. During the period of growth, the static lung volumes, as well as the functional pulmonary tests, increase to the time of physical maturity. Shortly after reaching this peak, however, there is a gradual reduction with age. Vital capacity, FEV 1.0 (the greatest volume of air that can be exhaled in the first second of a forced vital capacity test) and forced expiratory flow rate, all exhibit a linear decrease with age, starting between 20 and 30 years of age. While these volumes and rates are decreasing, the residual lung volume increases and the total lung capacity remains unchanged; thus, the ratio of the residual volume to the total lung capacity (RV/TLC) increases. In the early twenties, 18 to 22 percent of the total lung capacity is represented by the residual volume, but this increases to 30 percent, and higher, as the individual reaches 50 years of age. Smoking appears to accelerate this process.

The changes in these volumes and flow rates are matched by the changes in maximal ventilatory capacity during exhaustive exercise. Maximal expiratory ventilation ($\dot{V}E$ max) will increase with age to the point of physical maturity, and then will decrease during the aging process. From cross-sectional data for males, the $\dot{V}E$ max, for four- to six-year-old boys, will average about 40 liters/min, increase to between 110 and 140 liters/min at full maturity, and decrease to 60 and 80 liters/min for 60- to 70-year-olds. Females follow the same general pattern, although their absolute values are considerably lower for each age level, due, primarily, to their smaller stature.

These changes in pulmonary function are probably the result of a combination of factors. The most important factor is the loss in elasticity of the lung tissue and chest wall, which increases the work involved in breathing. The stiffening of the chest wall with age appears to be the major cause of reduction in lung function. Despite all these changes, the lungs still hold a remarkable reserve and adequate diffusion capacity to permit maximal exertion. During middle- and old-age, endurance training reduces the loss in elasticity of the lungs and chest wall. As a result, the decline in endurance capacity or aerobic capacity among masters athletes cannot be attributed to changes in mechanisms of external respiration.

As shown in Figure 16-5, a number of changes also occur in cardiovascular function as the

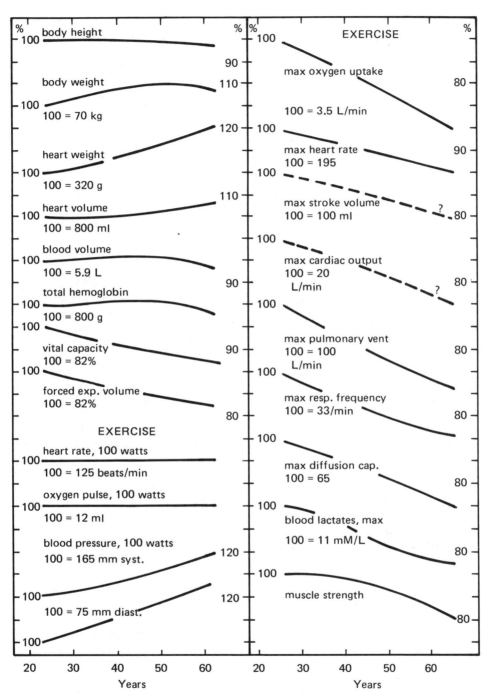

Figure 16-5 Variation in physical dimensions and physiological function with age (from Åstrand, 1967. By permission of the American Heart Association, Inc.).

individual ages. One of the most notable circulatory changes with training is a decrease in maximal heart rate. Whereas children frequently exceed 210 beats/min, the average 60-year-old has a maximal heart rate of approximately 160 beats/min. It has been estimated that the maximal heart rate decreases by slightly less than one beat per year as the individual ages. The average maximal heart rate for each age level can be estimated by using the following equation:

$$HR\ max = 220 - age$$

It should be recognized that this represents only an estimate of the mean, or average, value for the age. Individual values could deviate from this estimated value by ±20 beats per min, or more.

The reduction in maximal heart rate with age appears to be similar in both sedentary and athletic adults. At the age of 50 years, for example, normally active men have the same maximal heart rates as former and still-active distance runners. This reduction in maximal heart rate with age may be attributed to morphological and electrophysiological alterations in the SA node, as well as in the bundle of His, which could reduce the velocity by which the conduction of the cardiac impulse is transmitted (Lakatta, 1979). Heath, et al. (1981) have suggested that the decline in maximal heart rate is responsible for the decrease in $\dot{V}O_2$ max observed among masters athletes, although this theory is not supported by the recent data from Pollock, et al. (1987).

Maximum stroke volume and cardiac output values appear to decline with age (see Figure 16-5). However, the number of studies conducted and the number of subjects examined is quite limited. In fact, few data are available for middle-aged and older athletes. Studies on endurance runners have shown that the lower $\dot{V}O_2$ max observed in older athletes is the result of a lower maximal cardiac output, despite the fact that heart volumes of masters athletes are similar to those of young athletes. Saltin (1986) has reported that 51-year-old orienteers (distance runners) have a cardiac output that is about five liters per minute lower than young orienteers. This was mainly due to a lowering of their maximal heart rate and to a reduction in maximal stroke volume. Compared to sedentary, middle-aged men, the active orienteers of the same age had markedly higher maximal oxygen uptakes, mostly due to a larger stroke volume and therefore, a larger maximal cardiac output.

Peripheral (such as, leg) blood flow capacity is reduced with aging, despite the fact that the density of capillaries in the muscles remains unchanged. It is difficult to determine whether the decreases in stroke volume, cardiac output, and peripheral flow are directly the result of the aging process or the result of an increasingly sedentary life style, which leads to cardiovascular deconditioning. Recent studies would tend to suggest that both are involved, but the relative contribution of each is not known.

Studies of blood flow to the exercising muscles in older athletes reveals that there is a ten to 15 percent reduction at any given workload compared to well-trained young athletes. The lower leg blood flow in the middle-aged endurance runner (orienteers) appears to be compensated for by a greater oxygen extraction (arterial-venous difference for oxygen is wider). As a result, the oxygen uptake by the exercising muscle is similar at a given work intensity in both the young and older athlete. Why then, does maximal cardiac output and $\dot{V}O_2$ max decline with age?

One possible explanation may be related to the fact that aging causes an increase in peripheral resistance. As a result of a reduction in the elasticity and capacity for vasodilation of the arteries and arterioles, aging produces a rise in blood pressure at rest and during exercise. Although mean arterial pressure is slightly less in older athletes than in sedentary men, they still have greater peripheral resistance than younger athletes. As noted by Saltin (1986), stroke volume can be maintained among middle and aging adults who continue to train intensely. The fact that stroke volumes are lower in older, rather than in younger athletes, is due to an increase in afterload (peripheral resistance). Thus, the gradual decline in maximal cardiac output and oxygen uptake among aging masters athletes appears to be the result of restrictions placed on peripheral blood flow, rather than a reduction in the heart's pumping capacity.

The purpose of the basic pulmonary and cardiovascular adaptations that are made with varying levels of training is to accommodate the need of the exercising muscles for oxygen. Thus, the

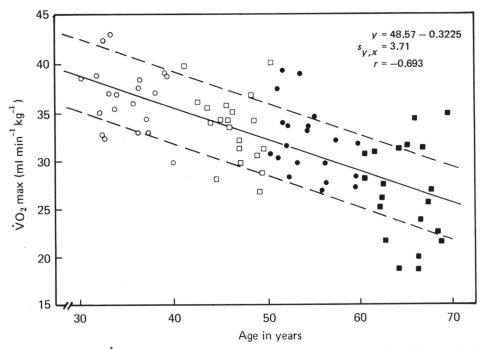

$$y = 48.57 - 0.3225$$
$$s_{y,x} = 3.71$$
$$r = -0.693$$

Figure 16-6 Decrease in $\dot{V}O_2$ max with age (from Adams, et al., 1972. Reproduced by permission of the publisher.).

decreases in pulmonary and cardiovascular function with age suggest that aerobic capacity, or $\dot{V}O_2$ max, experiences a similar decline with age. As noted earlier, Robinson (1938) demonstrated this phenomenon in a cross-sectional sample of boys and men ranging in age from six to 91 years. He found that $\dot{V}O_2$ max attained its peak value between 17 and 20 years of age and then decreased as a linear function of age (see Figure 16-4). Adams, McHenry, and Barnauer (1972) found a similar relationship between $\dot{V}O_2$ max and age in a large population of adult males (see Figure 16-6). Studies of girls and women have shown essentially the same trend, although the female starts her decline at a much younger age (refer to Chapter 17), probably due to an earlier assumption of a sedentary lifestyle.

Thus, the decline in endurance performance, aerobic capacity, and cardiovascular function are more the result of a decrease in activity, than to aging. A decrease in physical activity, a gain in

body weight, and aging changes in the cardiovascular system combine to produce a decline in $\dot{V}O_2$ max of about 9 percent per decade after the age of 25 years in healthy men in our society. If body composition and physical activity are kept constant, deterioration due to the aging process results in a decline in $\dot{V}O_2$ max of only about five percent/decade. Nevertheless, in later life (after 55 to 65 years), cardiovascular capacity is reduced as the result of a lower maximal heart rate.

Factors of Muscular Strength

In general, maximal muscular strength is achieved between the ages of 25 and 35 years. As in other measurements of human performance, there is a wide variation in individual performances. There are, for example, some individuals, who at 60 years of age exhibit greater strength than persons half their age. As noted in Figure 16-7, arm strength declines at a steady rate after the age of 30. It

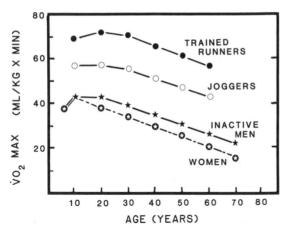

Figure 16–7 Arm muscle strength in male and female masters swimmers. Note the gradual decline in strength from about age 30 years.

should be noted, however, that some of the older swimmers shown in this figure were stronger than many of the younger men and women.

The cause for this decline in muscle strength, for the most part, can be accounted for by a large deterioration in muscle mass that occurs with aging. In the normally sedentary adult, these changes are characterized by decrements in the size and number of muscle fibers, an increase in body fat, and a reduction in the aerobic capacity of the muscle. These changes are substantially smaller, however, in the masters athlete, suggesting that a large part of the age-related decrements in muscle strength are a function of inactivity rather than aging.

Saltin (1986) noted that despite the reduction in muscle mass in aging men, the quality of the remaining muscle mass is well-maintained. The number of capillaries/unit area is similar in young and old endurance runners. Oxidative enzyme activities in the muscle of endurance-trained masters athletes are only ten to 15 percent lower than in young athletes, a 50 percent difference in maximal oxygen uptake. Thus, oxidative capacity in the skeletal muscle of elderly endurance-trained runners is only slightly less than young, elite runners suggesting that aging has little effect on the adaptability of skeletal muscle to endurance training.

Without regular physical activity there is a loss of muscle fibers from individual motor units, resulting in fewer fibers being available for force development to share the load of heavy exercise. Recent research has suggested that there is a selective loss of the fast-twitch fibers, thereby reducing muscle strength and power. In addition to the structural loss of contractile units, aging muscle is less excitable and requires a greater stimulus for contraction. It has been proposed that one factor responsible for the decline in muscle mass with aging is the result of an inability to retain muscle protein. With aging there is a gradual reduction in the hormonal controls on protein synthesis in the muscle, resulting in a gradual loss of muscle fibers. Indirect evidence suggests that regular physical activity stimulates protein retention, thereby delaying the strength losses seen with aging.

The neural controls of muscle are also affected by aging. With advanced years, there is a decline in the number of spinal cord axons and a decline in nerve conduction velocity. Studies have shown that with aging, there are large changes in the nervous system's capacity to process information and to activate the muscles. Specifically, aging affects the ability to detect a stimulus and process the information to produce a response. Simple and complex movements are slowed with aging, although persons who remain physically active are only slightly slower than young, active individuals.

It is apparent that aging has a detrimental effect on muscle strength and endurance, but active participation in sports will lessen the impact on performance. This is not to say that biological aging will be retarded by regular physical activity, although many of the decrements in physical work capacity can be markedly retarded by an active life-style.

Body Composition and Aging

The degree of fat accumulation with growth and aging depends on the dietary and exercise habits of the individual, in addition to heredity. While

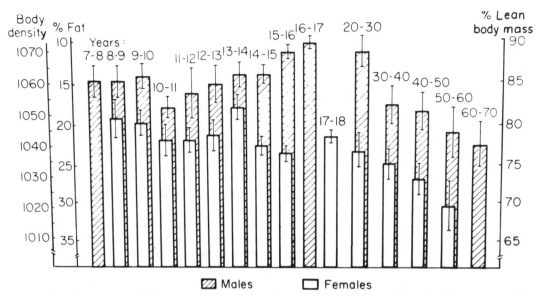

Figure 16-8 Changes in relative body fat with age for males and females (from Parizkova, 1974. Reproduced by permission of the publisher.).

heredity is unchangeable, diet and exercise can be manipulated to either increase or decrease the fat stores. At birth, the body weight is 10 to 12 percent fat, and by the time the individual reaches physical maturity, the fat content reaches 15 to 25 percent of the total body weight for males and females, respectively. Figure 16-8 illustrates the relationship between percent body fat and age for males and females. Both relative and absolute fat increase with age once physical maturity is reached. This is probably due to an increase in dietary intake, in addition to a decrease in the level of physical activity, although there is also a reduced ability to mobilize fat with age. Beyond the age of thirty, there is also a progressive decrease in the lean body weight, which is primarily the result of decreased muscle mass and reduced bone mineral content. Both of these decreases are, at least partially, the result of decreased levels of physical activity.

From the age of 20 through 70 years of age, normally active (sedentary) men and women experience a gradual increase in body weight. This occurs despite a gradual reduction in lean body tissue (muscle and bone). Consequently, body fat increases at a steady rate throughout life, as shown in the following example:

Age	Men	Women
20	14	20
30	17	23
40	20	26
50	22	28
60	25	30

As one might anticipate, the body fat content of masters athletes is significantly lower than age-matched, sedentary adult men and women. Competitive male (50-years-old) and female (43-years-old) swimmers, for example, have been reported to have 15 percent and 23 percent body fat, respectively. Highly-trained runners, on the other hand, have been observed to have only 11 percent and 18 percent fat at the average age of 45 years. Pollock, et al. (1974) have reported very low body fat levels on 40- to 75-year-old champion track athletes (see Table 16-3).

Table 16–3   Physical characteristics and body composition of American Champion Track Athletes between the ages of 40 and 75 years (from Pollock, et al., 1974).

Age (years)	Number	Height (cm)	Weight (kg)	Fat (%)	Training (miles/wk)
40–49	11	180.7	71.6	11.2	40.4
50–59	5	174.7	67.2	10.9	42.0
60–69	6	175.7	67.1	11.3	29.7
70–75	3	175.6	66.8	13.6	20.0

Although these values for both the runners and swimmers are lower than those reported for normal, sedentary adults of similar ages, masters athletes have substantially more body fat than younger competitors. Nevertheless, these lower body fat levels in the older athletes, compared to age-matched sedentary individuals, are undoubtedly the result of their higher rate of caloric expenditure, and conscious monitoring of their body weight.

Trainability of the Older Athlete

In the previous discussion it was shown clearly that despite the decrements associated with aging, middle-aged and older athletes are still capable of exceptional performances. Their ability to adapt to endurance and strength training is well-documented. Studies which have attempted to gauge the degree of adaptation to training in middle- and older-aged subjects have produced some conflict-

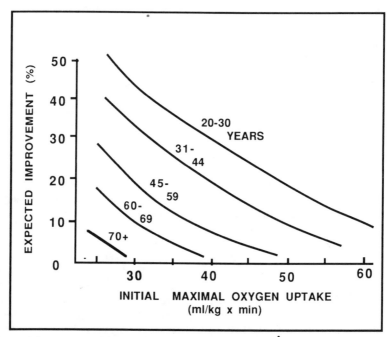

Figure 16–9   Potential improvements in maximal oxygen uptake ($\dot{V}O_2$ max) with physical conditioning relative to age and initial level of fitness.

ing results. It is generally agreed, however, that older individuals are not able to improve their strength and endurance capacities to the same extent as younger subjects.

Since the precise mechanisms responsible for triggering the body's adaptations to training are not understood, it is impossible to determine why aging reduces trainability. One might speculate that it is the combined result of age-related decrements in the neurological, muscular, and cardiorespiratory systems. Protein synthesis and hormonal regulation of growth and development are also altered with aging. These factors are known to be important in the body's adaptation to the physical stress of training.

Figure 16-9 illustrates the relationship between age and the percent improvement in maximal oxygen uptake that can be expected. The amount of improvement is dependent on the age of the individual and his or her initial level of fitness. When athletes already have a high $\dot{V}O_2$ max compared to others of similar age, they are unlikely to improve as much as younger individuals having the same initial fitness level. Thus, the degree of improvement seems to be less in persons who begin to train later in life. As an example, Benestad (1965) trained 13 men who ranged in age from 70 to 81 years. He found no improvement in their $\dot{V}O_2$ max (27 ml/kg $\times$ min^{-1}) after five to six weeks of endurance training, in spite of a significant decrease in the heart rate at a standard submaximal exercise task.

It has been suggested that middle- and older-aged individuals require more training to achieve the same training benefits as younger individuals. There are no data with human subjects to substantiate this theory. However, studies with animals have reported that it takes longer to train older rats to the same fitness level and they experience less muscle hypertrophy than younger animals during training. It has also been suggested that the rate of adaptation and recuperative powers are less in older individuals than in younger men and women. Again, we have only anecdotal evidence to support this contention.

It is possible that the rate and degree of adaptation to training may also be influenced by the lifelong activity habits of the individual. For those who have been inactive for many years, the ability to adapt to training may be reduced, compared to those who have actively trained and competed in sports throughout life. While there is limited evidence to support this concept, some longitudinal studies with a few runners and swimmers have shown that there is little decrease in aerobic capacity over a 26-year period when the athletes continued their training. Longitudinal data on a swimmer and a runner at the ages of twenty-four and fifty years are presented in Table 16-4. These two athletes experienced about a four percent decrease in $\dot{V}O_2$ max over that period compared to the normal, expected decline of 20.5 percent calculated from the data in Figure 16-6. Therefore, it appears that the losses in endurance normally associated with aging can be remarkably reduced with a continued, lifelong program of intense training.

Since regular physical activity is an important contributor to good health, it is logical to ask, Does training throughout middle and old age have an effect on longevity? While it is true that an endurance exercise program may reduce a number of the risk factors associated with cardiovascular disease, there is no direct evidence to prove that you will live longer if you exercise regularly. Even

Table 16-4 A comparison of maximal oxygen uptake (liters/min) and maximal heart rate (beats/min) values for two masters athletes at the ages of 24 and 50 years.

Athlete	24 years		50 years		Percent Change $\dot{V}O_2$ max
	$\dot{V}O_2$ max	HR max	$\dot{V}O_2$ max	HR max	
Runner	4.33	192	4.15	174	−4.2
Swimmer	4.25	196	4.09*	166*	−3.8

*Measured during swimming. All other measurements taken during treadmill running.

studies using animals have provided conflicting results. A study by Goodrick (1980) demonstrated that rats who exercised freely lived roughly 15 percent longer than sedentary animals, but a recent investigation by a group in St. Louis has shown no significant increase in the life span of rats who voluntarily ran on an exercise wheel (Holloszy, et al., 1985). The total percentage of early death among the animals who exercised was reduced; however, even though more of the active rats lived to old age, on the average, they still died at the same age as their sedentary counterparts. It was also interesting to note that in this latter study, the animals that had a restricted food intake and maintained a lower body weight lived ten percent longer than the freely eating sedentary rats. Of course, it is difficult to apply these findings to humans, but it does raise some interesting questions that may be relevant to our health and longevity.

SUMMARY

This chapter has outlined those physiological and body composition alterations that accompany the aging process. Most of these changes are illustrated in Figure 16-5, which summarizes data from a large number of studies. It appears that strenuous physical exercise and intense competition can be of considerable value to athletes of all ages, providing that the athletes have proper medical clearance and guidance and that the goals of competition are adjusted to serve the needs of the athlete. In spite of the negative effects of aging on the body, records of performance by masters athletes are exceptional, demonstrating that the body is capable of extensive adaptations late into life.

Training regimens for the masters athlete do not appear to differ from those used by younger sports participants. Although there are some indications that it takes more physical work to achieve maximal training benefits in the older athlete, it should be remembered that the rate of adaptation and recuperation from intense training is slower for middle- and older-aged adults. Consequently, the risk of injury and overstress may pose a limitation to training in these athletes.

Finally, the changes with aging that attack the cardiovascular system must be considered as a serious health risk among masters athletes who participate in events that place great stress on oxygen transport and cardiovascular function. This is not to suggest that masters competition is unhealthy nor that it places the healthy athlete at high risk. Rather, it is meant to emphasize the need for regular physical examinations, including an exercise stress electrocardiogram, even in apparently healthy men and women. At present, there is limited evidence to indicate that physical training will increase longevity, though it is known to reduce many of the risk factors known to be associated with cardiovascular disease. Hopefully, future research will provide greater insight into the role of lifelong activity and sports participation on health and longevity.

STUDY QUESTIONS

1. Describe the changes in strength and endurance records with aging.
2. What cardiovascular changes occur during aging? How do these changes affect maximal oxygen uptake?
3. What neurological changes occur during aging? How do they affect athletic performance?
4. Describe the trainability of the endurance masters athlete. How does training alter the biology of aging?
5. How does aging affect strength training?
6. What influence does aging and training have on body composition?
7. How does the respiratory system change with aging—VC, $FEV_{1.0}$, RV, RV/TLC and $\dot{V}E$ max?
8. Is it advisable for men and women over 40 years of age to begin engaging in competitive athletics? What precautions should be taken?
9. Describe the changes in $\dot{V}O_2$ max with age. How do trained individuals differ from untrained subjects?
10. Describe the changes in HR_{max} with age. How does training alter this relationship?
11. How does aging affect maximal stroke volume and maximal cardiac output? What mechanisms can potentially explain these changes?

12. How does aging affect muscle and the characteristics of muscle, for instance, muscle fiber composition?

REFERENCES

Adams, J. E. (1965). Injury to the throwing arm. *California Medicine, 102,* 127–132.

Adams, W. C., McHenry, M. M., & Bernauer, E. M. (1972). Multistage treadmill walking performance and associated cardiorespiratory responses of middle-aged men. *Clinical Science, 42,* 355–370.

Albinson, J. G., & Andrew, G. M. (1976). *Child in sport and physical activity.* Baltimore: University Park Press.

Anderson, K., & Hermansen, L. (1965). Aerobic work capacity in middle-aged Norwegian men. *Journal of Applied Physiology, 20,* 432–436.

Andersen, K. L., Shephard, R. J., Denolin, H., Varnauskas, E., & Masironi, R. (1971). *Fundamentals of exercise testing.* Geneva: World Health Organization.

Aniansson, A. (1980). Muscle function in old age with special reference to muscle morphology: Effect of training and capacity in activities of daily living. (Dissertation) Sweden: University of Goteborg.

Åstrand, I. (1960). Aerobic work capacity in men and women with special reference to age. *Acta Physiologica Scandinavica, 49,* (Suppl. 169), 11.

Åstrand, I. (1967). *Aerobic work capacity: Its relation to age, sex, and other factors.* American Heart Association Monograph, No. 15. New York.

Benestad, A. (1965). *Trainability of old men. Acta Medica Scandinavica, 178,* 321.

Child, J. S., Barnard, R. J., & Taw, R. L. (1984). Cardiac hypertrophy and function in master endurance runners and sprinters. *Journal of Applied Physiology, 57,* 176–181.

Corbin, C. B. (1973). *A textbook of motor development.* Dubuque, IA: William C. Brown.

Costill, D. L. (1986). *Inside running: Basics of sports physiology.* Indianapolis: Benchmark Press.

Costill, D. L., King, D., Hargreaves, M., & Holdren, A. (1984). The facts are in: Stress those sprint muscles and increase performance. *Swim Swim, 6,* 13–14.

deVries, H. A. (1974). *Physiology of exercise for physical education and athletics* (2nd ed.). Dubuque, IA: William C. Brown.

deVries, H. A. (1970). Physiological effects of an exercise training regimen upon men aged 52 to 88. *Journal of Gerontology 25,* 325–336.

Dill, D. B., Robinson, S., & Ross, J. C. (1967). A longitudinal study of sixteen champion runners. *Journal of Sports Medicine and Physical Fitness, 7,* 4–27.

Espenshade, A. S., & Eckert, H. M. (1967). *Motor development.* Columbus, OH: Charles E. Merrill Publishing Co.

Goodrick, C. L. (1980). Effects of long-term voluntary wheel exercise on male and female Wistar rats. 1. Longevity, body weight and metabolic rate. *Journal of Gerontology, 26,* 22–33.

Heath, G. W., Hagberg, J. M., Ehsani, A. A., & Holloszy, J. O. (1981). A physiological comparison of young and older endurance athletes. *Journal of Applied Physiology, 51,* 634–640.

Holloszy, J. O., Smith, E. K., Vining, M., & Adams, S. (1985). Effect of voluntary exercise on longevity of rats. *Journal of Applied Physiology, 59,* 826–831.

Lakatta, E. G. (1979). Alterations in the cardiovascular system that occur in advanced age. *Federation Proceedings, 38,* 163–167.

Larsson, L. (1978). Morphological and functional characteristics of the aging skeletal muscle in man. *Acta Physiologica Scandinavica, 457,* 36.

Orlander, J., & Aniansson, A. (1979). Effects of physical training on skeletal muscle metabolism and ultrastructure in 70- to 75-year-old men. *Acta Physiologica Scandinavica, 109,* 149–154.

Parizkova, J. (1974). Body composition and exercise during growth and development. In G. L. Rarick (Ed.), *Physical activity: Human growth and development.* New York: Academic Press.

Pollock, M. L., Miller, H. S., & Wilmore, J. H. (1974). Physiological characteristics of champion American track athletes 40 to 75 years of age. *Journal of Gerontology, 29,* 645–649.

Pollock, M. L., Miller, H. S., Linnerud, A. C., & Cooper, K. H. (1975). Frequency of training as a determinant for improvement in cardiovascular function and body composition of middle-aged men. *Archives of Physical Medicine and Rehabilitation, 56,* 141–145.

Pollock, M. L., Foster, C., Knapp, D., Rod, J. L., & Schmidt, D. H. (in press) Effect of age and training on aerobic capacity and body composition of master athletes. *Journal of Applied Physiology.*

Robinson, S. (1938). Experimental studies of physical fitness in relation to age. *Arbeitsphysiologie, 10,* 251–323.

Saltin, B., & Grimby, G. (1968). Physiological analysis of middle-aged and old former athletes. *Circulation, 38,* 1104–1115.

Saltin, B. (1986). The aging endurance athlete. In J. R. Sutton & R. M. Brock (Eds.), *Sports medicine for the mature athlete.* IN: Benchmark Press.

Seals, D. R., Hagberg, J. M., Hurley, B. F., Ehsani, A. A., & Holloszy, J. O. (1984). Endurance training in older men and women. 1. Cardiovascular responses to exercise. *Journal of Applied Physiology, 57,* 1024–1029.

Siegel, W., Blomquist, G., & Mitchell, J. H. (1970). Effects of a quantitated physical training program on middle-aged sedentary men. *Circulation, 41,* 19–29.

Spirduso, W. W. (1975). Reaction and movement time as a function of age and physical activity level. *Journal of Gerontology, 30,* 435.

Young, K., & Young, J. H. (1985). *Running records by age 1985.* Tucson: National Running Data Center, Inc.

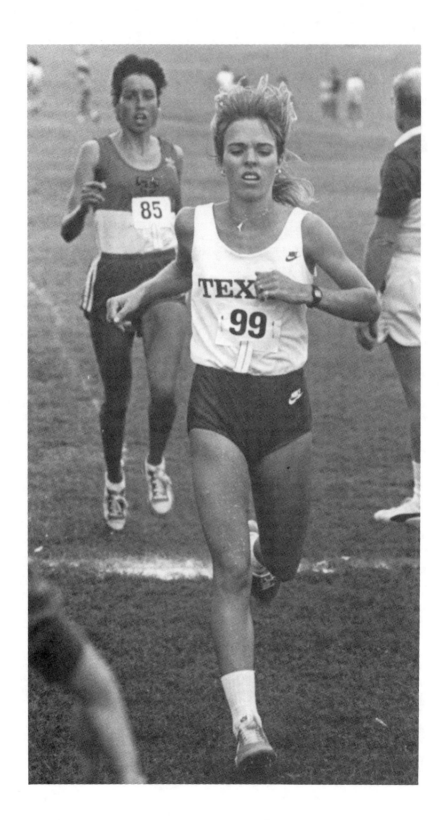

17

The Female Athlete

INTRODUCTION

The decade of the 1970s and the first half of the 1980s has produced considerable interest in the physical abilities and limitations of females, both in the work place and in the athletic arena. In the United States, passage of the Civil Rights Act of 1964 prohibited job discrimination on the basis of sex. The passage of the Women's Equal Rights Amendment of 1972, although never ratified, increased the awareness of women's rights under the law. Finally, the passage in 1972 of the U. S. Education Amendment, Title IX, forbids sex discrimination in any institution receiving federal funds. The first two legislative acts opened many employment opportunities for women that were previously unavailable. Women are now found in such occupations as commercial airline pilots, law enforcement officers, combat assignments in the military, telephone linemen, construction workers, and heavy equipment operators. This amendment also had a major impact on athletic programs in public and private schools at all grade levels. In the past, when compared to programs for boys and men, girls and women were denied the opportunity for quality athletic experiences. Title IX has accomplished much in a relatively short period of time, equalizing athletic opportunities for the sexes.

The sudden changes brought about by this federal legislation have created considerable confusion and many questions. Are girls and women physically capable of assuming these new roles as they take advantage of these new opportunities? Can girls and women physically cope with the rigors of high-level athletic competition? Can girls and women obtain the traditional benefits of exercise and sport that boys and men have enjoyed for centuries? Finally, can girls and women be trained for sport or conditioned for fitness using a format identical to that for boys and men, or are there special considerations that dictate a unique training or conditioning format? On the basis of world records in the year 1986, the male was 8.4 percent faster in the 100-meter dash, jumped 14.0 percent higher in the high jump, ran 11.0 percent faster in the 1,500-meter run, and swam 7.5 percent faster in the 400-meter freestyle swim. Do these differences result from biological differences between the sexes, or do they reflect the social and cultural restrictions that have been placed on the female during her preadolescent and adolescent development? The intent of this chapter is to probe the similarities and differences between males and females relative to their physique and body composition, as well as their physiological responses to acute exercise and physiological adaptations to chronic exercise.

319

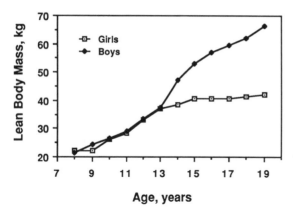

Figure 17-1 Changes in lean body mass with growth and aging (data from Forbes, 1972).

PHYSIQUE AND BODY COMPOSITION

It appears that differences between the sexes in height, weight, girths or circumferences, bone widths or diameters, and skinfold thicknesses do not exist until between 12 and 14 years of age, approximately at the time of puberty. Prior to puberty, there is a striking similarity between boys and girls of the same socioeconomic background for all indices of size and maturity. Lean body mass (LBM), estimated from ^{40}K assessment, in a study of 609 normal boys and girls between the ages of 7½ and 20½, showed no sex differences prior to adolescence, when LBM was expressed per unit of height (Forbes, 1972). Between 12 and 13 years of age, the LBM/height ratio begins to plateau in females, but continues to increase in males up to the age of 20 years. The LBM starts to peak in the male between 18 and 20 years of age and is approximately 1.4 times greater than the peak value attained by the female between 15 and 16 years of age. These changes with growth and age development are illustrated in Figure 17-1. Body density data from hydrostatic weighings are somewhat inconsistent with the preceding data, as females typically demonstrate lower body density values at all ages, including the preadolescent period, indicating a higher relative body fat. Somatotype data are generally lacking for the preadoles-

cent ages. The limited data that have been published indicate a similarity in somatotype between the sexes up to the age of 12 years, with girls exhibiting a slightly higher degree of endomorphy and a lesser degree of ectomorphy.

At puberty, rather major differences in body composition begin to develop between the sexes, due largely to the associated endocrine changes. Testosterone secretion by the testes, which stops at birth, is reinstituted at puberty, producing an increased deposition of protein in muscle, bone, skin, and other parts of the body. This ultimately results in the male adolescent being larger and more muscular than the female, characteristics which carry over into adulthood. Prior to puberty, the anterior pituitary gland is unable to secrete any gonadotrophic hormones. Thus, in the female, at the time when a sufficient quantity of follicle-stimulating hormone begins to be secreted from the anterior pituitary, the ovaries develop, and estrogen secretion begins. Estrogen has a significant influence on body growth, broadening the pelvis, increasing the size of the breasts, and proliferating the deposition of fat, particularly in the thighs and hips. Additionally, estrogen increases the growth rate of bone, allowing the ultimate bone length to be reached within two to four years following the onset of puberty. As a result, the female grows very rapidly for the first few years following puberty and then ceases to grow. The male has a much longer growth phase, allowing him to attain a greater height. As a result of the above endocrine changes at puberty, the male at full maturity is nearly 13 cm (5 in) taller, 14 to 18 kg (30 to 40 lb) heavier in total weight, 18 to 22 kg (40 to 50 lb) heavier in LBM, 3 to 6 kg (7 to 13 lb) lighter in fat weight, and 6 to 9 percentage units (15 percent versus 21 to 24 percent) less in relative body fat. With respect to somatotype at the age of 17 years, the female exhibits a substantially greater degree of endomorphy, while the male has a greater degree of mesomorphy and ectomorphy.

There are rather substantial sex differences in anthropometric measurements at maturity, as illustrated in Table 17-1. Men have broader shoulders, narrower hips, and a greater chest girth relative to total body size. Men also tend to carry body fat in the abdominal and upper regions of the body, while women pattern their fat in the hips and lower regions of the body.

Table 17-1 Anthropometric measurements for young and middle-aged men and women.

	Men			Women		
	Young		Middle-aged	Young		Middle-aged
	Wilmore and Behnke* (n = 133)	Pollock et al† (n = 95)	Pollock et al† (n = 84)	Wilmore and Behnke* (n = 128)	Pollock et al† (n = 83)	Pollock et al† (n = 60)
Skin folds (mm)						
Scapula	14.1	13.9	20.2	13.2	15.3	17.3
Triceps	7.9	13.6	18.5	12.8	18.8	22.2
Midaxillary	11.7	15.5	24.8	10.7	13.3	16.9
Chest		11.4	20.6		14.0	14.0
Suprailiac	19.3	15.2	22.0	17.2	15.3	17.3
Abdominal	16.0	20.6	30.0	15.1	22.8	29.6
Thigh	14.9	17.4	22.2	31.8	28.8	33.1
Knee	5.3			7.0	17.4	17.3
Circumferences (cm)						
Head	57.5			55.0		
Neck	38.5			31.8		
Shoulders	117.0	112.5	114.8	101.9	99.7	100.9
Chest	97.4	91.4	96.3	85.2	84.6	87.1
Bust				87.8	87.7	90.8
Abdomen	84.0	81.0	91.1	75.3	75.0	82.7
Hips	96.9	94.4	98.4	95.9	93.1	97.5
Thigh	58.0	57.1	59.0	57.0	56.5	57.6
Knee	37.7			36.1		
Calf	37.6	36.5	36.9	35.1	33.9	34.4
Ankle	22.7	22.1	22.1	21.1	20.8	20.8
Deltoid	36.3			30.7		
Biceps, flexed	33.2	32.6	34.0	27.2	27.0	28.6
Biceps, extended	29.1			25.0		
Forearm	27.6	28.3	29.2	23.5	23.8	24.4
Wrist	17.0	16.7	17.4	14.9	14.8	15.1
Diameters (cm)						
Head length	19.9			19.0		
Head width	15.5			14.9		
Biacromial	40.4	41.1	41.5	36.5	36.8	36.7
Bideltoid	47.6	46.9	47.4	42.1	41.4	41.8
Chest	29.3	31.8	33.0	25.8	27.8	28.6
Bi-iliac	28.4	29.6	31.4	28.4	29.9	31.2
Bitrochanteric	32.9	33.6	35.1	32.1	34.0	35.3
Knee	9.5	9.8	10.1	8.9	9.3	9.6
Ankle	7.1			6.3		
Elbow	7.0			6.0		
Wrist	5.6	5.9	6.0	4.9	5.1	5.2
Arm span	181.7			165.8		
Foot length	26.7			24.1		
Hand length	19.1			17.3		

*From Wilmore, J. H., & Behnke A. R. *Journal of Applied Physiology, 27,* 25, 1969 and *American Journal of Clinical Nutrition, 23,*267, 1970.
† From Pollock M. L., et al: *Journal of Applied Physiology, 38,*745, 1975 and *Journal of Applied Physiology, 40,*300, 1976.

Table 17-2 Relative body fat values for males and females of various ages.

Age Group, years	Relative Fat, percentage	
	Men	Women
15–19	13–16	20–24
20–29	15–20	22–25
30–39	18–26	24–30
40–49	23–29	27–33
50–59	26–33	30–36
60–69	29–33	30–36

With aging, both men and women tend to accumulate fat and decrease lean body mass starting in their mid-twenties. In one of the few longitudinal studies conducted, Forbes (1976) found an average decrease in LBM of approximately 3 kg per decade, or more than 0.6 lb per year. This data confirms previous cross-sectional data, which indicated a loss in LBM of 0.3 to 0.5 lb per year. This decline is associated with lower levels of physical activity and testosterone. Apparently, the concomitant increase in total body fat with aging is also associated with the general decline in physical activity, without an equivalent decrease in caloric intake. Table 17-2 illustrates the changes in relative body fat with aging for both sexes.

The normative data cited earlier in this section can be highly misleading. As an example, the average difference in relative body fat between young men and women ages 18 to 24 years, is six to ten percentage units, (13 to 16 percent for men versus 20 to 25 percent for women). At first, this difference was thought to be the result of sex-specific differences in fat depots, such as breast tissue and hips. However, subsequent research with female athletes, particularly women distance runners, indicates that these women were exceptionally lean, well below the average woman, and even below the average for young men. Many of the better runners were below ten percent body fat (see Figure 17-2). These low values can be the result of either a genetic predisposition toward leanness or the high-training mileage run by these women each week, which in some cases exceeded 100 miles per week. In any event, it is obvious that women can reduce their fat stores to levels well below those considered normal for women of this age.

Figure 17-2 provides an important illustration of the wide range of variability in the relative body fat values of women track and field athletes. Of the

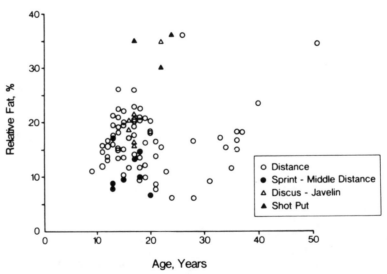

Figure 17-2 Relative body fat in female track and field athletes.

78 runners evaluated, 12 had relative fat values under ten percent. Two of these women were approximately six percent fat, and one of these two had started running because she was considered obese and wanted to use exercise in addition to diet to reduce her weight to a more normal level. She became enthusiastic with her running and eventually became a world record-holding, long-distance runner! Low levels of body fat are achievable by the female athlete, but there is now some concern that some of our female athletes are becoming too lean. This will be discussed in great detail at the conclusion of this chapter.

Differences between the sexes have also been noted for body fluids. In the newborn, total body water (TBW), expressed as a percentage of total body weight, is approximately 77 percent, with the extracellular water (ECW) and intracellular water (ICW) contributing 44 percent and 33 percent, respectively. By one year of age, the infant has achieved the adult fraction of TBW (58 to 64 percent), composed of approximately 25 percent ECW and 36 percent ICW. Sex differences are evident by the age of 18 years, with the TBW of females dropping to approximately 47 to 54 percent. This difference comes almost totally from the ICW, which is only 23 to 29 percent in the female. It is quite possible that the decreases in TBW and ICW are due to the increased levels of body fat, since adipose tissue contains only a small fraction of water and since both TBW and ICW are expressed relative to total body weight. Fluid levels are also altered considerably consequent to menstruation. Weight gains of between two and six pounds, resulting from fluid retention, are very common.

PHYSIOLOGICAL RESPONSES TO ACUTE EXERCISE

When males and females are exposed to an acute bout of exercise, whether it be an all-out run to exhaustion on the treadmill or a one-time attempt to lift the heaviest weight possible, there are characteristic responses that differentiate the sexes. These will be discussed very briefly.

Neuromuscular Responses

Females have typically been regarded as the weaker sex. In previous studies, females have been found to be 43 to 63 percent weaker than males in upper body strength, but only 25 to 30 percent weaker in lower body strength. Since there is a considerable size difference between the sexes, as noted in the previous section, several studies have expressed strength relative to body weight (absolute strength/body weight) or relative to LBM as a reflection of the muscle mass (absolute strength/LBM). When lower body strength is expressed relative to body weight there is still a 5 to 15 percent difference between the sexes. When expressed relative to LBM, however, the difference between the sexes disappears (see Figure 17–3). This indicates that the histological and biochemical qualities of muscle and its motor control properties are similar for males and females. Although the differences in upper body strength are reduced somewhat when expressed relative to total body weight and LBM, substantial differences remain. There are at least two possible explanations for the different findings in upper and lower body strength. First, the female has a higher percentage of her LBM below the waist. Second, and probably related, the female uses the muscle mass of her lower body to a much greater extent than she uses her upper body muscle mass, particularly when compared to patterns of use in males. Some women of normal body size have remarkable strength, exceeding even that of the average man. This points to the importance of neuromuscular recruitment and synchro-

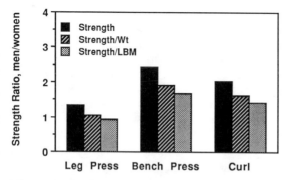

Figure 17–3 Strength values in males versus females, comparing absolute values and values scaled for body weight and lean body mass.

nization of motor-unit firing in determining ultimate levels of strength (see Chapter 7).

Recently, there has been a great deal of interest in muscle fiber typing. In the 1960s, researcher_ started using the muscle biopsy technique to investigate several aspects of muscle physiology. Through various staining techniques, it was possible to identify the different muscle fiber types, which led to an interest in how athletes of both sexes might differ in various sports. Within the past few years, biopsies have become more common among female athletes; this has led to a natural interest in the differences and similarities between males and females participating in the same sport or event. The classification system most commonly used identifies three basic fiber types: slow-twitch oxidative (Type I), fast-twitch oxidative (Type II_a), and a fast-twitch glycolytic (Type II_b). A Type II_c fiber has also been identified but will not be considered in this discussion. Men and women athletes in the same sport or event have similar distributions of fiber types, although the men appear to reach greater extremes (for instance, > 90 percent Type I or > 90 percent Type II), as well as to have larger fiber areas (see Table 1–1).

Cardiovascular Responses

When placed on a cycle ergometer, where the power output can be precisely controlled independently of body weight, males generally have a lower heart rate (HR) response at each level of submaximal exercise. However, maximal heart rate (HR max) does not appear to be different between the sexes. Since cardiac output $(\dot{Q})$ of both sexes is nearly identical for the same absolute power output, the lower HR response in males is associated with a higher stroke volume (SV). The enhanced SV in the male is primarily the result of at least three factors. First, the male has a larger heart and therefore a larger left ventricle, both advantages of a larger body size. Second, and also related to body size, the male has a greater blood volume. Third, the average male is typically better conditioned and will therefore exhibit the classic alterations (to be discussed in the next section) that are associated with physical training. When the power output is controlled to provide the same relative level of exercise, usually expressed as a fixed percentage of the maximal oxygen uptake ($\dot{V}O_2$ max), the HR of the female is still elevated compared to that of the male. At 50 percent of $\dot{V}O_2$ max, $\dot{Q}$, SV, and $\dot{V}O_2$ are generally less and the heart rate is slightly higher in women.

In one of the first studies to investigate the response of $\dot{Q}$ to exercise in boys and girls, Bar-Or and his associates (1971) exercised 29 girls and 27 boys, 10 to 13 years of age, at levels ranging from 40 to 70 percent of their respective $\dot{V}O_2$ max values. For a given $\dot{V}O_2$, the girls had a higher $\dot{Q}$, a higher HR, and a lower arteriovenous oxygen difference (a-$\bar{v}O_2$ difference). Stroke volume was higher in the boys at the low work loads, but was the same as that of the girls at the higher work loads. Becklake and her associates (1965) measured $\dot{Q}$ in males and females, between 20 and 85 years of age, at three different power outputs on the cycle ergometer. From the age of 20 to 39 years, $\dot{Q}$, HR, and SV were higher, and the a-$\bar{v}O_2$ difference was lower in the women at identical power outputs. For those 40 years of age or older, at the same power outputs the women had higher HR, similar $\dot{Q}$, and lower SV. Miyamura and Honda (1975) conducted a study of maximal cardiac output ($\dot{Q}$ max) responses to exercise in 233 males, 9 to 53 years of age, and 102 females, 9 to 20 years of age. While $\dot{Q}$ max was similar for boys and girls up to the age of 15 years, the males achieved values by 18 years of age that were approximately 30 percent higher than those of the females.

As stated above, the differences in SV response to exercise between males and females are primarily the result of differences in heart size, blood volume, and level of physical conditioning. In addition, the differences noted in a-$\bar{v}O_2$ difference are considered to be the result of a lower hemoglobin content in the female, resulting in a lower arterial oxygen content. This is an important consideration when discussing differences between the sexes in $\dot{V}O_2$ max.

Respiratory Responses

The differences between the sexes in their respiratory responses to exercise are largely the result of differences in body size. There appears to be little difference in breathing frequency when working at the same relative power output, although the female tends to breathe at a higher frequency at the same absolute power output. This latter response is probably due to the fact that the female is working at a higher percentage of her $\dot{V}O_2$ max. Tidal volume and ventilation volume are generally smaller in the female at both the same relative and absolute power outputs, up to and including maximal levels. While highly-trained male athletes have maximal ventilation volumes of 150 liters $\cdot$ min^{-1} and higher (some exceeding 250 liters $\cdot$ min^{-1}), most female athletes have maximal values below 125 liters $\cdot$ min^{-1}. Again, these differences in volume are closely associated with differences in body size.

Metabolic Responses

The $\dot{V}O_2$ max is regarded by most exercise scientists as the single best index of an individual's cardiorespiratory endurance capacity. For this reason, numerous studies have been conducted comparing $\dot{V}O_2$ max values of males and females, both trained and untrained. Åstrand (1952) conducted the first study comparing a large population of males and females, from four years of age up to adulthood. Subsequently, additional studies have been published confirming the original work of Åstrand and adding considerably to the data pool.

Before puberty, there are no significant differences in $\dot{V}O_2$ max between boys and girls when expressed relative to body weight (ml$\cdot$kg$^{-1}\cdot$ min^{-1}). The female tends to reach her peak $\dot{V}O_2$ max between the ages of 13 and 15 years, while the male does not reach his peak until 18 to 22 years of age. Beyond puberty, the $\dot{V}O_2$ max of the female is only 70 to 75 percent of that found in the normal male. These differences between the sexes with age were illustrated in Chapter 15 in Figures 15-8 and 15-9.

$\dot{V}O_2$ max differences between males and females must be interpreted carefully. In 1965, Hermansen and Andersen published a classic study indicating that there is considerable variability in $\dot{V}O_2$ max values within each sex and that there is considerable overlapping of values between sexes. Taking a group of males and females 20 to 30 years of age,

they compared the physiological responses to submaximal and maximal exercise of four subgroups: male athletes, male nonathletes, female athletes, and female nonathletes. First, for the same absolute level of work, they found that there was a tendency for athletes to have slightly higher $\dot{V}O_2$ values than nonathletes at submaximal levels and for males to have slightly higher values than females. Relative to body weight, average $\dot{V}O_2$ max values for the male athletes were 61 percent higher than those of male nonathletes, while those of the female athletes were 45 percent higher than those of female nonathletes. Values of male athletes were 29 percent higher than those of the female athletes, but the mean $\dot{V}O_2$ max of female athletes was 25 percent higher than the male nonathletes. From this study, Drinkwater (1973) calculated that 76 percent of the female nonathletes overlapped 47 percent of the male nonathletes and that 22 percent of the female athletes overlapped 7 percent of the male athletes. These data demonstrate the importance of considering both the level of physical conditioning in the sample and of looking beyond mean values to the extent of overlapping between samples that are being compared.

Since $\dot{V}O_2$ is the product of $\dot{Q}$ and a–$\bar{v}O_2$ difference, $\dot{V}O_2$ max represents that point during exhaustive exercise where the subject has maximized his or her oxygen delivery and utilization capabilities. Values range from less than 20 ml $\cdot$ kg$^{-1}\cdot$ min^{-1} in unfit, aging individuals, to values greater than 85 ml $\cdot$ kg$^{-1}\cdot$ min^{-1} in superbly-conditioned, endurance athletes. The highest value recorded in the literature for a male was 94 ml $\cdot$ kg$^{-1}\cdot$ min^{-1}, found in a champion Norwegian cross-country skier; the highest recorded female value was 77 ml $\cdot$ kg$^{-1}\cdot$ min^{-1} for a Russian cross-country skier.

In 1984, Drinkwater conducted an extensive review of the existing research literature relative to $\dot{V}O_2$ max values for females of varying age and athletic ability. While $\dot{V}O_2$ max values of males and females are similar up to the age of puberty, as discussed above, there is a question as to the validity of comparing the values of normal, non-athletic males and females beyond the age of 12 years. The data might reflect an unfair comparison of relatively sedentary females with relatively more active males. Thus, the differences would re-

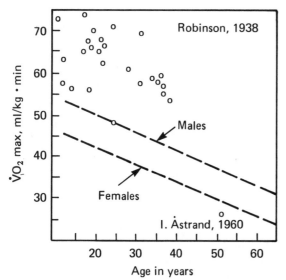

Figure 17-4 Maximal oxygen uptake values for female distance runners compared to normal untrained males and females (normal values for males obtained from Robinson, 1938, normal values for females obtained from Åstrand, 1960).

flect the level of conditioning, as well as possible sex differences. To overcome this potential problem, investigators began to look at highly-trained male and female athletes, with the assumption that the level of training would be similar for the sexes. Saltin and Åstrand (1967) compared $\dot{V}O_2$ max values of male and female athletes who participated on Swedish national teams. In comparable events, the men had 15 to 30 percent higher values. Wilmore and Brown (1974), in their study of 11 women long-distance runners of national and international caliber, found $\dot{V}O_2$ max values (mean = 59.1 ml $\cdot$ kg^{-1} $\cdot$ min^{-1}) that were considerably higher than those of the average female or male of similar age. Still, when compared to equally-trained male distance runners, the women had values 15.9 percent lower when expressed relative to body weight and 8.6 percent lower when expressed relative to LBM. The three best runners from this study had an average value of 67.4 ml $\cdot$ kg^{-1} $\cdot$ min^{-1}, which is similar to the average value of 70.3 ml $\cdot$ kg^{-1} $\cdot$ min^{-1} reported for nationally-ranked male marathon runners of similar

age. $\dot{V}O_2$ max values for males and females of different ages and in different sports have been presented in Appendix A. Further, $\dot{V}O_2$ max values for a group of elite, female distance runners are illustrated in Figure 17-4 and compared with values for normal, non-athletic males and females.

A number of studies have attempted to scale $\dot{V}O_2$ max values relative to height, weight, LBM, or limb volume in an attempt to more objectively compare male and female values. Several of these studies have shown that differences between the sexes disappear when $\dot{V}O_2$ max is expressed relative to fat-free body weight (LBM) or active muscle mass, but there are also studies that continue to demonstrate differences, even when one accounts for differences in body fat. Cureton and Sparling (1980) employed a novel approach to investigate this problem. They studied the submaximal and maximal responses to treadmill runs under various conditions in ten men and ten women who regularly engaged in distance running. The men were studied at normal weight and under an artificial condition where they had to run with external weight added to the trunk, so that the total percent of excess weight was equal to the percent fat of matched women. The women exercised only under normal weight conditions. Equating the sexes for excess weight reduced mean sex differences in treadmill run time by 32 percent, or 38 percent in the oxygen required per unit of fat-free weight in order to run at various submaximal speeds, and reduced $\dot{V}O_2$ max differences by 65 percent. They concluded that the greater sex-specific essential body fat stores of women is a major determinant of the sex differences in the metabolic responses to running. Finally, Davies (1971) found that when the $\dot{V}O_2$ max of 116 boys and girls was expressed relative to body weight, or to LBM, definite sex differences were observed. When expressed relative to the volume of the leg, however, these differences disappeared. Davies concluded that $\dot{V}O_2$ max is directly related to the active tissue involved in the exercise.

The lower hemoglobin level of females compared to males has also been proposed as a contributing factor to their lower $\dot{V}O_2$ max values. Cureton and his colleagues (1986) attempted to equate the hemoglobin concentrations of a group of ten men and eleven women who were active, but not highly trained. An amount of blood was withdrawn from men to equalize their hemoglobin concentrations to those of the women subjects. This significantly reduced the men's $\dot{V}O_2$ max values, but explained only a relatively small portion of the sex differences in $\dot{V}O_2$ max.

With respect to submaximal $\dot{V}O_2$ values, there appears to be little, if any difference between the sexes for the same absolute power output. It should be remembered, however, that at the same absolute submaximal load, women are usually working at a higher percentage of their $\dot{V}O_2$ max. As a result, blood lactate levels will be higher and the anaerobic or lactate threshold will occur at a lower absolute power output. Peak blood lactate values are generally higher in males but there is a paucity of data for female athletes who would be more inclined to exert themselves to higher values.

There is no obvious reason to expect differences between the sexes in peak blood lactate values. With respect to anaerobic or lactate threshold, there is only limited data available on females. It would appear, however, that anaerobic or lactate threshold values would be similar between equally trained males and females, providing the values were expressed in relative and not absolute terms. Anaerobic or lactate threshold appears to be related more to the mode of testing and to the state of training of the individual than to sex differences.

With the increase in popularity of distance running in the United States during the last fifteen years, an interesting theory was proposed that implied women were natural distance runners due to their inherently better ability to utilize fat as the energy substrate for endurance activity. Further, it was stated that with proper training, women might be even better distance runners than men because of their unique ability to mobilize and utilize free fatty acids, thus sparing glycogen. Costill and his colleagues put this theory to the test in 1979. Figure 17–5 illustrates the results of their study. They took muscle biopsies from the gastrocnemius muscle of 13 male and 12 female distance

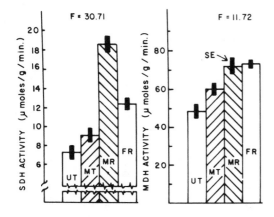

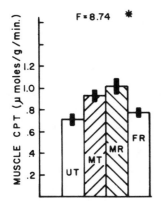

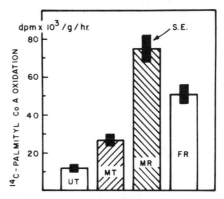

Figure 17–5 Enzyme activities from muscles of untrained (UT), moderately trained (MT), and highly-trained male (MR) and female runners (FR) demonstrating that highly-trained female runners matched for $\dot{V}O_2$ max and training mileage with male runners, do not exhibit an enhanced ability to utilize fat as a substrate (adapted from Costill, et al., 1979).

runners matched for $\dot{V}O_2$ max and training mileage. Although male and female runners had similar fiber types, male runners exhibited significantly greater activity of the muscle enzyme succinate dehydrogenase and carnitine palmitoyl transferase. They also found that male and female runners derive similar fractions of their energy from lipids during treadmill running at 70 percent $\dot{V}O_2$ max.

PHYSIOLOGICAL ADAPTATIONS TO CHRONIC EXERCISE

With physical training, there are substantial alterations in basic physiological function, both at rest and during exercise. This section will investigate how females adapt to chronic exercise, emphasizing those areas where their responses might be different from those of males.

Body Composition, Bone, and Connective Tissue

With exercise training, emphasizing either cardiorespiratory endurance activities or strength training, males and females both experience losses in total body weight, fat weight, and relative fat, in addition to gains in LBM. The gains in LBM are generally much less for females. The magnitude of change in body composition, with the exception of LBM, appears to be related more to the total energy expenditure associated with training activities, rather than to the participant's sex. Increases in LBM are of much greater magnitude in response to strength training than compared to endurance training.

Alterations in bone and connective tissue with training are not well understood. In general, studies on animals and limited studies on humans support an increase in the density of the weight-bearing long bones; this adaptation appears to be independent of sex, at least in young and middle-aged populations. There are exceptions to this which will be discussed in detail in the last section of this chapter. Connective tissue appears to be strengthened with endurance training; sex-specific differences in response have not been identified. There has been some concern that females are more susceptible to injury while participating in

physical activity and sport. This has been largely attributed to sex-specific differences in joint integrity, as well as to the strength of ligaments, tendons, and bones. Unfortunately, the research literature contributes little to confirming or denying the validity of such concerns. Where differences have been observed in the rate of injury, it is highly possible that the injury was related more to the level of conditioning than to the sex of the participant—those who are less fit are more prone to injury. This is an extremely difficult area in which to obtain objective data, but is nevertheless an important area that needs to be defined better.

Neuromuscular Adaptations

For a number of years, it was not considered appropriate to prescribe strength training programs for girls and women. During the 1960s and 1970s, it became evident that many of the better female athletes in the United States were not doing well in international competition and that this was mainly due to the fact that they were weaker than their competitors. Slowly, research demonstrated that females could gain considerable benefit from strength training programs and that strength gains were usually not accompanied by large increases in muscle bulk. One study compared the training responses of forty-seven women and twenty-six men who volunteered to participate in identical progressive resistance, weight-training programs. The program was conducted twice a week, 40 minutes per day, for a total of ten weeks. Bench press and leg press strength increased by 28.6 percent and 29.5 percent, respectively, in the females and 16.5 percent and 26.0 percent, respectively, in the males. There were only small increases in muscle girths in the females, while the males exhibited classic muscle hypertrophy (Wilmore, 1974). Thus, it is apparent that hypertrophy is neither a necessary consequence nor a prerequisite to gains in muscular strength. Several studies have confirmed these results.

From the above, it appears that the female has the potential to develop substantially higher levels of strength than those normally identified in the average, typically sedentary female. Will the female ever be able to attain the same levels of strength as the male for all major regions of the

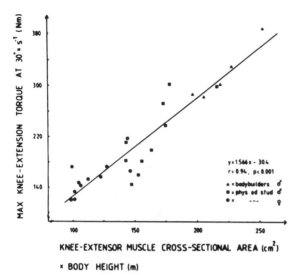

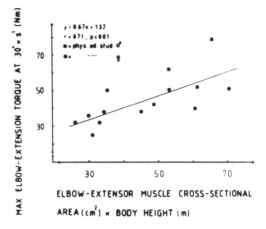

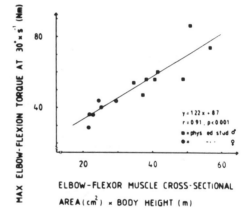

Figure 17-6 The relationship between muscle cross-sectional area times body height and maximal torque in the knee extensors, elbow extensors, and elbow flexors (adapted from Schantz, et al., 1983).

body? From the similarity of leg strength/weight ratios between the two sexes, it appears that the quality of muscle is the same, irrespective of sex. This was recently confirmed by computer tomography scans of the thigh of male and female physical education majors and male body builders (Schantz, et al., 1983). While the male students and body builders had much greater absolute levels of strength, there were no differences between the groups when strength was expressed per unit of muscle cross-sectional area (see Figure 17-6).

Because of the higher levels of testosterone, the male will continue to have a larger total muscle mass. If muscle mass is the major determinant of strength, then the male has a distinct advantage. If neural factors are as important, or even more important than size, then the potential for absolute strength gains in females is considerable. Since the basic mechanisms allowing the expression of greater levels of strength have not yet been clearly defined, it is premature to draw conclusions at this time.

Cardiovascular and Respiratory Adaptations

Major cardiovascular and respiratory adaptations accompany cardiorespiratory endurance training; these adaptations do not appear to be sex-specific. In a review article, Saltin and Rowell (1980) describe the classic cardiovascular, respiratory, and metabolic adaptations to physical activity and inactivity. With training, there are major increases in maximal $\dot{Q}$. Since HR max does not change with training, this increase in $\dot{Q}$ max is the result of a large increase in SV, which is the result of both a greater end-diastolic volume and a reduced end-systolic volume. The former is related to an increased blood volume and a more efficient venous return, while the latter is the result of a stronger myocardium (a stronger contraction). At submaximal levels of work, there is little or no change in $\dot{Q}$, although SV is considerably higher for the same absolute level of work. Consequently, HR for any given level of work is reduced. Resting HR can be reduced to 50 beats per min or less. Several female distance runners have had a resting HR below 36 beats $\cdot$ min^{-1}. This is considered a classic training response and corresponds to an exceptionally high stroke volume.

The increases in $\dot{V}O_2$ max which accompany cardiorespiratory endurance training will be discussed below, but are primarily the result of the large increases in $\dot{Q}$ max, with only small increases in a-$\bar{v}O_2$ difference. However, Saltin and Rowell state that the major limitation to $\dot{V}O_2$ max resides in the transport of oxygen to the working muscles. While $\dot{Q}$ is important in this respect, it is their position that the increases in maximal aerobic power that accompany training are attributed primarily to increased maximal muscle blood flow and muscle capillary density. There is no reason to suspect that females would differ in this response to training. In fact, Ingjer and Brodal (1978) have recently demonstrated that endurance-trained women have considerably higher capillary-to-fiber ratios than untrained women (1.69 and 1.11, respectively).

With respect to respiration, women experience considerable increases in maximal ventilation, which reflect increases in both tidal volume and breathing frequency. These changes are generally assumed to be unrelated to the increase in $\dot{V}O_2$ max.

Metabolic Adaptations

With cardiorespiratory endurance training, women experience the same relative increase in $\dot{V}O_2$ max that has been observed in men. The magnitude of increase is highly related to the initial level of fitness—those with low fitness levels prior to the start of training will generally experience a greater percentage increase. Each person, theoretically, has a genetically established upper limit of $\dot{V}O_2$ max which he or she cannot exceed, irrespective of the duration or intensity of training. Consequently, the closer one is to this upper limit, the more difficult it is to obtain large improvements

with subsequent training. Thus, it would be expected that most women would experience rather substantial improvements in $\dot{V}O_2$ max with endurance training, since they have relatively low initial values. From the research literature, women can improve their $\dot{V}O_2$ max by 10 to 30 percent with cardiorespiratory endurance training, the magnitude of change being dependent on the initial level of fitness, the intensity and duration of the individual exercise sessions, the frequency of sessions per week, and the length of the study.

Oxygen uptake at the same absolute submaximal work load does not appear to change, although several studies have reported decreases. Blood lactate levels are reduced for the same absolute submaximal work levels and peak lactate levels are generally increased. The anaerobic or lactate threshold does increase with training in men but this has not been verified in women. Finally, endurance training also improves the ability to utilize free fatty acids, an adaptation which is very important for glycogen sparing.

From the above, it would appear that the female responds to physical training in exactly the same manner as her male counterpart. While the adaptations to training may differ somewhat in magnitude (as in lean body weight), the trends do appear to be identical. This is an extremely important consideration when exercise is to be prescribed to a female population.

MOTOR SKILLS AND ATHLETIC ABILITY

With the exception of one activity, the softball throw for distance, boys and girls are quite similar in their performance of physical activities up to the ages of ten to 12 years. Tests of specific motor skills or general athletic ability show few differences between the sexes during this period of development. Past the age of 12 years, however, the male becomes considerably stronger, possesses greater muscular and cardiovascular endurance, and becomes more proficient in almost all motor skills. This phenomenon is illustrated in Figure 17-7 for selected motor skills.

From Figure 17-7 it is obvious that the female lags far behind the male at all ages in the softball throw, the female throwing only half of the

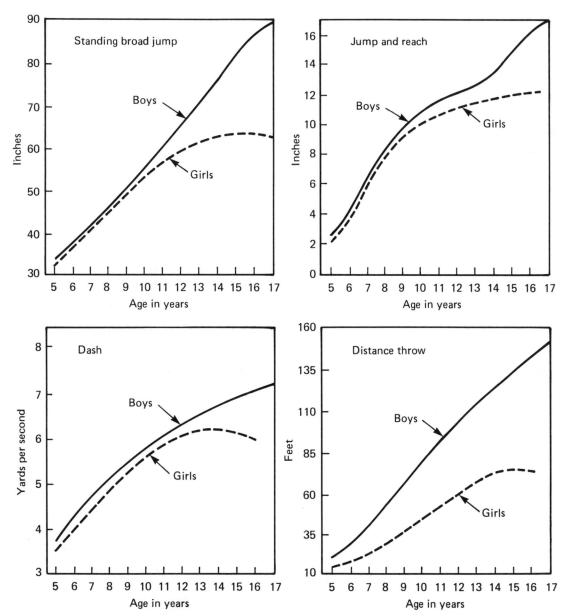

Figure 17-7 Performance of selected motor-skill test items for boys and girls between 5 and 16 years of age (from Espenschade & Eckert, 1974).

distance of the male at any particular age. In an unpublished study, Grimditch and Sockolov investigated why females perform so poorly in the softball throw. Postulating this difference to be the result of insufficient practice and experience, they recruited over 200 males and females from three to 20 years of age to throw the softball for distance with both the dominant and nondominant arms.

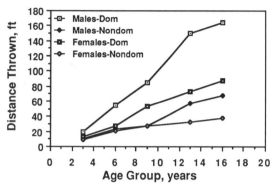

Figure 17-8   Softball throw for distance in males and females using the dominant and nondominant arms (from Grimditch & Sockolov, (1974) unpublished observations. University of California, Davis.

The results are illustrated in Figure 17-8. As they had theorized, there was absolutely no difference between the males and females for the nondominant arm, up to the age of 10 to 12 years, just as with each of the other motor skill tasks shown in Figure 17-7. Major differences at all ages were the results for the dominant arm, and this is in agreement with what had been reported previously. Thus, the softball throw for distance using the dominant arm appears to be biased by the previous experience and practice of the males. When the influence of experience and practice was removed by using the nondominant arm, this motor skill task was identical to each of the others.

Athletic performance differences were briefly discussed in the introduction to this chapter. The female is outperformed by the male in almost all sports, events, or activities. This is quite obvious in such activities as the shot put in track and field, where high levels of upper body strength are critical to successful performance. In the 400-meter freestyle, however, the winning time for the men in the 1924 Olympic games was 16 percent faster than that for the women, but this difference decreased to 11.6 percent in the 1948 Olympics, and to only 6.9 percent in the 1984 Olympics. The fastest female, 800-meter freestyle swimmer in 1979 swam faster than the world-record-holding male for the same distance in 1972! Therefore, in this

particular event, the gap between the sexes is narrowing, and there are indications that this is also true for other events and for other sports. Unfortunately, it is difficult to make valid comparisons, since the degree to which the sport, activity, or event has been emphasized is not constant, and other factors such as coaching, facilities, and training techniques have differed considerably between the sexes over the years. While the performance gap appears to be closing, it is far too early to predict whether it will ever close completely for any or all sports.

SPECIAL CONSIDERATIONS

While the sexes respond to acute exercise and adapt to chronic exercise in much the same manner, several additional areas must be considered, which are unique to the female.

Osteoporosis

There is evidence that maintaining a healthy lifestyle may retard one of the detrimental aging processes that is a major health concern for women, that of osteoporosis. **Osteoporosis** is characterized by an increase in bone porosity and a decrease in bone mineral content. These changes lead to an increase in the risk of fractures that typically begin in the late thirties and are accelerated 2 to 5 times that rate at the onset of menopause. Although there is still a good deal to discover concerning the etiology of osteoporosis, three major contributing factors in post-menopausal women include an overall reduction in calcium intake, estrogen deficiency, and a reduction in physical activity.

In addition to post-menopausal women, women with **amenorrhea** (failure to start menstruation, or discontinuation of normal menstruation) and those with anorexia nervosa, also suffer from osteoporosis due to a decreased calcium intake, a reduction in serum estrogen levels, or possibly both. Rigotti and associates (1984) assessed the skeletal mass of 18 women who were known anorexics and 28 normal controls by direct photon absorptiometry. They found that the patients with anorexia had significantly reduced bone densities compared to the controls. Cann and associates (1984) reported a substantially low bone mineral content (BMC) in six physically active women classified as having hypothalamic amenorrhea.

Drinkwater and associates (1984) compared radial and vertebral bone densities of 14 athletic women with amenorrhea, to 14 athletic women who were normally menstruating (eumenorrhea). They discovered that physical activity did not protect the amenorrheic group from significant bone density losses. When the amenorrheic group's bone density values were compared with an age-related regression equation, their values at a mean age of 29.4 years were equivalent to those of a woman 51.2 years of age. In a subsequent study, Drinkwater and her associates (1986) reported increases in vertebral bone mineral density in formerly amenorrheic women who resumed menstruation. Linnell and associates (1984) reported no significant difference in bone density in ten amenorrheic runners when compared to normal menstruating controls. It should also be noted that normally menstruating runners tend to exhibit higher bone mineral content values than those of normally menstruating non-running controls. Caution should be used when interpreting data such as those presented in this section, since there are confounding factors such as body composition, age, height, weight, and dietary intake which can all influence the interpretation of the results of these studies.

Although the precise mechanism of action is unknown, the lack of estrogen appears to play a major role in the development of osteoporosis. In the past, estrogen has been prescribed in an effort to reverse the degenerative effects of osteoporosis, but this therapy may be dangerous since it increases the risk of endometrial cancer. One should realize that the body's ability to absorb and maintain normal calcium levels is based not only on physiological but also nutritional factors. According to the National Health and Nutrition Examination Survey (HANES), 56 to 75 percent of the women surveyed consumed less than 75 percent of the Recommended Daily Allowance for calcium (800 mg). It has been proposed that increasing the calcium intake to between 1.5 and 2.0 grams/day would decrease the risk of osteoporosis. This approach, however, may not be as effective as once

hoped and this recommendation of an increased RDA for calcium remains controversial.

As of yet, there does not appear to be sufficient data to draw any firm conclusions on the effects of exercise and amenorrhea on osteoporosis. However, evidence certainly suggests that increased physical activity and adequate calcium intake, combined with an adequate caloric intake, is a sensible approach to maintaining the integrity of the skeletal system at any age.

Menstruation

Two questions which are foremost in the minds of many women, particularly women athletes, have to do with the influence of their menstrual cycle on athletic performance and the influence of their physical activity and competition on menstruation and childbirth. The question of childbirth will be discussed later. With respect to alterations in athletic performance during different phases of the menstrual cycle, there appears to be considerable individual variability. Some women have absolutely no noticeable change in their ability to perform at any one time in their monthly cycle, while others have considerable difficulty in the pre-flow and initial-flow phases. The limited research that has been conducted tends to suggest that performance ability is best in the immediate post-flow period, up to the 15th day of the cycle, with the first day of the cycle corresponding to the initiation of the flow or menstrual phase, and ovulation occurring on about the fourteenth day. The number of women who report impaired performance during the flow phase is approximately the same as those who experienced no difficulty. In fact, some women athletes have reportedly set world records during the flow phase.

With respect to the question concerning the influence of various training programs and intense competition on the menstrual cycle, the existing data is limited. Several long-term studies have been reported on former competitive swimmers, with findings suggesting that intense training at an early age has no serious consequences relative to future gynecological problems. However, athletes who have trained and competed intensely in such sports as figure skating, ballet dancing, gymnastics, cycling, and distance running have reported the absence of menses for months or even years, known as **secondary amenorrhea**. The prevalence of secondary amenorrhea, as well as **oligomenorrhea** (abnormally infrequent or scanty menses) among female athletes is not well-documented, but is estimated to be approximately five to 40 percent, or higher, depending on the sport or activity. These figures are considerably higher than the estimated two to three percent prevalence for amenorrhea and 10 to 12 percent prevalence for oligomenorrhea in the general population. The occurrence appears to be greater in those who are training many hours each day and in those who are working at high intensities. Another factor must be considered. Some have become pregnant during the period of amenorrhea, which indicates fertility is not always influenced by the absence of menstruation. This latter point is an important one, for many women assume that they have developed a simple but effective form of birth control.

Neither the cause nor the long-term consequences of secondary amenorrhea or oligomenorrhea are known. It is tempting to assume that exercise in itself is responsible for changes in menstrual dysfunction in female athletes, but the cause may be related to low levels of body weight or body fat, the acute effects of stress, or changes in the levels of circulating hormones. It has been known for some time that either excessive fatness, undernutrition, or both, are associated with amenorrhea. It has been suggested that a loss of one-third of one's body fat or a ten to 15 percent decrease in body weight will induce amenorrhea. The reason being that aromitization of androgens and estrogen takes place in adipose tissue and abdominal fat, and that any decrease in adipose tissue will influence the storage and metabolism of estrogen. More recently, investigators have challenged the theory that there is a critical body fat level that must be achieved and/or maintained to assure normal menses. A number of studies have now been published in which the relative body fat levels were compared and found to be identical in eumenorrheic (normally menstruating) and amenorrheic athletes.

Although many investigators have reported menstrual irregularities in athletes, it is apparently difficult to separate the effects of exercise per se from the effects of the physical and emotional stresses of intense training, the stress of excessive weight loss, hormonal alterations associated with exercise training, and a low body fat or low body weight which have all been associated with menstrual irregularities. Schwartz and associates (1981), in a descriptive study, showed that amenorrheic runners associate more stress with their training than do eumenorrheic runners. Bullen and associates (1985) attempted to induce amenorrhea in 28 untrained college women with an intense eight-week exercise program. Only four of the 28 subjects had normal menstrual cycles during the training period, the most significant factor being delayed menses, abnormal luteal function, and a loss of luteinizing hormone surge. Boyden and his associates (1983) trained 19 women for a period of 14 to 15 months in an attempt to induce amenorrhea. While none of the subjects became amenorrheic, 18 developed menstrual changes, mainly oligomenorrhea. Fortunately, athletically-induced amenorrhea is usually reversible during periods of reduced training, injury, or vacation.

Environmental Factors

Exercise in the heat, cold, or at altitude provides an additional stress or challenge to the body's adaptive abilities. Many early studies indicated that women are less tolerant of heat than men, particularly when physical work is involved. Much of this difference, however, is the result of lower levels of fitness in those women who were tested, since the men and women were tested at the same absolute rate of work. When the rate of work is adjusted relative to the individual's $\dot{V}O_2$ max, women respond in an almost identical manner to men. Women generally have lower sweat rates for the same exercise and heat stress, although they do possess a larger number of active sweat glands. When exposed to repeated bouts of heat stress, the body undergoes considerable adaptation (acclimatization) which enables it to survive future heat stress more efficiently. Recent evidence tends to indicate that males and females undergo similar reductions in the internal temperature thresholds for sweating and vasodilation, and an increase in the sensitivity of the sweating response per unit of increase in internal temperature following both physical training and heat acclimation. Any differences noted between the males and females were attributed to the initial differences in physical conditioning and not to the sex of the subject. With respect to cold exposure, women do have a slight advantage as a result of their higher levels of subcutaneous body fat. However, their smaller muscle mass will be a disadvantage in extreme cold, since shivering is the major adaptation for generating body heat—the greater the active muscle mass, the greater will be the subsequent generation of heat. An excellent review of the literature in this area was published in 1984 by Drinkwater.

Several studies have reported differences between the sexes in response to hypoxia, both at rest and during submaximal exercise. There is a decrease in $\dot{V}O_2$ max during hypoxic work, but the differences between men and women are small and do not seem to adversely affect the woman's ability to work at high altitude. Studies of maximal exercise at altitude demonstrate no difference in response between the sexes.

SUMMARY

There appears to be a substantial difference between the average female and the average male in almost all aspects of physical performance beyond the age of 10 to 12 years. Prior to this time, there are few, if any, differences between the sexes. What happens to the female once she reaches puberty? Is she physically over the hill, reaching her peak at a relatively early age, or are there other factors or circumstances which might account for her reduced physical capabilities? Recent studies on highly-trained female athletes suggest that the female is not appreciably different from her highly-trained male counterpart at ages beyond puberty. It appears that comparisons in the past between males and females beyond the age of puberty have been inappropriately contrasting relatively active males with relatively sedentary females. Somewhere between the ages of 10 and 12 years, the average female in the past has substituted the piano

for climbing trees, and sewing and cooking for chasing the boys down the street. Once you assume a sedentary lifestyle the basic components of general fitness deteriorate. Strength, muscular endurance, and cardiovascular endurance are lost, and body fat tends to accumulate. Similar trends can be noted for the male by the time he reaches 30 to 35 years of age, an age that corresponds to a reduction in his activity patterns. So, what appear to be dramatic biological differences between the sexes, in fact, may be related more to the cultural and social restrictions placed on the female after puberty, leading to an increasingly sedentary existence. The male generally starts reducing his activity levels ten to 20 years later.

With regard to the female athlete, there appears to be little difference between her and her male counterpart in terms of strength, endurance, and body composition, although women will always have slightly more body fat and considerably less total muscle mass. Strength of the lower extremities, when related to body weight, lean body weight, and the cross-sectional area of the involved muscle, is similar between the sexes. The male maintains a distinct superiority, however, in upper body strength, which is the result of his greater development of muscle mass in the upper body. Strength training, formerly condemned as a mode of training for women because of its supposed masculinizing effects, is now recognized as extremely valuable in developing the strength component, which has traditionally been the weakest link in the physiological profile of the female athlete.

Endurance capacity in the highly-trained female distance runner is approximately equal to the capacity of the highly-trained male distance runner when values are expressed relative to lean body weight. For the better female runners, $\dot{V}O_2$ max values are relatively close to those of male runners even when expressed relative to total body weight. Although the female has considerably less lean weight compared to the male, the female distance runner has a relative body fat similar to the male distance runner.

Because of these similarities, and because their needs are basically the same, there is little reason to advocate different training or conditioning programs on the basis of sex.

STUDY QUESTIONS

1. How do females compare with males with respect to body composition? How do comparisons of athletes differ from those of nonathletes?
2. To what levels can females reduce their relative (percent) body fat as a result of training?
3. How do men and women compare relative to upper body strength? Lower body strength? Relative to lean weight?
4. Why are there differences between upper and lower body strength in men and women?
5. What is the role of testosterone in the development of strength and lean weight?
6. What differences in $\dot{V}O_2$ max exist between normal males and females? Between highly trained males and females?
7. What cardiovascular differences exist between males and females with respect to submaximal exercise? Maximal exercise?
8. Why are male and female performances in motor skills similar up to the age of puberty, and yet considerably different once puberty has been attained?
9. How does the menstrual cycle influence athletic performance?
10. What are some of the possible reasons that women athletes in intensive training will, in some cases, stop menstruating for intervals of several months to several years or more?
11. What are the effects of amenorrhea on bone mineral? How does exercise training affect bone mineral?
12. How do females differ in their exercise response when exposed to intense heat and humidity? At altitude?

REFERENCES

Åstrand, I. (1960). Aerobic work capacity in men and women with special reference to age. *Acta Physiologica Scandinavica, 49* (suppl. 169).

Åstrand, P. O. (1952). *Experimental studies of physical working capacity in relation to age and sex.* Copenhagen: Munksgaard.

Bachmann, G. A., & Kemmann, E. (1982). Prevalence of oligomenorrhea and amenorrhea in a college population. *American Journal of Obstetrics and Gynecology, 144,* 98–102.

Bar-Or, O., Shephard, R. J., & Allen, C. L. (1971). Cardiac output of ten- to thirteen-year-old boys and girls during submaximal exercise. *Journal of Applied Physiology, 30,* 219–223.

Becklake, M. R., Frank, H., Dagenais, G. R., Ostiguy, G. L., & Guzman, C. A. (1965). Influence of age and sex on exercise cardiac output. *Journal of Applied Physiology, 20,* 938–947.

Boyden, T. W., Pamenter, R. W., Stanforth, P., Rotkis, T., & Wilmore, J. H. (1983). Sex steroids and endurance running in women. *Fertility and Sterility, 39,* 629–632.

Bullen, B. A., Skrinar, G. S., Beitins, I. Z., von Mering, G., Turnbull, B. A., & McArthur, J. W. (1985). Induction of menstrual disorders by strenuous exercise in untrained women. *New England Journal of Medicine, 312,* 1349–1353.

Cann, C. E., Martin, M. C., Genant, H. K., & Jaffe, R. B. (1984). Decreased spinal mineral content in amenorrheic women. *Journal of the American Medical Association, 251,* 626–629.

Costill, D. L., Fink, W. J., Getchell, L. H., Ivy, J. L., & Witzmann, F. A. (1979). Lipid metabolism in skeletal muscle of endurance-trained males and females. *Journal of Applied Physiology, 47,* 787–791.

Cureton, K. J., & Sparling, P. B. (1980). Distance running performance and metabolic responses to running in men and women with excess weight experimentally equated. *Medicine and Science in Sports and Exercise, 12,* 288–294.

Cureton, K., Bishop, P., Hutchinson, P., Newland, H., Vickery, S., & Zwiren, L. (1986). Sex differences in maximal oxygen uptake: Effect of equating haemoglobin concentration. *European Journal of Applied Physiology, 54,* 656–660.

Davies, C. T. M.(1971). Body composition in children: A reference standard for maximum aerobic power output on a stationary bicycle ergometer. In C. Thoren (Ed.), *Pediatric work physiology. Acta Pediatrica Scandinavica* (suppl.), *217,* 136–137.

Drinkwater, B. L. (1973). Physiological responses of women to exercise. *Exercise and Sport Sciences Reviews, 1,* 125–153.

Drinkwater, B. L. (1984). Women and exercise: Physiological aspects. *Exercise and Sport Sciences Reviews, 12,* 21–51.

Drinkwater, B. L., Folinsbee, L. J., Bedi, J. F., Plowman, S. A., Loucks, A. B., & Horvath, S. M. (1979). Response of women mountaineers to maximal exercise during hypoxia. *Aviation, Space, and Environmental Medicine, 50,* 657–662.

Drinkwater, B. L., Nilson, K., Chesnut, C. H., III, Bremner, W. J., Shainholtz, S., & Southworth, M. B. (1984). Bone mineral content of amenorrheic and eumenorrheic athletes. *New England Journal of Medicine, 311,* 277–281.

Drinkwater, B. L., Nilson, K., Ott, S., & Chesnut, C. H., III. (1986). Bone mineral density after resumption of menses in amenorrheic athletes. *Journal of the American Medical Association, 256,* 380–382.

Espenschade, A., & Eckert, H. (1974). Motor development. (1974, 1960). In Warren R. Johnson and E. R. Buskirk (Eds.), *Science and Medicine of Exercise and Sport* (2nd ed.), pp. 326–330. Copyright © 1974 by Warren R. Johnson and Elsworth R. Buskirk; copyright © 1960 by Warren R. Johnson. Reprinted by permission of Harper and Row Publishers, Inc.

Forbes, G. B. (1976). The adult decline in lean body mass. *Human Biology, 48,* 161–173.

Forbes, G. B. (1972). Growth of the lean body mass in man. *Growth, 36,* 325–338.

Forbes, G. B. (1972). Relation of lean body mass to height in children and adolescents. *Pediatric Research, 6,* 32–37.

Frisch, R. E. (1984). Body fat, puberty, and fertility. *Biological Review, 59,* 161–188.

Hermansen, L., & Andersen, K. L. (1965). Aerobic work capacity in young Norwegian men and women. *Journal of Applied Physiology, 20,* 425–431.

Ingjer, F., & Brodal, P. (1978). Capillary supply of skeletal muscle fibers in untrained and endurance-trained women. *European Journal of Applied Physiology, 38,* 291–299.

Linnell, S. L., Stager, J. M., Blue, P. W., Oyster, N., & Robertshaw, D. (1984). Bone mineral content and menstrual regularity in female runners. *Medicine and Science in Sports and Exercise, 16,* 343–348.

McCammon, R. W. (1970). *Human growth and development.* Springfield, IL: Charles C. Thomas.

Miyamura, M., & Honda, Y. (1975). Maximum cardiac output related to sex and age. *Japanese Journal of Physiology, 23,* 645–653.

Montoye, H. J., Willis, P. W., III, & Cunningham, D. A. (1968). Heart rate response to submaximal exercise: Relation to sex and age. *Journal of Gerontology, 23,* 127–133.

Nadel, E. R., Roberts, M. F., & Wenger, C. B. (1978). Thermoregulatory adaptations to heat and exercise: Comparative responses of men and women. In L. J. Folinsbee, et al., (Eds.), *Environmental stress,* (pp. 29–38). New York: Academic Press.

Pollock, M. L., Hickman, T., Kendrick, Z., Jackson, A., Linnerud, A. C., & Dawson, G. (1976). Prediction of body density in young and middle-aged men. *Journal of Applied Physiology, 40,* 300–304.

Pollock, M. L., Laughridge, E. E., Coleman, B., Linnerud, A. C., & Jackson, A. (1975). Prediction of body density in young and middle-aged women. *Journal of Applied Physiology, 38,* 745–749.

Rigotti, N. A., Nussbaum, S. R., Herzog, D. B., & Neer, R. M. (1984). Osteoporosis in women with anorexia nervosa. *New England Journal of Medicine, 311,* 1601–1606.

Robinson, S. (1938). Experimental studies of physical fitness in relation to age. *Arbeitsphysiologie, 10,* 251–323.

Saltin, B., & Åstrand, P. O. (1967). Maximal oxygen uptake in athletes. *Journal of Applied Physiology, 23,* 353–358.

Saltin, B., & Rowell, L. B. (1980). Functional adaptations to physical activity and inactivity. *Federation Proceedings, 39,* 1506–1513.

Schantz, P., Randall-Fox, E., Hutchison, W., Tyden, A., & Åstrand, P. O. (1983). Muscle fibre type distribution, muscle cross-sectional area and maximal voluntary strength in humans. *Acta Physiologica Scandinavica, 117,* 219–226.

Schwartz, B., Cumming, D. C., Riordan, E., Selye, M., Yen, S. S. C., & Rebar, R. W. (1981). Exercise-associated amenorrhea: A distinct entity? *American Journal of Obstetrics and Gynecology, 141,* 662–670.

Shangold, M. M. (1984). Exercise and the adult female: Hormonal and endocrine effects. *Exercise and Sport Sciences Reviews, 12,* 53–79.

Shangold, M. M. (1986). How I manage exercise-related menstrual disturbances. *Physician and Sportsmedicine, 14,* 113–120.

Stager, J. M. (1984). Reversibility of amenorrhea in athletes. *Sports Medicine, 1,* 337–340.

Vaccaro, P., Ostrove, S. M., Vandervelden, L., Goldfarb, A. H., & Clarke, D. H. (1984). Body composition and physiological responses of masters female swimmers twenty to seventy years of age. *Research Quarterly for Exercise and Sport, 55,* 278–284.

Wilmore, J. H. (1974). Alterations in strength, body composition, and anthropometric measurements consequent to a ten-week weight training program. *Medicine and Science in Sports, 6,* 133–138.

Wilmore, J. H. (1975). Inferiority of female athletes: Myth or reality. *Journal of Sports Medicine, 3,* 1–6.

Wilmore, J. H. (1979). The application of science to sport: Physiological profiles of male and female athletes. *Canadian Journal of Applied Sports Sciences, 4,* 103–115.

Wilmore, J. H. (1983). Body composition in sport and exercise: Directions for future research. *Medicine and Science in Sports and Exercise, 15,* 21–31.

Wilmore, J. H., & Behnke, A. R. (1969). An anthropometric estimation of body density and lean body weight in young men. *Journal of Applied Physiology, 27,* 25–31.

Wilmore, J. H., & Behnke, A. R. (1970). An anthropometric estimation of body density and lean body weight in young women. *American Journal of Clinical Nutrition, 23,* 267–274.

Wilmore, J. H., & Brown, C. H., (1974). Physiological profiles of women distance runners. *Medicine and Science in Sports, 6,* 178–181.

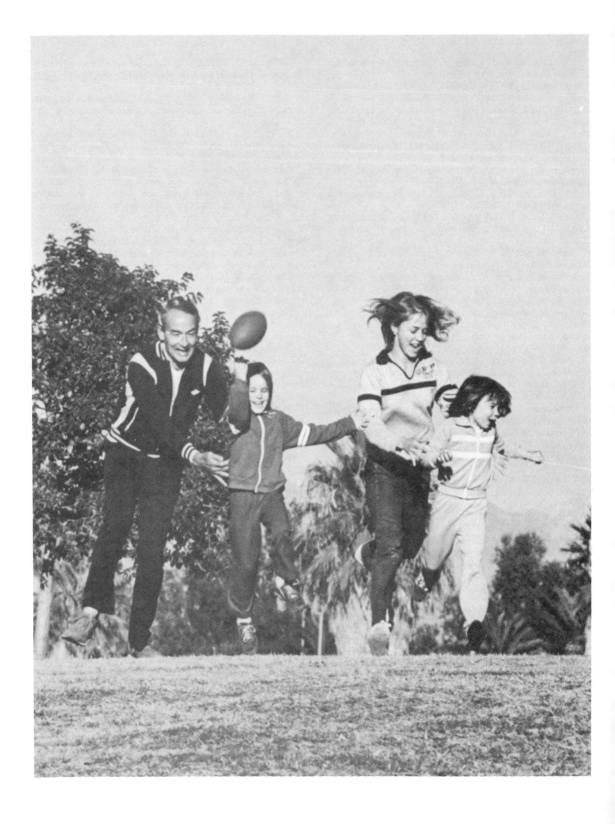

18

Physical Activity
for Health and Fitness

INTRODUCTION

Throughout the previous chapters of this book, emphasis has been almost totally focused on the relationship of physical activity to various aspects of athletic performance. Discussion has centered on such topics as the male and female athlete, the young and old athlete, the basic elements of athletic performance, the influence of the environment on performance, and the role of selected ergogenic aids. This final chapter will look briefly at the health-related aspects of physical activity, a topic of considerable importance to the athlete and non-athlete alike. How important is physical activity to the health, fitness, and general well-being of the average individual in today's world, with its emphasis on sedentary living? Can we, who have been designed for strenuous activity, successfully adapt to this newly-imposed sedentary life style?

DISEASES OF MODERN LIVING

Chronic and degenerative diseases of the cardiovascular and pulmonary systems are the major causes of serious illness and death in the United States. Cardiovascular disease alone affects more than 43.5 million Americans each year, resulting in nearly one million deaths, and costs the individual, government, and private industry over 72 billion dollars annually. While infectious diseases, such as influenza, tuberculosis, and pneumonia, were the major causes of death in the early 1900s, diseases of our modern life style, such as cancer, lung, and heart disease, have now attained the distinction of being the major causes of death. Cardiovascular disease, including heart disease and stroke, now kills almost as many Americans each year as all other causes of death combined, including infant mortality and accidents (see Figure 18-1 on page 340)!

Most individuals consider themselves to be healthy, until they experience some overt sign of illness. However, with chronic degenerative diseases, such as heart disease and cancer, the individual is generally unaware that the disease process is smoldering and slowly progressing from a minor affliction to one of major proportions. As one grows older, the frequency and rate of these undetected disease processes accelerate. Fortunately, early detection and proper treatment of the various chronic diseases can substantially reduce their intensity and the resulting number of deaths.

339

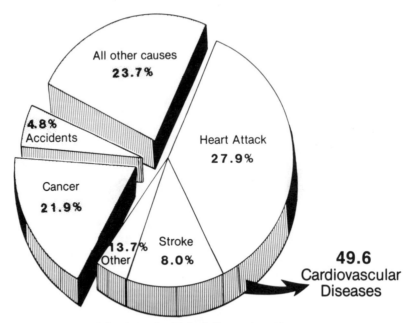

Figure 18-1   Leading causes of death in the United States in 1984.

Perhaps even more importantly, the alteration of factors associated with an increased risk for a particular disease can either prevent the development of that disease or delay its onset for many years. This would include changing dietary habits, increasing habitual physical activity, abstaining from the use of tobacco, moderating alcohol intake, getting proper sleep and rest, and improving the ability to handle psychological stress.

A discussion of each of the various chronic diseases would require considerably more space than is available in this chapter. Consequently, discussion has been limited to those two areas where physical activity is known to play a predominant role—heart disease and obesity. Both are now recognized to begin in childhood, thus, the preventive aspects are very important.

Heart Disease

As humans age, their coronary arteries (those arteries that supply the heart muscle itself) become progressively narrower as a result of fat being deposited along the inner wall of the artery (see Figure 18-2). This process of progressive narrowing is referred to as **atherosclerosis.** Kannel and Dawber (1972) have stated that atherosclerosis is not only a disease of the aged but that it is primarily a pediatric problem, since the pathologic changes that lead to atherosclerosis begin in infancy and progress during childhood. Fatty streaks, or lipid deposits, which are thought to be the probable precursors to atherosclerosis, are common in children by the age of three to five years. Enos, Holmes, and Beyer (1953) demonstrated that over 70 percent of autopsied Korean War combat casualities, with an average age of 22.1 years, already had at least moderately advanced coronary atherosclerosis. McNamara, et al. (1971) found evidence of coronary atherosclerosis in 45 percent of Vietnam war casualties, with five percent exhibiting severe manifestations of the disease.

Between the years 1900 and 1970, there was a threefold increase in the number of heart disease deaths per 100,000 population, ranking it as the number one cause of death in the United States.

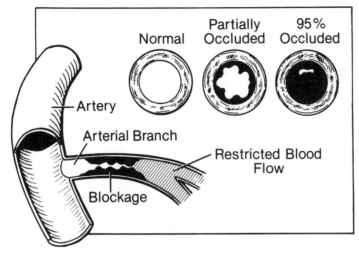

Figure 18-2   The progressive narrowing of a coronary artery.

This threefold increase is a relative increase, expressed in deaths per 100,000 population. Since the population of the United States has more than doubled over this 70-year period, the absolute number of deaths from heart disease has risen even more dramatically. It is presently estimated that cardiovascular disease, including heart disease which represents nearly 60 percent of all cardiovascular disease deaths, is identifiable in approximately 25 percent of the adult American population. Furthermore, heart disease has become the leading cause of death in men between the ages of 35 and 45 years. Heart disease has become a national tragedy!

How does atherosclerosis develop in the coronary arteries? First, the coronary arteries are composed of three distinct layers: the intima or inner layer, the media or middle layer, and the adventitia or outer layer. There is a thin layer of cells on the artery's innermost layer, the intima, which provides a protective coating between the blood flowing through the artery and the intimal layer. Local injury to these **endothelial cells,** or the **endothelium,** appears to initiate the process of atherosclerosis. For example, studies in primates have shown that scratching the inner lining of the coronary artery causes a sloughing off of the endothelial cells, exposing the subendothelial connective tissue.

Blood platelets are attracted to the site of injury and adhere to the subendothelial connective tissue. These platelets degranulate and release a substance referred to as platelet-derived growth factor (PDGF), which promotes the migration of smooth muscle cells from the medial layer into the intimal layer. The intimal layer normally contains few, if any, smooth muscle cells. A plaque forms at the site of injury, which is basically composed of smooth muscle cells, connective tissue, and debris. Eventually, lipids in the blood, specifically low-density lipoprotein cholesterol, become deposited in the plaque. This theory of atherosclerosis, which has evolved from the work of Dr. Russell Ross and his colleagues at the University of Washington, is illustrated in Figure 18-3 on page 342.

Risk Factors. Over the years, scientists have attempted to determine the basic etiology, or cause, of the atherosclerotic process. Several studies have been conducted that have closely observed selected members of communities for extensive periods of time. When a substantial number of deaths occur over a 25- to 35-year period, it is possible to group those individuals who died from heart attacks to determine what risk factors they possessed in common. While this approach does

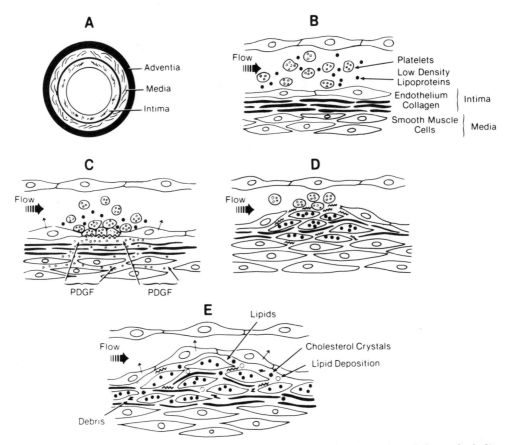

Figure 18–3   Changes in the arterial wall with injury, illustrating the disruption of the endothelium and the subsequent alterations.

not specifically define the actual causal mechanisms, it does provide the researcher with valuable insights into the disease process.

The factors identified in these long-term, longitudinal, population studies are referred to as **risk factors.** The factors associated with an increased risk for premature development of heart disease can be grouped into those over which the individual has no control, and those that can be altered through basic changes in life style. Those that are beyond the individual's control include heredity, sex, age, and race. Those factors that can be altered include elevated blood fats (cholesterol and triglycerides), elevated blood pressure (hypertension), cigarette smoking, obesity, diabetes, abnormalities of the electrocardiogram, anxiety and ten-

sion (stress), and physical inactivity. These risk factors are outlined in Table 18–1.

The primary risk factors, or those which have been conclusively shown to have a strong association with heart disease, include smoking, hypertension, and blood lipids. More recent data from research studies conducted in the 1980s indicate that diabetes and obesity could also be classified as primary, or major, risk factors. The classification of blood lipids in the high-risk category needs to be further defined. For many years, cholesterol and triglycerides were the only two lipids observed in these epidemiological studies. Conflicting data, and certainly conflicting opinions as to the importance of lipids, confused the public. More recently, scientists have started studying the manner in

Table 18–1 Coronary heart disease risk factors.

Primary Risk Factors	Secondary Risk Factors
Accepted	**Alterable**
Hypertension	Stress/
Elevated Blood	Personality Type
Lipids	Physical
LDL-C	Inactivity
Triglycerides	Abnormal Electro-
Smoking	cardiogram
Proposed	**Unalterable**
Diabetes	Age
Obesity	Male Gender
	Race
	Heredity

which lipids are carried in the blood. Since lipids, or fat, are insoluble in a fluid medium such as blood, they need to be packaged with a protein in order to be transported through the body. **Lipoproteins** are proteins that carry or transport the blood lipids. Two lipoproteins of major concern for heart disease are the low-density lipoprotein (LDL) and the high density lipoprotein (HDL). Paradoxically, high levels of LDL cholesterol (LDL-C) and low levels of HDL cholesterol (HDL-C) place you at an extremely high risk for an early heart attack (under the age of 60 years). Conversely, a high level of HDL-C and a low level of LDL-C place you at an extremely low risk for an early heart attack.

Therefore, it is not sufficient to look only at total cholesterol. It is possible to have moderately high levels of total cholesterol and be at a relatively low risk due to a combination of high concentration of HDL-C and low concentration of LDL-C, and to have moderately low levels of cholesterol and be at a relatively high risk due to a combination of relatively high concentration of LDL-C and low concentration of HDL-C. Why do these carriers of cholesterol have different responses? It is theorized that LDL-C is responsible for depositing cholesterol in the arterial wall, as was illustrated in

Figure 18–3. HDL-C, on the other hand, is regarded as a scavenger, removing cholesterol from the arterial wall and transporting it to the liver where it is metabolized.

Evidence is now available suggesting that these risk factors can be identified at an early age. Studies of college students indicate that coronary and stroke mortality rate can be predicted at this relatively young age. In a study of 96 boys, ages eight to 12 years (Wilmore & McNamara, 1974), 19.8 percent had cholesterol values in excess of the suggested, high-normal value of 200 mg/100 ml, 5.2 percent exhibited abnormal resting electrocardiograms, and 37.5 percent had in excess of 20 percent relative fat. Elevated blood pressure was not observed. In a later study (Wilmore, et al., 1982) of 13- to 15-year-old boys, similar data were reported. Both of these studies are summarized in Table 18–2 on page 344.

Role of Exercise. A number of research studies have identified inadequate physical activity as a risk factor in heart disease. Well over fifty studies have reported the incidence of heart attack in sedentary populations to be approximately twice to three times that found in men who are physically active, either in their jobs or in their recreational pursuits. These studies suggest that the clinical manifestations of the disease should be preventable if suitable activity programs are instituted early in life. Fox, Naughton, and Haskell concluded in 1971 that the existing evidence suggested, but fell short of actually proving, that habitual physical activity would be beneficial in the prevention of heart disease. As of 1986, sufficient evidence has accumulated to suggest a strong relationship, but which still falls short of directly proving a causal link between inactivity and increased risk for heart disease.

There are studies that also suggest that the patient who has survived a first heart attack will be less likely to have a second attack or die from a subsequent attack if he or she has been active in a cardiac rehabilitation program that has a strong emphasis on vigorous aerobic exercise. Studies at Washington University in St. Louis, Missouri have provided rather dramatic evidence that intense aerobic conditioning leads not only to substantial changes in the periphery (increased

Table 18-2 Coronary heart disease risk factor prevalence in boys, eight through fifteen years of age.

Risk Factor	8-to-12-year-olds (n = 96) percentage	13-to-15-year-olds (n = 308) percentage
Blood Lipids		
Total Cholesterol ≥ 200 mg/100 ml	20.0	11.0
HDL-C ≤ 36 mg/100 ml	—	14.6
Triglycerides ≥ 100 mg/100 ml	8.4	25.0
Blood Pressure		
Systolic > 90th percentile	0.0	13.0
Diastolic > 90th percentile	0.0	4.9
Smoking ≥ 10 cigarettes/day	0.0	0.0
Diabetic	0.0	1.3
Abnormal ECG	4.5	6.5
Relative Body Fat ≥ 25% fat	12.6	14.9
Maximal Oxygen Uptake ≤ 42 ml·kg^{-1}·min^{-1}	3.2	18.8
Family History MI ≤ 60 years of age	33.7	30.9
Presence of Risk Factors		
None	36.0	29.9
One	46.0	35.4
Two	14.0	22.1
Three	3.0	10.7
Four	1.0	1.9

muscle blood flow), but they have found indirect evidence that there may also be important changes in the heart itself, including possible increases in coronary blood flow, or blood flow to the heart.

A number of studies have also been conducted investigating the role of exercise in altering those risk factors associated with heart disease. While there is little direct evidence to support the contention that exercise reduces the number of smokers or the number of cigarettes smoked, there is a great deal of anecdotal information that suggests this is true. There is relatively strong data supporting the effectiveness of exercise for reducing blood pressure in those with mild-to-moderate hypertension. Exercise appears to have little or no effect in those with severe hypertension. Exercise possibly exerts its most beneficial effect on blood lipid levels. Endurance exercise apparently elevates HDL-C, although there have been studies that have reported little or no change, and even a decrease. Almost all studies, however, have shown the ratios of HDL-C/LDL-C and HDL-C/Total-C to be increased following endurance training. With respect to the remaining risk factors, exercise plays an important role in weight reduction and control, in the control of diabetes, and in reducing the negative effects of stress.

Finally, a case can be made for the importance of regular physical activity on the basis of those physiological changes that occur in response to exercise training. These were discussed in detail in Section B and will not be further discussed in this chapter, with one exception. A most important study was conducted at Boston University by Dr. Dieter Kramsch and his associates (1981). They studied the effects of moderate exercise training on the development of coronary artery disease in monkeys. The monkeys were divided into three groups: a control group eating normal low-fat monkey chow; a non-exercising group who ate an atherogenic diet known to induce heart disease; and an exercising group who ate the same atherogenic diet as the second group. The group that remained sedentary and consumed the atherogenic diet developed atherosclerosis, while the exercise-trained monkeys who consumed the atherogenic diet had an increase in the size of the coronary arteries (an increased inside diameter) and substantially less atherosclerosis. There was a two- to threefold larger cross-sectional area of the lumen of all of the major coronary vessels in the exercised compared to the sedentary monkeys. The left main coronary artery in a sedentary and an exercising monkey are illustrated in Figure 18–4.

From these data, it is impossible to state, unequivocally, that exercise will provide protection from a premature heart attack. The available evidence suggests that an increase in habitual physical activity is beneficial. Fox (1973) has concluded that the likely benefits of habitual physical activity will be more in the area of an improved quality of life than in life extension. Obviously, the identification of the preventive role of exercise in heart disease must await further study of a longitudinal nature. While this may take 50 years, or more, to resolve beyond a shadow of a doubt, it would be prudent to subscribe to the theory that physical activity is important until it is proven otherwise.

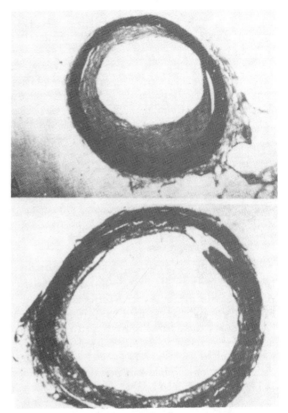

Figure 18–4 Comparison of the left main coronary artery in (A) sedentary versus (B) exercising monkeys (from Kramsch, et al., 1981. Reprinted by permission of The New England Journal of Medicine).

Obesity

Obesity and overweight constitute two of the most serious medical and health problems in the United States today. It is ironic that while millions of people are dying of starvation each year in all parts of the world, many Americans are dying as an indirect result of an overabundance of food. The prevalence of obesity and overweight in this country has increased dramatically over the past 25 years. Presently, as many as 10 million teenagers are overweight, representing about 20 percent of the total U. S. teenage population. For the adult population, 22.8 percent of American men (14.5 million) and 25.8 percent of American women (18.1 million) between the ages of 20 and 74 years are overweight. Further, for the same age range, 22 percent of American men (13.9 million) and 24 percent of American women (16.7 million) are obese (National Dairy Council, 1984). It has also been demonstrated that the average individual in this country will gain approximately one pound of additional weight each year after the age of 25. Such a seemingly small gain, however, results in 30 pounds of excess weight by the age of 55. Since the bone and muscle mass decreases by approximately one-half pound per year due to reduced physical activity, this means a 45-pound gain in fat over this 30-year period!

Overweight versus Obesity. What is the distinction between the terms overweight and obesity? Also, what is meant by the term ideal weight? First, **overweight** is defined as any body weight that exceeds the normal or standard weight for a particular individual, based on his or her age, height, and frame size. These values are established solely on the basis of population averages. It is quite possible to be overweight according to these standards and yet have a body fat content lower than normal. Football players have frequently been found to be overweight, while actually being much leaner than individuals of the same age, height, and frame size who are of normal or even underweight (see Chapter 10). There are also individuals who are not overweight by the standard tables, but who are, in fact, obese.

Obesity refers to the condition in which the total amount of body fat exceeds that considered optimal for a particular individual's body weight. This implies that the amount of body fat must be assessed much more accurately than can be guessed from the standard tables, which are based on height and frame size. The hydrostatic, or underwater, weighing technique is probably the most accurate of the clinical research techniques available for estimating body fat, but it is not practical for the assessment of the general population, due to the time and cost of each test. A much simpler technique, which is not as accurate as hydrostatic weighing but is much faster and less expensive, involves measuring with calipers the thickness of

two layers of skin plus the interposed layer of fat at several sites. Theoretically, the skinfold thickness will vary directly with the thickness of the underlying subcutaneous fat, which is related to the total body fat. The quantity of fat is normally expressed as a percentage of the individual's total body weight. Exact standards for allowable fat percentages have not been established. However, men with over 25 percent body fat and women with over 35 percent should be considered obese, while relative fat values of 20 to 25 percent in men and 30 to 35 percent in women should be considered borderline obesity.

The concept of **ideal weight** is closely related to these upper limits of body fat. It is felt that the average male should possess approximately 14 to 17 percent of his weight as fat and the average female approximately 21 to 24 percent. This will vary somewhat between individuals, but it does provide a realistic target to aim for. As an example, assume that a 180-pound man had 20 percent of his body weight as fat. He would possess 36 pounds of fat. The remaining weight, 144 pounds, is referred to as the lean body weight, or mass, and consists of bone, muscle, and other nonfat components. In order for this man to reach a level of 15 percent fat, he would have to lose 11 pounds, providing his lean body mass remained the same (see Table 18–3 for a summary of these calculations). This would give him a target, or ideal, weight of 169 pounds. Ideal weight is determined by dividing the lean body weight by the fraction of the total body weight that is desired to be lean. For 15 percent, the fraction would be .85, or 85 percent lean weight.

It should be clear that to identify those people who are obese, it is necessary to first determine the actual, or relative, fat content of the body. Simply referring to even the most sophisticated standard

Table 18–3   Calculating ideal or target weights.

Weight 180 lb   Relative fat 20%
Total fat = 20% × 180 lb = 36 lb
Lean body weight = 180 lb − 36 lb = 144 lb
Ideal relative fat 15%
Ideal weight = 144 ÷ .85 = 169 lb
Target weight loss = 180 lb − 169 lb = 11 lb

weight table is not sufficient to identify a large percentage of the obese population. It is quite possible to be obese by these criteria and still be within, or even below, the allowable limits established by these tables.

Etiology of Obesity. At one time, obesity was thought to be the result of basic hormonal imbalances in the blood, resulting from a failure of one or more of the endocrine glands. Later, it was believed that only a small fraction of the total obese population could be accounted for in this manner, and that it was gluttony, rather than glandular malfunction, that caused the majority of obesity problems. The results of more recent medical and physiological research show that obesity can be the result of any one, or a combination of many, factors. Its etiology is not as simple or straightforward as was once believed.

A number of recent experimental studies on animals have linked obesity to hereditary or genetic factors. Indirect studies suggest a similar link for humans. According to several studies (Mayer, 1972), only eight to nine percent of children with parents of normal weight were found to be obese, whereas 40 or 80 percent were considered to be obese when either or both parents, respectively, were obese. Recent studies by Dr. Albert Stunkard and his associates (1986) at the University of Pennsylvania have shown that concordance rates for different degrees of overweight were twice as high for monozygotic (identical) twins as for dizygotic (fraternal) twins, indicating a substantial genetic component to obesity.

Obesity has also been experimentally and clinically linked with both physiological and psychological trauma. Hormonal imbalances, emotional trauma, and alterations in basic homeostatic mechanisms have all been shown to be either directly or indirectly related to the onset of obesity. Environmental factors—cultural habits, inadequate physical activity, and improper diets—have also been shown to contribute to obesity.

Thus, obesity is of complex origin, and the specific causes undoubtedly differ from one person to the next. Recognizing this fact is important both in the treatment of existing obesity and in the application of measures to prevent its onset. To attribute obesity solely to gluttony is unfair and very damaging psychologically to obese individuals who are concerned and are attempting to correct their problem. Several studies have even shown that obese individuals actually eat less than normal individuals of similar sex and age, although their levels of physical activity are less.

Health Problems in Obesity. Obesity has been directly related to four different types of health problems: changes in various normal body functions, increased risk of developing certain diseases, detrimental effects on established diseases, and adverse psychological reactions.

Just as the cause of obesity varies from one individual to another, so do the prevalence and extent of changes in body function. However, there are certain trends that are specifically linked to obesity. Respiratory problems are quite common among the obese. They have difficulty in normal breathing, a greater incidence of respiratory infections, and a lower exercise tolerance. Lethargy, associated with increased levels of carbon dioxide in the blood, and polycythemia (increased red blood cell production) due to lowered arterial blood oxygenation, are also common results from obesity. These can lead to blood clotting (thrombosis), enlargement of the heart, and congestive heart failure. Hypertension and atherosclerosis have also been linked to obesity, as have metabolic and endocrine disorders, such as impaired carbohydrate metabolism and diabetes. Obesity has also been associated with an increased risk of gallbladder disease, digestive diseases, and nephritis. More importantly, the mortality rate of the obese is substantially higher for each of these diseases than for people of normal weight.

The effect of obesity on existing diseases is not clearly understood at the present time. Obesity can contribute to the further development of certain diseases, and weight reduction is usually prescribed as an integral part of the treatment of the disease. Conditions such as angina pectoris, hypertension, congestive heart failure, myocardial infarction, varicose veins, diabetes, and orthopedic problems would benefit from weight reduction.

It is possible that psychological problems actually cause obesity in a substantial percentage of the obese population. Further emotional or psychological problems can arise from the existence of the condition itself. There is definitely a social stigma to obesity in our society, which contributes substantially to the problems of those who are obese. Consequently, obese individuals may also need psychiatric assistance in their efforts to lose weight.

Treatment, Prevention, and Controls. On paper, weight control seems to be a very simple matter. The energy consumed by the body in the form of food must be equal to the energy expended by the body in physical activity. In both cases, the energy is expressed in calories. The body will normally maintain a balance between the caloric intake and the caloric expenditure. However, when this balance is upset, a loss or gain in weight will result. It appears that both weight losses and weight gains are basically dependent on only two factors—dietary and exercise habits—although there does appear to be a considerable degree of variability between individuals in the storage and expenditure of calories.

A reasonable, or sensible, weight loss would be no more than one to two pounds per week. Losses any greater than this should not be attempted, unless under direct medical supervision. By losing just one pound of fat a week, you will lose 52 pounds in only one year! Few people become obese that rapidly. Weight loss should be a long-term project. Research has demonstrated, and experience has proven, that rapid weight losses are usually short-lived and the original weight is quickly regained. Rapid weight losses are generally the result of large losses of body water. Since the body has built-in safety mechanisms to prevent an imbalance in body water levels, the water loss will, eventually, be replaced. Thus, the individual wishing to lose 20 pounds of fat is advised to attempt to attain this goal in a 6- to 12-month period.

Many special diets have been popular in recent years, such as the Drinking Man's Diet, the Beverly Hills Diet, the Cambridge Diet, the California Diet, Dr. Stillman's Diet, and Dr. Adkin's Diet. Each claims to be the ultimate in terms of effectiveness and comfort in weight loss. Likewise, each diet has its loyal following of confirmed believers who make a strong case for the superiority of their particular diet over the others. Is there a superior diet? Research has shown that many of these diets are effective, but *no one single diet has been shown*

to be any more effective than any other. Again, the important factor is the development of a caloric deficit, while maintaining a balanced diet that is complete in all respects with regard to vitamin and mineral requirements. The diet that meets these criteria, and is best suited to the comfort and personality of each individual, is the best diet. Several of the more popular diets have been considered unsafe, therefore considerable care must be taken when selecting a specific diet.

Several agents or aids have been advocated to assist in reducing caloric intake. Anorexigenic agents (agents used to decrease or suppress the appetite), such as amphetamines, have been prescribed with varying success, but they produce side effects such as insomnia, irritability, and tenseness, and they are addictive. Thyroid hormone has also been used, but its effectiveness is highly questionable and it produces side effects similar to the amphetamines. Human chorionic gonadotropin, a hormone derived from the urine of pregnant women, has been used to promote rapid weight loss. Daily injections of this hormone, in addition to a 500-kcal per day diet, supposedly produce a one-pound-per-day weight loss. Recent evidence, however, shows human chorionic gonadotropin to be no more effective than an injection of plain salt water. The weight that is lost appears to be strictly the result of the 500-kcal per day diet.

Diuretics have been suggested, but the resulting weight loss is almost entirely salt and water. Therefore, these should be used only for those patients who have problems with water retention or hyperhydration. Total fasting has been shown to be helpful in the initial stages of weight loss in highly-obese individuals, but hospitalization and close supervision of the patient is required. It must be emphasized that, regardless of their effectiveness, none of these agents or aids should be used except under the prescription and close supervision of a physician.

Surgical techniques are also used in the treatment of extreme obesity, but they are only used as a last resort, when other treatment procedures have failed and the obesity constitutes a life-threatening situation for the patient. Intestinal bypass surgery, where a rather large segment of the small intestine is bypassed, reducing the transit time of food in the intestine, is seldom used today due to serious complications associated with the operative procedure. Gastric bypass surgery, where the size of the stomach is surgically reduced, was then proclaimed as a simpler, more effective surgical procedure. Again, while the outcome of these surgeries was generally good, the risk of complications was high. More recently, gastric stapling to partition off part of the stomach, and the insertion of gastric balloons to reduce the size of the stomach, have been proposed as safer and more effective surgical techniques.

Behavior modification has been proposed as one of the most effective techniques for dealing with individuals with weight problems. By changing basic behavior patterns, many associated with eating, major weight losses have been achieved. Further, these weight losses appear to be much more permanent—the weight is less likely to be regained.

It has been a commonly held belief that exercise is of little help in programs of weight reduction and control. The classic examples are the statements that to lose one pound of fat, you must chop wood for seven hours, walk 35 miles, or climb a ten-foot staircase 1,000 times. These examples are intended to show the foolishness of trying to lose weight through exercise. It is also argued that the appetite increases as a result of exercise, and that this increase in caloric intake has the same, or greater, caloric value as the expenditure from the exercise itself. Both of these concepts have been proven false, as was discussed in Chapter 10. Inactivity is a major cause of obesity in the United States. In fact, inactivity may be a far more significant factor in the development of obesity than overeating! Thus, exercise must be recognized as an essential component in any program of weight reduction, or control.

When planning an exercise program, it is important to remember that one seldom obtains something for nothing. An effortless exercise program, of course, would be ideal but such a program would result in no significant changes. With the popularity of exercise increasing, there are many gimmicks, gadgets, and fads on the market. While some of these are legitimate and effective, many are of no practical value for either exercise or weight loss. Three such devices were recently evaluated to determine the legitimacy of their claims: the Mark II bust developer; the Astro-Trimmer exercise belt; and the Slim-Skins vacuum pants. These devices are illustrated in Figure 18–5. While rather remarkable claims were made in newspaper

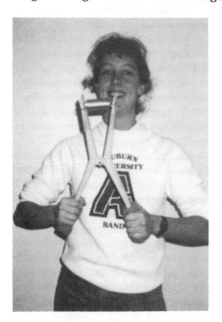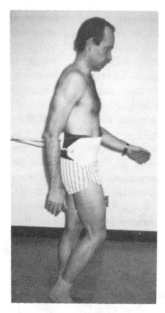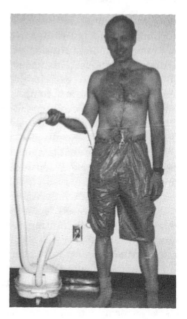

Figure 18–5 Illustration of three exercise devices: Mark II Bust Developer, Astro-Trimmer Exercise Belt, and Slim-Skins Vacuum Pants.

and magazine advertisements for each of these devices, they failed to produce any changes whatsoever when evaluated in tightly controlled scientific studies. To exercise efficiently and make substantial progress requires hard work and sweat.

THE PRESCRIPTION OF EXERCISE

From the preceding discussion, it is obvious that the sedentary nature of modern man has led to a number of health-related problems. Many of these problems can be either resolved or prevented by prescribing programs of routine physical activity for the young and old, alike. The exercise sciences have now progressed to the point where individualized exercise programs can be prescribed and tailored to the likes, needs, and physical capacity of the individual participant. The era of a single group program to fit people of all ages and capacities has come and gone. The individualized prescription of exercise is now a reality and is being used successfully throughout the United States.

Medical Clearance

Prior to beginning any exercise program, it is important that all individuals over thirty years of age have a complete physical examination by their private physicians. This should include a discussion of the proposed exercise program, in the event that there are medical complications that might make a particular activity or sport undesirable. As an example, patients who have elevated blood pressure should be cautioned to avoid activities that use isometric contractions. Isometric contractions tend to cause a considerable rise in blood pressure and usually result in a Valsalva maneuver in which the intra-abdominal and intrathoracic pressure are increased to the point of restricting the vena cava, thus limiting venous return to the heart. Both responses can lead to serious medical complications.

The physical examination should include a health and family history, a resting electrocardiogram and blood pressure assessment, and an exercise electrocardiogram performed on either a cycle ergometer or treadmill for those 45 years of age

and older. The stress electrocardiogram is extremely important, since between eight and 14 percent of the normal, asymptomatic adult population with normal resting electrocardiograms will demonstrate abnormalities in their electrocardiograms during or following exercise, which is indicative of coronary atherosclerosis. This does not preclude the participation of these individuals in an exercise program, but it does place them in a special, high-risk category in which exercise should be done under a physician's supervision.

Factors in Prescribing Exercise

Once an individual has been cleared by his or her physician, an exercise program can be prescribed. The exercise prescription involves four basic factors: mode or type of exercise, frequency of participation, duration of each exercise period, and intensity of the exercise bout. Each of these will be discussed individually.

Mode of Exercise. The prescribed exercise program should include, as its focus, a cardiovascular endurance activity. Traditionally, walking, jogging, running, hiking, and swimming have been the activities prescribed most frequently. Unfortunately, these activities do not appeal to everyone, so additional activities need to be identified that will promote similar cardiovascular endurance development. Recently, aerobic dance, bicycling, and tennis have been shown to improve endurance capacity. Strenuous activities, like handball and racquetball, probably have a significant endurance component, but this has not, as yet, been substantiated by research.

For these sports-type of activities, it is advisable to be preconditioned through one of the standard endurance activities, such as jogging, before undertaking serious competition. This introduces the concept of conditioning activities and maintenance activities. It is felt by some researchers, clinicians, and practitioners that in order to successfully compete in certain sports or activities, a basic preconditioning program is essential. Rather than using the sport or activity to get in shape, one would get in shape prior to participating in that sport or activity. If the activity required a moderate-to-high level of cardiovascular endurance, the individual would engage in a jogging, swimming, or bicycling program for several months, until his or her endurance capacity was increased to the necessary level, at which time the person would switch over to the sport. Conditioning activities would be used to bring the individual to the desired fitness level. The sport would then act as a maintenance activity to maintain the individual at that desired level of fitness. This is an important concept that should not be overlooked.

When selecting activities, it is important to match individuals with activities that they will enjoy and be willing to continue throughout life. Exercise must be regarded as a lifetime pursuit, for the benefits are soon lost once participation stops. Motivation is probably the single most important factor in a successful exercise program. Thus, selecting an activity that is fun, provides a challenge, and can provide the needed benefits are the most critical tasks in the exercise prescription process.

Exercise Frequency. The frequency of participation is an important factor to consider, but it is probably less critical than either the exercise duration or intensity. Research studies conducted on this aspect have shown that three to four days per week is an optimal frequency. This does not mean that five, or more, days per week will not give additional benefits, but simply that, for the health-related benefits, you are getting the best return for the amount of time invested. It is important that the individual limit exercise to three to four days per week, initially, and build up to five, or more, days per week, only if the individual enjoys what he or she is doing. All too often, an individual who starts out with great intentions and is highly motivated will exercise every day for the first few weeks, only to stop from utter fatigue. Obviously, additional days per week above the three- to four-day frequency are beneficial for weight loss purposes, but this level should not be encouraged until the exercise habit is firmly established.

Exercise Duration. Several studies have demonstrated improvement in cardiovascular conditioning with endurance exercise programs as brief as five to ten minutes per day. More recent research has indicated that 20 to 30 minutes per day is an optimal amount. Again, optimal is used here in the context of the greatest return for time invested, and the specified time refers to the time during which the individual is at his or her training heart rate (THR).

Exercise Intensity. The intensity of the exercise bout is undoubtedly the most critical aspect of the three factors, frequency, duration, and intensity. How hard does one have to push oneself? Ex-athletes immediately recall the exhaustive workouts they endured to condition themselves for their sport. Unfortunately, this concept gets carried over into the area of exercise for health. Evidence now suggests that a substantial training effect can be accomplished by training at between 45 and 80 percent of your aerobic capacity. There appears to be a training threshold above which a training response occurs. Some evidence suggests that training must be at a level that is at least 60 percent of capacity, and that training below this level results in little, if any cardiovascular benefit. More recent studies have found substantial improvements in aerobic capacity while training at levels as low as 45 percent of his or her aerobic capacity.

Dr. Ronald LaPorte, an epidemiologist from the University of Pittsburgh, has made the important observation that most studies that have reported health-related benefits from systematic exercise have been able to demonstrate these positive effects at relatively low levels of intensity, in fact substantially below those levels currently recommended for aerobic conditioning (ACSM Guidelines, 1986). It is quite possible that these lower levels of exercise might have considerable health benefits without changing aerobic capacity. This is a most important point that must be researched in the near future. It may be much easier to get more active participation in low intensity exercise from our predominantly sedentary American adult population.

Exercise intensity is quantified by having the individual exercise at his or her own, individualized, training heart rate (THR). The THR is established by determining one's exercise capacity on a maximal exercise stress test. A heart rate is then assigned which represents a set percentage of that capacity. A THR set at 75 percent of HR max

Table 18–4 Selected activities and their respective MET values.

Self-Care Activities		Housework Activities (*cont.*)	
Activity	*METS*	*Activity*	
Rest, supine	1.0	Making beds	3.0
Sitting	1.0	Ironing, standing	3.5
Standing, relaxed	1.0	Mopping	3.5
Eating	1.0	Wringing wash by hand	3.5
Conversation	1.0	Hanging wash	3.5
Dressing and undressing	2.0	Beating carpets	4.0
Washing hands and face	2.0	**Occupational Activities**	
Propulsion, wheelchair	2.0	*Activity*	*METS*
Walking, 2.5 mph	3.0	Sitting at desk	1.5
Showering	3.5	Writing	1.5
Walking downstairs	4.5	Riding in automobile	1.5
Walking, 3.5 mph	5.5	Watch repairing	1.5
Ambulation, braces and crutches	6.5	Typing	2.0
Housework Activities		Welding	2.5
Activity	*METS*	Radio assembly	2.5
Handsewing	1.0	Playing musical instrument	2.5
Sweeping floor	1.5	Parts assembly	3.0
Machine sewing	1.5	Bricklaying and plastering	3.5
Polishing furniture	2.0	Heavy assembly work	4.0
Peeling potatoes	2.5	Wheeling wheelbarrow 115 lb, 2.5 mph	4.0
Scrubbing, standing	2.5	Carpentry	5.5
Washing small clothes	2.5	Mowing lawn by handmower	6.5
Kneading dough	2.5	Chopping wood	6.5
Scrubbing floors	3.0	Shoveling	7.0
Cleaning windows	3.0	Digging	7.5

represents a level of only 60 to 65 percent of $\dot{V}O_2$ max, but this will be sufficient to initiate a substantial training response. Some clinicians actually measure $\dot{V}O_2$ up to, and including, $\dot{V}O_2$ max. They establish the THR by using the heart rate equivalent to a set fraction of the $\dot{V}O_2$ max. As an example, when the individual is tested, heart rate and $\dot{V}O_2$ data for each minute are obtained and plotted against each other. If a training level of 75 percent of $\dot{V}O_2$ max is used, the $\dot{V}O_2$ max at 75 percent is determined ($\dot{V}O_2$ max $\times$ 0.75) and the corresponding heart rate is selected as the THR.

More recently, exercise intensity has been established by setting a THR range rather than a set THR value. This is a much wiser method since exercising at a set percentage of $\dot{V}O_2$ max may place the individual above his or her lactate threshold, in which case it would be difficult to train for any extended duration. With the THR range concept, a low and high value are established that will assure a training response. Beginning at the low end of the THR range, progression is made until the individual feels comfortable.

The concept of THR is extremely valuable. There is a high correlation between heart rate and the work done by the heart. Heart rate alone is a good index of myocardial oxygen consumption, as well as coronary blood flow. If the THR concept is followed, the individual's heart will perform at the same level of work even though the metabolic cost of the work might vary considerably. When exercising at high altitudes or under extremes in

Table 18-4 (*continued*)

Physical-Conditioning Activities		Recreational Activities	
Activity	*METS*	*Activity*	*METS*
Level walking, 2 mph (1 mi in 30 min)	2.5	Painting, sitting	1.5
Level cycling, 5.5 mph		Playing piano	2.0
(1 mi in 10 min 54 sec)	3.0	Driving car	2.0
Level cycling, 6 mph (1 mi in 10 min)	3.5	Canoeing, 2.5 mph	2.5
Level walking, 2.5 mph (1 mi in 24 min)	3.5	Horseback riding, walk	2.5
Level walking, 3 mph (1 mi in 20 min)	4.5	Volleyball, 6-man recreational	3.0
Calisthenics	4.5	Billiards	3.0
Level cycling, 9.7 mph		Bowling	3.5
(1 mi in 6 min 18 sec)	5.0	Horseshoes	3.5
Swimming, crawl, 1 ft/sec	5.0	Golf	4.0
Level walking, 3.5 mph (1 mi in 17 min)	5.5	Cricket	4.0
Level walking, 4.0 mph (1 mi in 15 min)	6.5	Archery	4.5
Level jogging, 5.0 mph (1 mi in 12 min)	7.5	Ballroom dancing	4.5
Level cycling, 13 mph		Table tennis	4.5
(1 mi in 4 min 37 sec)	9.0	Baseball	4.5
Level running, 7.5 mph (1 mi in 8 min)	9.0	Tennis	6.0
Swimming, crawl, 2 ft/sec	10.0	Horseback riding, trot	6.5
Level running, 8.5 mph (1 mi in 7 min)	12.0	Folk dancing	6.5
Level running, 10.0 mph (1 mi in 6 min)	15.0	Skiing	8.0
Swimming crawl, 2.5 ft/sec	15.0	Horseback riding, gallop	8.0
Swimming crawl, 3.0 ft/sec	20.0	Squash rackets	8.5
Level running, 12 mph (1 mi in 5 min)	20.0	Fencing	9.0
Level running, 15 mph (¼ mi in 1 min)	30.0	Basketball	9.0
Swimming crawl, 3.5 ft/sec	30.0	Football	9.0
		Gymnastics	10.0
		Handball and paddleball	10.0

temperature, the heart rate will be greatly elevated if the individual attempts to maintain a set rate of work, for example, run at a 6-min per mile pace. With the THR concept, the individual simply does less work under these extreme environmental conditions to maintain the same heart rate (THR). This is a much safer approach to the training program.

The THR concept automatically accounts for improvement. As you become better conditioned, your heart rate decreases for the same level of work, or conversely, you must actually perform more work in order to reach your THR. Theoretically, as one becomes better conditioned, one must work harder, or perform more work each day in order to attain the same THR level.

Exercise intensity has also been prescribed on the basis of the MET system. The amount of oxygen consumed by your body is directly proportional to the energy you expend in physical activity. At rest, you use approximately 3.5 ml of oxygen per kilogram (2.2 lb) of body weight per minute. This resting metabolic rate is referred to as a MET. All activities can be classified by intensity according to their oxygen requirements. An activity that is rated as two METS would, therefore, require two times the resting oxygen consumption, or 7 ml $\cdot$ kg^{-1} $\cdot$ min^{-1}, and an activity that is rated at 4 METS would require approximately 14 ml $\cdot$ kg^{-1} $\cdot$ min^{-1}. A number of activities and their MET values are presented in Table 18-4. It should be noted that these values are only approximations, due to the variations in metabolic efficiency within and between individuals. This table can also be used to select activities to supplement the endurance program. The MET system is useful as a guideline, but it fails to account for changes in environmental conditions and it does not allow for changes in physical conditioning.

Ratings of perceived exertion (RPE) have also been proposed for use in the prescription of exercise intensity. Providing the individual knows how to accurately use the RPE scale, this system for monitoring exercise intensity shows considerable promise. Using the old Borg scale (rating scale of from six to 20), you would exercise at an intensity of from an RPE of 13 (somewhat hard) to an RPE of 15 (hard).

THE EXERCISE PROGRAM

Once medical clearance has been obtained and the exercise prescription determined, it is necessary to integrate all of the previously described information into a total exercise program. This is an integral part of the overall health-improvement plan. The program should be designed, specifically, on the basis of the results of the medical evaluation, as well as on the basis of exercise capacity, interests, and personal needs. It should be designed to develop a reasonable level of fitness for age, health status, occupation, and leisure-time interests. Once this level has been achieved, the program then becomes one of fitness maintenance. At this time, the amount of physical activity required will become less, since the amount of physical activity needed to stay at the ideal level of fitness is less than it takes to get there. Also, once the ideal, or optimal, level of fitness is reached, it is possible to safely and enjoyably participate in a much greater variety of exercises and active sports or games.

The Conditioning Program

Exercise capacity varies widely among individuals, even when they are of similar ages and physical builds. That is why each program is based upon your own, personal test results. The total time it will take you to perform the recommended program will vary between 30 and 45 minutes per session, depending on your present level of fitness and your personal goals.

The conditioning program consists of the following activities listed in the order in which they should be performed:

- A set of warm-up exercises
- An endurance conditioning period
- A set of flexibility exercises
- A set of strength exercises (optional)
- A cooling-down period

Warm-up Period. The exercise session should begin with low-intensity, calisthenic and stretching exercises. Such a warm-up period will increase both heart rate and breathing to provide for the efficient and safe functioning of the heart, blood vessels, lungs, and muscles during the more vigorous exercise that follows. A good warm-up will also reduce the amount of muscle and joint soreness that may be experienced during the early stages of the exercise program.

Endurance Development Activities. Physical activities that develop cardiovascular endurance are the heart of the exercise program. They are designed to improve both the capacity and efficiency of the cardiovascular and respiratory systems. Also, they are the types of exercises that are most useful in helping to control, or reduce, body weight.

Activities such as walking, jogging, running, cycling, swimming, dancing, and hiking are good endurance activities. Sports such as handball, basketball, tennis, and badminton are also good, providing they are pursued vigorously. Activities such as golf, bowling, and softball are generally of little value from the standpoint of developing cardiorespiratory endurance, but they are fun, have definite recreational value, and may have health-related benefits. Tables 18–5 to 18–9 illustrate a progressive walk-jog-run type of program.

Flexibility Development Activities. The flexibility exercises are supplementary to those exercises performed during the warm-up period and are intended for those who have poor flexibility, as well as muscle and joint problems, such as low back pain. These exercises are to be performed slowly,

Table 18–5 A walking program.

Step	Peak O_2 Value[a]	Workout Description	Time (min)	Miles
I	8.5	Walk 0.67 mi in 20 min	20	0.67
II	8.5	Walk 1 mi in 30 min	30	1.00
III	10.4	Walk 1.25 mi in 30 min	30	1.25
IV	12.0	Walk 1.50 mi in 30 min	30	1.50
V	14.0	Walk 1.75 mi in 30 min	30	1.75
VI	16.0	Walk 2.0 mi in 30 min	30	2.00

[a] $ml \cdot kg^{-1} \cdot min^{-1}$

as quick stretching movements are potentially dangerous and can lead to muscle pulls or spasms. At one time it was recommended that these exercises be performed prior to endurance conditioning activity. It is now recognized that muscles, tendons, ligaments, and joints are more adaptable and responsive to flexibility exercises when done after the endurance conditioning phase.

Strength Exercises. If an individual participates in a weight-training program, it is advisable to start with a weight that is exactly one-half of his or her maximum strength (1-RM). The individual should attempt to lift that weight ten consecutive times. If this can just barely be done, this is the correct weight to begin at. If more could have been done, go to the next highest weight for the

Table 18–6 A walking-jogging program.

Step	Peak O_2 Value[a]	Workout Description	Time (min)	Miles
I	17.2	Walk 2.25 mi in 30 min	30	2.25
II	24.5	Walk .25 mi in 3 min 45 sec Jog .25 mi in 3 min Repeat for 31 min	31	2.25
III	24.5	Walk .5 mi in 7 min 30 sec Jog .5 mi in 6 min Repeat for 34 min 30 sec	34.5	2.50
IV	24.5	Walk .25 mi in 3 min 45 sec Jog .75 mi in 9 min Walk .5 mi in 7 min 30 sec Repeat first two steps	33	2.50
V	24.5	Jog 1 mi in 12 min Walk .25 mi in 3 min 45 sec Repeat	31.5	2.50
VI	27.5	Walk .25 mi in 3 min 45 sec Jog 1 mi in 11 min Repeat for 33 min 15 sec	33.25	2.75

[a] $ml \cdot kg^{-1} \cdot min^{-1}$

Table 18-7 A jogging program.

Step	Peak O₂ Value[a]	Workout Description	Time (min)	Miles
I	27.5	Jog 1 mi in 11 min Jog .5 mi in 6 min Repeat	34	3.00
II	27.5	Jog 3 mi in 33 min	33	3.00
III	30.5	Jog 1 mi in 10 min Jog 1 mi in 11 min Jog 1 mi in 10 min	31	3.00
IV	30.5	Jog 3 mi in 30 min	30	3.00
V	33.5	Jog 1 mi in 9 min 15 sec Jog 1 mi in 10 min Jog 1 mi in 9 min 15 sec	28.5	3.00
VI	33.5	Jog 3 mi at 9 min 15 sec/mi	28	3.00

[a] $ml \cdot kg^{-1} \cdot min^{-1}$

Table 18-8 A jogging-running program.

Step	Peak O₂ Value[a]	Workout Description	Time (min)	Miles
I	33.5	Jog 3.25 mi at 9 min 15 sec/mi	30	3.25
II	36.5	Jog 3.375 mi at 8 min 30 sec/mi	29	3.38
III	36.5	Jog 3.5 mi at 8 min 30 sec/mi	30	3.50
IV	39.5	Jog-Run 3.5 mi at 8 min/mi	28	3.50
V	39.5	Jog-Run 3.75 mi at 8 min/mi	30	3.75
VI	39.5	Jog-Run 4.0 mi at 8 min/mi	32	4.00

[a] $ml \cdot kg^{-1} \cdot min^{-1}$

Table 18-9 A running program.

Step	Peak O₂ Value[a]	Workout Description	Time (min)	Miles
I	42.5	Run 4 mi at 7 min 30 sec/mi	30	4.00
II	42.5	Run 4.25 mi at 7 min 30 sec/mi	32	4.25
III	42.5	Run 4.38 mi at 7 min 30 sec/mi	33	4.38
IV	45.5	Run 4.5 mi at 7 min/mi	31.5	4.50
V	45.5	Run 4.75 mi at 7 min/mi	33.25	4.75
VI	45.5	Run 5 mi at 7 min/mi	35	5.00

[a] $ml \cdot kg^{-1} \cdot min^{-1}$

second set. If less than eight repetitions on the first set were completed, the weight lifted should be reduced to the next lowest level for the second set. Once a given weight results in fatigue by the eighth to tenth repetition, the correct starting weight has been found. Two or three sets of each lift should be performed per day, three days per week, in which eight to ten repetitions count as a single set. As strength is increased, more repetitions will be able to be done per set. Once fifteen repetitions can be achieved, it is time to increase to the next highest weight. This training technique is referred to as **progressive resistance exercise.** For those lifts where the maximum strength has not been determined, the process of selecting an initial weight is largely one of trial and error. Refer to Chapter 7 for more details on setting up a strength training program.

Cooling-down Period. Every exercise session should be concluded with a tapering down, or cooling-off, period. This is best accomplished by slowly reducing the intensity of the activity during the last several minutes of the workout. A slow, restful walk for several minutes keeps the blood from pooling in the extremities, and helps reduce the chances of developing muscle soreness. Stopping abruptly following an endurance bout of exercise causes blood to pool in the legs and may actually result in dizziness or fainting.

Recreational Activities

Recreational activities are an important part of any comprehensive physical activity program. While these activities are primarily for enjoyment and relaxation, many of them also contribute to fitness development as well. Activities such as hiking, tennis, handball, squash, and certain team sports fall into this category. Guidelines to be used in the selection of these activities include the following: (1) Can they be learned or performed with at least a moderate degree of success? (2) Do they include opportunities for social development? and (3) Are they varied enough to maintain continued interest?

Many excellent opportunities exist for those individuals who have no recreational hobbies or activities but who would like to become involved.

Local recreation centers or clubs, YMCAs, YWCAs, public schools, and community colleges offer instructional classes in a wide variety of activities for little or no cost. Often the entire family can participate in these classes—an added bonus to a total health-improvement program.

Several words of caution are necessary. First, you should not be carried away by competitive activities. While the competitive spirit is natural and healthy, it does occasionally tend to overpower one's common sense. Second, contact-type sports or activities should be avoided, except for the exceptional individual who is in a highly trained and conditioned state. Also, it is important to keep in mind that these are primarily recreational activities, only one aspect of the total physical activity program. Once one has attained a reasonable state of fitness, however, these activities may be adequate to keep one there.

SUMMARY

Patterns of modern living have channeled the average American into an increasingly sedentary existence. Man, however, was designed and built for movement, and it appears that, physiologically, he has not adapted well to this reduced level of activity. Regular exercise is necessary to develop and maintain an optimal level of good health, performance, and appearance. It can increase one's physical working capacity by increasing muscle strength and endurance, enhancing the function of lungs, heart, and blood vessels, increasing the flexibility of joints, and improving the efficiency or skill of movement. For many adults with sedentary occupations, physical activity provides an outlet for job-related tensions or mental fatigue. It also aids in weight control or reduction, improves posture, contributes to a youthful appearance, and increases general vitality. Active individuals appear to have fewer heart attacks than their less-active counterparts. Furthermore, if an active individual does suffer an attack, it probably will be less severe and his or her chances of survival are greater. Additionally, more than 50 percent of lower back pain or discomfort is due to poor muscle tone and flexibility of the lower back and to inadequate abdominal muscle tone. In many

Table 18–10 Physiological changes resulting from endurance-type physical conditioning.

Heart
Reduced resting heart rate
Reduced heart rate for standardized, submaximal exercise
Increased rate of heart rate recovery after standardized exercise
Increased blood volume pumped per heart beat (stroke volume)
Increased size of heart muscle (myocardial hypertrophy)
Increased blood supply to heart muscle
Increased strength of contraction (contractibility)

Blood Vessels and Blood Chemistry
Reduced resting systolic and diastolic arterial blood pressure
Reduced risk of hardening of the arteries (arteriosclerosis)
Reduced serum lipids, i.e., cholesterol, triglycerides
Increased blood supply to muscles
Increased blood volume
More efficient exchange of oxygen and carbon dioxide in muscles

Lungs
Increased functional capacity during exercise
Increased blood supply
Increased diffusion of respiratory gases
Reduced nonfunctional volume of lung (residual volume)

Neural, Endocrine, and Metabolic Function
Increased glucose tolerance
Increased enzymatic function in muscle cells
Reduced body fat content (adiposity)
Increased muscle mass (lean body mass)
Reduced strain resulting from psychological stress
Increased maximal oxygen uptake

instances, this disability could be prevented or corrected by proper exercise. And finally, much of the degeneration of bodily functions and structure associated with premature aging seems to be reduced by frequent participation in programs of proper exercise.

An individually prescribed exercise program to supplement the normal daily activities of most adults is essential for good health. There is a sound physiological basis for such a program. The physiological and medical benefits that generally occur as a result of an increased activity program are summarized in Table 18–10. The magnitude of change in each of these measurements is dependent on the types of activities pursued, their frequency and duration, and the intensity of the effort.

STUDY QUESTIONS

1. What are the major causes of death in the United States at this time?
2. What is atherosclerosis? How does it develop? At what age does it begin?
3. What are the basic risk factors for coronary artery disease?
4. What is the role of exercise in the prevention of coronary artery disease?
5. What is the difference between overweight and obesity?
6. What is ideal body weight? How is it determined?
7. What are some of the health-related problems associated with obesity?
8. What is the most effective treatment of obesity?
9. What role does exercise play in the prevention and treatment of obesity?
10. What are the basic steps in prescribing exercise?
11. What four factors must be considered in the exercise prescription?
12. Which of the above four factors is the most important?
13. Describe the components of a good exercise program.
14. How do you effectively motivate individuals to maintain regular exercise habits?

REFERENCES

American College of Sports Medicine. (1986). *Guidelines for exercise testing and prescription* (3rd ed.). Philadelphia: Lea & Febiger.

Amsterdam, E. A., Wilmore, J. H., & DeMaria, A. N. (1977). *Exercise in cardiovascular health and disease.* New York: Yorke Medical Books.

Bjorntorp, P. (1983). Physiological and clinical aspects of exercise in obese persons. *Exercise and Sport Sciences Reviews, 11,* 159-180.

Cooper, K. H. (1968). *Aerobics.* New York: M. Evans & Co.

Cooper, K. H. (1970). *The new aerobics.* New York: M. Evans & Co.

Cooper, M., & Cooper, K. H. (1972). *Aerobics for women.* New York: M. Evans & Co.

Daniels, J. , Fitts, R., & Sheehan, G. (1978). *Conditioning for distance running.* New York: John Wiley & Sons.

Dowell, R. T. (1983). Cardiac adaptations to exercise. *Exercise and Sport Sciences Reviews, 11,* 99-117

Enos, W. F., Holmes, R. H., & Beyer, J. (1953). Coronary disease among United States soldiers killed in action in Korea. *Journal of the American Medical Association, 152,* 1090-1093.

Faria, I. E., & Cavanagh, P. R. (1978). *The physiology and biomechanics of cycling.* New York: John Wiley & Sons.

Fixx, J. F. (1977). *The complete book of running.* New York: Random House.

Fixx, J. F. (1980). *Jim Fixx's second book of running.* New York: Random House.

Foss, M. L., & Garrick, J. G. (1978). *Ski conditioning.* New York: John Wiley & Sons.

Fox, S. M., III. (1973). Relationship of activity habits to coronary heart disease. In J. P. Naughton & H. K. Hellerstein (Eds.), *Exercise testing and exercise training in coronary heart disease.* New York: Academic Press.

Fox, S. M., III., Naughton, J. P., & Haskell, W. L. (1971). Physical activity and the prevention of coronary heart disease. *Annals of Clinical Research, 3,* 404-432.

Getchell, B. (1983). *Physical fitness: A way of life* (3rd ed.). New York: John Wiley & Sons.

Haskell, W. L. (1984). The influence of exercise on the concentrations of triglyceride and cholesterol in human plasma. *Exercise and Sport Sciences Reviews, 12,* 205-244.

Kannel, W. B., & Dawber, T. R. (1972). Atherosclerosis as a pediatric problem. *Journal of Pediatrics., 80,* 544-554.

Katch, F. I., & McArdle, W. D. (1983). *Nutrition, weight control, and exercise* (2nd ed.). Philadelphia: Lea & Febiger.

Kramsch, D. M., Aspen, A. J., Abramowitz, B. M.,

Kreimendahl, T., & Hood, W. B. (1981). Reduction of coronary atherosclerosis by moderate conditioning exercise in monkeys on an atherogenic diet. *New England Journal of Medicine, 305,* 1483-1489.

Kuntzleman, C. T. (1975) *Activetics.* New York: Peter H. Wyden Publisher.

Lowenthal, D. T., Bharadwaja, K., & Oaks, W. W. (1979). *Therapeutics through exercise.* New York: Grune & Stratton.

Mayer, J. (1968). *Overweight causes, cost, and control.* Englewood Cliffs, NJ: Prentice-Hall, Inc.

Mayer, J. (1972). *Human nutrition: Its physiological, medical, and social aspects.* Springfield, IL: Charles C. Thomas.

McNamara, J. J., Molot, M. A., Stremple, J. F., & Cutting, R. T. (1971). Coronary artery disease in combat casualties in Vietnam. *Journal of the American Medical Association, 216,* 1185-1187.

Naughton, J. P., & Bruhn, J. (1970, July). Emotional stress, physical activity, and ischemic heart disease. *Disease-A-Month,* pp. 3-34.

Naughton, J. P., & Hellerstein, H. K. (Eds.). (1973). *Exercise testing and exercise training in coronary heart disease.* New York: Academic Press.

Pollock, M. L. (1973). The quantification of endurance training programs. *Exercise and Sport Sciences Reviews, 1,* 155-188.

Pollock, M. L., & Schmidt, D. H. (Eds.). (1979). *Heart disease and rehabilitation.* Boston: Houghton Mifflin.

Pollock, M. L., Wilmore, J. H., & Fox, S. M. (1978). *Health and fitness through physical activity.* New York: John Wiley & Sons.

Pollock, M. L., Wilmore, J. H., & Fox, S. M. (1984). *Exercise in health and disease: Evaluation and prescription for prevention and rehabilitation.* Philadelphia: W. B. Saunders, Co.

Sharkey, B. J. (1984). *Physiology of fitness* (2nd ed.). Champaign, IL: Human Kinetics Publishers.

Stunkard, A. J., Foch, T. T., & Hrubec, Z. (1986). A twin study of human obesity. *Journal of the American Medical Association, 256,* 51-54.

Tipton, C. M. (1984). Exercise, training, and hypertension. *Exercise and Sport Sciences Reviews, 12,* 245-306.

Wilmore, J. H. (1986). *Sensible fitness.* Champaign, IL: Leisure Press.

Wilmore, J. H., Constable, S. H., Stanforth, P. R., Tsao, W. Y., Rotkis, T. C., Paicius, R. M., Mattern, C. M., & Ewy, G. A. (1982). Prevalence of coronary heart disease risk factors in thirteen- to fifteen-year-old boys. *Journal of Cardiac Rehabilitation, 2,* 223-233.

Wilmore, J. H., & McNamara, J. J. (1974). Prevalence of coronary heart disease risk factors in boys eight to twelve years of age. *Journal of Pediatrics, 84,* 527-533.

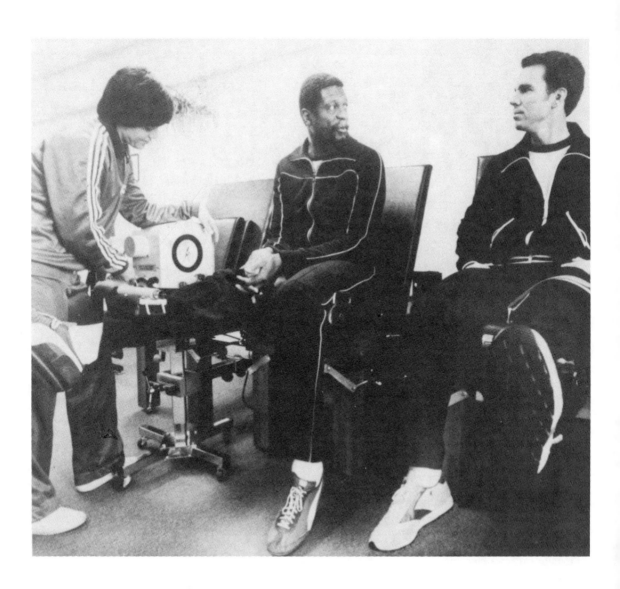

19

Assessing Human Performance

INTRODUCTION

The highly-skilled athlete, or the jogger on his or her daily run, does not perform or exercise in environments that are conducive to extensive monitoring of their physiological responses to exercise. While it is possible to monitor a few selected physiological parameters during exercise in a natural environment, there are many limitations on those variables that can be assessed accurately without disrupting performance. Telemetry and miniature tape recorders have been used to monitor heart rate and the electrocardiogram, respiration rate, skin and deep body temperature, and electromyography. More frequently, however, the person to be evaluated is brought into the laboratory where he or she can be studied in much greater depth under highly-controlled conditions.

This chapter will discuss various aspects of assessing human performance in both the highly-controlled laboratory situation as well as under semi-controlled conditions in the field. Discussion will be limited to those variables that have the most direct application to athletic performance, and will be focused in the areas of cardiorespiratory endurance capacity; strength, power and muscular endurance; anaerobic power, capacity, and threshold; flexibility; and body composition.

CARDIORESPIRATORY ENDURANCE CAPACITY

Exercise scientists agree that the best laboratory measure of cardiorespiratory endurance capacity is one's maximal oxygen uptake ($\dot{V}O_2$ max). In the research laboratory, oxygen uptake is measured directly while the individual exercises at increasing intensities on either the treadmill or cycle ergometer. While other types of ergometers can be used, the treadmill and cycle ergometers are by far the most common. With the increase in speed and/or grade on the treadmill, or in resistance on the cycle ergometer, there is a corresponding increase in the oxygen consumption. Eventually the maximum ability to deliver oxygen to the active muscle mass is reached, and the oxygen uptake will plateau as the rate of work continues to increase. Refer back to Figure 2–8 in which a highly-trained male distance runner and an untrained male were at or near exhaustion at the time when their oxygen uptake plateaued. The value achieved at this point of plateau is referred to as the maximal oxygen uptake or $\dot{V}O_2$ max (see Chapter 2 for a more detailed discussion). The substantially higher $\dot{V}O_2$ max of the distance runner allows him to run on the treadmill, the track, or on the road, at substantially higher speeds than the untrained individual. As we will discuss later in this section, field tests to predict $\dot{V}O_2$ max use this relationship when making predictions, assuming a linear relationship between speed and oxygen uptake exists.

Ergometers

When assessing cardiorespiratory endurance capacity, the type of ergometer selected for testing is an important factor. This will become quite clear later in this section when we discuss the concept of **specificity** as it relates to the choice of an ergometer. First, we will review the types of ergometers available, how they operate, and their respective strengths and weaknesses. Throughout this discussion, it is important for you to keep in mind that to obtain reproducible results on the same individual from one day to the next, and to be able to compare the responses of two or more individuals to the same rate of exercise, it is necessary to standardize either the total work performed or the rate at which that work is performed, or both. The physiological responses accurately track the rate of work, and when the rate of work increases or

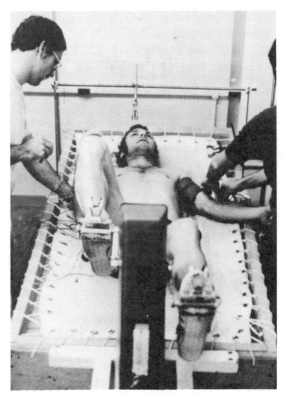

Figure 19-2 Supine cycle ergometry.

decreases, the physiological responses will be increased or decreased proportionally. With certain ergometric devices, it is difficult to control the rate of work within ±10 percent, which can lead to considerable variation in those physiological responses you are attempting to measure.

Cycle ergometers have been the primary ergometric device for a number of years, being used almost exclusively in the early research studies of exercise physiology. While they are still used extensively in both research and clinical settings, there has been a trend in the United States toward a more widespread use of treadmills. Cycle ergometers can be used in either the normal upright (see Figure 19-1) or supine position (see Figure 19-2).

Cycle ergometers generally operate on the basis of one of four principles: mechanical friction, electrical resistance, air resistance, and hydraulic fluid

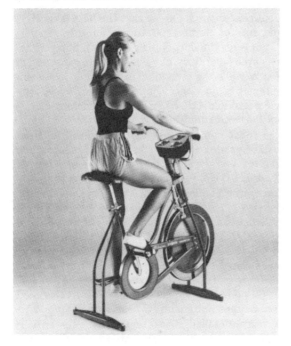

Figure 19-1 A cycle ergometer.

resistance. With mechanical friction devices, a belt encompassing a flywheel is tightened or loosened adjusting the resistance against which one pedals (see Figure 19–1). Mechanically-braked cycle ergometers are rate-dependent—the power output is dependent on the subject's pedal rate. Therefore, care must be taken to monitor the subject's pedal rate, as any variation in pedal rate will alter the desired power output, thus affecting the standardization of the test protocol. Usually, testing is conducted at pedal rates of 50 or 60 rpm, with a metronome used to assist the subject in maintaining a constant pedal rate. Competitive cyclists prefer a much higher rate of pedaling, for example, 80 to 100 rpm, due to the nature of their training and competition. Actual pedal revolutions are multiplied by the fixed distance the flywheel travels per revolution, and by the resistance, to obtain a precise calculation of power output.

$$\text{Power Output} = \text{rev/min} \times \text{distance/rev} \times \text{resistance}$$

As an example, if you pedal at 50 rev/min, the flywheel travels 6 meters/rev, and the resistance is 2.0 kilograms, then:

$$\text{Power Output} = 50 \text{ rev/min} \times 6 \text{ meters/rev} \times 2.0 \text{ kg,}$$
$$\text{Power Output} = 600 \text{ kilograms} \times \text{meters/minute}$$

Electrically-braked cycle ergometers are rate-independent, in that the power output is independent of the pedal rate. Viscous resistance is provided by a conductor which moves through a magnetic or electromagnetic field, with the strength of the field determining the resistance to pedaling. A feedback loop automatically increases the resistance as the pedal rate decreases, and decreases the resistance as the pedal rate increases, maintaining a constant power output.

Air resistance cycle ergometers (see Figure 19–3) are relatively new. The flywheel of a standard mechanically-braked ergometer is replaced by a wheel that contains a series of blades arranged in a manner similar to spokes on a wheel. The fan blades displace air as the wheel turns, with the resistance being directly proportional to the cube of the wheel's rpm, thus, as the pedal speed increases there is a corresponding increase in resistance.

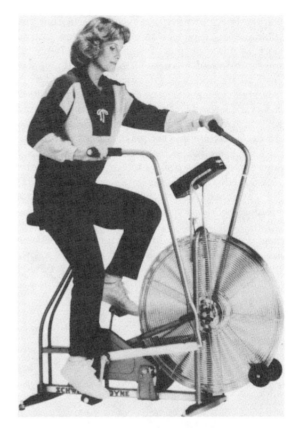

Figure 19–3 An air-braked cycle ergometer.

Cycle ergometers using hydraulic fluid to vary the resistance to pedaling have the capability to produce constant power outputs independent of pedal rate, and have the added advantage of sustaining power outputs up to, or in excess of, approximately 3,000 kpm/min.

There are many advantages to using cycle ergometers as opposed to other ergometric devices. The upper body is relatively immobile, allowing for greater accuracy in blood pressure determinations, rebreathing procedures for determining cardiac output, catheterizations, and blood sampling procedures. The mechanically-braked ergometers are relatively inexpensive, portable, the rate of work or power output can be accurately defined, and the task is weight independent (the rate of work can be set independently of your body weight). This last feature is important whenever investigating the submaximal responses to a standardized rate of work, or power output. As an example, a 15-pound weight loss resulting from an exercise training program will confound submaximal data derived from treadmill testing since the physiological responses to a standardized speed and grade on the treadmill will vary with the weight of the individual. With the cycle ergometer, the loss of weight will not alter the physiological responses to a standardized power output. The ability to have precisely definable power outputs is also important when predicting cardiorespiratory endurance capacity from submaximal rates of work.

There are certain disadvantages to cycle ergometers. First, an individual tends to become greatly limited by local leg muscle fatigue rather than total body fatigue. In addition, and probably

related to this factor of local fatigue, the peak or maximum values for certain physiological variables obtained on the cycle ergometer are frequently lower than comparable values obtained on a treadmill. This could be the result of a) localized fatigue; b) a reduction in venous return from the legs due to the longer period of contraction during cycling as opposed to running, thus reducing local arterial inflow through a reduction in cardiac output; or, c) a lower active muscle mass cycling when compared to treadmill exercise.

Treadmills (see Figure 19–4) have become the ergometer of choice for an increasing number of researchers and clinicians, particularly in the United States. Their principle of operation is relatively simple. A motor and pulley system drive a large belt on which you can either walk or run. Important features to consider when selecting a treadmill are the power requirements of the motor, the belt length and width, and the maximum attainable speed and grade. An underpowered motor will tend to drag, resulting in actual decreases in belt speed when the foot strikes the belt in the landing phase of the walk, jog, or run. This is particularly apparent with very heavy individuals. Belt length and width should be selected to accommodate both the maximum size of those who are to be tested, as well as their stride length. Treadmills that are too narrow or too short make it nearly impossible to test elite athletes. The maximum attainable speed and grade of the treadmill must be considered relative to the types of tests to be conducted and the protocols to be used—the increments in speed and/or grade.

There are a number of advantages to the use of treadmills. First, the treadmill is rate-independent, in that the individual either maintains the belt speed or is carried off the back of the treadmill. Thus, unlike most cycle ergometers, resistance and rate of pedaling do not have to be closely monitored. Treadmill walking is a very natural activity and individuals normally adjust to the skill required within one to two minutes. Treadmills generally provide the highest physiological values for the respective variables measured, $\dot{V}O_2$ max and maximal heart rate (HR max), when compared to other ergometric devices. While some athletes achieve higher values on ergometers that most closely approximate their mode of training or com-

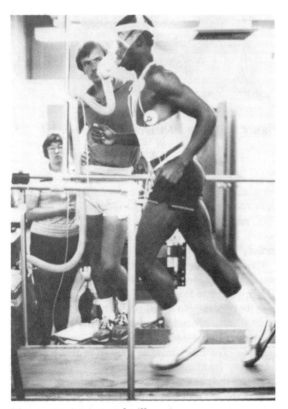

Figure 19–4 A treadmill.

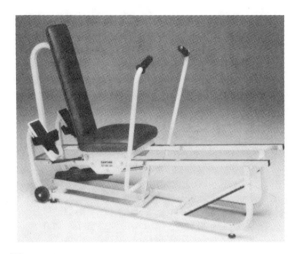

Figure 19-5   A rowing ergometer.

peting, the average individual will almost always achieve his or her highest values on the treadmill.

There are certain disadvantages in using treadmills. They are generally very expensive, when compared to other ergometric devices, bulky, and not very portable. Obtaining accurate blood pressure measurements is a problem during treadmill exercise. This is the result of both the noise associated with normal treadmill operation and the difficulty in obtaining accurate measurements once the

speed is such that the individual must switch from a brisk walk to a jog or run. Excessive upper body movement associated with brisk walking and jogging can result in considerable artifact in the electrocardiogram when the electrodes are not properly applied. This problem is further magnified by the heel strike.

One additional problem with treadmill testing concerns the use of the handrails. To maintain stability during testing, some subjects prefer to either hold on to the handrails, or to make light contact with the handrails. While this may be desirable with respect to safety and the subject's security, it is widely recognized that this substantially reduces the energy cost associated with any given rate of work. In other words, the subject is actually performing a lower rate of work than would be indicated by the speed and grade at which he or she is walking, jogging or running.

Other types of ergometers have been utilized for testing for specific or specialized purposes. The rowing ergometer (see Figure 19-5) was devised to test competitive oarsmen in an activity that more closely approximated their competitive task. The swimming flume (see Figure 19-6) was developed for the same purpose. Valuable research data have been obtained by instrumenting swimmers in a swimming pool and monitoring them during actual swimming. The problems of turns and a constantly

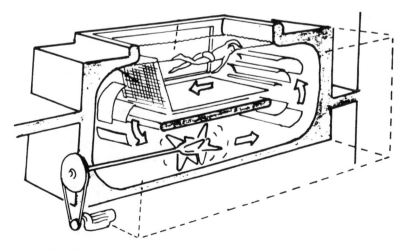

Figure 19-6   A swimming flume.

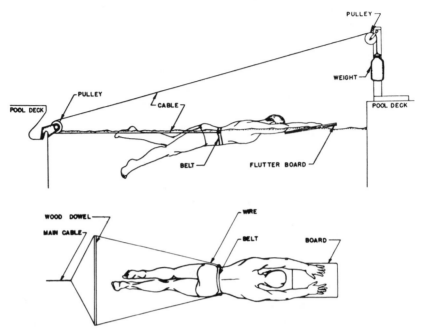

Figure 19-7 Tethered swimming.

moving swimmer led investigators to the use of tethered swimming (see Figure 19-7). With tethered swimming, the swimmer is attached to a harness which is connected to a rope, a series of pulleys, and a pan in which known weights are placed. Swimming begins at a pace that allows maintenance of proper positioning in the pool. As weights are added, a faster pace must be assumed to maintain this position. While important data have resulted from tethered swimming testing, the swimmer's technique is not at all similar to that used in free swimming. The swimming flume, while very expensive, has at least partially resolved this problem and has created new opportunities to investigate many aspects of swimming.

When selecting a mode of testing, it is important to recognize the concept of test specificity. As was mentioned earlier, most individuals will normally attain the highest $\dot{V}O_2$ max value when tested on a treadmill. However, it has now been clearly established that most athletes will perform better when tested on an ergometric device that most closely approximates their sport. Strømme and his associates (1977) tested 14 female and 10 male cross-country skiers, 8 elite male rowers, and 8 elite male cyclists while running to exhaustion on the treadmill, and during maximal performance at their specific sport activity, including uphill roll skiing, rowing in a single sculler, and uphill cycling on a treadmill. The $\dot{V}O_2$ max values were higher in almost every case when the athletes were tested on the sport-specific ergometer (see Figure 19-8). These results underscore the specific local adaptations that occur in response to training. For the average, untrained individual this would not be a factor. This point is further illustrated by the study of Magel and his associates (1975) who studied improvements in $\dot{V}O_2$ max with swim training (1 hr/day, 3 days/week, for 10 weeks), with subjects performing maximal treadmill running and tethered swimming tests, both before and after training. The swimming $\dot{V}O_2$ max increased by 11.2 percent following the ten week period of training, while the running $\dot{V}O_2$ max increased by only 1.5 percent, which was not a statistically significant change from the pre-training value. If only the treadmill had been used for testing in this study, the authors would have concluded that swim

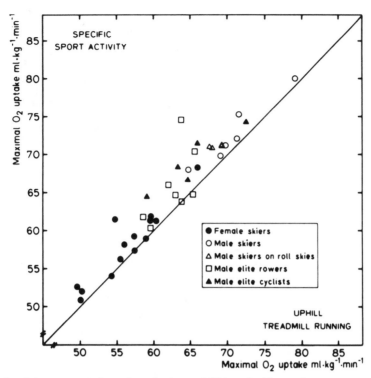

Figure 19-8 Maximal oxygen uptake values during uphill treadmill running versus sport-specific activities in selected groups of athletes (from Strømme, et al., 1977).

training, as defined by their training program, has no influence on increasing cardiorespiratory endurance capacity as represented by $\dot{V}O_2$ max. A more recent study by Gergley and his associates (1984) reported similar results, where $\dot{V}O_2$ max did not change following a swim training program when evaluated by treadmill, but increased by 18 percent when determined during tethered swimming.

Indirect Assessment of $\dot{V}O_2$ Max

The direct assessment of $\dot{V}O_2$ max requires expensive instrumentation, trained technicians, and a maximal effort on the part of the individual who is tested. Consequently, investigators have attempted to define simple submaximal tests which would provide accurate estimates of $\dot{V}O_2$ max, and could be administered to large numbers of individuals with a minimum of time and expense.

Techniques for the estimation of $\dot{V}O_2$ max from submaximal tests developed in the earliest studies used either a step test, or cycle ergometry. Due to difficulty in standardizing the step test, as discussed earlier in this chapter, most studies estimating $\dot{V}O_2$ max from submaximal exercise tests have used the cycle ergometer. Most of these tests have been based on the fact that heart rate and oxygen consumption are linearly related over a range of work rates varying in intensity from light to heavy. The underlying assumption is that the better-fit individual will achieve a higher rate of work for the same heart rate, and thus will be able to achieve a higher rate of work before reaching HR max. Several of the earlier tests defined cardiorespiratory endurance capacity as the maximum work intensity consistent with a steady state. The physical working capacity (PWC) at a set heart rate was one of the very first of these types of indirect tests. As an example, a PWC₁₇₀ test was a test that determined the rate of work necessary to maintain a heart rate response of 170 beats per minute. The more fit individual would have a much higher rate of work at this particular heart rate. The test developed by Åstrand and Ryhming in 1954 is possibly the most widely used of the indirect tests. In their test, $\dot{V}O_2$ max is estimated from a single, steady-state, heart-rate response to a fixed rate of work.

In 1982, the YMCA published a revision of their 1973 test protocol, in which they provide an estimate of $\dot{V}O_2$ max by extrapolation of the HR/power output curve to an age-adjusted predicted maximal heart rate. Assuming a constant metabolic efficiency, the predicted maximal power output is converted to an oxygen consumption expressed in liters/minute. This test procedure is outlined in Figure 19–9 with an example of a 40-year-old male with a predicted HR max of 180 beats per minute (220 − age). The estimated $\dot{V}O_2$ max of 3.2 liters/minute translates into a value of 40 ml $\cdot$ kg^{-1} $\cdot$ min^{-1} when divided by his body weight of 80 kilograms (3200 ml ÷ 80 kg).

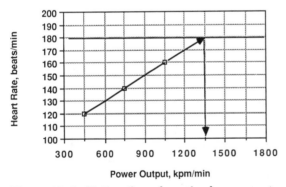

Figure 19–9 Estimation of maximal power output from heart rate and submaximal power output. Plot the heart rate response to three submaximal power outputs and extrapolate this line to an estimated maximal heart rate. The maximal power output is then estimated to be that power output corresponding to the maximal heart rate. Maximal oxygen uptake (liters/min) = Maximal power output (kpm/min) × 2.0 ml (adapted from Golding, et al., 1982).

Table 19–1 Estimation of maximal oxygen uptake from the 1.5-mile walk-jog-run test.

Time for 1.5 miles (min/sec)	Estimated $\dot{V}O_2$ max (ml/kg × min)
7:30 and under	75
7:31– 8:00	72
8:01– 8:30	67
8:31– 9:00	62
9:01– 9:30	58
9:31–10:00	55
10:01–10:30	52
10:31–11:00	49
11:01–11:30	46
11:31–12:00	44
12:01–12:30	41
12:31–13:00	39
13:01–13:30	37
13:31–14:00	36
14:01–14:30	34
14:31–15:00	33
15:01–15:30	31
15:31–16:00	30
16:01–16:30	28
16:31–17:00	27
17:01–17:30	26
17:31–18:00	25

In addition to estimating $\dot{V}O_2$ max from submaximal tests, it is also possible to use maximal tests. Several running tests have been proposed which have relatively high correlations with actual $\dot{V}O_2$ max values. Balke (1963) and Cooper (1968) developed all-out walk-jog-run tests to determine the maximum distance that can be attained in a fixed time—15 and 12 minutes, respectively. For administrative ease, these fixed-time tests were later translated into fixed-distance tests of 1.0 and 1.5 miles, and the time to complete the distance is then used as an estimate of $\dot{V}O_2$ max. These tests are appropriate for children and young adults, but not for middle-aged and older adults who may have underlying disease. Tables 19–1 and 19–2 provide estimates of $\dot{V}O_2$ max from the time to complete 1.5 miles and the distance covered in 12 minutes respectively.

Table 19–2 Estimation of maximal oxygen uptake from the 12-minute walk-jog-run test.

Distance (Miles)	Laps (¼-Mile Track)	Maximal Oxygen Consumption (ml/kg/min)
<1.0	<4	<25.0*
1.000	4	25.0*
1.030	...	26.0*
1.065	4¼	27.0*
1.090	...	28.2
1.125	4½	29.0
1.150	...	30.2
1.187	4¾	31.6
1.220	...	32.8
1.250	5	33.8
1.280	...	34.8
1.317	5¼	36.2
1.340	...	37.0
1.375	5½	38.2
1.400	...	39.2
1.437	5¾	40.4
1.470	...	41.6
1.500	6	42.6
1.530	...	43.8
1.565	6¼	45.0
1.590	...	46.0
1.625	6½	47.2
1.650	...	48.0
1.687	6¾	49.2
1.720	...	50.2
1.750	7	51.6
1.780	...	52.6
1.817	7¼	53.8
1.840	...	54.8
1.875	7½	56.0
1.900	...	57.0
1.937	7¾	58.2
1.970	...	59.2
2.000	8	60.2

*Insufficient data at these distances to make reliable comparisons.

STRENGTH, POWER, AND MUSCULAR ENDURANCE

Strength refers to the ability of the muscle, or a group of muscles, to exert or apply force. Usually, the term strength is used in the context of maximum force-producing capabilities. The individual who can successfully bench press a maximum of 200 pounds is twice as strong as the individual who can bench press a maximum of only 100 pounds. In the purest sense, however, this illustration is not totally accurate, as the result of a bench press is work, since work is defined as the product of force times distance (work = force · distance), not just force alone. A static or isometric contraction provides a more precise estimate of strength. In fact, strength is defined in absolute terms as the ability to develop force against an unyielding resistance in a single contraction of unrestricted duration. However, dynamic tests of functional strength are generally considered acceptable.

For the athlete, and possibly for the average person as well, power is the key component for most physical activity. **Power** is defined as work per unit time [power = {force · distance}/time]. Two male athletes who can bench press a maximum of 200 pounds have identical functional strength. However, if one is able to execute his maximum bench-press strength in half of the time, 1.0 second compared to 2.0 seconds, he would have twice the power of the other individual. While absolute strength is important for many activities, power is probably of even greater functional significance.

Muscular endurance refers to the ability of the muscle, or a group of muscles, to sustain repeated contractions, or to sustain a fixed or static contraction for an extended period of time. Muscular endurance is frequently equated with resistance to local muscular fatigue.

Laboratory Assessments

There is no universally accepted standard measure which is considered representative of total body muscular strength in the same manner that $\dot{V}O_2$ max is considered representative of cardiorespiratory endurance capacity. First, there appears to be a high degree of specificity associated with

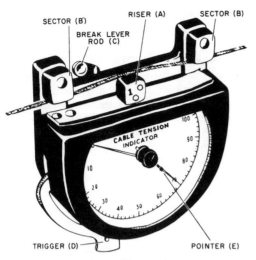
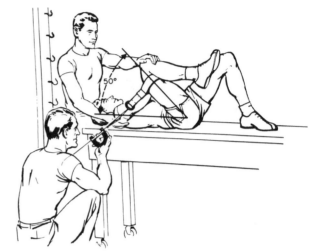

Figure 19-10 The cable tensiometer.

strength. A person with a high level of grip strength does not necessarily have high levels of upper or lower body strength. From several-factor analytic studies, it appears that strength of the total body is best reflected by strength assessment in each of three different areas: upper body, lower body and trunk.

Strength can be measured by any one of three types of devices: spring-type, pressure, and electrical. Spring-type devices include dynamometers, spring balances, and the cable tensiometer. The cable tensiometer is probably the most widely used of these three and is illustrated in Figure 19-10. A cable is attached to a hook fixed to a testing table. A sleeve-like attachment on the end of the cable allows the specific segment of the limb or the head, neck, or trunk to be fixed at a predetermined angle. The individual then exerts maximum force in a static contraction, and the cable tensiometer is able to detect the increased tension in the cable.

Pressure-type devices have used mercury, hydraulic fluid, or air as the transducer of force when assessing strength. Figure 19-11 illustrates a hydraulic fluid, pressure-type device. Coupled with microcomputers, these devices can provide detailed analyses of strength and power curves throughout the full range of motion. Electrical devices for assessing strength include wire strain

gauges and load cells, which are also a form of strain gauge.

The assessment of muscular endurance can also be accomplished with testing devices similar to

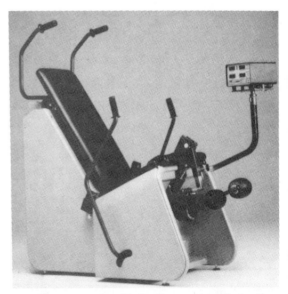

Figure 19-11 The HydraGym strength testing device.

those illustrated in Figure 19–11. While a number of protocols have been reported in the research literature, each protocol specifies a time period and a rate of contraction, and then defines muscular endurance by any one of a number of measurements that can be obtained from the resulting data. As an example, a popular test protocol for assessing knee extensor endurance has the individual perform a series of maximal knee extensor contractions at a rate of one repetition every two seconds for a period of 60 seconds. Endurance can be assessed by the total work performed over the sixty-second time interval, or by an index of work decrement from an average of the first few contractions to an average of the last few contractions. The latter measurement would be a more specific measure of endurance since total work would be related to the individual's initial level of strength, and interpretation of endurance could then be made only by comparisons with individuals with similar initial strength. The use of a work decrement index provides an excellent index of fatigue, which is considered to be the reciprocal of endurance.

Field Assessments

While there are no widely accepted field methods for assessing static strength, dynamic strength can be assessed accurately by the one-repetition maximum test (1-RM). For any given lift, (bench press, leg press, or two-arm curl), a series of trials are given to determine the greatest weight that can be lifted just once. For individuals who have no experience lifting weights, this test is conducted largely by trial and error. Start with a weight that can be lifted comfortably, and then add weight for each subsequent lift until the weight can be lifted correctly in just one time. If this weight can be lifted more than once, more weight should be added until a true 1-RM is established. The 1-RM assessment can be obtained for any one of a number of basic weight training exercises. Test batteries, however, usually select three or four exercises that represent the body's major muscle groups. Table 19–3 provides what have been considered to be optimal strength values for males and females, based on body weight, for four standard lifts: bench press, standing press, curl, and leg press. These values were derived to serve as guidelines, not absolute standards, since the data necessary for deriving standards are not available.

Muscular endurance has been measured in a number of different ways, including the greatest number of sit-ups one can perform in a fixed period of time, usually 30 or 60 seconds; the maximum number of push-ups, pull-ups, or bar-dips one can perform; or the length of time one can sustain a flexed arm hang. Most of these tests are a part of the AAHPERD Youth Fitness Test, the President's Council on Physical Fitness, and Sports' Youth Physical Fitness Test. Many of these tests penalize the participant who has long legs, short

Table 19–3 Optimal strength values for various body weights based on the 1-RM test.

Body Weight lb	Bench Press		Standing Press		Curl		Leg Press	
	Male	Female	Male	Female	Male	Female	Male	Female
80	80	56	53	37	40	28	160	112
100	100	70	67	47	50	35	200	140
120	120	84	80	56	60	42	240	168
140	140	98	93	65	70	49	280	196
160	160	112	107	75	80	56	320	224
180	180	126	120	84	90	63	360	252
200	200	140	133	93	100	70	400	280
220	220	154	147	103	110	77	440	308
240	240	168	160	112	120	84	480	336

arms, or a heavy body weight. Thus, we have suggested a simple test of endurance that attempts to standardize for these factors. It is suggested that one lift a fixed percentage of his or her maximum strength for any given lift, and that this fixed percentage be constant for all lifts—70 percent of the 1-RM has been suggested. One then lifts this weight as many times as possible until the point of fatigue or exhaustion is reached. Since this is a relatively new concept, norms or standards are not yet available.

ANAEROBIC POWER, CAPACITY, AND THRESHOLD

The anaerobic component of performance has been one of the most difficult to objectively quantify. Part of this difficulty stems from a basic lack of agreement among exercise and sport scientists as to how this component is defined. In fact, the use of different terminology to represent the same basic physiological concept, or the use of the same terminology to represent different physiological concepts, has added greatly to the confusion. The terms anaerobic power, anaerobic capacity, and anaerobic threshold have all been used interchangeably to denote the same physiological concept by some scientists, and have been used independently to describe separate physiological events or processes by other scientists. For purposes of this discussion, the following terminology will be adopted. **Anaerobic power** is defined as the peak power output attained in a short duration test of usually ≤ 30 sec. **Anaerobic capacity** is defined as the maximal work performed, or the maximal oxygen deficit, over a period of 30-sec to 2-min. **Anaerobic threshold** is defined as being identical in concept to lactate threshold—that rate of work, or percentage of $\dot{V}O_2$ max, corresponding to the initial increase in blood lactate above resting levels. For the purposes of this chapter, the term lactate threshold will be used.

Anaerobic Power

Several tests of anaerobic power have been developed. The Wingate Anaerobic Test has become the test of choice in most laboratories. This is a 30-second test in which one attempts to pedal at maximal rate against a high, constant resistance. The resistance is established on the basis of body weight. Once the resistance has been set, the individual is asked to begin pedaling as rapidly as possible, maintaining as high a rate as possible for the full 30-second test. Power output is computed for each 5-second period (power = resistance × revolutions/5 second × distance/revolution), and the peak power output selected as the highest power output achieved over the six 5-second periods. The test requires a cycle ergometer which can be accurately calibrated, a timing device, and a means of accurately counting the revolutions in a 5-second period. Bar-Or provides a detailed description of this test in his book, *Pediatric Sports Medicine for the Practitioner* (1983).

The Margaria-Kalamen leg power test represents an objective measure of lower body power. The test begins with the individual standing six meters in front of a series of steps. On command, the individual runs as quickly as possible up the stairs, stepping on every third step. A microswitch embedded in a rubber mat is placed on the third step and activates a timer when the subject hits this step. A second microswitch, which stops the timer when initial contact is made, is placed on the ninth step. The elapsed time represents the time required to move the body weight the vertical distance between the third and ninth steps. Power is then calculated by the formula:

$$\text{Power (kg} \times \text{m/sec)} = [\{\text{weight (kg)} \times \text{vertical distance (m)}\}/\text{elapsed time (sec)}]$$

Anaerobic Capacity

The Wingate Anaerobic Test has also been proposed as a test of anaerobic capacity. The mean power output, or total work accomplished in 30 seconds, is used to represent anaerobic capacity instead of using the peak power output. Hermansen has proposed the use of a 2-minute test to determine the maximal oxygen deficit, using this as an index of anaerobic capacity. Oxygen deficit is defined as the difference between the predicted and actual oxygen consumption during the 2-min all-out work bout.

Lactate Threshold

Lactate threshold has a very high relationship with distance running performance. In fact, lactate threshold appears to be the single best predictor of distance running success. For distances of 10-km or more, runners tend to run at a pace that closely corresponds to their pace on the treadmill; this corresponds to, or elicits, their lactate threshold. **Lactate threshold** is determined by taking consecutive blood samples during an exercise test, in which the power output is increased in step-wise increments of three to five minutes per step. Once steady-state has been achieved at each step or stage, a blood sample is drawn and analyzed for lactate concentration. Generally, lactate concentrations remain relatively stable at resting levels up to about 50 percent to 80 percent of $\dot{V}O_2$ max, at which point the concentrations begin to increase linearly with the increasing rate of work (refer back to Figure 3–8).

There are non-invasive techniques that can be used to estimate lactate threshold from respiratory measures. Several respiratory parameters undergo rather marked changes at the point determined to be the lactate threshold on the basis of direct blood lactate analyses. The ventilatory equivalent for oxygen ($\dot{V}E/\dot{V}O_2$) and end-tidal PO_2 tend to decrease during the lower rates of work in an incremental work-rate test. They both reach their lowest values and start to increase at the point of lactate threshold. To provide even greater accuracy, the systematic increase in $\dot{V}E/\dot{V}O_2$ should occur without a concomitant increase in $\dot{V}E/\dot{V}CO_2$. A break from linearity in the increase in $\dot{V}E$, indicating hyperventilation, and a break in linearity in the respiratory exchange ratio (RER = $\dot{V}O_2/\dot{V}CO_2$), have both been proposed as markers of lactate threshold. However, they do not appear to have the degree of sensitivity necessary to provide consistent results. Conconi and his colleagues (1982) have proposed a field test for the determination of lactate threshold that simply plots heart rate response to several constant paced running velocities. The point where there is a deflection in linearity between running speed and the heart rate response to that running speed, is highly correlated to lactate threshold, and is highly predictive of endurance running performance from 5,000 meters through the marathon (26.2 miles).

FLEXIBILITY

Flexibility refers to the range of motion, or to the looseness or suppleness of the body or specific joints, and reflects the interrelationships between muscles, tendons, ligaments, skin, and the joint itself. Flexibility is influenced by a number of factors. These include the level of activity and type of activity performed, with full range of motion promoting improved flexibility and limited range of motion leading to reductions in flexibility. Gender and age are factors, with females having greater flexibility than males, and with flexibility increasing up to young adulthood and then decreasing with aging. Finally, temperature is a factor, with flexibility increasing with heat and decreasing with cold. Flexibility also appears to be highly specific to the joint being evaluated. In other words, one can be highly flexible in one joint and have limited range of motion in another. Thus, testing for flexibility must reflect this specificity.

Flexibility of individual joints can be measured directly by goniometry. In its simplest form, a protractor-like device is used to measure the angle of the joint at both extremes in its range of motion, with the difference between these two joint angles representing the extent of joint movement. The amount of soft tissue around the joint greatly influences the accuracy of measurement, since the axis of the bones forming any one joint are not readily visible. This introduces a certain amount of subjectivity into the measurement technique.

More accurate measurements of flexibility can be made using two instruments devised specifically for flexibility assessment. The Leighton flexometer, illustrated in Figure 19–12, consists of a weighted 360-degree dial and a weighted pointer mounted in a case. The dial and pointer move independently and are both controlled by gravity. Both can be locked in position independently of each other. The segment is usually positioned at one extreme in the range of motion, the dial locked in position, and then the segment moved through the

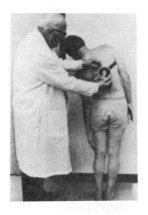
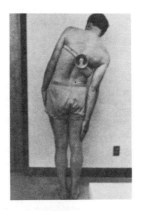
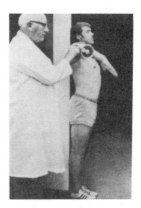
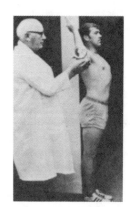

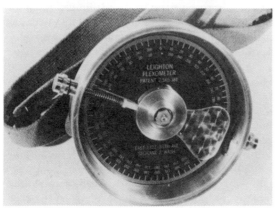

Figure 19–12   The Leighton flexometer.

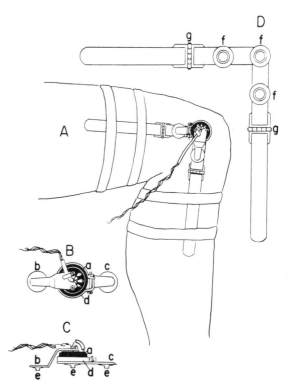

full range of motion. The pointer follows the movement of the segment, thus indicating the extent of joint movement in degrees. Since the length of limbs or segments is not a factor in this assessment, the device provides a more accurate estimate of flexibility than most other instruments or field tests.

A second device developed for measuring flexibility is the electrogoniometer, or the ELGON. The ELGON, illustrated in Figure 19–13, is a protractor-like device in which the protractor has been replaced by a potentiometer. The potentiometer provides an electrical signal that is directly proportional to the angle of the joint. This device can give continuous recordings during a variety of activities. The versatility of this unit allows a much

Figure 19–13   The ELGON (from Karporich and Sinning, 1971. Reproduced by permission of the publishers.).

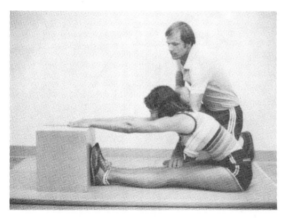

Figure 19-14 The sit-and-reach test for lower back and hamstring flexibility.

more accurate and realistic assessment of functional flexibility, or that degree of flexibility exhibited during actual physical activity.

There are a number of field tests that have been proposed for assessing flexibility. Probably the most popular test is the sit-and-reach test illustrated in Figure 19-14. With the sit-and-reach test, one sits on the floor with feet extended forward in front and pressed flat against a box that supports the measuring stick. With the back of the knees pressed flat against the floor, lean forward and extend the tips of your fingers as far forward as possible. The distance reached is recorded and serves as an index of lower back and hip flexibility. While tests such as the sit-and-reach test are adequate for providing a crude index of flexibility for mass screening, these tests do not allow for differences in limb length or for proportional differences between the legs and arms. If the individual has long arms and short legs, he or she will attain a good score on the sit-and-reach test even with limited or poor flexibility. Likewise, if one has short arms and long legs, he or she will be penalized and will find it nearly impossible to attain a good score. The sit-and-reach test, as described, can be modified to at least partially correct for the problem of limb length disproportionality. The test is started with the individual seated, back against a wall, and legs extended forward. An initial measure is obtained with the back pressed firmly against the wall and the arms extended forward. A measure

is then recorded in the standard forward stretch position, and the difference between the two scores is an index of hip, or lower back and hamstrings, flexibility. Hoeger has recently developed additional flexibility tests that can be measured in the field. These are described in his book, *Lifetime Physical Fitness and Wellness: A Personalized Program* (1986).

BODY COMPOSITION

For purposes of simplicity and convenience, the total body weight is divided into two components: the lean body weight and the fat weight. When working with body composition data, the following relationships are important.

$$\text{Total weight} = \text{Lean weight} + \text{Fat weight}$$
$$\text{Relative lean (percent)} = [(\text{Lean weight}/ \text{total weight}) \cdot 100]$$
$$\text{Relative fat (percent)} = [(\text{fat weight}/ \text{total weight}) \cdot 100]$$

Lean weight refers to that part of the total body weight that remains after all of the body fat is removed. Technically, the term fat-free weight is a more appropriate term. We will consider the two terms synonymous. The lean weight is composed of muscle, skin, bone, organs, and all other non-fat tissue. It can be assessed in a number of ways, but the most common is through densitometry, using the underwater weighing technique. The individual is weighed while totally submerged under water (see Figure 19-15 on page 376). The weight is measured when the individual has blown all of the air out of the lungs and only the residual volume remains. The residual volume is also assessed and is used to correct the underwater weight. In this way, the increased buoyancy resulting from the air trapped in the lungs is taken into account.

Several thousand years ago, Archimedes determined that a body immersed in a fluid experiences a loss in weight equal to the weight of the displaced fluid. In water, the weight of the displaced fluid can easily be converted to the volume of water that has been displaced; thus, the loss of weight in water is directly proportional to the volume of water that is displaced or to the volume of

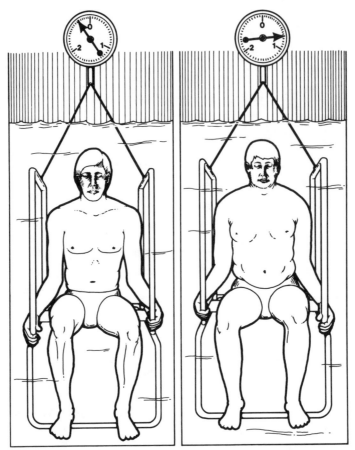

Figure 19–15 The underwater weighing technique illustrating two individuals with the same weight and height, but different body composition.

the body that displaces that water. Since density is equal to the ratio of mass to volume, or

$$\text{Density}_{body} = \text{mass or weight}_{body}/\text{volume}_{body,}$$

it is relatively simple to calculate the density of an individual's body. The density of fat is known, and the density of the lean tissue of the body has been calculated to be a relatively stable constant in chemically mature (post-adolescent) individuals. By knowing the density of the whole body, the fat, and the lean tissue, it is a simple calculation to determine the relative fat weight and relative lean weight of the body.

As an example, two athletes are exactly the same age, height, and weight, and are competing for the same position of middle linebacker on the university football team. Prior to the start of training camp these two athletes undergo a series of tests, including the underwater weighing technique for determining body composition. The results of the body composition analysis are shown in Table 19–4. From this analysis, it is obvious that Ken is right at his desired playing weight, while Dave is 19.1 pounds over his desired playing weight. This analysis would also indicate that Dave may be too light at his desired playing weight to play the middle linebacker position. He

Table 19–4 Comparison of underwater weighing in two athletes for determining body composition.

	Ken		Dave	
Height	74.0 in	188.0 cm	74.0 in	188.0 cm
Weight	205 lb	93.0 kg	205 lb	93.0 kg
Underwater weight		6.5 kg		5.0 kg
Volume (weight-underwater weight)		86.5 kg		88.0 kg
Density (mass or weight/volume)		1.075 gm/ml		1.057 gm/ml
Relative fat		10.5%		18.4%
Fat weight	21.4 lb	9.7 kg	37.7 lb	17.1 kg
Lean weight	183.6 lb	83.3 kg	167.3 lb	75.9 kg
Weight at 10 percent fat	204.2 lb	92.6 kg	185.9 lb	84.3 kg
Weight loss to achieve 10 percent fat	0.8 lb	0.4 kg	19.1 lb	8.7 kg

would have to emphasize an intensive weight training program to increase his lean weight.

While the underwater weighing technique has been considered the "gold standard" or criterion technique, other laboratory techniques have been used with varying degrees of success. These include helium dilution for determining total body volume, isotopic dilution for determining total body water, ^{40}K for determining lean body weight, radiography (X-rays) of the extremities for determining proportions of bone, muscle and fat, computer-assisted tomography (CAT scan) to observe cross-sections of extremity segments, nuclear magnetic resonance, total body electrical activity, and electrical impedance. The last technique, electrical impedance, became quite popular in the mid-1980s. While it is a simple and promising technique, its accuracy is still being determined.

The underwater weighing technique, itself, is subject to considerable error for certain populations. There is no problem in obtaining an accurate density of the whole body. The problem involves the conversion of this density into a percentage of body fat. To do this you must assume that fat and lean tissue have a constant, unvarying density. For fat, this is largely true, in that the density of fat is typically 0.9007 gm/cm^3 with little variation within or between individuals. For the lean tissue,

however, this becomes a problem. Because the lean tissue is composed of several different tissues, one must assume that the density of each of these tissues is constant, and that each represents a constant proportion of the total.

It is now well-accepted that the density of the lean tissue differs among populations. In children and adolescents, the body is not chemically mature, in that bone mineral is still increasing and total body water is decreasing. This results in a density of the lean tissue which is substantially less than that assumed in standard equations (1.100 gm/cm^3 assumed, 1.085 gm/cm^3 actual for a prepubescent child), and will lead to an overestimation of the relative body fat. Black athletes have been estimated to have a density of the lean tissue of 1.113 gm/cm^3 as opposed to the assumed value of 1.100 gm/cm^3. While this may not seem like a major difference, for a body density of 1.075 gm/cm^3 the relative body fat would be 10.5 percent using a constant of 1.100 versus 14.1 percent using a constant of 1.113 gm/cm^3. With aging, there is also a change in the composition of the lean tissue, for example, loss of bone mineral and muscle mass, which will result in an overestimation of one's body fat.

Field methods can be used to assess body composition. Equations have been developed to estimate body density, lean body weight, fat weight,

Table 19-5 Estimation of relative body fat, by percent*, in women from the sum of triceps, suprailiac, and thigh skinfolds (from Pollock, et al., 1980).

Age to the Last Year Sum of Skinfolds (mm)	Under 22	23 to 27	28 to 32	33 to 37	38 to 42	43 to 47	48 to 52	53 to 57	Over 58
23–25	9.7	9.9	10.2	10.4	10.7	10.9	11.2	11.4	11.7
26–28	11.0	11.2	11.5	11.7	12.0	12.3	12.5	12.7	13.0
29–31	12.3	12.5	12.8	13.0	13.3	13.5	13.8	14.0	14.3
32–34	13.6	13.8	14.0	14.3	14.5	14.8	15.0	15.3	15.5
35–37	14.8	15.0	15.3	15.5	15.8	16.0	16.3	16.5	16.8
38–40	16.0	16.3	16.5	16.7	17.0	17.2	17.5	17.7	18.0
41–43	17.2	17.4	17.7	17.9	18.2	18.4	18.7	18.9	19.2
44–46	18.3	18.6	18.8	19.1	19.3	19.6	19.8	20.1	20.3
47–49	19.5	19.7	20.0	20.2	20.5	20.7	21.0	21.2	21.5
50–52	20.6	20.8	21.1	21.3	21.6	21.8	22.1	22.3	22.6
53–55	21.7	21.9	22.1	22.4	22.6	22.9	23.1	23.4	23.6
56–58	22.7	23.0	23.2	23.4	23.7	23.9	24.2	24.4	24.7
59–61	23.7	24.0	24.2	24.5	24.7	25.0	25.2	25.5	25.7
62–64	24.7	25.0	25.2	25.5	35.7	26.0	26.7	26.4	26.7
65–67	25.7	25.9	26.2	26.4	26.7	26.9	27.2	27.4	27.7
68–70	26.6	26.9	27.1	27.4	27.6	27.9	28.1	28.4	28.6
71–73	27.5	27.8	28.0	28.3	28.5	28.8	28.0	29.3	29.5
74–76	28.4	28.7	28.9	29.2	29.4	29.7	29.9	30.2	30.4
77–79	29.3	29.5	29.8	30.0	30.3	30.5	30.8	31.0	31.3
80–82	30.1	30.4	30.6	30.9	31.1	31.4	31.6	31.9	32.1
83–85	30.9	31.2	31.4	31.7	31.9	32.2	32.4	32.7	32.9
86–88	31.7	32.0	32.2	32.5	32.7	32.9	33.2	33.4	33.7
89–91	32.5	32.7	33.0	33.2	33.5	33.7	33.9	34.2	34.4
92–94	33.2	33.4	33.7	33.9	34.2	34.4	34.7	34.9	35.2
95–97	33.9	34.1	34.4	34.6	34.9	35.1	35.4	35.6	35.9
98–100	34.6	34.8	35.1	35.3	35.5	35.8	36.0	36.3	36.5
101–103	35.3	35.4	35.7	35.9	36.2	36.4	36.7	36.9	37.2
104–106	35.8	36.1	36.3	36.6	36.8	37.1	37.3	37.5	37.8
107–109	36.4	36.7	36.9	37.1	37.4	37.6	37.9	38.1	38.4
110–112	37.0	37.2	37.5	37.7	38.0	38.2	38.5	38.7	38.9
113–115	37.5	37.8	38.0	38.2	38.5	38.7	39.0	39.2	39.5
116–118	38.0	38.3	38.5	38.8	39.0	39.3	39.5	39.7	40.0
119–121	38.5	38.7	39.0	39.2	39.5	39.7	40.0	40.2	40.5
122–124	39.0	39.2	39.4	39.7	39.9	40.2	40.4	40.7	40.9
125–127	39.4	39.6	39.9	40.1	40.4	40.6	40.9	41.1	41.4
128–130	39.8	40.0	40.3	40.5	40.8	41.0	41.3	41.5	41.8

*Percent fat calculated by the formula of Siri: Percent fat = $[(4.95/BD) - 4.5] \times 100$, where BD = body density.

Table 19-6 Estimation of relative body fat, by percent*, in men from the sum of chest, abdominal, and thigh skinfolds (from Pollock, et al., 1980).

Age to the Last Year Sum of Skinfolds (mm)	Under 22	23 to 27	28 to 32	33 to 37	38 to 42	43 to 47	48 to 52	53 to 57	Over 58
8–10	1.3	1.8	2.3	2.9	3.4	3.9	4.5	5.0	5.5
11–13	2.2	2.8	3.3	3.9	4.4	4.9	5.5	6.0	6.5
14–16	3.2	3.8	4.3	4.8	5.4	5.9	6.4	7.0	7.5
17–19	4.2	4.7	5.3	5.8	6.3	6.9	7.4	8.0	8.5
20–22	5.1	5.7	6.2	6.8	7.3	7.9	8.4	8.9	9.5
23–25	6.1	6.6	7.2	7.7	8.3	8.8	9.4	9.9	10.5
26–28	7.0	7.6	8.1	8.7	9.2	9.8	10.3	10.9	11.4
29–31	8.0	8.5	9.1	9.6	10.2	10.7	11.3	11.8	12.4
32–34	8.9	9.4	10.0	10.5	11.1	11.6	12.2	12.8	13.3
35–37	9.8	10.4	10.9	11.5	12.0	12.6	13.1	13.7	14.3
38–40	10.7	11.3	11.8	12.4	12.9	13.5	14.1	14.6	15.2
41–43	11.6	12.2	12.7	13.3	13.8	14.4	15.0	15.5	16.1
44–46	12.5	13.1	13.6	14.2	14.7	15.3	15.9	16.4	17.0
47–49	13.4	13.9	14.5	15.1	15.6	16.2	16.8	17.3	17.9
50–52	14.3	14.8	15.4	15.9	16.5	17.1	17.6	18.2	18.8
53–55	15.1	15.7	16.2	16.8	17.4	17.9	18.5	18.1	19.7
56–58	16.0	16.5	17.1	17.7	18.2	18.8	19.4	20.0	20.5
59–61	16.9	17.4	17.9	18.5	19.1	19.7	20.2	20.8	21.4
62–64	17.6	18.2	18.8	19.4	19.9	20.5	21.1	21.7	22.2
65–67	18.5	19.0	19.6	20.2	20.8	21.3	21.9	22.5	23.1
68–70	19.3	19.9	20.4	21.0	21.6	22.2	22.7	23.3	23.9
71–73	20.1	20.7	21.2	21.8	22.4	23.0	23.6	24.1	24.7
74–76	20.9	21.5	22.0	22.6	23.2	23.8	24.4	25.0	25.5
77–79	21.7	22.2	22.8	23.4	24.0	24.6	25.2	25.8	26.3
80–82	22.4	23.0	23.6	24.2	24.8	25.4	25.9	26.5	27.1
83–85	23.2	23.8	24.4	25.0	25.5	26.1	26.7	27.3	27.9
86–88	24.0	24.5	25.1	25.7	26.3	26.9	27.5	28.1	28.7
89–91	24.7	25.3	25.9	25.5	27.1	27.6	28.2	28.8	29.4
92–94	25.4	26.0	26.6	27.2	27.8	28.4	29.0	29.6	30.2
95–97	26.1	26.7	27.3	27.9	28.5	29.1	29.7	30.3	30.9
98–100	26.9	27.4	28.0	28.6	29.2	29.8	30.4	31.0	31.6
101–103	27.5	28.1	28.7	29.3	29.9	30.5	31.1	31.7	32.3
104–106	28.2	28.8	29.4	30.0	30.6	31.2	31.8	32.4	33.0
107–109	28.9	29.5	30.1	30.7	31.3	31.9	32.5	33.1	33.7
110–112	29.6	30.2	30.8	31.4	32.0	32.6	33.2	33.8	34.4
113–115	30.2	30.8	31.4	32.0	32.6	33.2	33.8	34.5	35.1
116–118	30.9	31.5	32.1	32.7	33.3	33.9	34.5	35.1	35.7
119–121	31.5	32.1	32.7	33.3	33.9	34.5	35.1	35.7	36.4
122–124	32.1	32.7	33.3	33.9	34.5	35.1	35.8	36.4	37.0
125–127	32.7	33.3	33.9	34.5	35.1	35.8	36.4	37.0	37.6

*Percent fat calculated by the formula by Siri: Percent fat = $[(4.95/BD) - 4.5] \times 100$, where BD = body density.

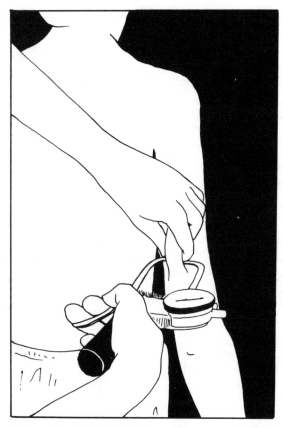

Figure 19–16   Skinfold fat assessment at the triceps site.

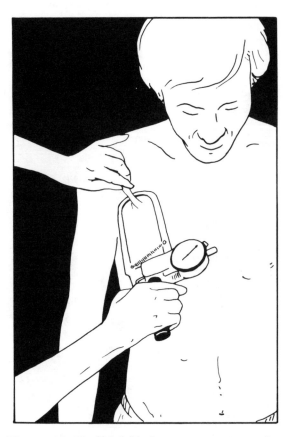

Figure 19–17   Skinfold fat assessment at the chest site.

and relative body fat from various combinations of bone diameters or widths, circumferences or girths, and skinfold thicknesses. Many of the initial equations have been found to be population-specific, in that they predict accurately only those populations that are similar in age, sex, nationality, and general physical fitness, to the population used in the initial study. It would not be appropriate to use an equation developed from a group of middle-aged, sedentary males for the evaluation of a group of male college athletes. The more recent equations have taken a different statistical approach in their generation, and they do appear to be more general in their application. Tables 19–5 and 19–6 on pages 378 and 379 provide estimates of relative body fat from the sum of three skin-

folds. The correct procedure for taking these skinfolds is illustrated in Figures 19–16 through 19–20, pages 380 to 382.

SUMMARY

This chapter has discussed various aspects of assessing human performance in both the highly-controlled laboratory situation, as well as under semi-controlled conditions in the field. The focus was on those variables that have the most direct application to human performance—cardiorespiratory endurance capacity; strength, power, and muscular endurance; anaerobic power, capacity, and threshold; flexibility; and body composition.

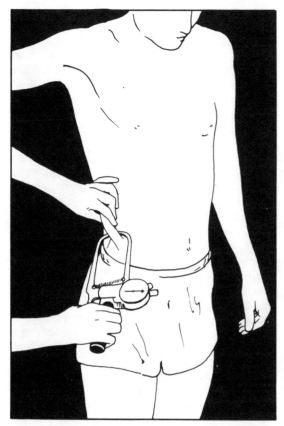

Figure 19–18 Skinfold fat assessment at the suprailiac site.

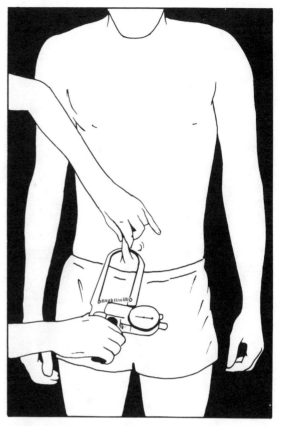

Figure 19–19 Skinfold fat assessment at the abdominal site.

The best laboratory measure of cardiorespiratory endurance capacity is maximal oxygen uptake ($\dot{V}O_2$ max). As exercise increases in intensity, one will eventually reach a point where oxygen uptake plateaus or decreases, even though the rate of work continues to increase, indicating that the limits of one's ability to provide oxygen to the working muscle have been reached. VO_2 max is highly specific to the type of ergometer used. So, when testing athletes, it is important to use an ergometer that most closely approximates the sport or activity of the athlete being tested. A number of field tests have been proposed to estimate $\dot{V}O_2$ max. Many of these are based on the fact that there is a linear relationship between heart rate and oxygen uptake. $\dot{V}O_2$ max can also be estimated from running tests, such as a 1.5-mile test for time or a 12-minute test for distance.

Strength, defined as the maximum force-producing capacity of a muscle usually during a static or isometric contraction, can be assessed directly in a laboratory using sophisticated electronic equipment. Simple field tests, such as the one repetition maximum (1-RM) or the greatest amount of weight that can be lifted just one time, appear to provide adequate measures of functional strength. Strength is not considered to be a generalizable factor, where the assessment of one muscle or muscle group will be representative of the total body. Therefore, at least three different areas should be assessed to provide a composite of total body strength—upper body, lower body, and trunk.

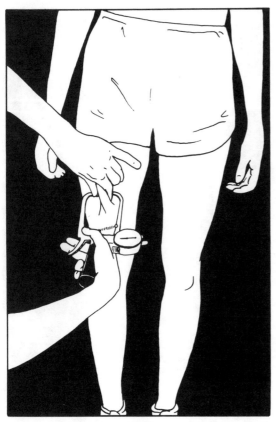

Figure 19–20 Skinfold fat assessment at the thigh site.

2-min duration. The Wingate Anaerobic Test is a 30-sec test in which one attempts to pedal at his or her maximal rate against a high, constant resistance. The highest rate of work for a given 5-sec segment is considered to be a measure of anaerobic power, and the total work performed in 30 sec would be a measure of anaerobic capacity. Anaerobic threshold, considered in this book to be identical in concept to lactate threshold, is assessed by directly measuring the blood lactate response to increasing rates of work. Lactate threshold is considered to be that rate of work, or that percentage of $\dot{V}O_2$ max, at which the lactate levels increase above resting levels.

Flexibility refers to the range of motion, or to the looseness or suppleness of the body or specific joints. It is not a generalizable factor, so those segments of the body considered important for a specific sport, or for health, should be assessed. Flexibility can be assessed with goniometers, flexometers, and by relatively simple field tests.

Body composition attempts to differentiate between the various tissues of the body that comprise the total body weight. In its simplest form, body weight is comprised of fat weight and fat-free or lean weight. Underwater weighing has been the standard method for determining body composition in the laboratory, although it can be used as a field test as well. A number of equations have been derived for estimating body composition from skinfolds, girths, and breadths.

Power, which is the rate of producing work, is perhaps the most important component for most athletic events. Power can be measured in the laboratory under highly-controlled conditions, but there are no accepted field tests to provide estimates of this component at this time. Muscular endurance refers to the ability of the muscle or muscle group to sustain static or dynamic contractions over time. A number of both laboratory and field tests are available to assess muscular endurance.

The anaerobic component of performance has been one of the most difficult to quantify. Anaerobic power is typically defined and measured as the peak power output attained in a short duration test of $\leq$ 30 sec. Anaerobic capacity is defined as the maximal work performed in a test of 30-sec to

STUDY QUESTIONS

1. Differentiate between cardiorespiratory endurance and muscular endurance.
2. What is the standard or criterion measurement of cardiorespiratory endurance capacity? How is it measured?
3. What type of ergometer would be most appropriate for testing a swimmer? A marathoner? A triathlete? A cyclist?
4. Discuss the relative merits of cycle ergometry versus treadmills for both submaximal and maximal testing.
5. Describe in detail three field tests for assessing $\dot{V}O_2$ max.

6. Describe how strength and power are assessed in both a laboratory setting and in the field.

7. How can you best measure muscular endurance in the laboratory? In the field?

8. Differentiate between anaerobic power, anaerobic capacity, and anaerobic threshold. Describe how each is measured in the laboratory.

9. Describe three methods of measuring flexibility. Describe a flexibility test battery for divers; for gymnasts.

10. How does body size differ from body build?

11. How does the underwater weighing allow one to determine body fat and fat-free, or lean, weight?

12. Describe other techniques for assessing body composition in the laboratory and their relative strengths and weaknesses.

13. What is the major limitation of the underwater weighing technique?

14. Describe the basis for field methods for assessing body composition using skinfolds, girths, and breadths.

REFERENCES

AAHPERD youth fitness test manual. (1976). Reston, VA: American Alliance for Health, Physical Education, Recreation, and Dance.

AAHPERD health related physical fitness test manual. (1980). Reston, VA: American Alliance for Health, Physical Education, Recreation, and Dance.

Åstrand, P. O., & Ryhming, I. (1954). A nomogram for calculation of aerobic capacity (physical fitness) from pulse rate during submaximal work. *Journal of Applied Physiology, 7,* 218–221.

Balke, B. (1963, April). A simple field test for the assessment of physical fitness. *Federal Aviation Agency, Aviation Medical Service.*

Bar-Or, O. (1983). *Pediatric sports medicine for the practitioner.* New York: Springer-Verlag.

Behnke, A. R., & Wilmore, J. H. (1974). *Evaluation and regulation of body build and composition.* Englewood Cliffs, NJ: Prentice-Hall.

Blair, S. N., Falls, H. B., & Pate, R. R. (1983). A new physical fitness test. *Physician and Sportsmedicine, 11* (#4), 77–83.

Brooks, G. A., & Fahey, T. D. (1984). *Exercise physiology: Human bioenergetics and its applications.* New York: John Wiley & Sons.

Conconi, F., Ferrari, M., Ziglio, P. G., Droghetti, P., & Codeca, L. (1982). Determination of the anaerobic thresh-old by a noninvasive field test in runners. *Journal of Applied Physiology, 52,* 869–873.

Cooper, K. H. (1968). A means of assessing maximal oxygen intake. *Journal of the American Medical Association, 203,* 201–204.

Davis, J. A. (1985). Anaerobic threshold: Review of the concept and directions for future research. *Medicine and Science in Sports and Exercise, 17,* 6–18.

Fox, E. L., & Mathews, D. K. (1981). *The physiological basis of physical education and athletics* (3rd ed.). New York: CBS College Publishing.

Froelicher, V. F. (1983). *Exercise testing and training.* New York: Le Jacq Publishing, Inc.

Gergley, T. J., McArdle, W. D., DeJesus, P., Toner, M. M., Jacobowitz, S., & Spina, R. J. (1984). Specificity of arm training on aerobic power during swimming and running. *Medicine and Science in Sports and Exercise, 16,* 349–354.

Golding, L. A., Myers, C. R., & Sinning, W. E. (1982). *The Y's way to physical fitness* (Revised). Chicago: National Board of YMCA.

Hoeger, W. W. K. (1986). *Lifetime physical fitness and wellness: A personalized program.* Englewood, CO: Morton Publishing Company.

Jackson, A. S., & Pollock, M. L. (1983). Generalized equations for predicting body density of men. *British Journal of Nutrition, 40,* 497–504.

Jackson, A. S., Pollock, M. L., & Ward, A. (1980). Generalized equations for predicting body density of women. *Medicine and Science in Sports and Exercise, 12,* 175–182.

Lohman, T. G. (1981). Skinfolds and body density and their relation to body fatness: A review. *Human Biology, 53,* 181–225.

MacDougall, J. D., Wenger, H. A., & Green, H. J. (1982). *Physiological testing of the elite athlete.* Canada: Canadian Association of Sport Sciences, Sport Medicine Council of Canada.

Magel, J. R., Foglia, G. F., McArdle, W. D., Gutin, B., Pechar, G. S., & Katch, F. I. (1975). Specificity of swim training on maximum oxygen uptake. *Journal of Applied Physiology, 38,* 151–155.

McArdle, W. D., Katch, F. I., & Katch, V. L. (1986). *Exercise physiology: Energy, nutrition, and human performance* (2nd ed.). Philadelphia: Lea & Febiger.

Perrine, J. J. (1968). Isokinetic strength. *Journal of Health, Physical Education, and Recreation, 39,* 40–44.

Pollock, M. L., & Jackson, A. S. (1984). Research progress in validation of clinical methods of assessing body composition. *Medicine and Science in Sports and Exercise, 16,* 606–613.

Pollock, M. L., Schmidt, D. H., & Jackson, A. S. (1980). Measurement of cardiorespiratory fitness and body composition in the clinical setting. *Comprehensive Therapy, 6,* 12–27.

Pollock, M. L., Wilmore, J. H., & Fox, S. M. (1984). *Exercise in health and disease: Evaluation and prescription for prevention and rehabilitation.* Philadelphia: W. B. Saunders.

Strømme, S. B., Ingjer, F., & Meen, H. D. (1977). Assessment of maximal aerobic power in specifically trained athletes. *Journal of Applied Physiology, 42,* 833–837.

Stull, G. A., & Clarke, D. H. (1979). Muscular strength testing and training. In *Proceedings of the first international conference on life style and health: Optimal health and fitness for people with physical disabilities,* pp. 195–214. Minneapolis, MN: University of Minnesota.

APPENDIX

Body Composition and
$\dot{V}O_2$ *Max Data for*
Male and Female Athletes
of Varying Ages

Body Composition Values in Male and Female Athletes.

Athletic Group or Sport	Sex	Age (yr)	Height (cm)	Weight (kg)	Relative Fat %	Reference
Baseball	male	20.8	182.7	83.3	14.2	Novak
	male	—	—	—	11.8	Forsyth
	male	26.0	185.4	87.5	16.2	Gurry
	male	27.3	185.8	86.4	12.6	Coleman
	male	27.4	183.1	88.0	12.6	Wilmore
Pitchers	male	26.7	188.1	89.8	14.7	Coleman
Infielders	male	27.4	183.1	83.2	12.0	Coleman
Outfielders	male	28.3	185.9	85.6	9.9	Coleman
Basketball	female	19.1	169.1	62.6	20.8	Sinning
	female	19.4	173.0	68.3	20.8	Vaccaro
	female	19.4	167.0	63.9	26.9	Conger
Centers	male	27.7	214.0	109.2	7.1	Parr
Forwards	male	25.3	200.6	96.9	9.0	Parr
Guards	male	25.2	188.0	83.6	10.6	Parr
Bicycling	male	—	180..3	67.1	8.8	Burke
	female	—	167.7	61.3	15.4	Burke
Canoeing/	male	23.7	182.0	79.6	12.4	Rusko
paddlers	male	20.1	179.9	76.3	10.4	Vaccaro
Dancing, ballet	female	15.0	161.1	48.4	16.4	Clarkson
General	female	21.2	162.7	51.2	20.5	Novak
Fencers	male	20.4	174.9	68.0	12.2	Vander
Football	male	19.3	186.8	93.1	13.7	Smith
	male	20.3	184.9	96.4	13.8	Novak
	male	—	—	—	13.9	Forsyth
Defensive	male	17–23	178.3	77.3	11.5	Wickkiser
Backs	male	24.5	182.5	84.8	9.6	Wilmore
Offensive	male	17–23	179.7	79.8	12.4	Wickkiser
Backs	male	24.7	183.8	90.7	9.4	Wilmore
Linebackers	male	17–23	180.1	87.2	13.4	Wickkiser
	male	24.2	188.6	102.2	14.0	Wilmore
Offensive	male	17–23	186.0	99.2	19.1	Wickkiser
Linemen	male	24.7	193.0	112.6	15.6	Wilmore
Defensive	male	17–23	186.6	97.8	18.5	Wickkiser
Linemen	male	25.7	192.4	117.1	18.2	Wilmore
Quarterbacks, Kickers	male	24.1	185.0	90.1	14.4	Wilmore
Golf	female	33.3	168.9	61.8	24.0	Crews
Gymnastics	male	20.3	178.5	69.2	4.6	Novak
	female	14.0	—	—	17.0	Parizkova
	female	15.2	161.1	50.4	13.1	Moffatt
	female	19.4	163.0	57.9	23.8	Conger
	female	20.0	158.5	51.5	15.5	Sinning

Body Composition Values in Male and Female Athletes.

Athletic Group or Sport	Sex	Age (yr)	Height (cm)	Weight (kg)	Relative Fat %	Reference
	female	23.0	—	—	11.0	Parizkova
	female	23.0	—	—	9.6	Parizkova
Ice Hockey	male	22.5	179.0	77.3	13.0	Rusko
	male	26.3	180.3	86.7	15.1	Wilmore
Jockeys	male	30.9	158.2	50.3	14.1	Wilmore
Orienteering	male	31.2	—	72.2	16.3	Knowlton
	female	29.0	—	58.1	18.7	Knowlton
Pentathalon	female	21.5	175.4	65.4	11.0	Krahenbuhl
Racketball	male	25.0	181.7	80.3	8.1	Pipes
Lightweight	male	21.0	186.0	71.0	8.5	Hagerman
	female	23.0	173.0	68.0	14.0	Hagerman
Rowing	male	25.6	192.0	93.0	6.5	Secher
Rugby	male	28.1	181.6	86.3	9.1	Maud
Skiing	male	25.9	176.6	74.8	7.4	Sprynarova
Alpine	male	16.5	173.1	65.5	11.0	Song
	male	21.0	178.0	78.0	9.9	Veicsteinas
	male	21.2	176.0	70.1	14.1	Rusko
	male	21.8	177.8	75.5	10.2	Haymes
	female	19.5	165.1	58.8	20.6	Haymes
Cross-country	male	21.2	176.0	66.6	12.5	Niinimaa
	male	22.7	176.2	73.2	7.9	Haymes
	male	25.6	174.0	69.3	10.2	Rusko
	female	20.2	163.4	55.9	15.7	Haymes
	female	24.3	163.0	59.1	21.8	Rusko
Nordic	male	21.7	181.7	70.4	8.9	Haymes
Combination	male	22.9	176.0	70.4	11.2	Rusko
Skijumping	male	22.2	174.0	69.9	14.3	Rusko
Soccer	male	26.0	176.0	75.5	9.6	Raven
US Junior	male	17.5	178.3	72.3	9.4	Kirkendahl
US Olympic	male	20.6	179.3	72.5	9.1	Kirkendahl
US Collegiate	male	20.0	175.3	72.4	10.9	Kirkendahl
US National	male	22.5	178.6	76.2	9.9	Kirkendahl
M I S L	male	26.9	177.3	74.5	10.5	Kirkendahl
Skating, Speed	male	21.0	181.0	76.5	11.4	Kusko
	male	—	181.0	73.6	9.0	Vanlugen
Figure	male	21.3	166.9	59.6	9.1	Niinimaa
	female	16.5	158.8	48.6	12.5	Niinimaa
Swimming	male	15.1	166.8	59.1	10.8	Vaccaro
	male	20.6	182.9	78.9	5.0	Novak
	male	21.8	182.3	79.1	8.5	Sprynarova
	female	19.4	168.0	63.8	26.3	Conger

Body Composition Values in Male and Female Athletes.

Athletic Group or Sport	Sex	Age (yr)	Height (cm)	Weight (kg)	Relative Fat %	Reference
Sprint	female	—	165.1	57.1	14.6	Wilmore
Middle Distance	female	—	166.6	66.8	24.1	Wilmore
Distance	female	—	166.3	60.9	17.1	Wilmore
Synchronized Swimming	female	20.1	166.2	55.8	24.0	Roby
Tennis	male	—	—	—	15.2	Forsyth
	male	42.0	179.6	77.1	16.3	Vodak
	female	39.0	163.3	55.7	20.3	Vodak
Track and Field	male	21.3	180.6	71.6	3.7	Novak
	male	—	—	—	8.8	Forsyth
Runners	male	22.5	177.4	64.5	6.3	Sprynarova
Distance	male	26.1	175.7	64.2	7.5	Costill
	male	26.2	177.0	66.2	8.4	Rusko
	male	26.2	177.1	63.1	4.7	Pollock
	male	40–49	180.7	71.6	11.2	Pollock
	male	47.2	176.5	70.7	13.2	Lewis
	male	55.3	174.5	63.4	18.0	Barnard
	male	50–59	174.7	67.2	10.9	Pollock
	male	60–69	175.7	67.1	11.3	Pollock
	male	70–75	175.6	66.8	13.6	Pollock
	female	19.9	161.3	52.9	19.2	Malina
	female	32.4	169.4	57.2	15.2	Wilmore
	female	37.8	165.1	54.1	15.5	Upton
	female	43.8	161.5	53.8	18.3	Vaccaro
Middle	male	20.1	178.1	71.9	6.9	Wilmore
Distance	male	24.6	179.0	72.3	12.4	Rusko
Sprint	female	20.1	164.9	56.7	19.3	Malina
	male	20.1	178.2	72.8	5.4	Wilmore
	male	46.5	177.0	74.1	16.5	Barnard
Cross-country	female	15.6	164.2	51.1	15.3	Butts
	female	15.6	163.3	50.9	15.4	Butts
Race Walking	male	26.7	178.7	68.5	7.8	Franklin
Discus	male	26.4	190.8	110.5	16.3	Wilmore
	male	28.3	186.1	104.7	16.4	Fahey
	female	21.1	168.1	71.0	25.0	Malina
Jumpers and Hurdlers	female	20.3	165.9	59.0	20.7	Malina
Shot put	male	22.0	191.6	126.2	19.6	Behnke
	male	27.0	188.2	112.5	16.5	Fahey
	female	21.5	167.6	78.1	28.0	Malina
Triathalon	male	—	—	—	7.1	Holly
	female	—	—	—	12.6	Holly

Body Composition Values in Male and Female Athletes.

Athletic Group or Sport	Sex	Age (yr)	Height (cm)	Weight (kg)	Relative Fat %	Reference
Volleyball	male	26.1	192.7	85.5	12.0	Puhl
	female	19.4	166.0	59.8	25.3	Conger
	female	19.9	172.2	64.1	21.3	Kovaleski
	female	21.6	178.3	70.5	17.9	Puhl
Weight Lifting	male	24.9	166.4	77.2	9.8	Sprynarova
Power	male	25.5	173.6	89.4	19.9	Hakkinen
	male	26.3	176.1	92.0	15.6	Fahey
Olympic	male	25.3	177.1	88.2	12.2	Fahey
Body Builders	male	25.6	176.9	87.6	13.4	Hakkinen
	male	27.6	178.8	88.1	8.3	Pipes
	male	29.0	172.4	83.1	8.4	Fahey
	female	27.0	160.8	53.8	13.2	Freedson
Wrestling	male	11.3	141.2	34.2	12.7	Sady
	male	15–18	172.3	66.3	6.9	Katch
	male	19.6	174.6	74.8	8.8	Sinning
	male	20.6	174.8	67.3	4.0	Stine
	male	22.0	—	—	5.0	Parizkova
	male	23.0	—	79.3	14.3	Taylor
	male	24.0	173.3	77.5	12.7	Hakkinen
	male	26.0	177.8	81.8	9.8	Fahey
	male	27.0	176.0	75.7	10.7	Gale

Maximal Oxygen Uptake ($ml \cdot kg^{-1} \cdot min^{-1}$) of Male and Female Athletes.

Athletic group or sport	Sex	Age (years)	Height (cm)	Weight (kg)	$\dot{V}O_2$ max	Reference
Baseball/	M	21	182.7	83.3	52.3	Novak
Softball	M	26	185.4	87.5	41.6	Gurry
	M	28	183.6	88.1	52.0	Wilmore
	F	19–23	—	—	55.3	Rubal
Basketball	F	19	167.0	63.9	42.3	Conger
	F	19	169.1	62.6	42.9	Sinning
	F	19	173.0	68.3	49.6	Vaccaro
Centers	M	28	214.0	109.2	41.9	Parr
Forwards	M	25	200.6	96.9	45.9	Parr
Guards	M	25	188.0	83.6	50.0	Parr
Bicycling	M	24	182.0	74.5	68.2	Gollnick
(competitive)	M	24	180.4	79.2	70.3	Hermansen

Maximal Oxygen Uptake (ml·kg^{-1}·min^{-1}) of Male and Female Athletes.

Athletic group or sport	Sex	Age (years)	Height (cm)	Weight (kg)	$\dot{V}O_2$ max	Reference
Bicycling (cont.)	M	25	180.0	72.8	67.1	Burke
(competitive)	M	—	180.3	67.1	74.0	Burke
	M	—	—	—	74.0	Saltin
	M	—	—	—	69.1	Strømme
	F	20	165.0	55.0	50.2	Burke
	F	—	167.7	61.3	57.4	Burke
Canoeing/	M	18	—	66.5	71.2	Tesch
Paddlers	M	19	173.0	64.0	60.0	Sidney
	M	20	179.9	76.3	60.1	Vaccaro
	M	22	190.5	80.7	67.7	Hermansen
	M	24	182.0	79.6	66.1	Rusko
	M	25	—	78.0	69.2	Tesch
	M	26	181.0	74.0	56.8	Gollnick
	F	18	166.0	57.3	49.2	Sidney
Dancing, Ballet	M	24	177.5	68.0	48.2	Cohen
	M	28	175.0	64.0	59.3	Mostardi
	M	29	177.0	69.0	56.0	Schantz
	F	15	161.1	48.4	48.9	Clarkson
	F	24	165.6	49.5	43.7	Cohen
	F	25	165.0	50.0	48.6	Mostardi
	F	28	164.0	51.0	51.0	Schantz
General	F	21	162.7	51.2	41.5	Novak
Fencing	M	20	174.9	68.0	50.2	Vander
Football	M	19	186.8	93.1	56.5	Smith
	M	20	184.9	96.4	51.3	Novak
Defensive backs	M	25	182.5	84.8	53.1	Wilmore
Offensive backs	M	25	183.8	90.7	52.2	Wilmore
Linebackers	M	24	188.6	102.2	52.1	Wilmore
Offensive line	M	25	193.0	112.6	49.9	Wilmore
Defensive line	M	26	192.4	117.1	44.9	Wilmore
Quarterbacks/ Kickers	M	24	185.0	90.1	49.0	Wilmore
Gymnastics	M	20	178.5	69.2	55.5	Novak
	F	15	161.1	50.4	45.2	Moffatt
	F	15	159.7	48.8	49.8	Hermansen
	F	19	163.0	57.9	36.3	Conger
Golf	F	33	168.9	61.8	34.2	Crews
Ice hockey	M	11	140.5	35.5	56.6	Cunningham
	M	22	179.0	77.3	61.5	Rusko
	M	24	179.3	81.8	54.6	Seliger
	M	26	180.1	86.4	53.6	Wilmore

Maximal Oxygen Uptake (ml·kg^{-1}·min^{-1}) of Male and Female Athletes.

Athletic group or sport	Sex	Age (years)	Height (cm)	Weight (kg)	V̇O₂ max	Reference
Jockey	M	31	158.2	50.3	53.8	Wilmore
Orienteering	M	25	179.7	70.3	71.1	Hermansen
	M	31	—	72.2	61.6	Knowlton
	M	52	176.0	72.7	50.7	Gollnick
	F	23	165.8	60.0	60.7	Hermansen
	F	29	—	58.1	46.1	Knowlton
Pentathlon	F	21	175.4	65.4	45.9	Krahenbuhl
Racketball/	M	24	183.7	81.3	60.0	Hermansen
Handball	M	25	181.7	80.3	58.3	Pipes
Rowing	M	—	—	—	65.7	Strømme
	M	23	192.7	89.9	62.7	Mickelson
	M	24	180.0	71.8	72.0	Secher
	M	25	189.9	86.9	66.9	Hermansen
	M	26	192.0	93.0	63.0	Secher
Heavyweight	M	23	192.0	88.0	68.9	Hagerman
Lightweight	M	21	186.0	71.0	71.1	Hagerman
	F	23	173.0	68.0	60.3	Hagerman
Rugby	M	28	181.6	86.3	45.9	Maud
Skating, Speed	M	—	181.0	73.6	64.4	van Ingen
	M	20	175.5	73.9	56.1	Maksud
	M	21	181.0	76.5	72.9	Rusko
	M	25	183.1	82.4	64.6	Hermansen
	F	20	168.1	65.4	52.0	Hermansen
	F	21	164.5	60.8	46.1	Maksud
Figure	M	21	166.9	59.6	58.5	Niinimaa
	F	17	158.8	48.6	48.9	Niinimaa
Skiing, Alpine	M	16	173.1	65.5	65.6	Song
	M	21	176.0	70.1	63.8	Rusko
	M	21	178.0	78.0	52.4	Veicsteinas
	M	22	178.5	77.6	63.1	Brown
	M	22	177.8	75.5	66.6	Haymes
	M	26	176.6	74.8	62.3	Sprynarova
	F	19	165.1	58.8	52.7	Haymes
Cross-country	M	21	176.0	66.6	63.9	Niinimaa
	M	23	176.2	73.2	73.0	Haymes
	M	25	180.4	73.2	73.9	Hermansen
	M	26	174.0	69.3	78.3	Rusko
	M	—	—	—	72.8	Strømme
	F	20	163.4	55.9	61.5	Haymes
	F	24	163.0	59.1	68.2	Rusko
	F	25	165.7	60.5	56.9	Hermansen
	F	—	—	—	58.1	Strømme

Maximal Oxygen Uptake (ml·kg^{-1}·min^{-1}) of Male and Female Athletes.

Athletic group or sport	Sex	Age (years)	Height (cm)	Weight (kg)	$\dot{V}O_2$ max	Reference
Nordic	M	23	176.0	70.4	72.8	Rusko
	M	22	181.7	70.4	67.4	Haymes
Ski jumping	M	22	174.0	69.9	61.3	Rusko
Soccer	M	26	176.0	75.5	58.4	Raven
US Junior	M	18	178.3	72.3	61.8	Kirkendall
Swimming	M	12	150.4	41.2	52.5	Cunningham
	M	13	164.8	52.1	52.9	Cunningham
	M	15	169.6	59.8	56.6	Cunningham
	M	15	166.8	59.1	56.8	Vaccaro
	M	20	181.4	76.7	55.7	Magel
	M	20	181.0	73.0	50.4	Charbonnier
	M	21	182.9	78.9	62.1	Novak
	M	21	181.0	78.3	69.9	Gollnick
	M	22	182.3	79.1	56.9	Sprynarova
	M	22	182.3	79.7	55.9	Cunningham
	F	12	154.8	43.3	46.2	Cunningham
	F	13	160.0	52.1	43.4	Cunningham
	F	15	164.8	53.7	40.5	Cunningham
Sprint	M	19	181.1	75.0	58.3	Shephard
Mid-distance	M	22	178.0	74.6	55.4	Shephard
Long-distance	M	21	179.0	74.9	65.4	Shephard
	F	19	168.0	63.8	37.6	Conger
Synchronized	F	20	166.2	55.8	43.2	Roby
Tennis	M	12	147.9	38.5	56.3	Buti
	M	42	179.6	77.1	50.2	Vodak
	F	12	150.9	42.9	52.6	Buti
	F	39	163.3	55.7	44.2	Vodak
Track and Field	M	21	180.6	71.6	66.1	Novak
Runners	M	22	177.4	64.5	64.0	Sprynarova
	M	23	177.0	69.5	72.4	Gollnick
Sprint	M	17–22	—	—	51.0	Thomas
	M	46	177.0	74.1	47.2	Barnard
Mid-distance	M	20	178.1	71.9	55.8	Wilmore
	M	25	180.1	67.8	70.1	Costill
	M	25	179.0	72.3	69.8	Rusko
Distance	M	10	144.3	31.9	56.6	Mayers
	M	17–22	—	—	65.5	Thomas
	M	26	177.1	63.1	76.9	Pollock
	M	26	176.1	64.5	72.2	Hermansen
	M	26	178.9	63.9	77.4	Costill
	M	26	177.0	66.2	78.1	Rusko
	M	27	178.7	64.9	73.2	Costill

Maximal Oxygen Uptake (ml·kg⁻¹·min⁻¹) of Male and Female Athletes.

Athletic group or sport	Sex	Age (years)	Height (cm)	Weight (kg)	V̇O₂ max	Reference
	M	32	177.3	64.3	70.3	Costill
	M	35	174.0	63.1	66.6	Costill
	M	36	177.3	69.6	65.1	Hagan
	M	40–49	180.7	71.6	57.5	Pollock
	M	55	174.5	63.4	54.4	Barnard
	M	50–59	174.7	67.2	54.4	Pollock
	M	60–69	175.7	67.1	51.4	Pollock
	M	70–75	175.6	66.8	40.0	Pollock
	M	—	—	—	72.5	Davies
	F	16	162.2	48.6	63.2	Burke
	F	16	163.3	50.9	50.8	Butts
	F	21	170.2	58.6	57.5	Hermansen
	F	25	165.7	52.3	59.8	Upton
	F	32	169.4	57.2	59.1	Wilmore
	F	38	165.1	54.1	55.5	Upton
	F	38	165.5	54.7	55.5	Upton
	F	44	161.5	53.8	43.4	Vaccaro
	F	—	—	—	58.2	Davies
Cross-country	F	16	163.3	50.9	50.8	Butts
Race Walking	M	27	178.7	68.5	62.9	Franklin
Jumpers	M	17–22	—	—	55.0	Thomas
Shot/Discus	M	17–22	—	—	49.5	Thomas
	M	26	190.8	110.5	42.8	Wilmore
	M	27	188.2	112.5	42.6	Fahey
	M	28	186.1	104.7	47.5	Fahey
Triathalon	M	—	—	—	72.0	Holly
	F	—	—	—	58.7	Holly
Volleyball	M	25	187.0	84.5	56.4	Conlee
	M	26	192.7	85.5	56.1	Puhl
	F	19	166.0	59.8	43.5	Conger
	F	20	172.2	64.1	56.0	Kovaleski
	F	22	183.7	73.4	41.7	Spence
	F	22	178.3	70.5	50.6	Puhl
Weight Lifting	M	25	171.0	81.3	40.1	Gollnick
	M	25	166.4	77.2	42.6	Sprynarova
Power	M	26	173.6	89.4	41.9	Hakkinen
	M	26	176.1	92.0	49.5	Fahey
Olympic	M	25	177.1	88.2	50.7	Fahey
Body Builder	M	26	176.9	87.6	50.8	Hakkinen
	M	27	178.8	88.1	46.3	Pipes
	M	29	172.4	83.1	41.5	Fahey
Wrestling	M	11	141.2	34.2	54.0	Sady
	M	21	174.8	67.3	58.3	Stine

Maximal Oxygen Uptake (ml·kg^{-1}·min^{-1}) of Male and Female Athletes.

Athletic group or sport	Sex	Age (years)	Height (cm)	Weight (kg)	$\dot{V}O_2$ max	Reference
Wrestling (*cont.*)	M	23	—	79.2	50.4	Taylor
	M	24	173.3	77.5	57.8	Hakkinen
	M	24	175.6	77.7	60.9	Nagel
	M	26	177.0	81.8	64.0	Fahey
	M	27	176.0	75.7	54.3	Gale

REFERENCES

Adams, J., Mottola, M., Bagnall, K. M., & McFadden, K. D. (1982). Total body fat content in a group of professional football players. *Canadian Journal of Applied Sports and Science, 7*, 36-40.

Åstrand, P. O., & Rodahl, K. (1986). *Textbook of work physiology* (3rd ed.). New York: McGraw-Hill Publishing Co.

Barnard, R. J., Grimditch, G. K., & Wilmore, J. H. (1979). Physiological characteristics of sprint and endurance Masters runners. *Medicine and Science in Sports, 11*, 167-171.

Bar-Or, O. (1975). Predicting athletic performance. *Physician and Sportsmedicine, 3* (#2), 80-85.

Behnke, A. R., & Wilmore, J. H. (1974). *Evaluation and regulation of body build and composition.* Englewood Cliffs, NJ: Prentice-Hall.

Bergh, U., Thorstensson, A., Sjodin, B., Hulten, B., Piehl, K., & Karlsson, J. (1978). Maximal oxygen uptake and muscle fiber types in trained and untrained humans. *Medicine and Science in Sports, 10*, 151-154.

Brown, C. H., & Wilmore, J. H. (1974). The effects of maximal resistance training on the strength and body composition of women athletes. *Medicine and Science in Sports, 6*, 174-177.

Brown, S. L., & Wilkinson, J. G. (1983). Characteristics of national, divisional, and club male alpine ski racers. *Medicine and Science in Sports and Exercise, 15*, 491-495.

Burke, E. J., & Brush, F. C. (1979). Physiological and anthropometric assessment of successful teenage female distance runners. *Research Quarterly, 50*, 180-187.

Burke, E. R. (1980). Physiological characteristics of competitive cyclists. *Physician and Sportsmedicine, 8* (#7), 78-84.

Burke, E. R., Cerny, F., Costill, D., & Fink, W. (1977). Characteristics of skeletal muscle in competitive cyclists. *Medicine and Science in Sports, 9*, 109-112.

Buti, T., Elliott, B., & Morton, A. (1984). Physiological and anthropometric profiles of elite prepubescent tennis players. *Physician and Sportsmedicine, 12* (#1), 111-116.

Butts, N. K. (1982). Physiological profile of high school female cross-country runners. *Physician and Sportsmedicine, 10*, 103-111.

Butts, N. K. (1982). Physiological profiles of high school female cross country runners. *Research Quarterly for Exercise and Sport, 53*, 8-14.

Charbonnier, J. P., Lacour, J. R., Riffat, J., & Flandrois, R. (1975). Experimental study of the performance of competition swimmers. *European Journal of Applied Physiology, 34*, 157-167.

Clarkson, P. M., Freedson, P. S., Keller, B., Carney, D., & Skrinar, M. (1985). Maximal oxygen uptake, nutritional patterns and body composition of adolescent female ballet dancers. *Research Quarterly for Exercise and Sport, 56*, 180-184.

Clement, D. B., Asmundson, C., Taunton, C., Taunton, J. E., Ridley, D., & Banister, E. W. (1979). The sport scientist's role in identification of performance criteria for distance runners. *Canadian Journal of Applied Sports Science, 4*, 143-148.

Coleman, A. E. (1981). Skinfold estimates of body fat in major league baseball players. *Physician and Sportsmedicine, 9* (#10), 77-82.

Conger, P. R., & Macnab, R. B. J. (1967). Strength, body composition, and work capacity of participants and nonparticipants in women's intercollegiate sports. *Research Quarterly, 38*, 184-192.

Conlee, R. K., McGown, C. M., Fisher, A. G., Dalsky, G. P., & Robinson, K. C. (1982). Physiological effects of power volleyball. *Physician and Sportsmedicine, 10* (#2), 93-97.

Costill, D. L. (1967). The relationship between selected physiological variables and distance running performance. *Journal of Sports Medicine, 7*, 61-66.

Costill, D. L. (1970). Metabolic responses during distance running. *Journal of Applied Physiology, 28*, 251-255.

Costill, D. L., Bowers, R., & Kammer, W. F. (1970). Skinfold estimates of body fat among marathon runners. *Medicine and Science in Sports, 2*, 93-95.

Costill, D. L., Daniels, J., Evans, W., Fink, W., Krahenbuhl, G., & Saltin, B. (1976). Skeletal muscle enzymes and fiber composition in male and female track athletes. *Journal of Applied Physiology, 40,* 149-154.

Costill, D. L., Fink, W. J., & Pollock, M. L. (1976). Muscle fiber composition and enzyme activities of elite distance runners. *Medicine and Science in Sports, 8,* 96-100.

Costill, D. L., Thomason, H., & Roberts, E. (1973). Fractional utilization of the aerobic capacity during distance running. *Medicine and Science in Sports, 5,* 248-252.

Costill, D. L., & Winrow, E. (1970). Maximal oxygen intake among marathon runners. *Archives of Physical and Medical Rehabilitation, 51,* 317-320.

Crews, D., Thomas, G., Shirreffs, J. H., & Helfrich, H. M. (1984). A physiological profile of ladies professional golf association tour players. *Physician and Sportsmedicine, 12* (#5), 69-76.

Cunningham, D. A., & Eynon, R. B. (1973). The working capacity of young competitive swimmers, 10-16 years of age. *Medicine and Science in Sports, 5,* 227-231.

Cunningham, D. A., Telford, P., & Swart, G. T. (1976). The cardiopulmonary capacities of young hockey players: Age 10. *Medicine and Science in Sports, 8,* 23-25.

Cureton, T. K. (1951). *Physical fitness of champion athletes.* Urbana, IL: University of Illinois Press.

Davies, C. T. M. (1971). Body composition in children: A reference standard for maximum aerobic power output on a stationary bicycle ergometer. In, Proceedings of the III International Symposium on Pediatric Work Physiology. *Acta Paediatrica Scandinavica* (Suppl) *217,* 136-137.

Davies, C. T. M., & Thompson, M. W. (1979). Aerobic performance of female marathon and male ultramarathon atheletes. *European Journal of Applied Physiology, 41,* 233-245.

deGaray, A. L., Levine, L., & Carter, J. E. L. (Eds). (1974). *Genetic and anthropological studies of Olympic athletes.* New York: Academic Press.

Drinkwater, B. L. (1973). Physiological responses of women to exercise. *Exercise and Sport Sciences Reviews, 1,* 125-153.

Drinkwater, B. L. (1984). Women and exercise: Physiological aspects. *Exercise and Sport Sciences Reviews, 12,* 21-51.

Edstrom, L., & Ekblom, B. (1972). Differences in sizes of red and white muscle fibers in vastus lateralis of musculus quadriceps femoris of normal individuals and athletes: Relation to physical performance. *Scandinavian Journal of Clinical Laboratory Investigation, 30,* 175-181.

Ekblom, B. (1986). Applied physiology of soccer. *Sports Medicine, 3,* 50-60.

Fahey, T. D., Akka, L., & Rolph, R. (1975). Body composition and $\dot{V}O_2$ max of exceptional weight-trained athletes. *Journal of Applied Physiology, 39,* 559-561.

Forsyth, H. L., & Sinning, W. E. (1973). The anthropometric estimation of body density and lean body weight of male athletes. *Medicine and Science in Sports, 5,* 174-180.

Franklin, B. A., Kaimal, K. P., Moir, T. W., & Hel-

lerstein, H. K. (1981). Characteristics of national-class race walkers. *Physician and Sportsmedicine, 9* (#9), 101-108.

Freedson, P. S., Mihevic, P. M., Loucks, A. B., & Girandola R. N. (1983). Physique, body composition, and psychological characteristics of competitive female body builders. *Physician and Sportsmedicine, 11* (#5), 85-93.

Gale, J. B., & Flynn, K. W. (1974). Maximal oxygen consumption and relative body fat of high-ability wrestlers. *Medicine and Science in Sports, 6,* 232-234.

Gollnick, P. D., Armstrong, R. B., Saubert, IV, C. W., Piehl, K., & Saltin, B. (1972). Enzyme activity and fiber composition in skeletal muscle of untrained and trained men. *Journal of Applied Physiology, 33,* 312-319.

Gurry, M., Pappas, A., Michaels, J., Maher, P., Shakman, A., Goldberg, R., & Rippe, J. (1985). A comprehensive preseason fitness evaluation for professional baseball players. *Physician and Sportsmedicine, 13* (#6), 63-74.

Hagan, R. D., Smith, M. G., & Gettman, L. R. (1981). Marathon performance in relation to maximal aerobic power and training indices. *Medicine and Science in Sports and Exercise, 13,* 185-189.

Hagberg, J. M., & Coyle, E. F. (1983). Physiological determinants of endurance performance as studied in competitive racewalkers. *Medicine and Science in Sports and Exercise, 15,* 287-289.

Hagerman, F. C., Hagerman, G. R., & Mickelson, T. C. (1979). Physiological profiles of elite rowers. *Physician and Sportsmedicine, 7* (#7), 74-83.

Hakkinen, K., Alen, M., & Komi, P. V. (1984). Neuromuscular, anaerobic, and aerobic performance characteristics of elite power athletes. *European Journal of Applied Physiology, 53,* 97-105.

Haymes, E. M., & Dickinson, A. L. (1980). Characteristics of elite male and female ski racers. *Medicine and Science in Sports and Exercise, 12,* 153-158.

Hermansen, L. (1973). Oxygen transport during exercise in human subjects. *Acta Physiologica Scandinavica,* (Suppl) *399,* 1-104.

Hermansen, L., & Andersen, K. L. (1965). Aerobic work capacity in young Norwegian men and women. *Journal of Applied Physiology, 20,* 425-431.

Holly, R. G., Barnard, R. J, Rosenthal, M., Applegate, E., & Pritikin, N. (1986). Triathlete characterization and response to prolonged strenuous competition. *Medicine and Science in Sports and Exercise, 18,* 123-127.

Katch, F. I., & Michael, E. D. (1971). Body composition of high school wrestlers according to age and wrestling weight category. *Medicine and Science in Sports, 3,* 190-194.

Kirkendall, D. T. (1985). The applied sport science of soccer. *Physician and Sportsmedicine, 13* (#4), 53-59.

Knowlton, R. G., Ackerman, K. J., Fitzgerald, P. I., Wilde, S. W., & Tahamont, M. V. (1980). Physiological and performance characteristics of United States championship class orienteers. *Medicine and Science in Sports and Exercise, 12,* 164-169.

Kovaleski, J. E., Parr, R. B., Hornak, J. E., & Roitman,

J. L. (1980). Athletic profile of women college volleyball players. *Physician and Sportsmedicine, 8* (#2), 112–118.

Krahenbuhl, G. S., Wells, C. L., Brown, C. H., & Ward, P. E. (1979). Characteristics of national and world class female pentathletes. *Medicine and Science in Sports, 11,* 20–23.

Lewis, S., Haskell, W. L., Klein, H., Halpern, J., & Wood, P. D. (1975). Prediction of body composition in habitually active middle-aged men. *Journal of Applied Physiology, 39,* 221–225.

Magel, J. R., & Faulkner, J. A. (1967). Maximum oxygen uptakes of college swimmers. *Journal of Applied Physiology, 22,* 929–933.

Maksud, M. G., Wiley, R. L., Hamilton, L. H., & Lockhart, B. (1970). Maximal $\dot{V}O_2$, ventilation, and heart rate of Olympic speed skating candidates. *Journal of Applied Physiology, 29,* 186–190.

Malina, R. M., Harper, A. B., Avent, H. H., & Campbell, D. E. (1971). Physique of female track and field athletes. *Medicine and Science in Sports, 3,* 32–38.

Malina, R. M., & Rarick, G. L. (1973). Growth, physique and motor performance. In G. L. Rarick (Ed). *Physical activity, human growth and development* (pp. 125–153). New York: Academic Press.

Maud, P. J., & Shultz, B. B. (1984). The U. S. national rugby team: A physiological and anthropometric assessment. *Physician and Sportsmedicine, 12* (#9), 86–99.

Mayers, N., & Gutin, B. (1979). Physiological characteristics of elite prepubertal cross-country runners. *Medicine and Science in Sports, 11,* 172–176.

Mickelson, T. C., & Hagerman, F. C. (1982). Anaerobic threshold measurements of elite oarsmen. *Medicine and Science in Sports and Exercise, 14,* 440–444.

Moffatt, R. J., Surina, B., Golden, B., & Ayres, N. (1984). Body composition and physiological characteristics of female high school gymnasts. *Research Quarterly for Exercise and Sport, 55,* 80–84.

Mostardi, R. A., Porterfield, J. A., Greenberg, B., Goldberg, D., & Lea, M. (1983). Musculoskeletal and cardiopulmonary characteristics of the professional ballet dancer. *Physician and Sportsmedicine, 11* (#12), 53–61.

Nagle, F. J., Morgan, W. P., Hellickson, R. O., Serfass, R. C., & Alexander, J. F. (1975). Spotting success traits in Olympic contenders. *Physician and Sportsmedicine, 3,* 31–36.

Nicholas, J. A., & Hershman, E. B. (Eds). (1984). *Profiling.* (Clinics in Sports Medicine, Volume 3, #1) Philadelphia: W. B. Saunders Company.

Niinimaa, V. (1982). Figure skating: What do we know about it? *Physician and Sportsmedicine, 10* (#1), 51–56.

Niinimaa, V., Dyon, M., & Shephard, R. J. (1978). Performance and efficiency of intercollegiate cross-country skiers. *Medicine and Science in Sports, 10,* 91–93.

Novak, L. P., Hyatt, R. E., & Alexander, J. F. (1968). Body composition and physiologic function of athletes. *Journal of the American Medical Association, 205,* 764–770.

Novak, L. P., Magill, L. A., & Schutte, J. E. (1978).

Maximal oxygen intake and body composition of female dancers. *European Journal of Applied Physiology, 39,* 277–282.

Parizkova, J. (1973). Body composition and exercise during growth and development. In G. L. Rarick (Ed.) *Physical activity, human growth and development.* New York: Academic Press. (pp. 97–124).

Parizkova, J., & Poupa, D. (1963). Some metabolic consequences of adaptation to muscular work. *British Journal of Nutrition, 17,* 341–345.

Parr, R. B., Wilmore, J. H., Hoover, R., Bachman, D., & Kerlan, R. K. (1978). Professional basketball players: Athletic profiles. *Physician and Sportsmedicine, 6* (#4), 77–84.

Pipes, T. V. (1979). Physiological characteristics of elite body builders. *Physician and Sportsmedicine, 7* (#3), 116–122.

Pipes, T. V. (1979). The racquetball pro: A physiological profile. *Physician and Sportsmedicine, 7* (#10), 91–94.

Pollock, M. L. (1973). The quantification of endurance training programs. *Exercise and Sport Sciences Reviews, 1,* 155–188.

Pollock, M. L. (1977). Submaximal and maximal working capacity of elite distance runners. Part I. Cardiorespiratory aspects. *New York Academy of Science, 301,* 310–322.

Pollock, M. L., Miller, H. S., & Wilmore, J. (1974). Physiological characteristics of champion American track athletes 40 to 75 years of age. *Journal of Gerontology, 29,* 645–649.

Prince, F. P., Hikida, R. S., & Hagerman, F. C. (1977). Muscle fiber types in women athletes and non-athletes. *Pflugers Archives, 371,* 161–165.

Puhl, J., Case, S., Fleck, S., & Van Handel, P. (1982). Physical and physiological characteristics of elite volleyball players. *Research Quarterly for Exercise and Sports, 53,* 257–262.

Raven, P. B., Gettman, L. R., Pollock, M. L., & Cooper, K. H. (1976). A physiological evaluation of professional soccer players. *British Journal of Sports Medicine, 10,* 209–216.

Roby, F. B., Buono, M. J., Constable, S. H., Lowdon, B. J., & Tsao, W. Y. (1983). Physiological characteristics of champion synchronized swimmers. *Physician and Sportsmedicine, 11* (#4), 136–147.

Rusko, H., Havu, M., & Karvinen, E. (1978). Aerobic performance capacity in athletes. *European Journal of Applied Physiology, 38,* 151–159.

Sady, S. P., Thomson, W. H., Berg, K., & Savage, M. (1984). Physiological characteristics of high-ability prepubescent wrestlers. *Medicine and Science in Sports and Exercise, 16,* 72–76.

Saltin, B., & Åstrand, P. O. (1967). Maximal oxygen uptake in athletes. *Journal of Applied Physiology, 23,* 353–358.

Schantz, P. G., & Åstrand, P. O. (1984). Physiological characteristics of classical ballet. *Medicine and Science in Sports and Exercise, 16,* 472–476.

Secher, N. H. (1983). The physiology of rowing. *Journal of Sports Science, 1,* 23-53.

Secher, N. H., Vaage, O., Jensen, K. & Jackson, R. C. (1983). Maximal aerobic power in oarsmen. *European Journal of Applied Physiology, 51,* 155-162.

Seliger, V., Kostka, V., Grusova, D., Kovac, J., Machovcova, J., Pauer, M., Pribylova, A., & Urbankova, R. (1972). Energy expenditure and physical fitness of ice-hockey players. *International Zeitschrift Angewandte Physiology, 30,* 283-291.

Shephard, R. J., Godin, G., & Campbell, R. (1974). Characteristics of sprint, medium, and long-distance swimmers. *European Journal of Applied Physiology, 32,* 99-103.

Sidney, K., & Shephard, R. J. (1973). Physiological characteristics and performance of the white-water paddler. *European Journal of Applied Physiology, 32,* 55-70.

Sinning, W. E. (1973). Body composition, cardiorespiratory function, and rule changes in women's basketball. *Research Quarterly, 44,* 313-321.

Sinning, W. E. (1974). Body composition assessment of college wrestlers. *Medicine and Science in Sports, 6,* 139-145.

Sinning, W. E., & Lindberg, G. D. (1972). Physical characteristics of college-age women gymnasts. *Research Quarterly, 43,* 226-234.

Smith, D. P., & Byrd, R. J. (1976). Body composition, pulmonary function and maximal oxygen consumption of college football players. *Journal of Sports Medicine, 16,* 301-308.

Song, T. M. K. (1982). Relationship of physiological characteristics to skiing performance. *Physician and Sportsmedicine, 10* (#12), 96-102.

Spence, D. W., Disch, J. G., Fred, H. L., & Coleman, A. E. (1980). Descriptive profiles of highly skilled women volleyball players. *Medicine and Science in Sports and Exercise, 12,* 299-302.

Sprynarova, S., & Parizkova, J. (1971). Functional capacity and body composition in top weight-lifters, swimmers, runners and skiers. *International Zeitschrift Angewandte Physiology, 29,* 184-194.

Stine, G., Ratliff, R., Shierman, G., & Grana, W. A. (1979). Physical profile of the wrestlers at the 1977 NCAA championships. *Physician and Sportsmedicine, 7* (#11), 98-105.

Strømme, S. B., Ingjer, F., & Meen, H. D. (1977). Assessment of maximal aerobic power in specifically trained athletes. *Journal of Applied Physiology, 42,* 833-837.

Tanner, J. M. (1964). *The physique of the Olympic athlete.* London: George Allen and Unwin Ltd.

Taylor, A. W., Brassard, L., Proteau, L., & Robin, D. (1979). A physiological profile of Canadian Greco-Roman wrestlers. *Canadian Journal of Applied Sport Sciences, 4,* 131-134.

Tesch, P., Piehl, K., Wilson, G., & Karlsson, J. (1976). Physiological investigations of Swedish elite canoe competitors. *Medicine and Science in Sports, 8,* 214-218.

Thorstensson, A., Larsson, L., Tesch, P., & Karlsson, J. (1977). Muscle strength and fiber composition in athletes and sedentary men. *Medicine and Science in Sports, 9,* 26-30.

Upton, S. J., Hagan, R. D., Lease, B., Rosentswieg, J., Gettman, L. R., & Duncan, J. J. (1984). Comparative physiological profiles among young and middle-aged female distance runners. *Medicine and Science in Sports and Exercise, 16,* 67-71.

Upton, S. J., Hagan, R. D., Rosentswieg, J., & Gettman, L. R. (1983). Comparison of the physiological profiles of middle-aged women distance runners and sedentary women. *Research Quarterly for Exercise and Sport, 54,* 83-87.

Vaccaro, P., Clarke, D. H., & Morris, A. F. (1980). Physiological characteristics of young well-trained swimmers. *European Journal of Applied Physiology, 44,* 61-66.

Vaccaro, P., Clarke, D. H., & Wrenn, J. P. (1979). Physiological profiles of elite women basketball players. *Journal of Sports Medicine, 19,* 45-54.

Vaccaro, P., Dummer, G. M., & Clarke, D. H. (1981). Physiological characteristics of female masters swimmers. *Physician and Sportsmedicine, 9* (#12), 75-78.

Vaccaro, P., Gray, P. R., Clarke, D. H., & Morris, A. F. (1984). Physiological characteristics of world class white-water slalom paddlers. *Research Quarterly for Exercise and Sport, 55,* 206-210.

Vaccaro, P., Morris, A. F., & Clarke, D. H. (1981). Physiological characteristics of masters female distance runners. *Physician and Sportsmedicine, 9* (#7), 105-108.

Vander, L. B., Franklin, B. A., Wrisley, D., Scherf, J., Kogler, A. A., & Rubenfire, M. (1984). Physiological profile of national-class national collegiate athletic association fencers. *Journal of American Medical Association, 252,* 500-503.

van Ingen Schenau, G. J., de Groot, G., & Hollander, A. P. (1983). Some technical, physiological and anthropometrical aspects of speed skating. *European Journal of Applied Physiology, 50,* 343-354.

Veicsteinas, A., Ferretti, G., Margonato, V., Rosa, G., & Tagliabue, D. (1984). Energy cost of and energy sources for alpine skiing in top athletes. *Journal of Applied Physiology, 56,* 1187-1190.

Vodak, P. A., Savin, W. M., Haskell, W. L., & Wood, P. D. (1980). Physiological profile of middle-aged male and female tennis players. *Medicine and Science in Sports and Exercise, 12,* 159-163.

Wickkiser, J. D., & Kelly, J. M. (1975). The body composition of a college football team. *Medicine and Science in Sports, 7,* 199-202.

Wilmore, J. H. (1974). Alterations in strength, body composition and anthropometric measurements consequent to a 10-week weight training program. *Medicine and Science in Sports, 6,* 133-138.

Wilmore, J. H. (1983). Body composition in sport and exercise: Directions for future research. *Medicine and Science in Sports and Exercise, 15,* 21-31.

Wilmore, J. H. (1984). The assesment of and variation in aerobic power in world class athletes as related to specific sports. *American Journal of Sports Medicine, 12,* 120–127.

Wilmore, J. H., & Bergfeld, J. A. (1979). A comparison of sports: Physiological and medical aspects. In R. H. Strauss (Ed.) *Sports medicine and physiology.* Philadelphia: W. B. Saunders.

Wilmore, J. H., & Brown, C. H. (1974). Physiological profiles of women distance runners. *Medicine and Science in Sports, 6,* 178–181.

Wilmore, J. H., Brown, C. H., & Davis, J. A. (1977). Body physique and composition of the female distance runner. *Annals of the New York Academy of Science, 301,* 764–776.

Wilmore, J. H., Parr, R. B., Haskell, W. L., Costill, D. L., Milburn, L. J., & Kerlan, R. K. (1976). Football pros' strengths—and CV weakness—charted. *Physician and Sportsmedicine, 4* (#10), 45–54.

Glossary of Terms

Acceleration: rate of change in velocity.

Acclimatization: adaptation to a particular environmental stress.

Acid-base balance: the proper balance of H and OH ions in the blood.

Acidosis: the situation in which the acid-base balance shifts to the acid side, due either to increased levels of unbuffered acids in the blood or to a reduction in the blood bicarbonates.

Actin: thin protein filament that acts with the protein filament myosin to allow muscle contraction.

Action potential: The change in the electrical potential across the cell or tissue membrane.

Acute: referring to something immediate or of short duration, e.g., a treadmill run to exhaustion would be an acute bout of exercise.

Adipose tissue: connective tissue in which fat is stored.

Adolescence: developmental period of time between the onset of puberty and the attainment of full physiological maturity.

ADP: adenosine diphosphate. A high energy phosphate compound from which ATP is synthesized.

Adrenal glands: endocrine glands located directly above each kidney, composed of the medulla (the hormones epinephrine and norepinephrine) and the cortex (cortical hormones).

Adrenaline: see epinephrine.

Adrenocorticotrophic hormone (ATCH): a pituitary hormone responsible for controlling the hormones released by the adrenal cortex.

Aerobic: in the presence of air or oxygen.

Aerobic power: synonomous with the terms maximal oxygen uptake, maximal oxygen consumption, and cardiovascular endurance capacity.

Afferent nerve: sensory nerve that carries impulses from the sensory receptors, e.g., skin, eyes, ears, to the central nervous system.

Agility: the ability to change directions rapidly while maintaining total body balance and awareness of body position.

Aldosterone: hormone from the adrenal cortex responsible for sodium retention.

Alkaline reserve: the amount of bicarbonate in the blood available for buffering acids.

Alkalosis: the situation in which the acid-base balance shifts to the alkaline, or basic, side.

Alveolar air: that air present in the alveoli which is involved in the exchange of gases with the blood in the pulmonary capillaries.

Alveoli: small air sacs, located at the termination of the pulmonary tree, in which the exchange of respiratory gases takes place with the blood in the adjacent capillaries.

Amino acids: the basic building blocks of protein.

Amphetamine: prescription drug that stimulates the central nervous system.

Anabolic steroid: a prescription drug that has the anabolic or growth-stimulating characteristics of the male androgen, testosterone. Frequently taken by athletes to increase body size and muscle bulk.

Anabolism: the building up of body tissue.

Anaerobic: in the absence of oxygen.

Anaerobic threshold: that point where the metabolic demands of exercise cannot be met totally by available aerobic sources and at which an increase in anaerobic metabolism occurs, as reflected by an increase in the blood lactate.

Androgen: male sex hormone from the testes, and, in limited amounts, from the adrenal cortex.

Anemia: inadequate number of red blood cells, or low hemoglobin levels, limiting oxygen transport.

Angina pectoris: chest pain associated with a lack of blood to the heart.

Angstrom: unit of measure equal to 10^{-8} cm.

Anorexia: inadequate appetite, which, if chronic, e.g., anorexia nervosa, can lead to eventual death.

Anoxia: inadequate oxygen in the blood or tissues.

Anthropometry: the study of body measurements.

Antidiuretic hormone: hormone from the posterior pituitary gland, which promotes water retention through its action on the kidney.

Arteriole: a small artery that regulates the flow of blood from the arteries to the capillaries.

Arteriosclerosis: loss of elasticity of the arteries, or hardening of the arteries. The precursor to various diseases of the cardiovascular system, e.g., stroke and coronary artery disease.

Artery: a vessel which transports blood away from the heart.

Aspartates: potassium and magnesium salts of aspartic acid.

Athlete's heart: an enlarged heart, typically found in endurance athletes, due, primarily, to hypertrophy of the left ventricle. It is no longer considered to be a pathological or diseased condition, as it once was.

ATP: adenosine triphosphate. A high-energy compound from which the body derives its energy.

Atrium: one of the chambers of the heart. The right atrium receives blood from the systemic circulation, and the left atrium receives blood from the pulmonary circulation.

Atrophy: loss of size, or mass, of body tissue, e.g., muscle atrophy with disuse.

Autonomic nervous system: that portion of the nervous system that controls involuntary activity, e.g., smooth muscle and the myocardium, and includes both sympathetic and parasympathetic nerves.

Axis cylinder: the central core of the axon of the nerve fiber.

Axon: the fiber-like extension of the nerve cell, which transmits the nerve impulse away from the cell body.

Balance: the ability to have complete control of the body as it is moved through space.

Basal metabolic rate (BMR): the rate of body metabolism under the most optimal conditions of quiet, rest, and relaxation. The lowest rate of metabolism compatible with life.

Blood pressure: the force that blood exerts against the walls of the blood vessels or heart.

Body density: the density of the body is equal to the body weight divided by the body volume.

Bronchiole: small terminal branch of the bronchus.

Bronchus: the subdivision of the trachea, as it splits into two branches.

Buffer: a substance in the blood that combines with either acids or bases to maintain a constant acid-base, or pH, balance.

Calorie: a unit of heat energy defined as the amount of heat required to raise the temperature of one kilogram of water 1°C, from 15 to 16°C.

Calorimeter: a device for measuring the heat production of the body or of specific chemical reactions.

Capillaries: the smallest vessels in the vascular system which connect the arterioles and venules, where all exchanges of gases or materials between the circulatory system and the tissues or lungs take place.

Carbohydrate: a food substance that includes various sugars and starches and is found in the body in the form of glucose and glycogen.

Cardiac: relating to the heart, e.g., cardiac muscle and cardiac output.

Cardiac muscle: the myocardium, or muscle, of the heart.

Cardiac output: output, or volume, of blood pumped by the heart per minute. The product of heart rate and stroke volume.

Cardiovascular endurance capacity: the term used to define overall body endurance, or stamina. See aerobic power or maximal oxygen uptake.

Catabolism: the tearing down, or destruction, of body tissue.

Catalyst: a chemical substance that initiates or accelerates a chemical action without being altered as a result of the action.

Central nervous system: that division of the nervous system that includes the brain and spinal cord.

Cerebellum: the hindbrain, responsible for the smooth coordination of body movements.

Cerebral cortex: the portion of the brain that contains the primary and supplementary motor areas which control all movement patterns of a voluntary nature.

Cerebrum: the large forebrain.

Cholesterol: a lipid or fatty substance essential for life and found in various tissues and fluids. Elevated levels in the blood have been associated with an increased risk of cardiovascular disease.

Chronic: referring to something of an extended or long-term nature, e.g., physical training program of six months' duration.

Cinematography: the use of films to analyze movement.

Circuit training: selected exercises or activities performed in sequence, as rapidly as possible.

Collagen: a protein substance found in bones, cartilage, and white fibrous tissues.

Concentric contraction: a muscular contraction in which shortening of the muscle occurs.

Conditioned reflex: a nervous reflex pattern that is learned.

Conduction: transfer of heat or cold through direct contact with an object or medium.

Connective tissue: specialized tissue, such as ligaments and tendons, that connects various body structures.

Convection: the transfer of heat or cold from a body to a moving liquid or gas.

Coordination: the act of movement in an organized, controlled, and precise manner.

Coronary arteries: those arteries that supply the heart muscle or myocardium.

Cortex: refers to the outer layer, e.g., cerebral cortex is the outer layer of the brain.

Cortisol: a hormone from the adrenal cortex.

Creatine phosphate: an energy-rich compound, which plays a critical role in providing energy for muscular contraction.

Dead space: the volume of the various parts of the respiratory system in which no gas exchange occurs.

Dehydration: loss of body fluids.

Dendrite: the projection of the nerve cell that transmits impulses toward the cell body.

Diaphragm: the major muscle of respiration, which separates the thorax from the abdomen.

Diastole: the relaxation phase of each cardiac cycle, immediately following the contraction, or systole, of the heart.

Diastolic pressure: the lowest pressure of the arterial blood against the walls of the vessels or heart resulting from the diastole of the heart.

Diuretic: a substance that increases kidney function leading to a loss of body fluids through frequent urination.

Dynamometer: a device for measuring muscular strength.

Dyspnea: labored breathing.

Eccentric contraction: lengthening of the muscle under tension, as when lowering a heavy object.

Ectomorphy: one of three categories of the somatotype in which the body is rated for the degree of linearity.

Edema: filled with fluid.

Effective blood volume: that volume of blood available to supply the exercising muscles.

Efferent nerve: also referred to as a motor nerve or motoneuron. Conducts impulses from the central nervous system to the various end organs, such as muscle.

Electrocardiogram (ECG): a recording of the electrical activity of the heart.

Electrocardiograph: an instrument that picks up and produces a record of the electrical activity of the heart.

Electromyogram (EMG): a recording of the elec-measure joint angles and changes in joint angles.

Electrolyte: any solution that conducts electricity by means of its ions.

Electromyogram (EMG): A recording of the electrical activity of a muscle or a group of muscles.

Endocrine gland: a ductless gland that produces and/or releases hormones directly into the blood stream.

Endomorphy: one of three categories of the somatotype in which the body is rated for corpulence or obesity.

Endurance: the ability to resist fatigue. Includes

muscular endurance, which is a local or specific endurance, and cardiovascular endurance, which is a more general, total body endurance.

Enzyme: an organic catalyst that speeds the velocity of specific chemical reactions.

Epinephrine: one of the hormones of the adrenal medulla. Also referred to as adrenaline.

Epiphysis: that part of the long bone that ossifies separately before uniting with the main shaft, or diaphysis, of the bone.

Ergogenic aid: substance or phenomenon that elevates or improves physical performance.

Ergograph: an instrument or device used for recording muscular work.

Ergometer: a device for exercising the subject in a manner in which the physical work performed can be measured, e.g., bicycle ergometer.

Estrogen: female sex hormone.

Evaporation: the loss of heat through the conversion of the water in sweat to a vapor.

Exercise prescription: individualizing the exercise program on the basis of the duration, frequency, intensity, and mode of exercise.

External respiration: the process of bringing air into the lungs and the resulting exchange of gas between the alveoli and the capillary blood.

Fartlek training: speed play, where the athlete varies his or her pace at will from fast sprints to slow jogging; normally performed in the country, using hills.

Fascia: connective tissue surrounding and connecting muscle.

Fast-twitch muscle fiber: one of several types of muscle fibers that have low oxidative capacity, high glycolytic capacity, and are associated with speed or power activities.

Fat: a food substance that is composed of gylcerol and fatty acids.

Fatigue: inability to continue work, due to any one or a combination of factors.

Fatty acid: along with glycerol, the product of the breakdown of fats.

Fat weight: absolute amount of body fat. Fat weight plus lean body weight equals total body weight.

Flexibility: the range of movement of a specific joint or a group of joints, influenced by the associated bones and boney structures, muscles, tendons, and ligaments.

Glucagon: a hormone from the pancreas that acts to increase blood glucose, or sugar, levels.

Glucose: a simple sugar which is transported in the blood and metabolized in the tissues.

Glycerol: a substance that combines with fatty acids to form fat.

Glycogen: the storage form of carbohydrates in the body, found predominantly in the muscles and liver.

Glycogen loading: manipulating exercise and diet to optimize the total amount of glycogen stored in the body.

Glycogenolysis: the metabolic breakdown of glycogen.

Glycolysis: breakdown of glycogen to lactic acid.

Golgi tendon organ: a proprioceptor located in series with muscle tendons.

Gonads: endocrine glands responsible for reproduction; the testes in males and ovaries in females.

Growth hormone (GH): a pituitary hormone responsible for contolling tissue growth. Also referred to as somatotrophic hormone.

Heat cramp: severe cramping of the skeletal muscles, due to excessive dehydration and the associated salt loss.

Heat exhaustion: a disorder due to an excessive heat load on the body, characterized by breathlessness, extreme tiredness, dizziness, and rapid pulse, and usually associated with a decrease in sweat production.

Heat stroke: the most serious heat disorder, characterized by a body temperature above 105°F, cessation of sweating, and total confusion or unconsciousness, which can lead to death.

Hematocrit: the relative contribution, or percentage, of the blood cells to the total blood volume.

Hemoconcentration: used in reference to an apparent increase in red blood cell number due to a plasma volume reduction, i.e., there is a relative, but not an absolute, increase.

Hemoglobin: iron pigment of the red blood cell that has a high affinity for oxygen.

Hormone: a chemical substance produced or released by one of the endocrine glands, which is transported by the blood to a specific target organ.

Hyperemia: an excessive amount of blood in a part of the body.

Hyperglycemia: elevated levels of glucose, or sugar, in the blood.

Hyperplasia: increase in size, due to an increased number of cells.

Hypertension: abnormally high blood pressure, usually defined in adults as a systolic pressure in excess of 140 mmHg and/or diastolic pressure in excess of 90 mmHg.

Hyperthermia: overheating.

Hypertrophy: increase in the size, or mass, of an organ or body tissue.

Hyperventilation: breathing rate and/or tidal volume increased above levels necessary for normal function.

Hypoglycemia: abnormally low blood glucose, or sugar, levels.

Hypotension: an abnormally low blood pressure.

Hypothalamus: that region of the brain involved in controlling or releasing many of the hormones of the pituitary gland.

Hypoxia: a lack of oxygen in the blood or tissues.

Inhibition: negative nervous control to restrict, or limit, the amount of force generated.

Innervation ratio: the ratio of the number of muscle fibers per motoneuron.

Insulin: a hormone produced by the pancreas that assists in the control of the blood sugar, or glucose, levels.

Internal respiration: the exchange of gases between the blood and tissues.

Interval training: training program that alternates bouts of heavy or very heavy work with periods of rest or light work.

In vitro: functioning outside of, or detached from, the body.

In vivo: functioning within the body.

Ion: an electrically charged atom or group of atoms.

Ischemia: a temporary deficiency of blood to a specific area of the body.

Isokinetic contraction: contraction in which the muscle generates force against a variable resistance where the speed of movement is maintained constant.

Isometric contraction: contraction in which the muscle generates force, but there is no observable movement, e.g., pushing against a building.

Isotonic contraction: contraction in which the muscle generates force against a constant resistance and movement results, either shortening (concentric) or lengthening (eccentric).

Kinesthesis: a sense, or awareness, of body position.

Lactic acid: the end product of glycolysis, or anaerobic metabolism.

Latent period: period of time between the stimulus and the response to that stimulus.

Lean body weight: determined by subtracting the fat weight from the total body weight. That weight of the body which is not fat, e.g., bone, muscle, skin, organ weights, etc.

Ligament: connective tissue that binds bone to bone, to maintain the integrity of a joint.

Lipid: fat, or fat-like, substance.

Manometer: an instrument for measuring pressure.

Maximal oxygen consumption: see maximal oxygen uptake.

Maximal oxygen intake: see maximal oxygen uptake.

Maximal oxygen uptake ($\dot{V}O_2$ max): the best physiological index of total body endurance. Also referred to as aerobic power, maximal oxygen intake, maximal oxygen consumption, and cardiovascular endurance capacity.

Menstruation: the periodic cycle in the uterus associated with preparation of the uterus to receive a fertilized egg.

Mental practice: mental rehearsal of the athletic event or sport.

Mesomorphy: one of three categories of the somatotype in which the body is rated for the degree of muscularity.

Metabolism: the sum total of the energy-producing and -absorbing processes in the body, i.e., the energy used by the body.

Micron: unit of measure equal to 0.001 mm.

Mitochondria: energy-producing bodies within the cell.

Motor area, or motor cortex: that area of the cerebral cortex which controls voluntary muscle movement.

Motor end plate: where the efferent or motor nerve attaches to the muscle fiber.

Motor nerve, or motoneuron: motor, or efferent, nerve which transmits impulses to muscles.

Motor unit: the motor nerve and the group of muscle fibers it supplies.

Muscle fiber: the structural unit of muscle. A single cell with multiple nuclei composed of a number of smaller units called myofibrils.

Muscle spindle: a sensory receptor located in the muscle itself, which senses changes in muscle tension.

Myelin sheath: the inner covering of the medullated nerve fiber.

Myocardium: the muscle of the heart.

Myofibril: the small elements which comprise the muscle fiber, composed of the proteins actin and myosin.

Myoneural junction: the junction between the muscle fiber and its nerve.

Myosin: a muscle protein that acts with actin, another muscle protein, to allow the muscle to contract.

Neurilemma: the outermost covering of a nerve fiber.

Neuron: the nerve cell; the basic structural unit of the nervous system. Conducts nervous impulses to and from various parts of the body.

Nitrogen narcosis: "rapture of the deep." A condition which is caused by breathing air underwater at depths where the partial pressure of nitrogen increases until it has a narcotic-like effect on the central nervous system, leading to distortions in judgment and sometimes to serious injury or death.

Norepinephrine: a hormone produced by the adrenal medulla and, also, a chemical transmitter substance at peripheral sympathetic nerve endings.

Obesity: an excessive amount of body fat. The state of being overfat.

One-repetition maximum (1-RM): the greatest amount of weight that can be lifted just one time.

Ossification: process of calcification or hardening of the bone during the growth process.

Overload: stressing the body or parts of the body to levels above that normally experienced.

Oxygen debt: the quantity of oxygen above normal resting levels used in the period of recovery from any specific exercise or muscular activity.

Oxygen poisoning: caused by breathing concentrations of oxygen for long periods of time during deep dives, resulting in visual distortion, confusion, rapid and shallow breathing, and convulsions.

Pacinian corpuscle: a proprioceptor located in muscle and tendon sheaths adjacent to joints.

Pancreas: an endocrine gland that produces both the hormones insulin and glucagon, which control blood glucose, or sugar, levels.

Parasympathetic nervous system: a major subdivision of the autonomic nervous system whose fibers arise from the midbrain, medulla, or sacral region of the spinal cord.

Parathormone: hormone produced by the parathyroid glands, which assists in controlling calcium and phosphorus levels.

Parathyroids: endocrine glands that are located on or embedded in the thyroid glands and that produce parathormone.

Pericardium: the fibrous sac that encapsulates the heart.

Periosteum: the fibrous membrane that surrounds bone.

Peripheral nervous system: that part of the nervous system that lies outside the central nervous system, i.e., spinal cord and brain.

pH: a system for expressing the degree of acidity or alkalinity of a solution, in which a value of 7.0 is neutral, greater than 7.0 alkaline, and less than 7.0, acidic.

Plasma: the liquid fraction of the whole blood.

Ponderal index: defined as height divided by the cube root of weight.

Power: the product of force and velocity. This is probably far more important than absolute strength alone.

Precapillary sphincter: small band of smooth muscle controlling the flow of blood to the true capillaries.

Progressive overload: gradually increasing the training stimulus in a systematic manner.

Progressive resistance exercise (PRE): the resistance used in training is progressively increased systematically as the body adapts to the training stimulus.

Proprioceptor: a sensory receptor sensitive to pressure, stretch, tension, pain, etc.

Protein: a food substance formed from amino acids.

Pulse: periodic expansion of the artery, resulting from the systole of the heart.

Pulse pressure: the mathematical difference between the systolic and diastolic pressures.

Radiation: the transfer of heat through electromagnetic waves.

Reaction time: the period of time between the presentation of a stimulus and the subsequent reaction to that stimulus.

Reciprocal inhibition: the inhibition of the antagonist muscles, which allows the agonists to move.

Reflex: an automatic, involuntary, unlearned response to a given stimulus.

Relative body fat: the ratio of fat weight to total body weight, expressed as a percentage.

Relative humidity: a ratio expressing the degree of moisture in the surrounding air.

Repetition running: similar to interval training but with long work intervals and long periods of recovery.

Residual volume: that volume of air remaining in the lung following a maximal expiration. Vital capacity plus residual volume equal total lung capacity.

Respiration: the exchange of gases at both the level of the lung and tissue.

Respiratory exchange ratio (R or RER): the ratio of carbon dioxide expired to oxygen consumed, at the level of the lungs.

Respiratory quotient (RQ): the ratio of the carbon dioxide produced in the tissues to the oxygen consumed by the tissues.

Ruffini receptor: a proprioceptor located in the joint capsule.

Sarcolemma: the membrane surrounding the muscle fiber.

Sarcomere: the functional contractile unit of muscle, which is a part of the myofibril.

Sarcoplasm: the fluid portion of the muscle fiber, or the muscle protoplasm.

Sarcoplasmic reticulum: network of tubules and vesicles within muscle fibers, which are necessary to allow excitation of the muscle fibers.

Sensory nerve: afferent or sensory nerves transmit impulses from the sensory organs to the central nervous system.

Skeletal muscle: muscle controlling skeletal movement that is normally under voluntary control.

Slow-twitch muscle fiber: one of several types of muscle fibers that have high oxidative capacity, low glycolytic capacity, and are associated with endurance type activities.

Smooth muscle: involuntary muscle, such as that which lines blood vessels and the gastrointestinal tract.

Somatic nervous system: the voluntary nervous system, including both cranial and spinal nerves.

Somatogram: a chart on which somatotypes are plotted.

Somatotrophic hormone: a hormone released by the pituitary gland that influences growth. Also referred to as STH, or growth hormone (GH).

Somatotype: the characterization of the body physique in an objective and systematic manner.

Sphygmomanometer: an instrument used to measure arterial blood pressure.

Spirometer: an instrument used to measure the various lung volumes and dynamic lung function.

Strength: the ability of a muscle to exert force.

Stroke volume: the volume of blood pumped per contraction of the ventricle.

Sympathetic nervous system: a major division of the autonomic nervous system.

Synapse: the junction between two neurons.

Systole: the contraction phase of the cardiac cycle.

Systolic pressure: the greatest pressure in the vessels or heart during a cardiac cycle, resulting from the systole.

Tendon: connective tissue that attaches muscle to bone.

Testosterone: the predominant male androgen.

Thyroid gland: an endocrine gland located at the base of the neck, which produces several hormones regulating total body metabolism.

Thyroid-stimulating hormone: a pituitary hormone which controls the thyroid gland's release of thyroxin.

Thyroxin: a hormone produced by the thyroid gland, which assists in the control of total body metabolism.

Tidal volume: the amount of air inspired or expired during a normal breathing cycle.

Tonus: that quality of a muscle which gives it firmness in the absence of a voluntary contraction.

Total lung capacity: the sum of the vital capacity and the residual volume.

Valsalva maneuver: increased intraabdominal

and intrathoracic pressure created by holding the breath and attempting to compress the contents of the abdominal and thoracic cavities.

Vasopressin hormone: a pituitary hormone which controls blood vessel diameter.

Vein: a vessel that transports blood back to the heart.

Velocity: speed, or the rate, of movement.

Ventilation: movement of air into and out of the lungs.

Ventricle: a chamber of the heart that expels, or pumps, blood into the lungs (right ventricle) or into the systemic circulation (left ventricle).

Venule: a small vein that provides the link between capillaries and veins.

Vestibular receptor: a proprioceptor located in the ear.

Viscosity: that quality of a fluid that describes its flow characteristics. Water has a low viscosity, while honey has a high viscosity.

Vital capacity: the greatest volume of air that can be expired following the deepest possible inspiration.

Work: the product of force and distance.

Index